COGNITIVE THERAPY
OF ANXIETY DISORDERS

Cognitive Therapy of Anxiety Disorders

Science and Practice

DAVID A. CLARK
AARON T. BECK

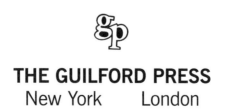

THE GUILFORD PRESS
New York   London

Library of Congress Cataloging-in-Publication Data

Clark, David A., 1954-
    Cognitive therapy of anxiety disorders: science and practice / David A. Clark and Aaron T. Beck.
        p. ; cm.
    Includes bibliographical references and index.
    ISBN 978-1-60623-434-1 (hardcover: alk. paper)
    1. Anxiety disorders—Treatment.   2. Cognitive therapy.   I. Beck, Aaron T.   II. Title.
    [DNLM: 1. Anxiety Disorders—therapy.   2. Cognitive Therapy—methods.
WM 172 C592c 2010]
    RC531.C535 2010
    616.85′22—dc22

                                                                              2009027597

To my wife, Nancy, and our daughters,
Natascha and Christina, with sincere love
for your steadfast interest, support, and understanding

D. A. C.

To my wife, Phyllis,
our children, Roy, Judy, Daniel, and Alice,
and our grandchildren,
Jodi, Sarah, Andy, Debbie, Eric, Ben, Sam, and Becky,
with love

A. T. B.

About the Authors

David A. Clark, PhD, is Professor of Psychology at the University of New Brunswick, Canada. He has published seven books, including *Intrusive Thoughts in Clinical Disorders: Theory, Research, and Treatment*; *Cognitive-Behavioral Therapy for OCD*; and *Scientific Foundations of Cognitive Theory and Therapy of Depression,* as well as over 100 articles and chapters on various aspects of cognitive theory and therapy of depression and anxiety disorders. Dr. Clark is a Fellow of the Canadian Psychological Association, a Founding Fellow of the Academy of Cognitive Therapy, and a recipient of the Academy's Aaron T. Beck Award for significant and enduring contributions to cognitive therapy. He is an Associate Editor of the *International Journal of Cognitive Therapy* and maintains a private practice.

Aaron T. Beck, MD, is University Professor Emeritus of Psychiatry, School of Medicine, University of Pennsylvania, and the founder of cognitive therapy. He has published 21 books and over 540 articles in professional and scientific journals. Dr. Beck is the recipient of numerous awards, including the Albert Lasker Clinical Medical Research Award in 2006, the American Psychological Association Lifetime Achievement Award in 2007, the American Psychiatric Association Distinguished Service Award in 2008, and the Robert J. and Claire Pasarow Foundation Award for Research in Neuropsychiatry in 2008. He is President of The Beck Institute for Cognitive Therapy and Research and Honorary President of the Academy of Cognitive Therapy.

Preface

The intricacies of anxiety have continued to capture the attention of some of the world's greatest scientists, scholars, and critical thinkers. In 1953 Rollo May stated in *Man's Search for Himself* that the "middle of the twentieth century is more anxiety-ridden than any period since the breakdown of the Middle Ages" (p. 30). If this statement characterized the last century, is it not even more applicable to the dawn of the 21st century with all the social, political, and economic threats that besiege us? Despite an end to the cold war, an era of relative global stability and cooperation, and an unprecedented rise in economic prosperity and technological advances, many in the Western world live in a state of perpetual threat and uncertainty. According to the National Institute of Mental Health (2003) approximately 40 million American adults (18%) suffer from an anxiety disorder, with serious mental illness, including the anxiety disorders, costing an estimated $193 billion in lost personal earnings (Kessler et al., 2008). No wonder the search for highly effective and accessible treatments for the anxiety disorders has become a major health initiative for most developed countries.

Twenty-five years ago, coauthor Aaron T. Beck published *Anxiety Disorders and Phobias: A Cognitive Perspective* with Gary Emery and Ruth Greenberg. In the first part of that book, Beck introduced a cognitive model of anxiety disorders and phobias that represented a significant reconceptualization of the etiology, nature, and treatment of anxiety (Beck, Emery, & Greenberg, 1985). At that time, research on the cognitive features of anxiety was scant, and so much of the theoretical scaffolding was, by necessity, based on clinical observation and experience. Since key aspects of the cognitive model of anxiety had not yet been investigated, some of the treatment recommendations described in the second half of the book have not stood the test of time. However, the last 20 years has witnessed a virtual explosion in basic information-processing research on the cognitive model of anxiety, the development of disorder-specific cognitive models and treatment protocols for the major anxiety disorders, and dozens of treatment outcome studies demonstrating the efficacy of cognitive therapy of anxiety. In light of the unprecedented advances in our understanding and treatment of the cognitive basis of anxiety, a comprehensive, updated, and reformulated presentation of the cognitive model of anxiety was needed so the model could be understood within the context of contemporary research findings. This book, then, was born out of this necessity. In addition, we believe that a single volume containing a detailed comprehensive treatment handbook for cognitive therapy is timely in order to encourage greater use by clinicians of evidence-based psychotherapy for the anxiety disorders.

The book is divided into three parts. Part I consists of four chapters on the reformulated cognitive model of anxiety and its empirical status. Chapter 1 discusses the distinctions between fear and anxiety and provides a rationale for taking a cognitive perspective on anxiety. Chapter 2 presents a reformulation of the generic cognitive model of anxiety based on the original model (Beck et al., 1985) that was later refined by Beck and Clark (1997). Twelve key hypotheses of the model are presented in Chapter 2, and the vast empirical research relevant to these hypotheses is critically reviewed in Chapters 3 and 4. The literature review spans hundreds of studies conducted in key research centers in Western Europe and North America, confirming our perception that the main tenets of the cognitive model of anxiety have achieved a broad basis of empirical support.

The cognitive therapy approach has been applied to a wide range of psychiatric and personality conditions. Thus, Part II consists of three chapters that explain how the basic elements of cognitive therapy are used to alleviate anxiety. Chapter 5 reviews several standardized measures of anxious symptoms and cognition that are useful for assessment and treatment evaluation and provides a detailed explanation for producing a cognitive case formulation of anxiety. Chapters 6 and 7 present a step-by-step description for implementing various cognitive and behavioral intervention strategies for reduction of anxious symptoms. Case illustrations, suggested therapy narratives, and clinical resource materials are provided in all three chapters as training tools in cognitive therapy.

The final section, Part III, consists of five chapters that present disorder-specific adaptations of cognitive therapy for panic disorder, social phobia, generalized anxiety disorder, obsessive–compulsive disorder, and posttraumatic stress disorder. We excluded specific phobias because there have been fewer developments on the cognitive aspects of phobia since its presentation in Beck et al. (1985), and exposure-based treatment is still considered the main treatment approach for reduction of phobic responses. Each of the disorder-specific chapters presents a cognitive model tailored to that disorder and a review of the empirical research that addresses key hypotheses of each model. In addition, the chapters offer disorder-specific case conceptualizations and cognitive therapy strategies that target unique symptom features of each disorder. In essence, Part III consists of five minitreatment manuals for complex anxiety disorders.

To assist therapists in explaining cognitive concepts and strategies to their clients, we are in the process of developing a companion client workbook that will match the organization and themes of the present book and will offer explanations for key aspects of the therapy, homework exercises, and record-keeping forms.

We are indebted to a large contingent of renowned experts in the anxiety disorders whose theoretical contributions, innovative and rigorous research, and clinically astute treatment insights are responsible for the significant advances that we have presented in this volume. In particular we acknowledge the notable contributions to cognitive theory and therapy of anxiety of Drs. Martin Antony, Jonathan Abramowitz, David Barlow, Thomas Borkovec, Brendan Bradley, Michelle Craske, David M. Clark, Meredith

Coles, Michel Dugas, Edna Foa, Mark Freeston, Randy Frost, Richard Heimberg, Stefan Hofmann, Robert Leahy, Colin MacLeod, Andrew Mathews, Richard McNally, Karen Mogg, Christine Purdon, Stanley Rachman, Ronald Rapee, John Riskind, Paul Salkovskis, Norman Schmidt, Robert Steer, Gail Steketee, Steven Taylor, and Adrian Wells. Furthermore, we wish to acknowledge with gratitude the tenacity and meticulousness of Michelle Valley, who laboriously revised and validated all the references, and to past and current graduate students, Mujgan Altin, Anna Campbell, Gemma Garcia-Soriano, Brendan Guyitt, Nicola McHale, Adriana del Palacio Gonzalez, and Adrienne Wang for their research and thoughtful discussions on cognitive aspects of anxiety. We also appreciate the partial financial support for publication costs from the University of New Brunswick Busteed Publication Fund. Finally we are grateful for the encouragement, guidance, advice, and support of the staff at The Guilford Press, especially Jim Nageotte, Senior Editor, and Jane Keislar, Assistant Editor.

Contents

PART I

COGNITIVE THEORY AND RESEARCH ON ANXIETY

Cognitive therapy is a theory-driven psychotherapy with a strong commitment to scientific empiricism. Its defining characteristics are not found in a set of unique intervention strategies but rather in its cognitive conceptualization of psychopathology and the therapeutic change process. Thus articulation of the cognitive model as well as the derivation of testable hypotheses and their empirical evaluation are critical to determining its construct validity. Similar to the organization of earlier primary treatment manuals of cognitive therapy, this book begins with a focus on the theoretical and empirical foundation of cognitive therapy for anxiety. Chapter 1 discusses phenomenology, diagnostic features, and the cognitive perspective on fear and anxiety. Chapter 2 presents the reformulated generic or transdiagnostic cognitive model of anxiety and its hypotheses, whereas Chapter 3 provides a critical evaluation of the prodigious experimental literature relevant to key aspects of the cognitive model. This section concludes with Chapter 4, which focuses on empirical evidence for cognitive vulnerability to experience heightened states of intense and persistent anxiety.

Chapter 1

Anxiety

A Common but Multifaceted Condition

Love looks forward, hate looks back, anxiety has eyes
all over its head.
—MIGNON MCLAUGHLIN (American journalist, 1915–)

Anxiety is ubiquitous to the human condition. From the beginning of recorded history, philosophers, religious leaders, scholars, and more recently physicians as well as social and medical scientists have attempted to unravel the mysteries of anxiety and to develop interventions that would effectively deal with this pervasive and troubling condition of humanity. Today, as never before, calamitous events brought about by natural disasters or callous acts of crime, violence, or terrorism have created a social climate of fear and anxiety in many countries around the world. Natural disasters like earthquakes, hurricanes, tsunamis, and the like have a significant negative impact on the mental health of affected populations in both developing and developed countries with symptoms of anxiety and posttraumatic stress showing substantial increases in the weeks immediately following the disaster (Norris, 2005).

Elevated levels of anxiety and other posttraumatic symptoms spike in the first few weeks after acts of terrorism, war, or other large-scale acts of community violence. In 5–8 weeks after the September 11, 2001, terrorist attacks on the World Trade Center towers in New York City, symptoms of posttraumatic stress disorder (PTSD) doubled (Galea et al., 2002). An Internet-based survey ($N = 2,729$) found that 17% of individuals outside New York City reported PTSD symptoms 2 months after 9/11 (Silver, Holman, McIntosh, Poulin, & Gil-Rivas, 2002). The National Tragedy Study, a telephone survey of 2,126 Americans, found that 5 months after the 9/11 terrorist attacks month, 30% of Americans reported difficulty sleeping, 27% felt nervous or tense, and 17% indicated they worried a great deal about future terrorist attacks (Rasinski, Berktold, Smith, & Albertson, 2002). The Gallup Youth Survey of American teenagers conducted 2½ years after 9/11 found that 39% of teens were either "very" or "somewhat" worried that they or someone in their families will become a victim of terrorism (Lyons, 2004).

Although large-scale threats have their greatest impact on the psychological morbidity of individuals directly affected by the disaster in the weeks immediately following the traumatic event, their wider effects are evident months and years later in the heightened concerns and worries of a significant proportion of the general population.

Fear, anxiety, and worry, however, are not the exclusive domain of disaster and other life-threatening experiences. In the majority of cases anxiety develops within the context of the fluctuating pressures, demands, and stresses of daily living. In fact anxiety disorders represent the single largest mental health problem in the United States (Barlow, 2002), with more than 19 million American adults having an anxiety disorder in any given year (National Institute of Mental Health, 2001). Approximately 12–19% of primary care patients meet diagnostic criteria for an anxiety disorder (Ansseau et al., 2004; Olfson et al., 1997). Moreover, antidepressants and mood stabilizers are the third most prescribed pharmacotherapy class, having 2003 global sales of $19.5 billion (IMS, 2004). Thus millions of people worldwide mount a daily struggle against clinical anxiety and its symptoms. These disorders cause a significant economic, social and health care burden for all countries, especially in developing countries that face frequent social and political upheavals and high rates of natural disaster.

This chapter provides an overview of the diagnosis, clinical features, and theoretical perspectives on the anxiety disorders. We begin by examining definitional issues and the distinction between fear and anxiety. The diagnosis of anxiety disorders is then considered with particular attention to the problem of comorbidity, especially with depression and substance abuse disorders. A brief review of the epidemiology, course, and consequence of anxiety is presented, and contemporary biological and behavioral explanations for anxiety are considered. The chapter concludes with arguments for the validity of a cognitive perspective for understanding the anxiety disorders and their treatment.

ANXIETY AND FEAR

The psychology of emotion is rich with diverse and opposing views on the nature and function of human emotions. All emotion theorists who accept the existence of basic emotions, however, count fear as one of them (Öhman & Wiens, 2004). As part of our emotional nature, fear occurs as a healthy adaptive response to a perceived threat or danger to one's physical safety and security. It warns individuals of an imminent threat and the need for defensive action (Beck & Greenberg, 1988; Craske, 2003). Yet fear can be maladaptive when it occurs in a nonthreatening or neutral situation that is misinterpreted as representing a potential danger or threat. Thus two issues are fundamental to any theory of anxiety: how to distinguish fear and anxiety, and how to determine what is a normal versus an abnormal reaction.

Defining Fear and Anxiety

Many different words in the English language relate to the subjective experience of anxiety such as "dread," "fright," "panic," "apprehension," "nervous," "worry," "fear," "horror," and "terror" (Barlow, 2002). This has led to considerable confusion and inaccuracy in the common use of the term "anxious." However, "fear" and "anxiety" must be clearly distinguished in any theory of anxiety that hopes to offer guidance for research and treatment of anxiety.

In his influential volume on the anxiety disorders, Barlow (2002) stated that "fear is a primitive alarm in response to present danger, characterized by strong arousal and action tendencies" (p. 104). Anxiety, on the other hand, was defined as "a future-oriented emotion, characterized by perceptions of uncontrollability and unpredictability over potentially aversive events and a rapid shift in attention to the focus of potentially dangerous events or one's own affective response to these events" (p. 104).

Beck, Emery, and Greenberg (1985) offered a somewhat different perspective on the differentiation of fear and anxiety. They defined fear as a cognitive process involving "the *appraisal* that there is actual or potential danger in a given situation" (1985, p. 8, emphasis in original). Anxiety is an emotional response triggered by fear. Thus fear "is the appraisal of danger; anxiety is the unpleasant feeling state evoked when fear is stimulated" (Beck et al., 1985, p. 9). Barlow and Beck both consider fear a discrete, fundamental construct whereas anxiety is a more general subjective response. Beck et al. (1985) emphasize the cognitive nature of fear and Barlow (2002) focuses on the more automatic neurobiological and behavioral features of the construct. On the basis of these considerations, we offer the following definitions of fear and anxiety as a guide for cognitive therapy.

Clinician Guideline 1.1

Fear is a primitive automatic neurophysiological state of alarm involving the **cognitive appraisal** of imminent threat or danger to the safety and security of an individual.

Clinician Guideline 1.2

Anxiety is a complex cognitive, affective, physiological and behavioral response system (i.e., **threat mode**) that is activated when anticipated events or circumstances are deemed to be highly aversive because they are perceived to be unpredictable, uncontrollable events that could potentially threaten the vital interests of an individual.

A couple of observations can be derived from these definitions. Fear as the basic automatic appraisal of danger is the core process in all the anxiety disorders. It is evident in the panic attacks and acute spikes of anxiousness that people report in specific situations. Anxiety, on the other hand, describes a more enduring state of threat or "anxious apprehension" that includes other cognitive factors in addition to fear such as perceived aversiveness, uncontrollability, uncertainty, vulnerability (helplessness), and inability to obtain desired outcomes (see Barlow, 2002). Both fear and anxiety involve a future orientation so that "what if?" questions predominate (e.g., "What if I 'bomb' this job interview?", "What if my mind goes blank during the speech?", "What if my heart palpitations trigger a heart attack?").

The distinction between fear and anxiety can be illustrated by Bill, who suffers from obsessive–compulsive disorder (OCD) due to a fear of contamination and so engages in compulsive washing. Bill is hypervigilant about the possibility of encountering "dangerous" contaminants, and so he avoids many things that he perceives as possible contamination. He is in a continual state of high arousal and subjectively feels nervous and apprehensive due to repetitive doubts of contamination (e.g., "What if I become contaminated?"). This cognitive–behavioral–physiological state, then, describes anxiety. If Bill touches a dirty object (e.g., the doorknob in a public building) he quickly experiences fear, which is the perception of imminent danger (e.g., "I've touched this dirty doorknob. A cancer patient may have recently touched it. I could contract cancer and die."). Thus we describe Bill's immediate response to the doorknob as "fear," but his almost continuous negative affective state as "anxiety." Anxiety, then, is of greater concern for those individuals who seek treatment for a heightened state of "nervousness" or agitation that causes considerable distress and interference in daily living. Consequently it is anxiety and its treatment that is the focus of the present volume.

Normal versus Abnormal

It would be difficult to find someone who hasn't experienced fear or felt anxious about an impending event. Fear has an adaptive function that is critical to the survival of the human species by warning and preparing the organism for response against life-threatening dangers and emergencies (Barlow, 2002; Beck et al., 1985). Moreover, fears are very common in childhood, and mild symptoms of anxiety (e.g., occasional panic attacks, worry, social anxiety) are frequently reported in adult populations (see Craske, 2003, for review). So, how are we to distinguish abnormal from normal fear? At what point does anxiety become excessive, so maladaptive that clinical intervention is warranted?

We suggest five criteria that can be used to distinguish abnormal states of fear and anxiety. It is not necessary that all these criteria be present in a particular case, but one would expect many of these characteristics to be present in clinical anxiety states.

1. *Dysfunctional cognition.* A central tenet of the cognitive theory of anxiety is that abnormal fear and anxiety derive from a false assumption involving an erroneous danger appraisal of a situation that is not confirmed by direct observation (Beck et al., 1985). The activation of dysfunctional beliefs (schemas) about threat and associated cognitive-processing errors leads to marked and excessive fear that is inconsistent with the objective reality of the situation.

For example, the sight of a loose Rotweiller charging toward you with teeth bared and raised fur on a lonely country road would likely elicit the thought "I am in grave danger of being attacked; I better get out of here fast." The fear experienced in this situation is perfectly normal, because it involves a reasonable deduction based on an accurate observation of the situation. On the other hand, anxiety elicited by the sight of a toy poodle dog held on a leash by its owner is abnormal: the threat mode is activated (e.g., "I'm in danger") even though direct observation indicates this is a "nonthreatening" situation. In this latter case we would suspect that the person has a specific animal phobia.

2. *Impaired functioning.* Clinical anxiety will directly interfere with effective and adaptive coping in the face of a perceived threat, and more generally in the person's daily social or occupational functioning. There are instances in which the activation of fear results in a person freezing, feeling paralyzed in the face of danger (Beck et al., 1985). Barlow (2002) notes that rape survivors often report physical paralysis at some point

during the attack. In other cases the fear and anxiety may lead to a counterproductive response that actually increases risk of harm or danger. For example, a woman anxious about driving after being involved in a rear-end collision would constantly check her rear-view mirror and so pay less attention to the traffic in front of her, increasing the chance that she would cause the very accident she feared.

It is also recognized that clinical fear and anxiety usually interfere in a person's ability to lead a productive and fulfilling life. Consequently, in the *Diagnostic and Statistical Manual of Mental Disorders* (DSM-IV-TR; American Psychiatric Association [APA], 2000), marked distress or "significant interference with the person's normal routine, occupational (or academic) functioning, or social activities or relationships" (p. 449) is one of the core diagnostic criteria for most of the anxiety disorders.

3. *Persistence.* In clinical states anxiety persists much longer than would be expected under normal conditions. Recall that anxiety prompts a future-oriented perspective that involves the anticipation of threat or danger (Barlow, 2002). As a result, the person with clinical anxiety can feel a heightened sense of subjective apprehension by just thinking about an impending potential threat, regardless of whether it eventually materializes. Thus it is not uncommon for anxiety-prone individuals to experience elevated anxiety on a daily basis over many years.

4. *False alarms.* In anxiety disorders one often finds the occurrence of false alarms, which Barlow (2002) defines as "marked fear or panic [that] occurs in the absence of any life-threatening stimulus, learned or unlearned" (p. 220). A spontaneous or uncued panic attack is one of the best examples of a "false alarm." The presence of panic attacks or intense fear in the absence of threat cues or very minimal threat provocation would suggest a clinical state.

5. *Stimulus hypersensitivity.* Fear is a "stimulus-driven aversive response" (Öhman & Wiens, 2004, p. 72) to an external or internal cue that is perceived as a potential threat. However, in clinical states fear is elicited by a wider range of stimuli or situations of relatively mild threat intensity that would be perceived as innocuous to the nonfearful individual (Beck & Greenberg, 1988). For example, most people would be quite fearful about approaching a Sydney funnelweb spider, which has the most lethal spider venom in the world for humans. On the other hand, a spider phobic patient was referred to our clinical practice who exhibited intense anxiety, even panic attacks, at the sight of a spider web produced by the smallest, most harmless Canadian household spider. Clearly the number of spider-related stimuli that elicits a fear response in the phobic individual is far greater than the spider-related stimuli that would elicit fear in the nonphobic individual. In the same way individuals with an anxiety disorder would interpret a broader range of situations as threatening compared to individuals without an anxiety disorder. Clinician Guideline 1.3 presents five questions to determine if a person's experience of fear or anxiety is sufficiently exaggerated and pervasive to warrant further assessment, diagnosis, and possible treatment.

Clinician Guideline 1.3

1. Is fear or anxiety based on a false assumption or faulty reasoning about the potential for threat or danger in relevant situations?

2. Does the fear or anxiety actually interfere in the person's ability to cope with aversive or difficult circumstances?

3. Is the anxiety present over an extended period of time?

4. Does the individual experience false alarms or panic attacks?

5. Is fear or anxiety activated by a fairly wide range of situations involving relatively mild threat potential?

ANXIETY AND THE PROBLEM OF COMORBIDITY

Over the last several decades clinical research on anxiety has recognized that the older term "anxiety neurosis" had limited heuristic value. Most theories and research on anxiety now recognize that there are a number of specific subtypes of anxiety that cluster under the rubric "anxiety disorders." Even though these more specific anxiety disorders share some common features such as the activation of fear in order to detect and avoid threat (Craske, 2003), there are important differences with implications for treatment. Thus the present volume, like most contemporary perspectives, will focus on specific anxiety disorders rather than treat clinical anxiety as a single homogenous entity. Table 1.1 lists the core threat and cognitive appraisal associated with the five DSM-IV-TR anxiety disorders discussed in this book (for similar summary, see Dozois & Westra, 2004).

Psychiatric classification systems like DSM-IV assume that mental disorders like anxiety consists of more specific disorder subtypes with diagnostic boundaries that sharply demarcate one type of disorder from another. However, a large body of epidemiological, diagnostic, and symptom-based research has challenged this categorical approach to psychiatric nosology, offering much stronger evidence for the dimensional nature of psychiatric disorders like anxiety and depression (e.g., Melzer, Tom, Brugha, Fryers, & Meltzer, 2002; Ruscio, Borkovec, & Ruscio, 2001; Ruscio, Ruscio, & Keane, 2002).

One of the strongest challenges to the categorical perspective is the evidence of extensive symptom and disorder comorbidity in both anxiety and depression—that is, the cross-sectional co-occurrence of one or more disorders in the same individual (Clark, Beck, & Alford, 1999). Only 21% of respondents with a lifetime history of disorder had only one disorder in the National Comorbidity Survey (NCS; Kessler et al., 1994), a National Institute of Mental Health (NIMH) epidemiological study of mental disorders involving a randomized nationally representative sample of 8,098 Americans who were administered the Structured Clinical Interview for DSM-III-R. Based on a sample of 1,694 outpatients from the Philadelphia Center for Cognitive Therapy evaluated between January, 1986, and October, 1992, only 10.5% of those with a primary mood disorder and 17.8% with panic disorder (with or without agoraphobia avoidance) had a "pure diagnosis" without Axis I or II comorbidity (Somoza, Steer, Beck, & Clark, 1994). Clearly then, diagnostic comorbidity is the norm rather than the exception, with *prognostic comorbidity*, in which one disorder predisposes an individual to the development of other disorders (Maser & Cloninger, 1990) also important to consider in the pathogenesis of psychiatric conditions.

Numerous clinical states have reported a high rate of diagnostic comorbidity within the anxiety disorders. For example, a large outpatient study ($N = 1,127$) found that

TABLE 1.1. Core Features of Five DSM-IV-TR Anxiety Disorders

Anxiety disorder	Threatening stimulus	Core appraisal
Panic disorder (with or without agoraphobia)	Physical, bodily sensations	Fear of dying ("heart attack"), losing control ("going crazy") or consciousness (fainting), having further panic attacks
Generalized anxiety disorder (GAD)	Stressful life events or other personal concerns	Fear of possible future adverse or threatening life outcomes
Social phobia	Social, public situations	Fear of negative evaluation from others (e.g., embarrassment, humiliation)
Obsessive–compulsive disorder (OCD)	Unacceptable intrusive thoughts, images, or impulses	Fear of losing mental or behavioral control or otherwise being responsible for a negative outcome to self or others
Posttraumatic stress disorder (PTSD)	Memories, sensations, external stimuli associated with past traumatic experiences	Fear of thoughts, memories, symptoms, or stimuli associated with the traumatic event

two-thirds of anxiety disorder patients had another current Axis I disorder, and over three-fourths had a lifetime comorbid diagnosis (Brown, Campbell, Lehman, Grisham, & Mancill, 2001). Individuals with an anxiety disorder, then, are much more likely to have at least one or more additional disorders than would be expected by chance (Brown et al., 2001).

Comorbid Depression

Anxiety disorders are more likely to co-occur with some disorders than with others. Much of the research on comorbidity has focused on the relationship between anxiety and depression. Approximately 55% of patients with an anxiety or depressive disorder will have at least one additional anxiety or depressive disorder, and this rate jumps to 76% when considering lifetime diagnoses (Brown & Barlow, 2002). In the Epidemiologic Catchment Area (ECA) study individuals with a major depression were 9 to 19 times more likely to have a coexisting anxiety disorder than individuals without major depression (Regier, Burke, & Burke, 1990). Fifty-one percent of anxiety disorder cases in NCS had major depressive disorder, and this increased to 58% for lifetime diagnoses (Kessler et al., 1996). Moreover, anxiety disorders are more likely to precede depressive disorders than the reverse, although the strength of this sequential association does vary across specific anxiety disorders (Alloy, Kelly, Mineka, & Clements, 1990; Mineka, Watson, & Clark, 1998; Schatzberg, Samson, Rothschild, Bond, & Regier, 1998). Results from the ECA survey waves indicated that simple phobia, obsessive–compulsive disorder (OCD), agoraphobia, and panic attacks were associated with increased risk for major depression 12 months later (Goodwin, 2002).

Research into comorbidity has important clinical implications for the treatment of all psychological disorders. Clinical depression comorbid with an anxiety disorder is associated with a more persistent course of disturbance, greater symptom severity, and greater functional impairment or disability (Hunt, Slade, & Andrews, 2004; Kessler & Frank, 1997; Kessler et al., 1996; Olfson et al., 1997; Roy-Byrne et al., 2000). In addition, anxiety disorders with a comorbid depression show a poorer treatment response, higher relapse and recurrence rates, and greater service utilization than cases of pure anxiety (Mineka et al., 1998; Roy-Byrne et al., 2000; Tylee, 2000).

Comorbid Substance Use

Substance use disorders, especially use of alcohol, are another category of conditions that are often seen in the anxiety disorders. In their review Kushner, Abrams, and Borchardt (2000) concluded that presence of an anxiety disorder (except simple phobia) doubles to quadruples the risk of alcohol or drug dependence, with anxiety frequently preceding the alcohol use disorder and contributing to its persistence, although alcohol misuse can also lead to anxiety. Even at subthreshold diagnostic levels, individuals with an anxiety condition are significantly more likely to use drugs and alcohol than nonclinical controls (Sbrana et al., 2005).

It is evident that a special relationship exists between alcohol use disorders and anxiety. Compared with mood disorders, anxiety disorders more often precede substance use disorders (Merikangas et al., 1998), leading to the assumption that anxious individuals must be "self-medicating" with alcohol. However, this "self-medicating" assumption was not supported in a 7-year prospective study in which alcohol dependence was as likely to increase risk of developing a subsequent anxiety disorder as was the reverse temporal relationship (Kushner, Sher, & Erickson, 1999). Kushner and colleagues concluded that anxiety and alcohol problems likely have reciprocal and interacting influences that will lead to an escalation of both anxiety and problem drinking (Kushner, Sher, & Beitman, 1990; Kushner et al., 2000). The end result can be a "downward self-destructive spiral" leading to helplessness, depression, and increased risk for suicide (Barlow, 2002).

Comorbidity within Anxiety Disorders

The presence of one anxiety disorder significantly increases the probability of having one or more additional anxiety disorders. In fact, pure anxiety disorders are less frequent than comorbid anxiety. In their large clinical study, Brown, DiNardo, Lehmann, and Campbell (2001) found that comorbidity for another anxiety disorder ranged from 27% for specific phobia to 62% for posttraumatic stress disorder (PTSD). Generalized anxiety disorder (GAD) was the most common secondary anxiety disorder, followed by social phobia. For PTSD, which had the highest comorbid rate for another anxiety disorder, panic disorder and GAD were the most common secondary anxiety conditions. Social phobia and GAD tended to precede many of the other anxiety disorders. Analysis of lifetime diagnoses revealed even higher rates for occurrence of a secondary anxiety disorder.

Clinician Guideline 1.4

A case conceptualization of anxiety should include a broad diagnostic assessment that covers investigation of comorbid conditions, especially major depression, alcohol abuse, and other anxiety disorders.

PREVALENCE, COURSE, AND OUTCOME OF ANXIETY

Prevalence

The anxiety disorders are the most prevalent form of psychological disturbance (Kessler, Chiu, Demler, & Walters, 2005). Epidemiological studies of adult community samples have been remarkably consistent in documenting a 25–30% lifetime prevalence rate for at least one anxiety disorder. For example the 1-year prevalence for any anxiety disorder in the NCS was 17.2%, compared with 11.3% for any substance abuse/dependence and 11.3% for any mood disorder (Kessler et al., 1994). The NCS lifetime prevalence, which includes all individuals who ever experienced an anxiety disorder, was 24.9%, but this may be an underestimate because OCD was not assessed. In a recent replication of the NCS (NCS-R), involving a nationally representative sample of respondents (*N* = 9,282) interviewed between 2001 and 2003, 12-month prevalence for any anxiety disorder was 18.1% and estimated lifetime prevalence was 28.8%, findings that are remarkably similar to the first NCS (Kessler et al., 2005; Kessler, Berglund, Demler, Robertson, & Walters, 2005).

National surveys conducted in other Western countries like Australia, Great Britain, and Canada have also reported high rates of anxiety disorders in the general population, although the actual prevalence rates vary slightly across studies because of different interview methodologies, diagnostic decision rules, and other design factors (Andrews, Henderson, & Hall, 2001; Jenkins et al., 1997; Canadian Community Health Survey, 2003). The World Health Organization (WHO) World Mental Health Survey Initiative found that anxiety was the most common disorder in every country except the Ukraine (7.1%), with 1-year prevalence ranging from 2.4% in Shanghai, China, to 18.2% in the United States (WHO World Mental Health Survey Consortium, 2004).

Anxiety disorders are also common in childhood and adolescence, with 6-month prevalence rates ranging from 6% to 17% (Breton et al., 1999; Romano, Tremblay, Vitaro, Zoccolillo, & Pagani, 2001). The most frequent disorders are specific phobia, GAD, and separation anxiety (Breton et al., 1999; Whitaker et al., 1990). Some disorders like social phobia, panic, and generalized anxiety significantly increase during adolescence, whereas others like separation anxiety show a decrease (Costello, Mustillo, Erkanli, Keeler, & Angold, 2003; Kashani & Orvaschel, 1990). Girls suffer higher rates of anxiety disorders than boys (Breton et al., 1999; Costello et al., 2003; Romano et al., 2001), comorbidity between anxiety and depression is high (Costello et al., 2003), and anxiety disorders that arise during childhood and adolescence often persist into early adulthood (Newman et al., 1996).

Individuals suffering from anxiety disorders often first come to the attention of family physicians in primary care settings because of unexplained physical symptoms like noncardiac chest pain, palpitations, faintness, irritable bowel syndrome, vertigo, and dizziness. These complaints may reflect an anxiety condition such as panic disorder (see discussion by Barlow, 2002). Moreover, patients with anxiety disorders seek out medical advice in disproportionate numbers. Studies of primary care patients find that 10–20% have a diagnosable anxiety disorder (Ansseau et al., 2004; Olfson et al., 1997, 2000; Sartorius, Ustun, Lecrubier, & Wittchen, 1996; Vazquez-Barquero et al., 1997). Sleath and Rubin (2002) found that anxiety was mentioned in 30% of visits to a university medical clinic family practice. Anxiety disorders, then, place a considerable burden on health service resources.

A large percentage of the general adult population experiences occasional or mild symptoms of anxiety. There is some evidence that individuals are at increased risk for developing a full-blown anxiety disorder if they experience panic attacks, sleep disturbance, or have obsessional concerns that are not sufficiently frequent or intense to meet diagnostic criteria (i.e., subclinical forms), or have high anxiety sensitivity (see Craske, 2003). Worry, the cardinal feature of GAD, is reported by a majority of nonclinical individuals who express concerns with work (or school), finances, family, and the like (e.g., Borkovec, Shadick, & Hopkins, 1991; Dupuy, Beaudoin, Rhéaume, Ladouceur, & Dugas, 2001; Tallis, Eysenck, & Mathews, 1992; Wells & Morrison, 1994). Problems with sleep are reported by 27% of British women and 20% of British men (Jenkins et al., 1997). In the U.S. 1991 National Sleep Foundation Survey, 36% of participants had occasional or chronic insomnia (Ancoli-Israel & Roth, 1999). Other studies indicate that 11–33% of nonclinical students and community adults have experienced at least one panic attack in the last year (Malan, Norton, & Cox, 1990; Salge, J. G. Beck, & Logan, 1988; Wilson et al., 1992). Thus symptoms of anxiety and its disorders are prevalent problems that threaten the physical and emotional well-being of a significant number of people in the general population.

Clinician Guideline 1.5

Given the high rate of anxiety disorders and symptoms in the general population, clinical assessment should include specification of symptom frequency and intensity as well as measures that enable differential diagnosis between disorders.

Gender Differences

Women have a significantly higher incidence of most anxiety disorders than men (Craske, 2003), with the possible exception of OCD, where the rates are approximately equal (see Clark, 2004). In the NCS women had a lifetime prevalence of 30.5% for any anxiety disorder, compared with 19.5% for men (Kessler et al., 1994). Other community-based and epidemiological studies generally have confirmed a 2:1 ratio of women to men in prevalence of anxiety disorders (e.g., Andrews et al., 2001; Jenkins et al., 1997; Olfson et al., 2000; Vazquez-Barquero et al., 1997). Since these gender differences were found in community-based surveys, the preponderance of anxiety disorders in women cannot be attributed to greater service utilization. In a critical review of research on gender differences in the anxiety disorders, Craske (2003) concluded that women may have higher rates of anxiety disorders because of an increased vulnerability such as (1) higher negative affectivity; (2) differential socialization patterns in which girls are encouraged to be more dependent, prosocial, empathic but less assertive and controlling of everyday challenges; (3) more pervasive anxiousness as evidenced by less discriminating and more overgeneralized anxious responding; (4) heightened sensitivity to reminders of threat and contextual threat cues; and/or (5) tendency to engage in more avoidance, worry, and rumination about potential threats.

Cultural Differences

Fear and anxiety exist in all cultures but their subjective experience is shaped by culture-specific factors (Barlow, 2002). Comparing the prevalence of anxiety across different cultures is complicated by the fact that our standard diagnostic classification system, DSM-IV-TR (APA, 2000), is based on American conceptualizations and experiences of anxiety that may not have high diagnostic validity in other cultures (van Ommeren, 2002). Cross-cultural generalizability is not necessarily improved by using the WHO's classification of anxiety disorders, the International Classification of Diseases—Tenth Revision (ICD-10), because of the dominance of the European-influenced Western experience (World Health Organization, 1992). Thus our standard diagnostic and assessment approaches to anxiety may overemphasize aspects of anxiety that are prominent in the European Western experience and omit significant expressions of anxiety that are more culture-specific.

Barlow (2002) concluded in his review that apprehension, worry, fear, and somatic arousal are common in all cultures. For example, a large community survey of 35,014 adult Iranians found that 20.8% had anxiety symptoms (Noorbala, Bagheri-Yazdi, Yasamy, & Mohammad, 2004). Even in remote rural or mountainous regions of developing countries where modern industrial amenities and pressures are minimal, the occurrence of anxiety and panic disorders is similar to rates reported in Western community surveys (Mumford, Nazir, Jilani, & Yar Baig, 1996). Nevertheless, countries do appear to have different population rates of the anxiety disorders. The WHO World Mental Health Surveys found that 1-year prevalence of DSM-IV anxiety disorders ranged from a low of 2.4%, 3.2%, and 3.3% in Shanghai, Beijing, and Nigeria, respectively, to 11.2%, 12%, and 18.2% in Lebanon, France, and the United States, respectively (WHO World Mental Health Survey Consortium, 2004). This broad variability in prevalence rates raises the possibility that culture may influence the actual rate of anxiety disorders across countries, although methodological differences across sites cannot be ruled out as an alternative explanation for the differences.

There is substantial evidence that culture does play a significant role in the expression of anxious symptoms. Barlow (2002) noted that somatic symptoms appear more prominent in emotional disorders in most countries other than those of the European-influenced West. Table 1.2 presents a select number of culture-bound syndromes with a significant anxiety component.

Clinician Guideline 1.6

Assessment for anxiety should include a consideration of the individual's culture and social/familial environment and their influence on the development and subjective experience of anxiety.

Persistence and Course

In contrast to major depression, anxiety disorders are often chronic over many years with relatively low remission but more variable rates of relapse after complete recovery (Barlow, 2002). The Harvard–Brown Anxiety Disorder Research Program (HARP), an 8-year prospective study, found that only one-third to one-half of patients with social phobia, GAD, or panic disorder achieved full remission (Yonkers, Bruce, Dyck, & Keller, 2003).[1] The Zurich Cohort Study found that nearly 50% of individuals with an initial

---

[1] Although these remission rates are very low, especially for social phobia and panic disorder, they probably overestimate the true remission rates for the anxiety disorders since 80% of the subjects had some form of pharmacological treatment over the 8-year follow-up.

TABLE 1.2. Select Culture-Bound Syndromes in Which Anxious Symptoms Play a Prominent Role

Syndrome name	Description	Country
dhat	Severe anxiety about the loss of semen through nocturnal emissions, urination, or masturbation. (Sumathipala, Siribaddana, & Bhugra, 2004)	Males in India, Sri Lanka, China
koro	Sudden and intense fear that one's sexual organs will retract into the abdomen eventually causing death. (APA, 2000)	Mainly occurs in males in south and east Asia
pa-leng	Morbid fear of the cold and wind in which the individual worries about further loss of body heat that could eventually lead to death. The person wears several layers of clothes even on warm days to keep out wind and cold. (Barlow, 2002)	Chinese cultures
taijin kyofusho	An intense fear that one's body parts or functions are displeasing, offensive, or embarrassing to other people by their appearance, odor, facial expressions, or movements. (APA, 2000).	Japan

anxiety disorder later developed depression alone or depression comorbid with anxiety at a 15-year follow-up (Merikangas et al., 2003). A Dutch longitudinal study of 3,107 older individuals found that 23% of subjects with an initial DSM-III anxiety disorder continued to meet criteria 6 years later, whereas another 47% suffered from subclinical anxiety (Schuurmans et al., 2005). It is evident the anxiety disorders persist for many years when not treated (Craske, 2003). Given that the majority of these disorders have their onset in childhood and adolescence (Newman et al., 1996), the chronic nature of anxiety is a significant component of its overall disease burden.

Clinician Guideline 1.7

Consider the chronicity of anxiety and its influence on the development of other conditions when conducting a cognitive assessment. We can expect that early onset and a more persistent course would be more challenging for treatment.

Consequences and Outcome

The presence of an anxiety disorder, or even just anxious symptoms, is associated with a significant reduction in quality of life as well as in social and occupational functioning (Mendlowicz & Stein, 2000). In a meta-analytic review of 23 studies, Olatunji, Cisler, and Tolin (2007) found that all individuals with anxiety disorders experienced significantly poorer quality of life outcomes compared with control samples, and overall quality of life impairment was equivalent across the anxiety disorders. Individuals with an anxiety disorder have an increase in number of work loss days (Kessler & Frank, 1997; Olfson et al., 2000), more disability days (Andrews et al., 2001; Marcus, Olfson, Pincus, Shear, & Zarin, 1997; Weiller, Bisserbe, Maier, & LeCrubier, 1998), and elevated rates of financial dependence in the form of disability payments, chronic unemployment, or welfare payments (Leon, Portera, & Weissman, 1995). Anxiety also tends to reduce the quality of life and social functioning in patients with a comorbid chronic medical illness (Sherbourne, Wells, Meredith, Jackson, & Camp, 1996). Olfson et al. (1996) even found that primary care patients who did not meet diagnostic criteria for GAD, panic, or OCD but had symptoms of these disorders reported significantly more days of lost work, marital distress, and visits to a mental health professional. The negative impact of anxiety disorders in terms of distress, disability, and utilization of services can be even greater than for individuals whose main problem is a personality disorder or substance abuse (Andrews, Slade, & Issakidis, 2002). In fact, individuals with panic disorder evidence significantly lower social and role functioning in daily activities than patients with a chronic medical illness like hypertension (Sherbourne, Wells, & Judd, 1996).

Individuals with a diagnosable anxiety disorder make more visits to mental health professionals and are more likely to consult with their general practitioners for psychological problems compared with nonclinical controls (Marciniak, Lage, Landbloom, Dunayevich, & Bowman, 2004; Weiller et al., 1998). A large-scale study of employed Americans found that individuals with anxiety disorders were significantly more likely than the nonclinical control group to visit medical specialists, more likely to use inpatient services, and more likely to visit emergency rooms (Marciniak et al., 2004; see also Leon et al., 1995, for similar results). However, the majority of individuals with an anxiety disorder never receive professional treatment, and even fewer come to the attention of mental health practitioners (Coleman, Brod, Potter, Buesching, & Rowland, 2004; Kessler et al., 1994; Olfson et al., 2000). Family physicians, for example, are particularly poor at recognizing anxiety, with at least 50% of anxiety disorders missed in primary care patients (Wittchen & Boyer, 1998).

Given the adverse personal and social effects of anxiety disorders, the economic costs of anxiety are substantial in both the direct costs of services and the indirect costs of lost productivity. Self-reported anxiety in one American study accounted for an estimated 60.4 million days per year in lost productivity, which is equivalent to the level of lost productivity associated with the common cold or pneumonia (Marcus et al., 1997). Greenberg et al. (1999) estimated the annual cost of anxiety disorders at $42.3 billion in 1990 U.S. dollars, whereas Rice and Miller (1998) found that the economic costs of anxiety were greater than for schizophrenia or the affective disorders.[2]

Clinician Guideline 1.8

Given the significant morbidity associated with anxiety, the negative impact of the disorder on work/school productivity, social relations, personal finances, and daily functioning must be included in the clinical assessment.

---

[2]There is evidence that a significant offset of the costs of anxiety can be achieved by early detection and treatment (Salvador-Carulla, Segui, Fernández-Cano, & Canet, 1995). Health economic studies have consistently shown that cognitive-behavioral therapy (CBT) for anxiety disorders is cheaper than medication and produces significant reduction in health care costs (Myhr & Payne, 2006). As the most common of the mental disorders, anxiety inflicts a significant human and social cost on our society, but increased provision of cognitive and cognitive-behavioral treatment could reduce the personal and economic costs of these disorders.

BIOLOGICAL ASPECTS OF ANXIETY

Anxiety is multifaceted, involving diverse elements of the physiological, cognitive, behavioral, and affective domains of human function. Table 1.3 lists the symptoms of anxiety divided into the four functional systems involved in an adaptive response to threat and danger (Beck et al., 1985, 2005).

The automatic physiological responses that typically occur in the presence of threat or danger are considered *defensive responses*. These responses, seen in the fear-eliciting contexts of both animals and humans, involve autonomic arousal that prepares the organism to deal with danger by fleeing (i.e., flight) or by directly confronting the danger (i.e., fight), a process known as the "fight-or-flight" response (Canon, 1927). The behavioral features primarily involve escape or avoidance as well as safety-seeking responses. The cognitive variables provide the meaningful interpretation of our internal state as that of anxiety. Finally the affective domain is derived from cognitive and physiological activation, and constitutes the subjective experience of feeling anxious. In the following sections, we briefly discuss the physiological, behavioral, and emotional aspects of anxiety. The cognitive features of anxiety are the focus of subsequent chapters.

Psychophysiology

As evident from Table 1.3, many of the symptoms of anxiety are physiological in nature, reflecting activation of the sympathetic (SNS) and parasympathetic (PNS) nervous systems. Activation of the SNS is the most prominent physiological response in anxiety, and it leads to hyperarousal symptoms such as constriction of the peripheral blood vessels, increased strength of the skeletal muscles, increased heart rate and force of contraction, dilation of the lungs to increase oxygen supply, dilation of the pupils for possible improved vision, cessation of digestive activity, increase in basal metabolism, and increased secretion of epinephrine and norepinephrine from the adrenal medulla (Brad-

---

TABLE 1.3. Common Features of Anxiety

Physiological symptoms

(1) Increase heart rate, palpitations; (2) shortness of breath, rapid breathing; (3) chest pain or pressure; (4) choking sensation; (5) dizzy, lightheaded; (6) sweaty, hot flashes, chills; (7) nausea, upset stomach, diarrhea; (8) trembling, shaking; (9) tingling or numbness in arms, legs; (10) weakness, unsteady, faintness; (11) tense muscles, rigidity; (12) dry mouth

Cognitive symptoms

(1) fear of losing control, being unable to cope; (2) fear of physical injury or death; (3) fear of "going crazy"; (4) fear of negative evaluation by others; (5) frightening thoughts, images, or memories; (6) perceptions of unreality or detachment; (7) poor concentration, confusion, distractible; (8) narrowing of attention, hypervigilance for threat; (9) poor memory; (10) difficulty in reasoning, loss of objectivity

Behavioral symptoms

(1) avoidance of threat cues or situations; (2) escape, flight; (3) pursuit of safety, reassurance; (4) restlessness, agitation, pacing; (5) hyperventilation; (6) freezing, motionless; (7) difficult speaking

Affective symptoms

(1) nervous, tense, wound-up; (2) frightened, fearful, terrified; (3) edgy, jumpy, jittery; (4) impatient, frustrated

ley, 2000). All of these peripheral physiological responses are associated with arousal but cause various perceptible symptoms such as trembling, shaking, hot and cold spells, heart palpitations, dry mouth, sweating, shortness of breath, chest pain or pressure, and muscle tension (see Barlow, 2002).

The role of PNS excitation, which causes a conservation of certain physiological responses, has not been as well researched in anxiety. The PNS is involved in symptoms like tonic immobility, drop in blood pressure, and fainting, which are a type of "conservation-withdrawal" response strategy (Friedman & Thayer, 1998). The effects of PNS stimulation include decreased heart rate and force of contraction, constricted pupils, relaxed abdominal muscles, and constriction of the lungs (Bradley, 2000). Moreover, research on heart rate variability in panic attacks indicates that the cardiovascular activity associated with anxiety should not be seen simply in terms of excessive SNS activation but also reduced compensatory PNS excitation. Thus the PNS probably plays a greater role in anxiety than previously considered.

Barlow (2002) concluded that one of the most robust and enduring findings in the past 50 years of psychophysiological research is that chronically anxious individuals exhibit a persistently elevated autonomic arousal level often in the absence of an anxiety-producing situation. For example, Cuthbert et al. (2003) reported significantly elevated heart rate base levels for panic and specific phobias but not social phobia or posttraumatic stress disorder (PTSD) groups. Other researchers, however, have linked anxiety (or neuroticism) to excess autonomic lability and reactivity rather than to enduring tonic levels of activation (Costello, 1971; Eysenck, 1979). Craske (2003) proposed that heightened cardiovascular reactivity might be a predisposing factor for panic disorder such that a tendency to experience intense and acute autonomic activation could increase the salience and therefore threat attributed to bodily sensations.

Empirical support for autonomic differences between anxious and nonanxious controls in response to stressful or threatening stimuli has not been consistently obtained across studies (Barlow, 2002). Freidman and Thayer (1998) also noted that psychophysiological findings of *reduced* heart rate and electrodermal variability challenge the view that anxiety is characterized by excessive autonomic lability and reactivity. Nevertheless, anxious individuals do show a slower decline in their physiological response to stressors (i.e., slow habituation), but this is probably due to their higher initial baseline arousal level (Barlow, 2002). In addition Lang and colleagues found greater physiological arousal to fear-relevant imagery in snake phobic individuals, but reactivity was less evident in those with panic (Cuthbert et al., 2003; Lang, 1979; Lang, Levin, Miller, & Kozak, 1983). Together these results suggest that heightened physiological reactivity to fear stimuli may be greatest in specific phobic conditions but less evident in other anxiety states like panic disorder or PTSD. However, a heightened basal arousal level and slower habituation rate might be seen more consistently across various anxiety disorders, thereby providing the physiological basis for chronically anxious individuals to misinterpret their persistent state of hyperarousal as evidence of an anticipated threat or danger.

Recent psychophysiological research suggests that individuals with chronic anxiety exhibit *diminished autonomic flexibility* in response to stressors (Noyes & Hoehn-Saric, 1998). This is characterized by a weak but sustained response to stressors, indicating a poor habituation trajectory. In a study of heart rate reactivity under baseline, relaxation, and worry conditions, Thayer, Friedman, and Borkovec (1996) found that individuals with GAD or those actively engaged in worry had lower cardiac vagal control, which supports the view that GAD is characterized by autonomic inflexibility.

In sum it would appear that important psychophysiological features of anxiety such as elevated basal arousal level, slower habituation, and diminished autonomic flexibility might contribute to the misinterpretation of threat that is the core cognitive feature of anxiety. However, a different physiological response pattern may distinguish phobia, panic disorder, and GAD, which prevents generalizing research findings across the anxiety disorders. Furthermore, it is unclear whether the anxiety state is primarily an excess of SNS activation and a withdrawal of vagal activity, or if SNS activity is depressed and PNS activity remains normal under the conditions of daily living (see Mussgay & Rüddel, 2004, for discussion).

Clinician Guideline 1.9

Assessment of anxiety disorders must include a thorough evaluation of the type, frequency, and severity of physiological symptoms experienced during acute anxiety episodes, as well as the patient's interpretation of these symptoms. Baseline as well as patterns of physiological reactivity should be assessed using diaries and daily rating scales.

Genetic Factors

There is considerable empirical evidence that anxiety runs in families (see Barlow, 2002, for review). In a meta-analysis of family and twin studies for panic disorder, GAD, phobias, and OCD, Hettema, Neale, and Kendler (2001) concluded there is significant familial aggregation for all four disorders, with the strongest evidence for panic disorder. Across all disorders, estimates of heritability ranged from 30 to 40%, leaving the largest proportion of the variance due to individual environmental factors. Even at the symptomatic level, heritability accounts for only 27% of the variability by predisposing individuals to general distress, with environmental factors determining the development of specific anxiety or depressive symptoms (Kendler, Heath, Martin, & Eaves, 1987).

Barlow (2002) raised the possibility that a separate genetic transmission might be evident for anxiety and panic. In a structural equation modeling of diagnostic data collected on a large female twin sample, Kendler et al. (1995) found separate genetic risk factors for major depression and GAD (i.e., anxiety), on the one hand, and for acute, short-lived anxiety like phobias and panic, on the other. An earlier study also found a common genetic diathesis for major depression and GAD with disorder-specificity determined by exposure to different life events (Kendler, Neale, Kessler, Heath, & Eaves, 1992a).

There is less evidence that individuals inherit specific anxiety disorders and stronger empirical support for inheritance of a general vulnerability to develop an anxiety disorder (Barlow, 2002). This nonspecific vulnerability for anxiety could be neuroticism, high trait anxiety, negative affectivity, or what Barlow, Allen, and Choate (2004) called a "negative affect syndrome." Vulnerable individuals might show a stronger (or at least more sustained) emotional response to aversive or stressful situations. However, environmental and cognitive factors would interact with this genetic predisposition to determine which of the specific anxiety disorders is experienced by a particular individual.

Clinician Guideline 1.10

A diagnostic interview should include questions about the prevalence of anxiety disorders in first-degree relatives.

Neurophysiology

In the last decade rapid advances have been made in our understanding of the neurobiological basis of fear and anxiety. One important finding that has emerged is the central role of the amygdala in emotional processing and memory (see discussion by Canli et al., 2001). Human and nonhuman research indicates that the amygdala is involved in the emotional modulation of memory, the evaluation of stimuli with affective significance, and the appraisal of social signals related to danger (see Anderson & Phelps, 2000). Research on auditory fear conditioning by LeDoux (1989, 1996, 2000) has contributed most to implicating the amygdala as the neural substrate for the acquisition of conditioned fear responses. LeDoux (1996) concluded that the amygdala is the "hub in the wheel of fear" (p. 170), that it is "in essence, involved in the appraisal of emotional meaning" (p. 169).

LeDoux (1989) contends that one of the most important tasks of the emotional brain is to evaluate the affective significance (e.g., threat vs. nonthreat) of mental (thoughts, memories), physical, or external stimuli. He proposed two parallel neural pathways in the amygdala's processing of fear stimuli. The first pathway involves direct transmission of a conditioned fear stimulus through the sensory thalamus to the lateral nucleus of the amygdala, bypassing the cortex. The second pathway involves transmission of fear stimulus information from the sensory thalamus through the sensory cortex and on to the lateral nucleus. Within the amygdala region the lateral nucleus, which receives inputs in fear conditioning, innervates the central nucleus that is responsible for the expression of the conditioned fear response (see also Davis, 1998). Figure 1.1 illustrates the two parallel pathways of LeDoux's conditioned fear reaction system.

LeDoux (1996) draws a number of implications from his dual pathway of fear. The more direct thalamo–amygdala path (called "the low road") is quicker, more rudimentary, and occurs without thinking, reasoning, and consciousness. The thalamo–cortical–amygdala path (labeled "the high road") is slower but involves more elaborative processing of the fear stimulus because of extensive involvement of higher cortical regions of the brain. Although LeDoux (1996) discusses the obvious evolutionary advantage of an automatic, preconscious neural basis to information processing of fear stimuli, his research demonstrated that the cortical pathway is necessary for fear conditioning to more complex stimuli (i.e., when the animal must discriminate between two similar tones in which only one is paired with the unconditioned stimulus [UCS]).

The central role of the amygdala in fear is entirely consistent with its neuroanatomical connections. It has multiple output projections via the central nucleus to the hypothalamus, hippocampus, and upward to various regions of the cortex, as well as downward to various brainstem structures involved in autonomic arousal and neuroendocrine responses associated with stress and anxiety like the periaqueductal gray region (PAG), the ventral tegmental area, the locus ceruleus, and the raphe nuclei (Barlow, 2002). All of these neutral structures have been implicated in the experience of anxiety, including the bed nucleus of the stria terminalis (BNST; Davis, 1998), which may be the most important neural substrate of anxiety (Grillon, 2002).

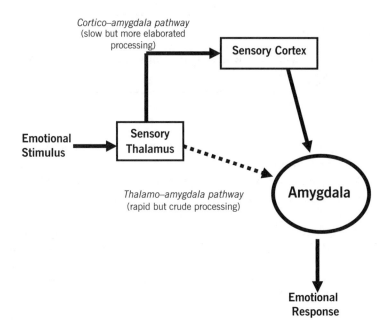

FIGURE 1.1. LeDoux's parallel neural pathways in auditory fear conditioning.

The role of conscious cognitive processing in fear is a much debated issue in light of LeDoux's research suggesting a rapid and rudimentary noncortical thalamo–amygdala pathway in the processing of conditioned fear. In fact LeDoux (1996) found that fear-relevant stimuli can be implicitly processed by the amygdala through the subcortical thalamo–amygdala pathway without conscious representation. Neuroimaging studies have found that fearful or negatively valenced stimuli are associated with relative increases in regional cerebral blood flow (rCBF) in the secondary or associative visual cortex and relative reductions in rCBF in the hippocampus, prefrontal, orbitofrontal, temporopolar, and posterior cingulated cortex (e.g., see Coplan & Lydiard, 1998; Rauch, Savage, Alpert, Fishman, & Jenike, 1997; Simpson et al., 2000). These findings have been interpreted as evidence that fear can be preconscious without the occurrence of higher cognitive processing.

Evidence for a subcortical, lower order pathway to immediate conditioned fear processing should not divert attention away from the critical role that attention, reasoning, memory, and subjective appraisal or judgments play in human fear and anxiety. LeDoux (1996) found that the thalamo–cortico–amygdala pathway was activated in more complex fear conditioning. Moreover, the amygdala has extensive connections with the hippocampus and cortical regions, where it receives inputs from cortical sensory processing areas, the transitional cortical area, and the medial prefrontal cortex (LeDoux, 1996, 2000). LeDoux emphasizes that the hippocampal system involving explicit memory and the amygdala system involving emotional memory will be activated simultaneously by the same stimuli and will function at the same time. Thus cortical brain structures involved in *working memory*, such as the prefrontal cortex and the anterior cingulate and orbital cortical regions, and structures involved in long-term *declarative memory*, like the hippocampus and temporal lobe, are implicated with amygdala-dependent emotional arousal to provide the neural basis to the subjective (conscious) experience of fear (LeDoux, 2000). The neural substrates of cognition, then, can be expected to play a critical role in the type of fear acquisition and persistence that characterizes complex human fears and anxiety disorders. This is supported by various neuroimaging studies that found differential activation of various medial prefrontal and frontotempororbital regions of the cortex (e.g., Connor & Davidson, 1998; Coplan & Lyiard, 1998; Lang, Bradley, & Cuthbert; 1998; McNally, 2007; van den Heuvel et al., 2004; Whiteside, Port, & Abramowitz, 2004).

In their review Luu, Tucker, and Derryberry (1998) argued that fear-relevant mental representations of the cortex influence emotional functioning not only at the later stage of fear expression and responsivity, but cortical influence can also serve an anticipatory function even before sensory information is physically available. The authors conclude that "with our highly evolved frontal networks, we humans are capable of cognitively mediating our actions, and of inhibiting the more reflexive responses triggered by limbic and subcortical circuits" (Luu et al., 1998, p. 588). This sentiment was recently echoed in a review paper by McNally (2007a) in which he concludes that activation in the medial prefrontal cortex can suppress conditioned fear acquisition that is mediated by the amygdala. Thus prefrontal executive functions (i.e., conscious cognitive processes) can have fear-inhibiting effects that involve learning new inhibitory associations or "safety signals" that suppress fear expression (McNally, 2007a). Frewen, Dozois, and Lanius (2008) concluded in their review of 11 neuroimaging studies of psychological interventions for anxiety and depression that CBT alters functioning in brain regions such as the dorsolateral, ventrolateral, and medial prefrontal cortices; anterior cingulate; posterior cingulate/precuneus; and the insular cortices that are associated with problem solving, self-referential and relational processing, and regulation of negative affect. Clearly, then, the extensive involvement of higher order cortical regions of the brain in emotional experiences is consistent with our contention that cognition plays an important role in the production of anxiety and that interventions like cognitive therapy can effectively inhibit anxiety by engaging cortical regions responsible for higher order reasoning and executive function.

Neurotransmitter Systems

Neurotransmitter systems such as the benzodiazepine–gamma-aminobutyric acid (GABA), noradrenergic, and serotonergic, as well as the corticotropin-releasing hormonal pathway, are important to the biology of anxiety (Noyes & Hoehn-Saric, 1998). The serotonergic neurotransmitter system has become of increasing interest in research on anxiety and panic. Serotonin acts as a neurochemical break on behavior, with blockage of serotonin receptors in humans associated with anxiety (Noyes & Hoehn-Saric, 1998). Although low levels of serotonin have been implicated as a key contributor to anxiety, direct neurophysiological evidence is mixed on whether abnormalities in serotonin can be found in anxiety disorders like GAD compared to controls (Sinha, Mohlman, & Gorman, 2004). The serotonergic system projects to diverse areas of the brain that regulate anxiety like the amygdala, septo-hippocampal, and prefrontal cortical regions and so may have a direct influence on anxiety or an indirect influence by altering the function of other neurotransmitters (Noyes & Hoehn-Saric, 1998; Sinha et al., 2004).

A subgroup of the inhibitory transmitter GABA contains benzodiazepine receptors that enhance the inhibitory effects of GABA when benzodiazepine molecules bind to these receptor sites (Gardner, Tully, & Hedgecock, 1993). Evidence that generalized anxiety may be due to a suppressed benzodiazepine-GABA system comes from the anxiolytic effects of benzodiazepine drugs (e.g., lorazepam [Ativan], alprazolam [Xanax]), which appear to have their clinical effectiveness by enhancing benzodiazepine-GABA inhibition (Barlow, 2002).

Corticotropin-releasing hormone (CRH) is a neurotransmitter that is primarily stored in the hypothalamic paraventricular nuclei (PVN). Stressful or threatening stimuli can activate certain brain regions like the locus ceruleus, amygdala, hippocampus, and prefrontal cortex, which then releases CRH. CRH then stimulates secretion of adrenocorticotropic hormone (ACTH) from the anterior pituitary gland and other pituitary–adrenal activity that results in increased production and release of cortisol (Barlow, 2002; Noyes & Hoehn-Saric, 1998). The CRH, then, not only mediates endocrine responses to stress but also other broad brain and behavioral responses that play a role in the expression of stress, anxiety, and depression (Barlow, 2002). Overall, then, abnormalities at the neurotransmitter level appear to have anxiogenic or anxiolytic effects that play an important contributory role in heightened physiological states that characterize fear and anxiety. However, the exact nature of these abnormalities is still unknown. Table 1.4 provides a summary of the biological aspects of anxiety that might underlie the cognitive features of these disorders discussed later in this volume.

Clinician Guideline 1.11

Discuss the neural basis of anxiety when educating the client about the cognitive model of anxiety. The rationale for cognitive therapy should include a discussion of how the higher order cortical centers of the brain involved in memory, reasoning, and judgment can "override" or inhibit subcortical emotional brain structures, thereby reducing the subjective experience of anxiety.

TABLE 1.4. **Biological Concomitants of Cognition in Anxiety**

Biological factors	Cognitive sequelae
• Elevated tonic autonomic activation	• Increased salience of threat-related stimuli
• Slower habituation rate	• Sustained attention to threat
• Diminished autonomic flexibility	• Reduced ability to shift attention
• Genetic predisposition for negative emotionality	• Hypervalent schemas of threat and danger
• Subcortical fear potentiation	• Preconscious fear stimulus identification and immediate physiological arousal
• Extensive cortical afferent and efferent pathways to subcortical emotion-relevant circuitry	• Cognitive appraisal and memory influence fear perception and modulates fear expression and action

BEHAVIORAL THEORIES

Over several decades experimental psychologists grounded in learning theory have demonstrated that fear responses can be acquired through an associative learning process. Theoretical and experimental work from this perspective has focused on the physiological and behavioral responses that characterize an anxious or fearful state. Early learning theory focused on the acquisition of fears or phobic reactions through classical conditioning.

Conditioning Theories

According to classical conditioning, a neutral stimulus, when repeatedly associated with an aversive experience (unconditioned stimulus [UCS] that leads to the experience of anxiety (unconditioned response [UCR]), becomes associated with the aversive experience, it acquires the capability to elicit a similar anxiety response (conditioned response [CR]) (Edelmann, 1992). The emphasis in classical conditioning is that human fears are acquired as a result of some neutral stimulus (e.g., visit to a dentist's office) coming into association with some previous anxiety-provoking experience (e.g., a highly painful and terrifying experience at the dentist office when a child). Although numerous experimental studies over the past 80 years have demonstrated that fears can be acquired in the laboratory by repeatedly pairing a neutral stimulus (e.g., tone) with an unconditioned stimulus (e.g., mildly aversive electric shock), the model could not provide a credible explanation for the remarkable persistence of human fears in the absence of repeated UCS–CS pairings (Barlow, 2002).

Mowrer (1939, 1953, 1960) introduced a major revision to the conditioning theory in order to better account for avoidance behavior and the persistence of human fears. Referred to as "two-factor theory," it became a widely accepted behavioral account of the etiology and persistence of clinical fears and anxiety states throughout the 1960s and early 1970s (e.g., Eysenck & Rachman, 1965). Although no longer considered a tenable theory of anxiety, the two-factor theory is important for two reasons. First, many of the behavioral interventions that have proven so effective in the treatment of anxiety disorders had their origins in the two-factor model. And second, our current cognitive models of anxiety were in large part born out of the criticisms and inadequacies of the two-factor theory.

Figure 1.2 provides an illustration of how the two-factor theory might be used to explain Freud's case study of Little Hans (Freud, 1909/1955). Little Hans was a 5-year-old Austrian boy who developed a fear that a horse would bite him, and so experienced considerable anxiety whenever he ventured outside for fear of seeing a horse. The onset of the "horse phobia" occurred after he witnessed a large "bus-horse" fall down and violently kick its feet in an effort to get up. Little Hans then became frightened that horses, particularly those pulling carts, would fall down and bite him. (Of course Freud interpreted the real source of Little Han's phobia as his repressed sexual affection for his mother and hostility toward his father that became transposed [displaced] onto horses.)

In the two-factor model, the first stage of fear acquisition is based on classical conditioning. Little Hans experiences a traumatic event: seeing a large horse fall to the street and thrash about violently (UCS). This elicits a strong fear response (UCR), so that the sight of horses (CS) through association with the UCS is now capable of elic-

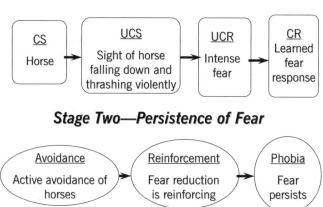

FIGURE 1.2. A two-factor theory of fear acquisition explanation of Freud's case study of Little Hans.

iting a CR (fear response). However, fear persistence is explained at the second stage because of extensive avoidance of the CS. In other words, Little Hans stays indoors and so avoids the sight of horses (the CS). Because avoidance of horses ensures that Little Hans will not experience fear or anxiety, the avoidance behavior is negatively reinforced. Avoidance is maintained because fear reduction is a powerful secondary reinforcer (Edelmann, 1992). Furthermore, because he stays indoors, Little Hans fails to learn that horses do not regularly fall down (i.e., he does not experience repeated CS-only presentations that would lead to extinction).

By the late 1970s serious problems were raised with the two-factor model explanation for human phobias (Rachman, 1976, 1977; see also Davey, 1997; Eysenck, 1979). First, classical conditioning assumes that any neutral stimulus can acquire fear-eliciting properties if associated with a UCS. However, this assumption was not supported in aversive conditioning experiments in which some stimuli (e.g., pictures of spiders and snakes) produced a conditioned fear response much more easily than other stimuli (e.g., pictures of flowers or mushrooms; for review, see Öhman & Mineka, 2001). Second, many individuals who develop clinical phobias can not recall a traumatic conditioning event. Third, there is considerable experimental and clinical evidence of nonassociative learning of fears through vicarious observation (i.e., witnessing someone else's trauma) or informational transmission (i.e., when threatening information about specific objects or situations is conveyed to the individual). Fourth, people often experience traumatic events without developing a conditioned fear response (Rachman, 1977). Again the two-factor model requires considerable refinement to explain why only a minority of individuals develop phobias in response to a traumatic experience (e.g., painful dental work). And finally, the two-factor theory has difficulty explaining the epidemiology of phobias (Rachman, 1977). For example, fear of snakes is much more common than dental phobia, and yet many more people experience the pain of dental work than are bitten by snakes.

Although various refinements were proposed, it became clear that the two-factor theory of conditioning was unable to explain the development and persistence of human fears and anxiety disorders. Many behavioral psychologists concluded that cognitive constructs were needed to provide an adequate account of the development and maintenance of anxiety, even phobic states (e.g., Brewin, 1988; Davey, 1997). A variety of cognitive concepts were proposed (e.g., expectancies, self-efficacy, attentional bias, or threat-related schemas) as mediators between the occurrence of a fear-eliciting stimulus and the anxious response (see Edelmann, 1992). Not all behavioral psychologists, though, embraced cognitive mediation as a causal mechanism in the development of anxiety. An example of a more "noncognitive" perspective is the fear module proposed by Öhman and Mineka (2001).

The Fear Module

Öhman and Mineka (2001) state that because fear evolved as a defense against predators and other threats to survival, it involves a *fear module* composed of behavioral, psychophysiological, and verbal-cognitive components. A fear module is defined as "a relatively independent behavioral, mental, and neural system that is specifically tailored to help solve adaptive problems encountered by potentially life-threatening situations in the ecology of our distant forefathers" (Öhman & Mineka, 2001, p. 484).

They discuss four characteristics of the fear module. First, it is *selectively sensitized* to respond to stimuli that are evoluntionarily prepotent because they posed particular threats to the survival of our ancestors. They reviewed a large experimental literature that demonstrated selective association in human aversive conditioning in which individuals evidence better conditioning and greater resistance to extinction for phylogenetic stimuli (e.g., slides of snakes or spiders) than for ontogenetic materials (e.g., slides of houses, flowers, or mushrooms). Öhman and Mineka (2001) concluded that (1) evolutionarily prepared fear-relevant stimuli have preferential access to the human fear module and (2) selective association of these prepared stimuli is largely independent of conscious cognition.

A second characteristic of the fear module is its *automaticity*. Öhman and Mineka (2001) state that because the fear module evolved to deal with phylogenetic threats to survival, it can be automatically activated without conscious awareness of the triggering stimulus. Evidence for automatic preconscious activation of fear includes physiological fear response (e.g., SCR) to fear stimuli that are not consciously recognized, continued conditioned fear response to nonreportable stimuli, and the acquisition of a conditioned fear response to fear-relevant stimuli that were not amenable to conscious awareness.

A third feature is *encapsulation*. The fear module is assumed to be "relatively impenetrable to other modules with which it lacks direct connections" (Öhman & Mineka, 2001, p. 485) and so will tend to run its course once activated with few possibilities that other processes can stop it (Öhman & Wiens, 2004). Even though the fear module is relatively impenetrable to conscious influences, Öhman and Mineka argue that the fear module itself can have a profound influence by biasing and distorting conscious cognition of the threat stimulus. In support of their contention of the independence of the fear module from the influence of conscious cognition, Öhman and Weins (2004) cite evidence that (1) masking of stimuli affects conscious appraisals but not conditioned responses (SCRs), (2) instructions that alter explicit UCS–CS expectancies do not affect conditioned response to biological fear-relevant stimuli, (3) individuals can acquire conditioned fear responses to masked stimuli outside conscious awareness, and (4) conditioned fear responses to masked stimuli can affect conscious cognition in the form of expectancy judgments.

A final characteristic is its *specific neural circuitry*. Öhman and Mineka (2001) consider the amygdala the central neural structure involved in the control of fear and fear learning and contend that fear activation (i.e., emotional learning) occurs via LeDoux's (1996) subcortical, noncognitive thalamo–amygdala pathway, whereas cognitive learning occurs via the hippocampus and higher cortical regions. The authors contend that the amygdala has more afferent than efferent connections to the cortex and so has more influence on the cortex than the reverse. Based on this view of the neural structure of the fear module, they conclude that (1) nonconscious activation of the amygdala occurs via a neural route that does not involve the cortex, (2) this neural circuitry is specific to fear, and (3) any conscious cognitive processes associated with fear are a consequence of the activated fear module (i.e., amygdala) and thus play no causal role in fear activation. Thus biased appraisals and beliefs are a product of automatic fear activation and the production of psychophysiological and reflexive defensive responses (Öhman & Weins, 2004). Exaggerated beliefs in danger may play a role in maintaining anxiety over time but they are the consequence rather than the cause of fear.

Clinician Guideline 1.12

Given the substantial evidence concerning the importance of learning in the development of anxiety, the clinician should explore with patients past anxiety-related learning experiences (e.g., trauma, life events, exposure to threat-related information).

THE CASE FOR COGNITION

Öhman and Mineka's (2001) perspective on fear and anxiety is at variance with the cognitive perspective advocated by Beck and colleagues (Beck et al., 1985, 2005; Beck & Clark, 1997; D. M. Clark, 1999). Although they acknowledge that cognitive phenomena should be targeted in treatment because they play a key role in the longer term maintenance of anxiety, they still consider anxious thinking, beliefs, and processing biases a consequence of fear activation. Öhman and Mineka (2001) do not consider conscious cognition critical in the pathogenesis of fear itself, which is contrary to the conceptualization of fear that we offered earlier in this chapter. This noncognitive view of fear is evident in other learning theorists like Bouton, Mineka, and Barlow (2001), who argue that interoceptive conditioning in panic disorder occurs without conscious awareness and is quite independent of declarative knowledge systems. Nevertheless, we consider cognitive appraisal a core element of fear and critical to understanding the etiology, persistence, and treatment of anxiety disorders. This view is based on several arguments.

Existence of Preconscious Cognition

Critics of cognitive models tend to overemphasize conscious awareness when discussing cognition, arguing that the substantial experimental evidence of conditioned fear responses without conscious awareness fails to support basic tenets of the cognitive perspective (e.g.,, Öhman & Mineka, 2001). However, there is equally robust experimental research demonstrating preconscious, automatic cognitive and attentional processing of fear stimuli (see MacLeod, 1999; Wells & Matthews, 1994; Williams, Watts, MacLeod, & Mathews, 1997). Thus the cognitive perspective on anxiety is misrepresented when cognition is characterized only in terms of conscious appraisal.

Cognitive Processes in Fear Acquisition (i.e., Conditioning)

Öhman and Mineka (2001) argue that cognitive processes are a consequence of fear activation and so play little role in their acquisition. However, over the last three decades many learning theorists have argued that cognitive concepts must be incorporated into conditioning models to explain the persistence of fear responses. Davey (1997), for example, reviews evidence that outcome expectancies as well as one's cognitive representation of the UCS will influence the strength of the fear CR in response to a CS. In other words, CRs increase or decrease in strength depending on how the person evaluates the meaning of the UCS or trauma (see also van den Hout & Merckelbach, 1991). According to Davey (1997), then, cognitive appraisal is a key element in Pavlovian fear conditioning.

It has long been recognized that outcome expectancies (i.e., expectations that in a particular situation a certain response will lead to a given outcome) play a critical role in aversive conditioning (e.g., Seligman & Johnston, 1973; de Jong & Merckelbach, 2000; see also experiments on covariation bias by de Jong, Merckelbach, & Arntz, 1995; McNally & Heatherton, 1993). In his influential review paper Rescorla (1988) argued that modern learning theory views Pavlovian conditioning in terms of learning the relations among events (i.e., associations) that must be perceived and that are complexly represented (i.e., memory) by the organism. For most behaviorally oriented clinical researchers, then, the acquisition and elicitation of fear and anxiety states will involve learning contingencies that recognize the influence and importance of various cognitive mediators (for further discussion, see van den Hout & Merckelbach, 1991).

Conscious Cognitive Processes Can Alter Fear Responses

Öhman and Mineka (2001) contend that the fear module is impenetrable to conscious cognitive control. However, this view is difficult to reconcile with empirical evidence that cognitive or informational factors can lead to a reduction in fear (see discussion by Brewin, 1988). Even with exposure-based interventions, which are directly derived from conditioning theory, there is evidence that long-term habituation of fear responses requires conscious directed attention and processing of the fear-relevant information (Foa & Kozak, 1986). Brewin (1988) succinctly makes a case for the influence of cognition on fear responses, stating that "a theory that assigns a role to conscious thought processes is necessary to explain how people can alternately frighten and reassure themselves by thinking different thoughts, test out a variety of different coping responses, set goals and reward or punish themselves depending on the outcome, etc." (p. 46).

The Amygdala Is Not Specific to Fear

A central argument of Öhman and Mineka (2001) is that a direct thalamus–amygdala link in fear activation and emotional learning accounts for the automaticity of the fear module and so is dissociable from declarative acquisition of information via the hippocampus. Thus activation of the amygdala begins a fear response which then leads to more complex cognition and memory processes via projections to the hippocampus and higher cortical brain regions (see also Morris, Öhman, & Dolan, 1998).

Although experimental research has been quite consistent in showing amygdaloid activation in the processing of fearful stimuli, there is evidence that the amygdala may also be involved in other emotional functions such as the appraisal of the social and emotional significance of facial emotions (Adolphs, Tranel, & Damasio, 1998; Anderson & Phelps, 2000). Neuroimaging studies suggest greater activation occurs in the prefrontal cortex, amygdala, other midbrain structures, and the brainstem when processing any generally negative, arousing emotional stimuli, which suggests that the amygdala and other structures involved in emotional processing may not be specific to fear but rather to the valence of emotional stimuli (e.g., Hare, Tottenham, Davidson, Glover, & Casey, 2005; Simpson et al., 2000; see also amygdala activation when processing sad film excerpts, Lévesque et al., 2003). In addition the amygdala is responsive to positively valenced stimuli, although this response seems to be more variable and elaborative in nature than the fixed, automatic response seen to fear expressions (Somerville, Kim, Johnstone, Alexander, & Whalen, 2004; see also Canli et al., 2002). Thus there is experimental evidence that the amygdala may not be the seat of anxiety specifically but an important neural structure of emotion processing more generally (see also Gray & McNaughton, 1996).

Other neuroimaging research suggests that the amygdala can be influenced by cognitive processes mediated by higher cortical regions of the brain. McNally (2007a) reviewed evidence that the medial prefrontal cortex can suppress conditioned fear acquired via activation of the amygdala. For example, in one study perceptual processing of threatening pictorial scenes was associated with a strong bilateral amygdala response that was attenuated by cognitive evaluation of the fear stimuli (Hariri, Mattay, Tessitore, Fera, & Weinberger, 2003). Together these findings suggest that conscious cognitive processes mediated by other cortical and subcortical regions of the brain have an important influence on the amygdala and together provide an integrated neural account of the experience of fear.

Role of Higher Order Cortical Regions in Fear

The critical issue for a cognitive perspective on anxiety is whether conscious cognitive processes play a sufficiently important role in the propagation and amelioration of anxiety to warrant an emphasis at the cognitive level. As discussed previously, there is considerable neurophysiological evidence that higher cortical regions of the brain are involved in the type of human fear and anxiety responses that are the target of clinical interventions. LeDoux (1996) has shown that the hippocampus and related areas of the cortex involved in the formation and retrieval of memories are implicated in more complex contextual fear conditioning. It is this type of conditioning that is particularly relevant to the formation and persistence of anxiety disorders. Moreover, LeDoux (1996, 2000) notes that the subjective feeling associated with fear will involve connections between the amygdala and the prefrontal cortex, anterior cingulate, and orbital cortical regions, as well as the hippocampus. From a clinical perspective, it is the subjective experience of anxiety that brings individuals to the attention of clinicians, and it is the elimination of this aversive subjective state that is the main criteria for judging treatment success. In sum, it is apparent that the neural circuitry of fear is consistent with a prominent role for cognition in the pathogenesis of anxiety.

SUMMARY AND CONCLUSION

In many respects anxiety is a defining feature of contemporary society and the tenacity of its clinical manifestations represents one of the greatest challenges facing mental health research and treatment. The pervasiveness, persistence, and deleterious impact of anxiety disorders have been well documented in numerous epidemiological studies. In this chapter, a number of issues in the psychology of anxiety disorders were identified. One of the most basic confusions arises from the definition of anxiety and its relation to fear. Taking a cognitive perspective, we defined fear as the automatic appraisal of imminent threat or danger, whereas anxiety is the more enduring subjective response to fear activation. The latter is a more complex cognitive, affective, physiological, and behavioral response pattern that occurs when events or circumstances are interpreted as representing highly aversive, uncertain, and uncontrollable threats to our vital interests. Fear, then, is the basic cognitive process underlying all the anxiety disorders. However, anxiety is the more enduring state associated with threat appraisals, and so the treatment of anxiety has become a major focus in mental health.

Another fundamental issue associated with anxiety is the differentiation between normal and abnormal states. Although fear is necessary for survival because it is essential for preparing the organism for response to life-threatening dangers, fear is clearly maladaptive when present in the anxiety disorders. Once again a cognitive perspective can be helpful in identifying the boundaries between normal anxiety or fear, and their clinical manifestations. Fear is maladaptive and more likely associated with an anxiety disorder when it involves an erroneous or exaggerated appraisal of danger, causes impaired functioning, shows remarkable persistence, involves a false alarm, and/or creates hypersensitivity to a wide range of threat-related stimuli. The challenge for practitioners is to offer interventions that "dampen down" or normalize clinical anxiety so it becomes less distressing and interfering in daily living. The elimination of all anxiety is neither desirable nor possible, but its reduction to within the normal range of human experience is the common goal of treatment regimens for anxiety disorders.

Anxiety states are multifaceted, involving all levels of human function. There is a significant biological aspect to anxiety, with particular cortical and subcortical neural structures playing a critical role in emotional experience. This strong neurophysiological element gives anxiety states a sense of urgency and potency that makes modification difficult. At the same time anxiety is often acquired through the organism's interaction with the environment even though this learning process may occur outside awareness and beyond rational consideration. And yet cognitive mediation such as expectancies, interpretations, beliefs, and memories play a critical role in the development and persistence of anxiety. As a subjective experience, anxiety may feel like a storm that surges and recedes throughout the day. Relief from this state of personal turmoil can be a potent motivator even when it elicits response patterns, such as escape and avoidance, that are ultimately counterproductive to the vital interests of the individual.

Despite its complexity, we have argued in this chapter that cognition plays a key role in understanding both normal and abnormal states of anxiety. The essence of maladaptive anxiety is a faulty or exaggerated interpretation of threat to an anticipated situation or circumstance that is perceived to have significance for the person's vital resources. In the last two decades substantial progress has been made in elucidating the cognitive structures and processes of anxiety. Based on the cognitive model of anxiety first proposed by Beck et al. (1985), this book presents a more refined, elaborated, and extended cognitive formulation that incorporates major advances made within cognitive-clinical research of anxiety. A systematic evaluation of the empirical status of this reformulation is presented along with theory-driven strategies for cognitive assessment and treatment. In subsequent chapters disorder-specific cognitive theories, research, and treatment are presented for the major forms of anxiety disorders: panic disorder, social phobia, GAD, OCD, and PTSD. It is our contention that the cognitive perspective continues to hold much promise for the advancement of our understanding of anxiety and the provision of innovative treatment approaches.

Chapter 2

The Cognitive Model of Anxiety

In cognitive therapy for anxiety and depression patients are taught a very basic idiom: "The way you think affects the way you feel." This simple statement is the cornerstone of cognitive theory and therapy of emotional disorders, and yet individuals often fail to recognize how their thoughts affect their mood state. Given the experience of intense and uncontrollable physiological arousal often present during acute anxiety, it is understandable why those who suffer with it may not recognize its cognitive basis. Notwithstanding this failure in recognition, cognition does play an important mediational function between the situation and affect, as indicated in this diagram:

Triggering Situation → Anxious Thought/Appraisal → Anxious Feeling

Individuals usually assume that situations and not cognitions (i.e., appraisals) are responsible for their anxiety. Take, for example, how you feel in the period before an important exam. Anxiety will be high if you expect the exam to be difficult and you doubt your level of preparation. On the other hand, if you expect the exam to be quite easy or you are confident in your preparation, anxiety will be low. The same holds true for public speaking. If you evaluate your audience as friendly and receptive to your speech, your anxiety will be lower than if you evaluate the audience as critical, bored, or rejecting of your talk. In each example it is not the situation (e.g., writing an exam, giving a speech, or having a casual conversation) that determines the level of anxiety, but rather how the situation is appraised or evaluated. It is the way we think that has a powerful influence on whether we feel anxious or calm.

The cognitive perspective can help us understand some apparent contradictions in anxiety disorders. How is it possible for a person to be so anxious over an irrational and highly improbable threat (e.g., that I might suddenly stop breathing), and yet react with ease and no apparent anxiety in the face of more realistic dangers (e.g., developing lung cancer from a chronic nicotine addiction)? What accounts for the highly selective and situationally specific nature of anxiety? Why is anxiety so persistent despite repeated nonoccurrences of the anticipated danger?

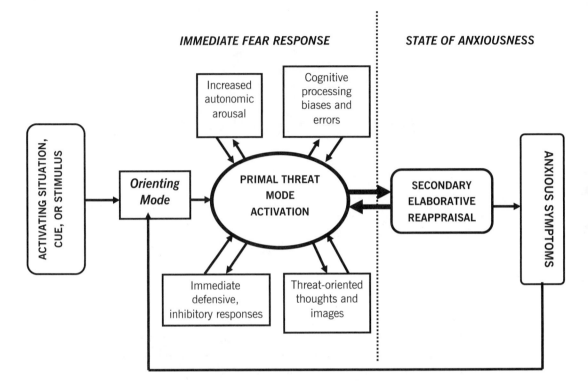

FIGURE 2.1. Cognitive model of anxiety.

In this chapter we examine the nature and persistence of anxiety. We present the cognitive model of anxiety as an explanation for one of the most important and perplexing questions faced by mental health researchers and practitioners: *Why does anxiety persist despite the absence of danger and the obvious maladaptive effects of this highly aversive emotional state?* The chapter begins with an overview of the cognitive model (Figure 2.1) followed by a discussion of its central tenets, a description of the model, analysis of the cognitive basis of normal and abnormal anxiety, and a statement of key cognitive hypotheses.

OVERVIEW OF THE COGNITIVE MODEL OF ANXIETY

Anxiety: A State of Heightened Vulnerability

The cognitive perspective on anxiety centers on the notion of *vulnerability*. Beck, Emery, and Greenberg (1985) defined *vulnerability* "as a person's perception of himself as subject to internal or external dangers over which his control is lacking or is insufficient to afford him a sense of safety. In clinical syndromes, the sense of vulnerability is magnified by certain dysfunctional cognitive processes" (pp. 67–68).

In anxiety this heightened sense of vulnerability is evident in individuals' biased and exaggerated appraisals of possible personal harm in response to cues that are neutral or innocuous. This *primary appraisal of threat* involves an erroneous perspective in which the probability that harm will occur and the perceived severity of the harm are greatly overestimated. Rachman (2004) noted that fearful individuals are much more likely to overestimate the intensity of threat, which then leads to avoidance behavior. At the same time anxious individuals fail to perceive the safety aspects of threat-evaluated situations and tend to underestimate their ability to cope with the anticipated harm or danger (Beck et al., 1985, 2005). This *secondary elaborative reappraisal*, however, occurs immediately as a result of the primary threat appraisal, and in anxiety states it amplifies the initial perception of threat. Thus the intensity of an anxiety state depends on the balance between one's initial appraisal of threat and the secondary appraisal of coping ability and safety. The level or intensity of anxiety can be expressed in the following manner:

> High Anxiety = ↑ threat probability/severity + ↓ coping and safety
> Low Anxiety = ↓ threat probability/severity + ↑ coping and safety
> Moderate Anxiety = ↔ threat probability/severity + ↔ coping and safety

Beck and Greenberg (1988) noted that the perception of danger sets off an "alarm system" involving primal behavioral, physiological, and cognitive processes that evolved to protect our species from physical harm and danger (see also Beck, 1985). Behavioral mobilization to deal with the danger might involve a fight-or-flight response (escape or avoidance), but it could also consist of other instrumental behaviors like calling for assistance, taking a defensive stance, or negotiating to minimize the danger (Beck et al., 1985, 2005). Autonomic arousal and other physiological responses that occur during threat vulnerability are important aspects of this early reflexive defense system. The presence of anxiety activates behavioral mobilization to deal with perceived threat. Although this primal behavioral mobilization evolved as a rapid and efficient response to physical danger, it can impair actual performance when activated in benign situations or the complex, diffusely stressful circumstances of contemporary society. Mobilization of the primal defense system can also have adverse effects when it is interpreted as signaling a serious disorder such as when the person with panic disorder misinterprets an elevated heart rate as a possible myocardial infarct (Beck et al., 1985; D. M. Clark & Beck, 1988).

A second type of behavioral response often seen in anxiety states as a result of a perception of threat is immobility in situations where active coping might increase the actual or imagined danger (Beck et al., 1985). Signs of this immobility response may be evident as freezing, feeling faint, or feeling "woozy." It is associated with the cognitive perspective of being totally helpless. The immobility response is apparent in social anxiety, such as when a highly anxious person feels faint when attempting to deliver a public speech.

Despite the importance of behavioral mobilization and physiological arousal, it is the initial primary appraisal of threat combined with a secondary appraisal of personal inadequacy and diminished safety that are responsible for instigating anxiety. In this sense faulty cognition is necessary but not sufficient for generating a state of anxiety. The cognitive model of anxiety is rooted within an information-processing perspective, in which emotional disturbance occurs because of an excess or deficient functioning of the cognitive apparatus. Previously we defined *information processing* as "the structures, processes, and products involved in the representation and transformation of meaning based on sensory data derived from the external and internal environment" (D. A. Clark et al., 1999, p. 77).

Anxiety, then, is the product of an information-processing system that interprets a situation as threatening to the vital interests and well-being of the individual. In this case a "threatening" meaning is generated and applied to the situation. The centrality of threat meaning-assignment (i.e., information processing) is nicely illustrated in an example provided by Beck et al. (1985, 2005). Most individuals could easily walk across a plank that is 6 inches wide without fear, if it were placed 1 foot off the ground. However, raise the plank 100 feet off the ground, and most individuals would become intensely afraid and refuse to walk the plank. What accounts for the different emotional experiences in these two situations is that individuals evaluate walking a plank 100 feet above the ground as highly dangerous. They also doubt whether their balance could be maintained, and might actually experience dizziness and unsteadiness should they venture a few inches onto the plank. Although the plank is at different heights, their ability to elicit fear or anxiety depends on the perception of danger. Likewise perceptions of danger are central to clinical states of anxiety. The cognitive model views clinical anxiety as a reaction to an inappropriate and exaggerated evaluation of personal vulnerability derived from a faulty information-processing system that misconstrues neutral situations or cues as threatening. This is entirely consistent with the definitions of fear and anxiety proposed in Chapter 1. Based on the concept of vulnerability, Figure 2.1 illustrates the structures, processes, and products of the information-processing system that are involved in the experience of anxiety.

Clinician Guideline 2.1

Correcting faulty appraisals of threat and secondary appraisals of vulnerability is a fundamental approach in cognitive therapy considered necessary for the reduction of anxiety.

Automatic and Strategic Processing

The cognitive model readily acknowledges that both automatic and strategic processes are involved in anxiety (see Beck & Clark, 1997). Table 2.1 presents the defining characteristics of automatic and strategic or controlled processing first outlined in Beck and Clark (1997).

At the cognitive level, automatic processing in anxiety has been most clearly demonstrated in the preconscious attentional bias for threat-related stimuli evidenced in emotional Stroop and dot probe experiments (Macleod, 1999). Findings from implicit memory tests suggest the presence of an automatic memory bias for negative information in anxiety disorders (Coles & Heimberg, 2002; Williams et al., 1997). Classical conditioning research has demonstrated the acquisition of conditioned fear responses (e.g., a skin conductance response) to masked fear-relevant stimuli presented outside conscious awareness, indicating that fear learning can occur as an automatic, preconscious process (Öhman & Wiens, 2004). LeDoux's (1996) research has documented the acquisition of auditory fear responses in rodents via the subcortical thalamo–amygdala pathway that bypasses the higher cortical centers for thinking, reasoning, and con-

TABLE 2.1. Characteristics of Automatic and Strategic Processing

Automatic processing	Strategic (controlled) processing
• Effortless	• Effortful
• Involuntary	• Voluntary
• Unintentional	• Intentional
• Primarily preconscious	• Fully conscious
• Fast, difficult to terminate or regulate	• Slow, more amenable to regulation
• Minimal attentional processing capacity	• Requires a lot of attentional processing
• Capable of parallel processing	• Relies on serial processing
• Stereotypic, involving familiar and highly practiced tasks	• Can deal with novel, difficult, and unpracticed tasks
• Low level of cognitive processing with minimal analysis	• Higher levels of cognitive processing involving semantic analysis and synthesis

sciousness. Clearly, then, certain cognitive, neurophysiological, and learning processes that are critical to the experience of anxiety occur at the automatic-processing level.

Although automatic processes are important to anxiety, one should not overlook the central role played by the slower, more elaborative, and strategic processes in the persistence of anxiety. Threat-biased judgments, reasoning, memory, and thinking are critical parts of the subjective experience of anxiety that motivates individuals to seek treatment. We should not overlook the importance of worry, anxious rumination, threat images, and traumatic memories if we want to understand the anxiety disorders. In fact controlled strategic processing allows us to interpret novel and complex information. McNally (1995) concluded that, because of its meaning-assignment capabilities, strategic, elaborative processing is required for the anxious person to misinterpret innocuous situations as threatening. Moreover, any particular cognitive task involves a mixture of automatic and strategic processing, so a specific aspect of information processing should not be rigidly dichotomized as automatic or strategic, but rather as reflecting more of one type of processing than another (see McNally, 1995). Furthermore, involuntariness rather than preconsciousness (i.e., outside conscious awareness) is the key feature of automaticity in anxiety states (McNally, 1995; Wells & Matthews, 1994).

In the cognitive model (Figure 2.1) the initial orientation toward threat involves a predominantly automatic, preconscious process. Activation of the *primal threat mode* (i.e., the primary appraisal of threat) will be largely automatic because of the necessity for rapid and efficient evaluation of a potential threat for the survival of the organism. (The term *mode* refers to a cluster of interrelated schemas organized to deal with particular demands that pertain to one's vital interests, survival, and adaptation [Beck, 1996; Beck et al., 1985, 2005; Clark et al., 1999].) However, some strategic, controlled processing must occur even at this stage of the immediate threat response because of our conscious, subjective experience of distress associated with the threat appraisal. As we engage in secondary appraisal of coping resources, the presence or absence of safety, and the reappraisal of the initial threat, this aspect of information processing will be much more controlled, strategic, and elaborative. Even at this secondary stage responsible for a sustained anxiety response, processing will not be entirely strategic as evident in processes such as worry and anxious rumination.

Clinician Guideline 2.2

Cognitive therapy teaches individuals to be more aware of their immediate threat appraisals and to correct maladaptive secondary cognitive processes.

CENTRAL TENETS OF THE COGNITIVE MODEL OF ANXIETY

A number of propositions derived from the cognitive perspective guided the development of the cognitive model (see Figure 2.1). These propositions were first articulated in the original cognitive model of anxiety (Beck et al., 1985, 2005) and are elaborated in the sections below (see Table 2.2 for a definition of the basic tenets).

TABLE 2.2. Central Tenets of the Cognitive Model of Anxiety

Exaggerated threat appraisals

Anxiety is characterized by an enhanced and highly selective attention to personal risk, threat, or danger that is perceived as having a serious negative impact on vital interests and well-being.

Heightened helplessness

Anxiety involves an inaccurate evaluation of personal coping resources, resulting in an underestimation of one's ability to cope with a perceived threat.

Inhibitory processing of safety information

Anxiety states are characterized by inhibited or highly restricted processing of safety cues and information that convey diminished likelihood and severity of a perceived threat or danger.

Impaired constructive or reflective thinking

During anxiety more constructive, logical, and realistic elaborative thinking and reasoning are difficult to access and so are ineffectively utilized for anxiety reduction.

Automatic and strategic processing

Anxiety involves a mixture of automatic and strategic cognitive processes that are responsible for the involuntary and uncontrollable quality of anxiety.

Self-perpetuating process

Anxiety involves a vicious cycle in which heightened self-focused attention on the signs and symptoms of anxiety will itself contribute to an intensification of subjective distress.

Cognitive primacy

The primary cognitive appraisal of threat and the secondary appraisal of personal vulnerability can generalize such that a broader array of situations or stimuli are misperceived as threatening and various physiological and behavioral defensive responses are inappropriately mobilized to deal with the threat.

Cognitive vulnerability to anxiety

Increased susceptibility to anxiety is a result of enduring core beliefs (schemas) about personal vulnerability or helplessness and the salience of threat.

Exaggerated Threat Appraisals

We previously introduced the concept of exaggerated threat appraisal as a primary, core feature of anxiety. The process of appraising or evaluating external or internal cues as potential threat, danger, or harm to personal vital resources or well-being involves a rapid, automatic, and highly efficient cognitive, physiological, behavioral, and affective defensive system that evolved to protect and ensure the survival of the organism. Many writers have noted the obvious evolutionary significance of a cognitive system primed to rapidly and selectively scan the environment for anything that might pose a physical danger to our primordial ancestors (Beck, 1985; D. M. Clark & Beck, 1988; Craske, 2003; Öhman & Mineka, 2001). Threat is rapidly appraised in terms of its temporal/physical proximity or intensifying nature (i.e., "threat imminence" [Craske, 2003] or "looming vulnerability" [Riskind & Williams, 2006]), probability of occurrence, and severity of outcome. Together these evaluated characteristics of the stimulus will result in the initial assignment of a *threat value*.

This primary assignment of threat value is inherent in all experiences of anxiety. In the cognitive model this initial, relatively automatic threat appraisal is due to activation of the primal threat mode (see Figure 2.1). The appraisal of threat will involve various cognitive processes and structures including attention, memory, judgment, reasoning, and conscious thought. This is illustrated in the following example. Imagine an individual running along a fairly isolated country road. He suddenly hears the bark of a dog in the yard of a house he is approaching. Instantly his muscles tighten, his pace quickens, his breathing and heart rate accelerate. These responses to the barking dog are triggered by a very rapid initial threat appraisal that just barely registers in the runner's conscious awareness: "Am I in danger of an attack?" The situation will be assigned a high threat value if the runner is close to the house in question, thinks there is high probability that the dog is not leashed, and assumes the dog is large and vicious (high severity). On the other hand, the runner might assign a low threat value with increased distance from the dog, or if he concludes that the dog is probably leashed or simply a friendly household pet. An immediate threat appraisal, then, will be apparent in all experiences of both normal and abnormal anxiety states. In clinical anxiety, the primary threat appraisal is exaggerated and disproportionate to the actual threat value of an event.

Clinician Guideline 2.3

Cognitive therapy focuses on helping clients recalibrate exaggerated threat appraisals and increase their tolerance for risk and uncertainty related to their anxious concerns.

Heightened Helplessness

A secondary appraisal of personal resources and coping ability involves a more conscious, strategic evaluation of one's ability to respond constructively to perceived threat. This appraisal occurs at the secondary elaborative phase of the cognitive model (see Figure 2.1). This secondary appraisal will involve Bandura's (1977, 1989) concepts of self-efficacy ("Do I have the ability to deal with this threat"?) and outcome expectancy ("What is the likelihood that my efforts will reduce or eliminate the threat?"). Positive self-efficacy and outcome expectation could lead to a reduction in anxiety, especially if the person's initial efforts to deal with the threat appeared successful. On the other hand, low perceived self-efficacy and a negative outcome expectation would lead to a heightened state of helplessness and greater feelings of anxiety.

Although secondary appraisal of coping resources is triggered by the primary threat appraisal, both will occur almost simultaneously as a highly reciprocal and interactive cognitive evaluation (Beck et al., 1985, 2005). As noted previously, the intensity of anxiety will depend on the degree of threat in relation to one's perceived capacity to cope with the danger. In our case of the runner hearing a barking dog, anxiety would be minimized if he recalled previous positive experiences of dealing with dogs, or if he remembered he was carrying a can of pepper spray. In clinical anxiety individuals have a heightened sense of helplessness in the face of certain perceived threats and so conclude they are unable to deal with the anticipated danger.

Clinician Guideline 2.4

Increasing self-confidence to deal with threat and uncertainty is an important objective of cognitive therapy of anxiety.

Inhibitory Processing of Safety

Beck (1985) noted that anxiety is not only characterized by a selective enhanced processing of danger but also a selective suppression of information that is incongruent with perceived danger. D. M. Clark and Beck (1988) included underestimated rescue factors (what others can do to help) as a cognitive error that will contribute to an exaggerated evaluation of threat in anxiety. It is suggested that in anxiety disorders the immediate and automatic formation of a threat appraisal based on activation of threat schemas will so bias the information-processing system toward detecting and evaluating threat, that any information incongruent with threat schemas will be filtered out, even ignored. As a result any corrective information, which could lead to a reduction in the threat value assigned to the situation, is lost and the anxiety persists. So, in our example, a runner intensely anxious about the barking dog may fail to notice a fence around the property, thus reducing the chance that the dog will charge out onto the road. This apparent inability to process the safety aspects of a situation is clearly seen in the anxiety disorders such as the speech-anxious person who fails to process cues from a receptive audience, or the test-anxious student who has successfully answered the most difficult questions.

Another consequence of inhibited processing of safety cues is that the person may seek inappropriate ways to secure safety or avoid danger. The person with agoraphobia may only venture outside with certain family members because this appears to reduce the chance of a panic attack, or the individual with contamination obsessions may develop certain compulsive rituals to reduce anxiety and secure a sense of safety from the prospect of contamination. Salkovskis (1996b) noted that safety-seeking behavior and avoidance may contribute to the persistence of anxiety, because both prevent disconfirmation that the perceived threat is benign or will not occur. Thus in health anxiety the person may spend many hours searching the Internet for information that would confirm that a particular skin rash is benign and not a sign of melanoma. However, in this case the safety-seeking behavior (i.e., reassurance seeking) may be particularly maladaptive and a potent contributor to anxiety because the individual fails to find conclusive evidence to disconfirm the threat attributed to the skin rash. Another form of disconfirmation bias occurs when the person with panic disorder, for example, engages in controlled breathing (safety-seeking behavior) whenever he feels tightness in the throat and fears suffocation. In this case the controlled breathing prevents the person from learning that the throat sensation will not lead to the catastrophic outcome of suffocation.

Clinician Guideline 2.5

Improved processing of safety cues that disconfirm perceived threats is an important element in cognitive therapy of anxiety disorders.

Impaired Constructive or Reflective Thinking

During anxious states constructive modes of thinking are less accessible. This means that slower, more logical and effortful deductive reasoning involving a more complete and balanced processing of a situation's threat potential is more difficult to achieve. This more constructive, reflective approach to threat is under conscious control and so takes more time and effort because it involves not only a more complete evaluation of the threat and safety features of a situation, but it also requires selection of instrumental behaviors for dealing with anxiety. Beck et al. (1985, 2005) noted that this constructive mode of thinking may be an alternative *anxiety-reduction system* to the anxiety-potentiating, automatic primal threat process. However, this reasoned, elaborative cognitive orientation appears lost to individuals who are intensely anxious. The predominance of the primal threat mode appears to inhibit access to constructive mode thinking. Beck (1996) stated that once an automatic or primal mode of thinking is activated, it tends to dominant information processing until the activating circumstance disappears.

The relative inaccessibility of constructive thinking contributes to the persistence of anxiety. Beck (1987) argued that a key factor in the experience of panic is the inability to realistically appraise (i.e., apply tests, draw on past experiences, generate alternative explanations) a specific physical sensation (e.g., chest pain) in any way other than from a catastrophic perspective. It is the existence of impaired reflective thinking that is a key entry point for cognitive therapy of anxiety. Clients are taught cognitive restructuring skills as a means of developing a more constructive cognitive perspective on perceived threat.

Clinician Guideline 2.6

Cognitive therapy seeks to improve access to and the effectiveness of reflective thinking to counter immediate faulty threat appraisals.

Automatic and Strategic Processing

We have already considered how automatic and strategic processes are evident at various facets of the cognitive basis of anxiety. Automatic processing will be more apparent in the early primary appraisal of threat involving activation of the primal threat mode, whereas controlled strategic processing will be more evident at the secondary elaborative phase of threat reappraisal, coping resources, and safety seeking. Given this mix of automatic and controlled processing, one question that emerges is whether more effortful and voluntary reflection really can have a significant effect on reducing anxiety.

As previously noted, there is considerable empirical evidence from conditioning experiments that acquired fear responses can be reduced via social transmission of information (e.g., see discussion by Brewin, 1988). Moreover, information on the predictability and controllability of future threat, danger, or other negative events determines in large part the presence or absence of anxious apprehension (Barlow, 2002). Furthermore, personal and clinical experience supports the assertion that conscious controlled cognition can have a significant anxiety-reducing effect. In our everyday lives we have all had experiences of correcting an initial feeling of anxiousness through controlled, effortful, and logical reanalysis of the perceived threat. So experimental and anecdotal evidence is consistent with the assertion in cognitive therapy that therapeutic interventions, like cognitive restructuring, that rely on controlled effortful thought processes can significantly contribute to anxiety reduction.

The presence of reflexive, automatic cognitive processing in anxiety does mean that experiential or behavioral interventions, such as direct exposure to the fear stimulus, will be needed in addition to controlled cognitive interventions to reduce anxiety. Exposure-based treatment strategies are important because they enable a deeper, more generalized and stronger activation of threat schemas and provide opportunities to gather direct disconfirming evidence against the high threat value initially assigned by the anxious patient (for related discussion, see Foa & Kozak, 1986). These kinds of behavioral experiences also become powerful tools for building self-confidence in one's ability to deal with the anticipated threat. Chapter 6 discusses cognitive interventions at the strategic processing level, and Chapter 7 presents various behavioral exercises used to provide disconfirming evidence for threat.

Clinician Guideline 2.7

Strategic cognitive processing interventions and more behavioral, experiential exercises are used to modify immediate threat appraisals and reduce heightened states of anxiety.

Self-Perpetuating Process

An anxiety episode can last from a few minutes to many hours. In fact some patients with GAD complain that they are never really free of anxiety. So the persistence of anxiety must be seen as a vicious cycle or a self-perpetuating process. Once the anxiety program is activated, it tends to be self-perpetuating through a number of processes. First, self-focused attention is enhanced during anxiety states so that individuals become acutely aware of their own anxiety-related thoughts and behaviors. This heightened attention to the symptoms of anxiety will intensify one's subjective apprehension. Second, the presence of anxiety can impair performance in certain threatening situations, such as when the speech-anxious person goes blank or starts to perspire profusely. Attention to these symptoms could easily interfere with the person's ability to deliver the speech.

In the final analysis the anxious person interprets the presence of anxiety itself as a highly threatening development that must be reduced as quickly as possible in order to minimize or avoid its "catastrophic effects." In this case the person literally becomes "anxious about being anxious." D. M. Clark and colleagues have developed cognitive models and interventions for panic, social phobia, and PTSD that emphasize the deleterious effects of misinterpreting the presence of anxious symptoms in a catastrophic (or at least highly negative) manner (D. M. Clark, 1996, 2001; D. M. Clark & Ehlers, 2004). This self-perpetuating characteristic of anxiety, then, indicates that any intervention designed to interrupt the cycle must deal with any threat-related appraisals of anxious symptoms themselves.

Clinician Guideline 2.8

Correcting misinterpretations of anxious symptoms is another important component of cognitive therapy for anxiety disorders.

Cognitive Primacy

The cognitive model asserts that the central problem in anxiety disorders is the activation of hypervalent threat schemas that present an overly dangerous perspective on reality and the self as weak, helpless, and vulnerable (Beck et al., 1985, 2005). From a cognitive perspective, an initial rapid and involuntary stimulus evaluation of threat occurs in the early phase of anxiety. It is within this framework that we view cognition as primary in the acquisition and maintenance of fear responses. Furthermore, because of the primacy or importance of cognition, we propose that some shift in the cognitive conceptualization of threat is needed before any reduction in anxiety can be expected. Without treatment, the repeated appraisal and reappraisal of threat and vulnerability will lead to a generalization of the anxiety program so that it encompasses a broader array of eliciting situations.

Clinician Guideline 2.9

Changing the cognitive evaluation of threat and vulnerability is necessary to reverse the generalization and persistence of anxiety.

Cognitive Vulnerability to Anxiety

There are individual differences in susceptibility or risk for anxiety disorders. Individuals are at increased risk for anxiety because of certain genetic, neurophysiological, and learning histories that are causal factors in the anxiety disorders (see Chapter 1). However, the cognitive model also asserts that particular enduring schemas involving rules and assumptions about danger and helplessness may predispose an individual to anxiety. See Chapter 4 for discussion of cognitive, personality, and emotional factors that may be contributors to the etiology of anxiety.

DESCRIPTION OF THE COGNITIVE MODEL

The cognitive model depicted in Figure 2.1 is divided into an early, immediate phase of fear response, followed by a slower, more elaborative processing phase that determines the persistence or termination of the anxious state. Our discussion of the cognitive model will proceed from the far left of the diagram to the end product at the far right. Although this allows us to provide a systematic presentation of the cognitive model, in reality all structures and processes involved in anxiety are activated almost simultaneously, and all are so interrelated that reciprocal feed forward and feedback loops are clearly evident throughout the anxiety program.

Activating Situations, Events, and Stimuli

Environmental factors are important in the cognitive model because anxiety is a response to an internal or external stimulus that triggers an appraisal of threat. In this sense the model is more consistent with a *diathesis–stress* perspective in which particular situations or cues (the stress) activate the anxiety program in individuals with an enduring propensity to generate primary appraisals of threat (the diathesis). Although it is possible for anxiety to occur spontaneously, as in panic attacks that occur "out of the blue," the more usual pattern is situation- or cue-activated anxiety.

The types of situations that can trigger anxiety are not randomly distributed. Activating situations or stimuli will differ according to the type of anxiety disorder with, for example, social situations as relevant triggers in social phobia, stimuli that trigger memories of a past trauma relevant to PTSD, and circumstances perceived as elevating risk of panic attacks relevant to panic disorder. Although the situations that provoke anxiety are personally idiosyncratic and highly diverse even within specific anxiety disorders, a stimulus will only activate the anxiety program if it is perceived as a threat to one's vital interests (Beck et al., 1985, 2005). This threat may be symbolic or hypothetical, as evident in GAD, or it could be perceived as real, such as when the person with agoraphobia believes that going to a store could trigger such intense panic that a heart attack and death could ensue.

Beck et al. (1985, 2005) conceptualized vital interests in terms of highly valued goals or personal strivings within the social or individual domains. "Sociality" (later termed "sociotropy") refers to goals that involve the establishment and maintenance of close, satisfying, and self-affirming relationships with others, whereas "individuality" (i.e., "autonomy") refers to goals relevant for gaining a personal sense of mastery, identity, and independence. Furthermore, these goals can be expressed in either the public or the private sphere. From this a classification of vital interests can be constructed that enables a better understanding of how situations might be interpreted in a threatening manner (see Table 2.3).

TABLE 2.3. Classification of Threats to Personal Concerns

Domain	Sociotropy	Autonomy
Public concerns	Disapproval	Defeat
	Disregard	Defection
	Separation	Depreciation
	Isolation	Thwarting
Private concerns	Abandonment	Disability
	Deprivation	Malfunction
	Disapproval	Illness
	Rejection	Death

Note. Based on Beck, Emery, and Greenberg (1985).

Personal strivings or goals of a social nature (sociotropy) within the public sphere focus on our relationships within larger social settings (e.g., an audience, being in class or at work, attending a party) that provide a sense of belonging, acceptance, approval, and affirmation, whereas the same social strivings in the private sector refer to our more intimate dyadic social relations (e.g., life partners, children, parents) that provide nurturance, love, empathy, and understanding. Individual personal goals within the private sphere are concerned with achieving self-sufficiency, mastery, independence, and competence, whereas individuality (autonomy) within the public realm deals with competition and comparison where other people become instruments to achieve personal goals and standards. Sociotropy and autonomy are understood from the perspective of the individual, so it is the perception of acceptance, approval, independence, or competence that is important, not some "objective" standard of whether or not a person has met his or her goals. Also individuals will differ in the value or importance of certain strivings for their own self-worth (for further discussion of sociotropy and autonomy, see Beck, 1983; D. A. Clark et al., 1999).

It is clear how a situation could be perceived as highly threatening if it is thought not only to interfere or prevent the satisfaction of valued personal strivings but, even much worse, result in a personally painful negative state of affairs (e.g., isolation, rejection, defeat, even death). For example, individuals concerned with the approval of others might feel particularly anxious if they perceive social cues of possible disapproval or criticism in a particular social setting. On the other hand, individuals who highly value good health and optimum functioning of their mind and body (autonomous strivings in the private sphere) could perceive any indication of possible disease or death a serious threat to their own survival. Any of the perceived threats common to the anxiety disorders, like loss of control or death in panic disorder and negative evaluation of others in social phobia, can be understood in terms of threat to one's vital interests in the public or private spheres of sociality and autonomy.

Clinician Guideline 2.10

Determining each individual's vital interests in the social and autonomous domains is important for understanding development of the exaggerated personal threat evaluations that underlie the anxiety condition.

Orienting Mode

Beck (1996) first proposed a cluster of schemas called the *orienting mode* that provides a very rapid initial perception of a situation or stimulus. The orienting mode operates on a matching basis such that these schemas are activated if the features of a situation match the orienting template. The template for the orienting mode may be quite global, simply reflecting the valence and possible personal relevance of a stimulus. That is, the orienting mode may be biased toward detection of negative and personally relevant stimuli. We would also expect that depression and anxiety may not be differentiated at the level of the orienting mode, with an orienting negativity bias evident in both disorders.

The orienting mode operates at the preconscious, automatic level and provides an almost instantaneous perception of negative stimuli that could represent a possible threat to the organism's survival. Moreover, the orienting mode is perceptually rather than conceptually driven. It is "an early warning detection system" that identifies stimuli and assigns an initial processing priority. Further, attentional resources will be diverted to situations or stimuli detected by the orienting mode. Because the function of the orienting mode is the basic survival of the organism, it is a very rapid, involuntary, and preconscious stimulus-driven registration process. At this stage stimulus detection is global and undifferentiated, primarily identifying the valence of stimuli (negative, positive, neutral) and its potential personal relevance. Furthermore, the orienting mode may be biased toward detection of emotional stimuli more generally (MacLeod, 1999). Thus in the anxiety disorders, the orienting mode is excessively tuned toward detection of negative emotional information that will subsequently be interpreted as threatening once the primal threat mode is activated. This preconscious attentional bias means that the anxious person has an automatic tendency to selectively attend to negative emotional material, thus making deactivation of the anxiety program more difficult.

Primal Threat Mode Activation

The detection of possible threat-relevant negative emotional information by the orienting schemas will result in a simultaneous automatic activation of threat-related schemas called the *primal threat mode*. Activation of these schemas will result in the production of a primary threat appraisal. We use the term "primal" in this context because this cluster of interrelated schemas is concerned with the basic evolutionary objectives of the organism: *to maximize safety and to minimize danger.* For this reason the primal threat-relevant schemas tend to be rigid, inflexible, and reflexive. They are an automatic "rapid response" system that enables the immediate detection of threat so the organism can set about maximizing safety and minimizing danger. Once activated, the primal threat mode tends to capture most of our attentional resources and dominates the information-processing system so that slower, more elaborative, and reflective modes of thinking are blocked. That is, once activated, threat schemas become hypervalent and dominant, making it difficult for the anxious person to process anything but threat. The simultaneous and immediate activation of the orienting and primal threat schemas are evident in our previous example of the runner. Subjectively the runner feels a sudden tension and anxiousness at hearing the dog bark. What has happened between the dog bark and the tension is an orientation toward the sound of the dog and the automatic primary appraisal "Could this be danger?" due to activation of primal threat schemas.

TABLE 2.4. Schemas of the Primal Threat Mode

Type of schema	Function
Cognitive-conceptual	Represents appraisals of threat and danger to personal well-being, and absence or reduced likelihood of safety
Behavioral	Represents early defensive behaviors (mobilization, immobility, escape, avoidance)
Physiological	Represents perceived autonomic arousal, physical sensations
Motivational	Represents aims of moving away; a desire to minimize unpredictability, lack of control, and unpleasantness
Affective	Represents subjective feelings of nervousness, agitation

The primal threat mode consists of different types of schemas all aimed at maximizing safety and minimizing danger. Table 2.4 lists the different schemas of the threat mode and their function.

Cognitive-Conceptual Schemas

These schemas represent beliefs, rules, and assumptions that are relevant to making inferences and interpretations of threat. Activation of the cognitive-conceptual schemas of the primal threat mode results in the primary appraisals of threat. They enable the selection, storage, retrieval, and interpretation of information in terms of degree of threat to one's vital resources. They also represent information about the self in terms of vulnerability to threat as well as specific beliefs about the dangerousness of certain experiences or situations in the external or internal environments.

Behavioral Schemas

Behavioral schemas consist of response disposition codes and action readiness programs that enable a very quick and automatic early defensive response to threat. Most often this will involve behavioral mobilization such as the fight-or-flight response regularly seen in anxiety states. However, the behavioral schemas of the primal threat mode also enable persons to perceive and evaluate their initial behavioral response. Behavioral responses that are considered effective in immediately reducing threat will be reinforced and utilized on future occasions, whereas behavioral responses that do not lead to immediate anxiety or threat reduction will tend to be discarded.

Physiological Schemas

These schemas represent information pertinent to autonomic arousal and other physical sensations. Physiological schemas are involved in the processing of proprioceptive stimuli and allow individuals to perceive and evaluate their physiological responses (D. A. Clark et al., 1999). Anxiety states are often associated with heightened perceptions of physiological arousal, which can make the situation seem even more threatening. In panic disorder the interpretation of certain physical sensations (e.g., elevated heart rate, chest pain, breathlessness) may actually constitute the primary appraisal of threat. In other anxiety disorders, like social phobia, PTSD, or OCD, perceived elevation of autonomic arousal and the physical symptoms of anxiousness can be interpreted as confirmation of threat. It is the physiological schemas of the threat mode that are responsible for anxious persons' threat appraisals of their heightened physical state.

Motivational Schemas

These schemas are closely related to the behavioral domain and involve representations of our aims and intentions relevant to threat. Thus motivational schemas involve beliefs and rules about the importance of moving away from threat or danger and of reducing the unpredictability and aversiveness of situations. Moreover, loss of control is a state that one is highly motivated to avoid under conditions of threat. Activation of the motivational schemas of the primal threat mode, then, is responsible for the sense of urgency anxious individuals feel in trying to escape or avoid a perceived threat and reduce their anxiety.

Affective Schemas

These schemas are involved in the perception of feeling states and so are integral to the subjective experience of emotion. The affective schemas play an important functional role in the survival of the organism by ensuring that attention is diverted to a potential threat and that some form of corrective action is taken (Beck, 1996). Activation of threat mode affect schemas, then, produces the emotional experience individuals report when in states of anxiety: increased nervousness, tension, agitation, feeling "on edge."

Clinician Guideline 2.11

Utilize cognitive and behavioral interventions in cognitive therapy to reduce the accessibility and dominance of primal threat schemas, which are considered central to the experience of anxiety.

Consequences of Threat Mode Activation

As depicted in Figure 2.1, the relatively automatic activation of the primal threat mode sets in motion a complex psychological process that does not end simply with a primary appraisal of threat. Four additional processes can be identified that help define the immediate fear response: increased autonomic arousal, immediate defensive and inhibitory responses, cognitive processing biases and errors, and threat-oriented automatic thoughts and images. Each of these four processes is bidirectional with primal mode activation responsible for their initial occurrence, but once active these processes feed back in a manner that strengthens the primary threat appraisal.

Heightened Autonomic Arousal

Threat mode activation involves an appraisal of the heightened autonomic arousal that characterizes anxiety states. Beck et al. (1985, 2005) stated that subjective anxiety is proportional to perceived estimate of danger. Thus the greater the appraised danger, the more likely that increased autonomic arousal will be given a threatening interpretation. Highly anxious individuals often experience heightened physiological arousal as an aversive state that confirms the initial appraisal of threat. Thus reduction of arousal can be a prime motivation for anxious individuals. In this way a negative, threatening interpretation of one's increased physiological state can augment the already hypervalent threat mode.

Defensive Inhibitory Responses

Activation of the primal threat mode will lead to very rapid, reflexive self-protective responses involving escape, avoidance (fight or flight), freeze, faint, and the like. Beck et al. (1985, 2005) noted that these responses tend to be relatively fixed, preprogrammed, and automatic. They are "primal" in the sense of being more innate than the complex acquired responses associated with more elaborative processes. In the anxiety disorders, these very immediate defensive and inhibitory responses are evident as an almost instantaneous response to a threat appraisal. For example, individuals with long-standing OCD often report that their performance of a compulsive ritual in response to an anxiety-provoking obsession can be so automatic that they are hardly aware of what they are doing until they are well into the ritual. Beck et al. (1985, 2005) also recognized that the occurrence of these protective or defensive behaviors can also reinforce primal mode activation. They noted that these behaviors often impair performance, thus elevating the threatening nature of the situation. Thus the socially anxious individual might automatically look away when talking to another person, which makes it more difficult to have an engaging conversation.

Cognitive Processing Errors

Threat mode activation is "primal" in the sense that it is a relatively automatic, nonvolitional, and reflexive system for dealing with basic issues of survival. Thus one of the cognitive by-products of this type of activation is a narrowing of attention on to the threatening aspects of a situation. Cognitive processing, then, becomes highly selective, involving the amplification of threat and the diminished processing of safety cues. Certain cognitive errors are evident such as *minimization* (underestimates the positive aspects of personal resources), *selective abstraction* (primary focus on weaknesses), *magnification* (views flaws as a serious shortcoming), and *catastrophizing* (mistakes or threat have disastrous consequences). In anxiety these cognitive errors are manifested primarily as exaggerated estimates of the proximity, probability, and severity of potential threat. Obviously with this type of cognitive processing dominant, the anxious individual finds it extremely difficult to generate alternative, more constructive modes of thinking about the situation.

Automatic Threat-Relevant Thoughts

Finally, activation of the primal threat mode will produce automatic thoughts and images of threat and danger. These thoughts and images have an automatic quality to them because they tend to be nonvolitional and intrude into the stream of consciousness. They are characterized as (1) transient or state-dependent, (2) highly specific and discrete, (3) spontaneous and involuntary, (4) plausible, (5) consistent with one's current emotional state, and (6) biased representation of reality (Beck, 1967, 1970, 1976). Because automatic thoughts reflect the person's current concerns, in anxiety disorders they reflect themes of threat, danger, and personal vulnerability and so are hypothesized to be content-specific to each of the anxiety disorders. In anxiety states the occurrence of threat-relevant automatic thoughts and images will capture attention and in that way reinforce activation of the primal threat mode.

Clinician Guideline 2.12

The adverse cognitive, behavioral, and physiological effects of threat mode activation are a primary focus of intervention in cognitive therapy of anxiety disorders. Teach patients alternative strategies to reduce the negative impact of the threat mode.

Secondary Elaboration and Reappraisal

The quick automatic production of an immediate fear response via activation of the primal threat mode triggers a secondary, compensatory process involving much slower, more elaborative, and more effortful information processing. This secondary reappraisal phase always occurs with threat activation. Whether this secondary elaborative processing leads to an increase or reduction in anxiety depends on a number of factors. The information processing that occurs at this more conscious, controlled level will feed back into the threat mode to enhance or reduce its activation strength. In the anxiety disorders this more constructive, reflective, and balanced thinking rarely attains sufficient plausibility to present an alternative to primal threat mode activation. Below we discuss five cognitive phenomena associated with secondary elaborative processing.

Evaluation of Coping Resources

A key aspect of secondary reappraisal involves the effortful evaluation of one's ability to cope with the perceived threat. This is a strategic mode of thinking that is predominantly under voluntary and intentional control. However, in anxiety disorders the primal threat mode activation so skews one's elaborative thought processes that any consideration of coping resources leads to an enhanced sense of vulnerability.

Beck et al. (1985, 2005) discussed a number of aspects of coping evaluation relevant to anxiety. The first is a more global self-appraisal that produces self-confidence or an increased sense of personal vulnerability. *Self-confidence* is "an individual's positive appraisal of his assets and resources in order to master problems and deal with threat" (Beck et al., 1985, p. 68). Self-confidence will be associated with high self-efficacy and an expectation of success (Bandura, 1977). In anxiety states, however, individuals perceive their coping resources as insufficient. A vulnerability cognitive set is reinforced, which causes individuals to interpret incoming information in terms of their weaknesses rather than their strengths. A second aspect of coping evaluation concerns whether individuals believe they lack important skills to deal with the situation. The person in our running example would experience an immediate reduction in anxiety if she recalled previous training in dealing with dog attacks. In addition the presence of self-doubt, uncertainty, and novel or ambiguous contexts can intensify a sense of vulnerability. Presence of these contextual factors can mean that a cognitive set of "self-confidence" is replaced by a "vulnerability" set (Beck et al., 1985, 2005).

One consequence of a negative evaluation of one's coping ability is that perceived lack of competence may cause a person to act tentatively or to withdraw from a threatening situation (Beck et al., 1985, 2005). Such tentativeness can impair one's performance in the situation, which only exacerbates its threatening nature (e.g., the socially anxious person trying to initiate a conversation). The anticipation of possible incompetence and subsequent injury may inhibit approach behaviors and trigger withdrawal. This automatic inhibition reflects a continual alteration between "confident mobility and fearful immobility" (Beck et al., 1985, p. 73). The resulting dilemma can be described in the following manner: "Anxiety in this instance is an unpleasant signal to stop forward progress. If the person stops or retreats, his anxiety decreases. If he advances, it increases. If he makes a conscious decision to proceed, he may be able to override the primal inhibitory reaction" (Beck et al., 1985, p. 72).

Clinician Guideline 2.13

Correcting maladaptive evaluations and beliefs about personal vulnerability, risk, and coping resources associated with anxious concerns is an important focus in cognitive therapy of anxiety.

Search for Safety Cues

Beck and Clark (1997) argued that the search for safety cues is another important process that takes place at the secondary elaborative reappraisal phase. Rachman (1984a, 1984b) introduced the concept of "safety signals" to explain the discordance that can be found between fear and avoidance (i.e., fear without avoidance and avoidance behavior in the absence of fear). Rachman proposed that in agoraphobia, for example, the intensity of threat is primarily a function of perceived access to and speed of return to safety. Thus the absence of reliable safety signals can leave the person in a chronic state of anxiety, with the presence of anxiety eliciting a more vigorous search for safety cues. The end result, however, is that the anxious person's attempts are often ineffective, especially in the long term. This is because safety is defined narrowly as an immediate reduction in anxiety rather than as a long-term coping strategy. Thus the person with panic disorder and agoraphobic avoidance might sit next to the exit in a theater, seek the company of close friends on an outing, or carry tranquilizers as a means of procuring an immediate sense of safety. However, all of these strategies are based on a dysfunctional belief that "there is great danger out there and I can't deal with it alone." In the end anxiety is characterized by a preoccupation with immediate safety but an unfortunate reliance on inappropriate safety-seeking strategies.

Clinician Guideline 2.14

Emphasize the elimination of safety-seeking behavior in cognitive therapy of anxiety disorders.

Constructive Mode Thinking

The presence of strategic elaborative thinking provides an opportunity for more constructive, reality-based reappraisal of perceived threat. It is possible that problem-solving strategies could be considered during secondary elaboration rather than more immediate reflexive responses aimed at self-protection or escape. Access to more realistic coping resources is represented by schemas of the *constructive mode*. Constructive mode schemas are primarily acquired through life experiences and promote productive activities aimed at increasing (not protecting) the vital resources of the individual (D. A. Clark et al., 1999). Our ability to engage in reflective thought, to be self-conscious and evaluative of our own thoughts (i.e., metacognition), to problem-solve, and to reevaluate a perspective based on contradictory evidence is attributable to activation of the constructive schemas.

Beck et al. (1985, 2005) proposed that anxiety is characterized by two systems, one of which is an automatic primal *inhibitory system* that occurs in response to primal threat mode activation. This system tends to be immediate and reflexive, and is aimed at self-protection and defense. A second system, called the *anxiety reduction system*, is slower, more elaborative, and processes more complete information about a situation. The presence of anxiety can motivate a person to mobilize the more strategic processes of anxiety reduction.

The problem in anxiety disorders, however, is that the initial automatic reflexive (inhibitory) system activated by the primal threat mode tends to dominate information processing and block access to more elaborative anxiety-reducing strategies represented in the constructive schemas. Once the inhibitory system aimed at self-protection and immediate threat reduction is activated, it is very difficult for the highly anxious person to shift to more reflective, constructive thinking. One of the aims of cognitive therapy is to help the anxious patient engage in more constructive mode thinking as a means of achieving longer term reduction of anxiety.

Clinician Guideline 2.15

Encourage the development of constructive mode thinking in anxious patients to achieve more enduring reduction in anxiety.

Initiation of Worry

Beck and Clark (1997) proposed that worry is a product of the secondary, elaborative reappraisal process triggered by primal threat mode activation (see p. 393 for a definition of worry). In nonanxious states worry can be an adaptive process that leads to effective problem solving. It is anchored in constructive mode thinking in which the individual arrives at realistic solutions based on a careful analysis of contradictory evidence. A minimal amount of anxiety may be experienced as the person considers the possibility of negative outcomes and the consequences of ineffective coping. However, the anxiety is not based in primal threat mode activation and so, if anything, it serves to motivate the individual toward action.

For the highly anxious individual worry takes on pathological features that do not lead to effective problem solving but rather to an escalation of the initial threat appraisal. Here the worry becomes uncontrollable and almost exclusively focused on negative, catastrophic, and threatening outcomes. Because of the domination of threat mode thinking in the anxiety disorders, any constructive aspects of worry are blocked and the narrow focus on negative outcomes potentiates the appraisal of threat. Thus worry in the anxiety disorders, especially GAD, can become a self-perpetuating elaborative cycle that intensifies the anxious state and is perceived as confirmation of the person's initial appraisal of threat.

Clinician Guideline 2.16

Since worry is a common feature of all anxiety disorders, interventions that focus directly on worry reduction are a major feature of cognitive therapy of anxiety.

Reappraisal of Threat

One outcome of secondary elaborative thinking is a more conscious, effortful reevaluation of the threatening situation. In nonanxious states this may result in a diminished state of anxiety as the person downgrades the probability and severity of anticipated threat in light of contradictory evidence. Moreover, recognition of safety features in the environment and a reappraisal of coping strategies may lead to a reduced sense of vulnerability. In this case elaborative processing can result in a reduction in anxiety.

In the anxiety disorders secondary elaborative thinking is dominated by the threat mode and so is biased toward confirming the dangerousness of situations. An increased sense of personal vulnerability is reinforced by this elaborative thinking and the realistic safety features of the situation are overlooked. Worry and anxious rumination support the anxious person's initial automatic appraisal of threat. In this way, secondary elaborative cognitive processes are responsible for the persistence of anxiety, whereas primal threat mode activation is responsible for the immediate fear response of the anxiety program.

Clinician Guideline 2.17

Cognitive therapy seeks to help clients process disconfirming evidence that will lead to a reevaluation of threat as less probable, severe, or imminent.

NORMAL AND ABNORMAL ANXIETY: A COGNITIVE PERSPECTIVE

In our description of the cognitive model, we focused primarily on pathological anxiety. As noted earlier, fear can be adaptive and anxiety is a common experience in everyday life. So, how does the cognitive model explain the difference between normal and abnormal anxiety? This is an important consideration for clinical practitioners as well as researchers. After all, our goal as therapists is to normalize the experience of anxiety. Thus what is the nature of normal cognitive processing of anxiety? Table 2.5 summarizes a few key differences at the automatic and elaborative phases of information processing that characterize nonclinical and clinical anxiety.

Automatic Cognitive Processes in Normal Anxiety

Given the automatic and involuntary nature of the immediate fear response, it is obvious that individuals who do not suffer an anxiety disorder have a distinct advantage over clinical samples. In normal anxiety, the orienting mode is not as primed for the detection of negative self-referent stimuli as in the anxiety disorders. In nonclinical states, the detection of negative stimuli will still be given attentional priority, but the range of stimuli that would be identified as negative and potentially self-relevant would be narrower. In fact, Mogg and Bradley (1999a) reviewed evidence that less anxious individuals show attentional avoidance of low threat stimuli whereas highly anxious individuals show enhanced attention to low, and especially moderately, threatening stimuli (see also

TABLE 2.5. Cognitive Differences between Normal and Abnormal Anxiety Predicted by the Cognitive Model

Phase of processing	Abnormal anxiety	Normal anxiety
Orienting mode	• Heightened sensitivity to negative stimuli	• More balanced sensitivity to the detection of positive and negative stimuli
Primal threat activation	• Exaggerated primary appraisal of threat • Negative evaluation of autonomic arousal • Presence of threat-related processing biases and errors • Frequent and salient automatic thoughts and images of threat • Initiation of automatic, inhibitory self-protective behaviors	• More appropriate, reality-based appraisal of threat • Views arousal as an uncomfortable but not a threatening state • Attention not as narrowly focused on threat; fewer cognitive errors • Fewer and less salient anxious thoughts and images • Delay in inhibitory self-protective behaviors as more elaborative coping responses are considered
Secondary elaborative reappraisal	• Focus on weakness; low self-efficacy and negative outcome expectancy • Poor processing of safety cues • Inaccessibility of constructive mode thinking • Uncontrollable, threat-oriented worry • Initial threat estimation is enhanced	• Focus on strength; high self-efficacy and positive outcome expectancy • Better processing of safety cues • Ability to access and utilize constructive mode thinking • More controlled and reflective, problem-oriented worry • Initial threat estimation is diminished

Wilson & MacLeod, 2003). Because the orienting mode in nonclinical individuals does not show the heightened sensitivity to negative stimuli, the anxiety program is less often activated in nonclinical than in clinical individuals.

When the anxiety program is activated in nonclinical individuals, we propose qualitative differences in primal threat mode activation compared with anxious patients. Nonclinical individuals are less likely to exhibit a preconscious attentional bias for threat, and so their initial appraisals of threat are less exaggerated and more appropriate to the situation at hand. In normal anxiety, threat appraisals will more accurately reflect the consensually recognized threat value associated with internal or external situations. For example, the panic disorder patient misinterprets chest pain as a heart attack, whereas the nonclinical individual might interpret the chest pain as only remotely indicative of heart disease and instead more likely due to recent strenuous physical activity.

In normal anxiety states, activation of the threat mode does not have the same negative processing effects that are evident in the anxiety disorders. For example, autonomic arousal will be perceived as uncomfortable but not dangerous. Thus nonclinical persons are more likely to view their aroused state as tolerable and not requiring immediate relief. Furthermore, both automatic and more strategic attentional processes are not as narrowly focused on threat, so nonclinically anxious individuals make fewer cognitive errors as they process both the threatening and the nonthreatening aspects of a situation. The automatic reflexive inhibitory behaviors aimed at self-protection (fight/flight, escape) that are so prominent in the anxiety disorders are delayed in nonclinical states. This gives opportunity for more elaborative and strategic cognitive processes to reconsider the situation and execute a more adaptive, controlled response. The end result is that even during times of anxiousness, nonclinical individuals will have fewer and less salient intrusive and uncontrollable automatic thoughts and images of threat.

Secondary Elaborative Cognitive Processing in Normal Anxiety

The greatest differences between clinical and nonclinical anxiety are evident in the secondary, strategic controlled processes responsible for the persistence of anxiety. For the clinical individual further elaboration results in a persistence and even escalation of anxiety, whereas the same processes result in reduction and possible termination of the anxiety program for the nonclinical person.

One of the most important differences at the elaborative phase is that nonclinical individuals have a more balanced understanding of their personal strengths and coping resources whereas clinical individuals tend to focus on their weaknesses and deficiencies. In nonclinical individuals this leads to high self-efficacy and expectancy of a successful or positive outcome. For individuals with anxiety disorders, negative evaluation of their coping resources intensifies a sense of personal vulnerability and helplessness.

Second, we expect that nonclinical individuals are better able to recognize and comprehend the safety cues in a situation compared to those with anxiety disorders. This will allow them to arrive at a more complete understanding of their circumstances and a more realistic assessment of its threat potential. Third, the nonclinical individual will have greater access to constructive mode thinking so that initial threat appraisals can be reevaluated in the light of more rational, evidenced-based reasoning. In the anxiety disorders, this type of rational, reflective thought is blocked by the hypervalent threat schemas.

A fourth consideration is the quality of worry that occurs at the elaborative phase. Normal anxiety is characterized by a more controlled, reflective, and problem-oriented type of worry. The worry of a nonclinical person may lead to the generation of possible solutions to a particular problem. The pathological worry in the anxiety disorders is less controllable, more persistent, and more focused on the immediate threat of the situation. Worry in the anxiety disorders appears to intensify anxiety, whereas the worry in nonclinical states may motivate an individual to take constructive action. The final result is that processes at the elaborative phase may lead to diminished threat estimation in normal anxiety, but to an intensification of the initial threat appraisal in the anxiety disorders. In this way secondary elaborative cognitive processes are responsible for the persistence of anxiety in abnormal states but for a controlled management and eventual reduction of the anxiety program in normal conditions.

The cognitive perspective on normal and abnormal anxiety has direct implications for the treatment of anxiety disorders. As cognitive therapists, our focus should be on the elaborative strategic processes involved in secondary reappraisal. Teachman and Woody (2004) concluded that experimental evidence supports the view that strategic elaborative processing can override implicit or automatic cognitive processes and behavior. This is the challenge for cognitive therapists

---

Clinician Guideline 2.18

Shift the secondary elaborative processing and reappraisal in anxiety disorders from one of threat enhancement to one of threat reduction, as seen in nonclinical states.

HYPOTHESES OF THE COGNITIVE MODEL

Table 2.6 presents 12 primary hypotheses derived from the cognitive model of anxiety. Although many other hypotheses can be formulated from the cognitive perspective, we believe these 12 hypotheses represent critical aspects of the model that provide an empirical test of its validity. These hypotheses were derived from the central tenets of the model (see Table 2.2) as well as the two-phase structure outlined in Figure 2.1. Chapters 3 and 4 provide an extensive review of the empirical support for each of the hypotheses.

SUMMARY AND CONCLUSION

It is 25 years since the cognitive model of anxiety was first introduced by Beck and colleagues (Beck et al., 1985). In this chapter we presented a reformulation of that model, which incorporates the considerable progress made in our understanding of the cognitive contributors to the pathogenesis of anxiety. The last two decades have represented an exceptionally productive period of cognitive-clinical research on the anxiety disorders and their treatment. In light of these developments a number of modifications, elaborations, and clarifications were made to the cognitive model.

TABLE 2.6. Hypotheses of the Cognitive Model of Anxiety

Hypothesis 1: Attentional threat bias

Highly anxious individuals will exhibit an automatic selective attentional bias for negative stimuli that are relevant to threats of particular vital concerns. This automatic selective attentional threat bias will not be present in nonanxious states.

Hypothesis 2: Diminished attentional processing of safety

Anxious individuals will exhibit an automatic attentional shift away from safety cues that are incongruent with their dominant threat concerns, whereas nonanxious individuals will show an automatic attentional shift toward safety cues.

Hypothesis 3: Exaggerated threat appraisals

Anxiety is characterized by an automatic evaluative process that exaggerates the threatening valence of relevant stimuli in comparison to the actual threat valence of the stimuli. Nonanxious individuals will automatically evaluate relevant stimuli in a less threatening manner that approximates the actual threat value of the situation.

Hypothesis 4: Threat-biased cognitive errors

Highly anxious individuals will commit more cognitive errors while processing particular threatening stimuli as reflected in biased estimates of the proximity, probability, and severity of potential threat. The reverse pattern will be evident in nonanxious states where a cognitive processing bias for nonthreat or safety cues is present.

Hypothesis 5: Negative interpretation of anxiety

Highly anxious individuals will generate more negative and threatening interpretations of their subjective anxious feelings and symptoms than individuals experiencing low levels of anxiety.

Hypothesis 6: Elevated disorder-specific threat cognitions

Anxiety will be characterized by an elevated frequency, intensity, and duration of negative automatic thoughts and images of selective threat and danger in comparison to nonanxious states or other types of negative affect. Furthermore, each of the anxiety disorders is characterized by a particular thought content relevant to its specific threat.

Hypothesis 7: Ineffective defensive strategies

Highly anxious individuals will exhibit less effective immediate defensive strategies for diminishing anxiety and securing a sense of safety relative to individuals experiencing low levels of anxiety. In addition highly anxious individuals will evaluate their defensive abilities in threatening situations as less effective than nonanxious individuals.

Hypothesis 8: Facilitated threat elaboration

A selective threat bias will be evident in explicit and elaborated cognitive processes such that in anxiety memory retrieval, outcome expectancies, and inferences to ambiguous stimuli will show a preponderance of threat-related themes relative to nonanxious individuals.

Hypothesis 9: Inhibited safety elaboration

Explicit and controlled cognitive processes in anxiety will be characterized by an inhibitory bias of safety information relevant to selective threats such that memory retrieval, outcome expectancies, and judgments of ambiguous stimuli will evidence fewer themes of safety in comparison to nonanxious individuals.

(cont.)

TABLE 2.6. *(cont.)*

Hypothesis 10: Detrimental cognitive compensatory strategies

In high anxiety worry has a greater adverse effect by enhancing threat salience, whereas worry in low anxiety states is more likely to be associated with positive effects such as the initiation of effective problem solving. In addition, other cognitive strategies aimed at reducing threatening thoughts, such as thought suppression, distraction, and thought replacement, are more likely to exhibit paradoxical effects (i.e., rebound, increased negative affect, less perceived control) in high than in low anxious states.

Hypothesis 11: Elevated personal vulnerability

Highly anxious individuals will exhibit lower self-confidence and greater perceived helplessness in situations relevant to their selective threats compared to nonanxious individuals.

Hypothesis 12: Enduring threat-related beliefs

Individuals vulnerable to anxiety can be distinguished from nonvulnerable persons by their preexisting maladaptive schemas (i.e., beliefs) about particular threats or dangers and associated personal vulnerability that remain inactive until triggered by relevant life experiences or stressors.

The present formulation places a much greater emphasis on the automatic, involuntary cognitive processes involved in the initial fear response. Although the original cognitive model recognized that some of the mechanisms of anxiety were more innate and automatic, the current model provides a more elaborated and fine-grained description of the automatic cognitive processes in anxiety. As the initial fear response, these automatic processes, such as preconscious attentional threat bias, immediate threat evaluation, and inhibitory processing of safety cues, are the catalyst for the more protracted state of anxiety that follows. Activation of threat-related schemas remains a core feature of the cognitive model of anxiety but is now seen as responsible for maintaining an automatic threat-processing bias and its negative consequences. Thus schematic change is still viewed as crucial to the therapeutic effectiveness of cognitive therapy for the anxiety disorders.

Beck et al. (1985) focused much of their original discussion on the conscious, elaborative cognitive processes and structures of anxiety. The present model offers further clarification of the role of these elaborative, strategic processes in the persistence of anxiety. Activation of secondary, elaborative reappraisal processes, such as a conscious evaluation of one's coping resources, search for safety cues, attempts at more constructive or reflective thinking, and worry about and deliberate reappraisal of threat, determine the persistence of an anxious state. If a person concludes from this elaborative processing that a significant personal threat or danger is highly probable and her ability to establish a sense of safety through effective coping is minimal, than a state of persistent anxiety will ensue. On the other hand, anxiety will be reduced or eliminated if the perceived probability and/or severity of threat are lowered, increased confidence in adaptive coping is established, and a sense of personal safety is restored. Based on this model, cognitive therapy focuses primarily on modification of these secondary, elaborative cognitive processes through specific cognitive and behavioral interventions that shift the patient's perspective from one of possible imminent threat to one of probable personal safety. A change in secondary elaborative processing will reduce the propensity for automatic threat processing and decrease the activation threshold for threat-related schemas.

The therapeutic strategy described in this book is theory-driven. In subsequent chapters we discuss various cognitive restructuring and exposure-based interventions derived from the cognitive model that can be used to modify the faulty cognitive and behavioral processes that maintain anxiety. The basic premise is that anxiety reduction depends on a change in the faulty cognitive processes and structures of anxiety. In the last part of the book, a disorder-specific cognitive model and treatment protocol is proposed for each of the major anxiety disorders, which draws on the basic propositions of the generic or "transdiagnostic" model described in this chapter. However before considering these therapeutic applications, the next two chapters discuss the empirical support and unresolved issues associated with our cognitive formulation for vulnerability and persistence of clinical anxiety.

Chapter 3

Empirical Status
of the Cognitive Model of Anxiety

Since the emergence of the cognitive model in the early 1960s (Beck, 1963, 1964, 1967), an emphasis on empirical verification has been important to its development and elaboration. The scientific basis of the model rests on constructs and hypotheses that are sufficiently precise to enable their support or disconfirmation in the laboratory (D. A. Clark et al., 1999). In this chapter and the next, we present a review of the empirical status of the cognitive model of anxiety based on the 12 hypotheses presented in Table 2.6. We begin in this chapter with the initial three hypotheses that refer to core cognitive attributes of primal threat mode activation. The next section discusses empirical support for the cognitive, physiological, and behavioral products involved in the immediate fear response (i.e., Hypotheses 4 to 7). The final section of this chapter reviews empirical findings that are relevant to the persistence of anxiety (i.e., Hypotheses 8 to 10), that is, the secondary elaboration and reappraisal phase of the model. Hypotheses 11 and 12 will be discussed in the next chapter on cognitive vulnerability to anxiety because they deal with the etiology of anxiety.

IMMEDIATE FEAR RESPONSE: THREAT MODE ACTIVATION

Hypothesis 1. Attentional Threat Bias

Highly anxious individuals will exhibit an automatic selective attentional bias for negative stimuli that are relevant to threats of particular vital concerns. This automatic selective attentional threat bias will not be present in nonanxious states.

After 20 years of experimental research it is now clear that anxiety disorders are characterized by a preconscious, automatic selective attentional bias for emotionally threatening information (for reviews, see D. M. Clark, 1999; Macleod, 1999; Mogg &

Bradley, 1999a, 2004; Wells & Matthews, 1994; Williams et al., 1997). Because human attentional capacity is limited, some stimuli will capture attentional resources and others will be ignored. The presence of an attentional bias for threat is expected to cause an increased propensity to experience anxiety (McNally, 1999). Below we organized our review of the attentional research around three types of experimentation; emotional Stroop, dot probe detection, and stimulus identification.

Emotional Stroop

In order to experimentally investigate attentional bias in anxiety, clinical researchers have borrowed and then modified various information-processing tasks from cognitive experimental psychology. One of the most popular of these experimental paradigms has been the emotional Stroop task. Based on the classic Stroop color-naming paradigm (Stroop, 1935), participants are asked to name as quickly as possible the color of emotionally threatening (e.g., "disease," "cancer," "embarrassed" "disaster," "dirty," "inferior") and nonthreatening (e.g., "upward," "network," "leisure," "secure") words printed in blue, yellow, green, or red and to disregard the meaning of the word. Typically, anxious but not nonanxious individuals take longer to name the printed color of threat words compared with nonthreat words (e.g., Bradley, Mogg, White, & Millar, 1995; Mathews & Klug, 1993; Mathews & MacLeod, 1985; Mogg, Mathews, & Weinman, 1989; Mogg, Bradley, Williams, & Mathews, 1993). This longer color-naming latency suggests that anxious individuals exhibit preferential allocation of attention to the threat meaning of the word (Mogg & Bradley, 2004). Thus the extent of interference in color-naming response by the meaning of the word is assumed to reflect attentional bias for threat.

The emotional Stroop threat interference effect has been found in all five of the anxiety disorders discussed in this volume: panic disorder (e.g., Buckley, Blanchard, & Hickling, 2002; Lim & Kim, 2005; Lundh, Wikström, Westerlund, & Öst, 1999; McNally, Riemann, & Kim, 1990); OCD (e.g., Kyrios & Iob, 1998; Lavy, van Oppen, & van den Hout, 1994); social phobia (e.g., Becker, Rinck, Margraf, & Roth, 2001; Hope, Rapee, Heimberg, & Dombeck, 1990); PTSD (e.g., J. G. Beck, Freeman, Shipherd, Hamblen, & Lackner, 2001; Bryant & Harvey, 1995); and GAD (e.g., Bradley et al., 1995; Mogg, Bradley, Millar, & White, 1995). Moreover, threat interference effects significantly correlate in the low to moderate range with state and symptom anxiety measures (e.g., MacLeod & Hagan, 1992; Mathews, Mogg, Kentish, & Eysenck, 1995; Spector, Pecknold, & Libman, 2003) and become more apparent as the threat stimulus intensity increases from mild to severe intensity (Mogg & Bradley, 1998). In addition, the best discrimination of attentional bias in high trait and nonclinically anxious individuals versus low anxiety individuals might be with weak to moderately threatening cues in which the nonanxious person would show no preferential bias for threat (Mathews & Mackintosh, 1998).

The most consistent and robust interference effects are found with words that are semantically related to the current emotional concerns of the anxious person (Mathews & Klug, 1993); this content-specificity seems particularly pronounced in OCD, social phobia, and PTSD (J. G. Beck et al., 2001; Becker et al., 2001; Buckley et al., 2002; Foa, Ilai, McCarthy, Shoyer, & Murdock, 1993; Hope et al., 1990; Kyrios & Iob, 1998; Lavy et al., 1994; Mattia, Heimberg, & Hope, 1993; Spector et al., 2003). However, the attentional bias in GAD and, to a lesser extent, panic may be more emotionally oriented and thus elicited by any negative emotional stimuli, and in some cases, even positive information (e.g., Becker et al., 2001; Bradley, Mogg, White, & Millar, 1995; Buckley et al., 2002; Lim & Kim, 2005; Lundh et al., 1999; Martin, Williams, & Clark, 1991; McNally et al., 1994; Mogg et al., 1993; Mogg, Bradley, Millar, & White, 1995).

To investigate the automaticity of attentional threat bias, researchers modified the emotional Stroop task to include subliminal (below conscious awareness) and supraliminal (above conscious awareness) conditions. In these studies individual threat and nonthreat words are presented very briefly (20 milliseconds or less) followed by a mask, which usually involves a string of random letters presented in the same location as the word. In some studies participants are asked to name the color of the word whereas in other studies they are asked to name the color of the background of the word. In the supraliminal condition the words remain unmasked on the screen until a color-naming response is made. Figure 3.1 provides an illustration of the modified emotional Stroop task.

In a number of studies anxious patients exhibited significantly slower color-naming latencies to subliminal threat words, suggesting that selective attention to threat occurs at the automatic preconscious level (e.g., Bradley et al., 1995; Kyrios & Iob, 1998; Lundh et al., 1999; Mogg et al., 1993). Since this threat interference effect was found on both subliminal and supraliminal trials within the same study, it suggests that attentional bias for threat involves both automatic and elaborative cognitive processes (e.g., Bradley et al., 1995; Lundh et al., 1999; Mogg et al., 1993).

Another important issue addressed in the emotional Stroop research is the relation of attentional threat bias to state and trait anxiety. MacLeod and Rutherford (1992) reported that automatic attentional threat bias is most influenced by an interaction between state and trait anxiety. They compared nonclinical high and low trait-anxious students on a modified emotional Stroop task and found that the high trait-anxious students under stress (tested 1 week before exams) showed greater subliminal Stroop interference for threat, whereas stress did not enhance threat interference for the low trait-anxious students. In the supraliminal condition both high and low trait-anxious students showed intentional avoidance of threat words. Other studies have also found that increased stress and arousal are associated with greater attentional bias, especially in high trait or fearful individuals (Chen, Lewin, & Craske, 1996; Mogg, Mathews, Bird, & MacGregor-Morris, 1990; Richards, French, Johnson, Naparstek, & Williams, 1992; see McNally, Riemann, Louro, Lukach, & Kim, 1992, for contrary findings). However, the effects of state and trait anxiety on attentional bias may be more complicated than first thought. High trait anxious individuals exhibit a preconscious, automatic attentional bias for threat, but unlike clinical samples, this attentional bias may be sensitive to negative valence more generally rather than to specific threat content (e.g., Fox, 1993; Mogg & Marden, 1990). In addition, elevated state anxiety may lead to greater automatic threat bias in high trait anxiety individuals (interaction effect), but at the more elaborative, strategic level, stress may have independent effects on attentional threat bias. MacLeod and Hagan (1992) suggested that nonclinical individuals may be able to strategically modify their automatic threat bias, thereby eliminating any differential interference effects in the supraliminal condition. Anxious patients, on the other hand, may fail to strategically modify their preconscious attentional threat bias so that threat differences continue to emerge at the elaborative stage of information processing.

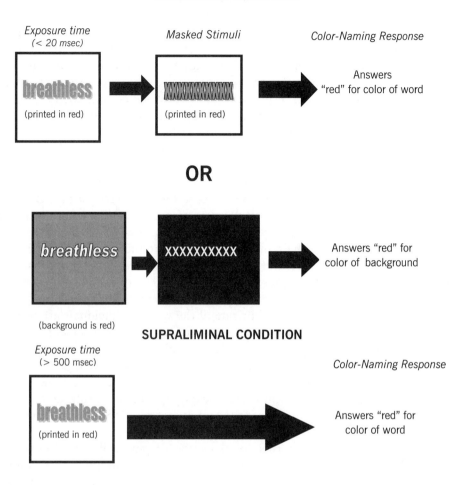

FIGURE 3.1. Illustration of the subliminal and supraliminal conditions in a modified emotional Stroop task.

Finally, results of an emotional Stroop experiment on PTSD led to the conclusion that an elevation in stress or arousal might enhance automatic threat bias whereas anticipation of a more potent threat might suppress attentional bias (Constans, McCloskey, Vasterling, Brailey, & Mathews, 2004).

There is some evidence that treatment responders do show a significant decline in the interference effects of disorder-specific threat words whereas treatment nonresponders show no change in Stroop interference (Mathews et al., 1995; Mattia, Heimberg, & Hope, 1993; Mogg, Bradley, Millar, & White, 1995). In sum, there is consistent evidence that preferential allocation toward threatening cues occurs at a preconscious, automatic level of information processing in both clinically anxious and high trait-anxious individuals. The emotional Stroop findings are less consistent when it comes to demonstrating attentional biases at the slower, elaborative level of information processing.

Unfortunately, interpretation of the Stroop findings is hindered by limitations in its methodology. It is possible that slower color naming could be due to diverting attention away from threatening words rather than because of enhanced attention to the meaning of the word (MacLeod, 1999). Also longer reaction times to threatening words could be due to the interfering effects of an emotional reaction to the word (e.g., startle response), or because of mental preoccupation with themes related to the word (Bögels & Mansell, 2004). Because of these potential response biases (see Mogg & Bradley, 1999a), probe detection tests have surpassed the emotional Stroop task as the preferred experimental paradigm for investigating attentional bias in anxiety.

Dot Probe Detection

The dot probe detection experiment is able to assess hypervigilance for threat in terms of both facilitation and interference with dot detection without the effects of response bias (MacLeod, Mathews, & Tata, 1986). In this task a series of word pairs is presented so that one word is in the upper half and the other word in the lower half of a computer screen. The trial begins with a central fixation cross presented for approximately 500 milliseconds, followed by a brief presentation (500 milliseconds) of a word pair. On critical trials a threat and neutral word pair are presented followed by the appearance of a dot in the location formerly occupied by one of the words. Individuals are instructed to press a key as quickly as possible when they see the dot. Hundreds of word pair trials are usually presented with many involving filler neutral–neutral word pairs.

A number of dot probe experiments have demonstrated an attentional threat bias in clinically anxious patients but not in nonanxious controls. Anxious patients mainly with a primary diagnosis of GAD exhibit significantly quicker dot probe detection after physically and socially threatening words (MacLeod et al., 1986; Mogg, Bradley, & Williams, 1995; Mogg, Mathews, & Eysenck, 1992). Attentional vigilance for threat has also been found in panic disorder for detection of physically threatening words (Mathews, Ridgeway, & Williamson, 1996), OCD for contamination words (Tata, Leibowitz, Prunty, Cameron, & Pickering, 1996), and social phobia for negative social evaluation cues (Asmundson & Stein, 1994). Vassilopoulos (2005), however, found that socially anxious students showed vigilance for all emotional words (positive and negative) at short exposure intervals (200 milliseconds) but avoidance of the same word stimuli at longer intervals (500 milliseconds). In addition, negative findings have also been reported, with GAD patients failing to show attentional vigilance for threatening words or angry faces (Gotlib, Krasnoperova, Joormann, & Yue, 2004; Mogg et al., 1991; see also Lees, Mogg, & Bradley, 2005, for negative results with high health-anxious students).

Researchers have employed a *visual dot probe task* in which probe detection is measured to pairs of pictorial stimuli involving angry versus neutral facial expressions as a more valid representation of social evaluative threat (Mogg & Bradley, 1998). However, visual dot probe has produced inconsistent results. While some researchers have reported an initial selective vigilance (quicker probe detection) to angry or hostile facial expressions at short intervals only (e.g., Mogg, Philippot, & Bradley, 2004), other researchers failed to find vigilance for threatening or angry faces in analogue or even clinical social anxiety groups (Gotlib, Kasch, et al., 2004; Pineles & Mineka, 2005), and others have even reported an opposite finding, with high social anxiety characterized by a significant avoidance of emotional faces (Chen, Ehlers, Clark, & Mansell, 2002; Mansell, Clark, Ehlers, & Chen, 1999). One possibility is that social phobia involves an initial attentional vigilance for social evaluation followed by an avoidance of social threat stimuli once more elaborative processing occurs (Chen et al., 2002; see findings by Mogg et al., 2004).

Dot probe experiments have been used to investigate cognitive vulnerability to anxiety by determining if high trait anxiety is characterized by speeded detection of threat stimuli. The most consistent finding is that high trait-anxious individuals exhibit quicker probe detection to threatening words or faces compared to low-trait anxious individuals, especially at shorter exposure intervals (Bradley, Mogg, Falla, & Hamilton, 1998; Mogg & Bradley, 1999b; Mogg, Bradley, Miles, & Dixon, 2004; Mogg et al., 2000, Experiment 2). Other studies, however, have reported entirely negative findings for trait anxiety, concluding that hypervigilance for threat was due to state anxiety (or immediate stress) either alone or in interaction with trait anxiety (e.g., Bradley, Mogg, & Millar, 2000; Mogg et al., 1990).

It is likely that these inconsistent findings occur because attentional bias in anxiety involves both hypervigilance and avoidance of threat stimuli (Mathews & Mackintosh, 1998; Mogg & Bradley, 1998). Generally hypervigilance for threat has been more apparent during brief exposures when preconscious automatic processes predominate and at higher levels of threat intensity. Avoidance of threat stimuli more likely occurs at longer exposure intervals when more elaborative processing comes into effect and with mildly threatening stimuli. This vigilance-avoidance pattern may be particularly evident in specific fears, with high trait anxiety characterized by initial vigilance for threat without subsequent avoidance (Mogg et al., 2004; see Rohner, 2002, for contrary findings). However, Rohner (2002) did not confirm this distinction between anxiety and fear.

In a study that directly examined the effects of varying levels of threat intensity, Wilson and MacLeod (2003) compared probe detection times of high and low trait-anxious students to very low, low, moderate, high, and very high anger facial expressions paired with a neutral face. All participants failed to show attentional bias to the very low threat stimuli, attentional avoidance of mildly threatening faces, and attentional vigilance at the most intensely threatening stimuli. Interestingly, group differences in attentional deployment were only apparent with the moderately threatening faces where only high trait-anxious group showed quicker detection of threatening than neutral faces. Others have also found that attentional bias for threat increases with stimulus threat value (Mogg et al., 2004; Mogg et al., 2000). In a more recent study high trait-anxious individuals showed clear evidence of facilitated attention and impaired disengagement from high threat at 100 milliseconds but attentional avoidance at 200 or 500 milliseconds (Koster, Crombez, Verschuere, Van Damme, & Wiersema, 2006). Finally, in an attentional training experiment by MacLeod, Rutherford, Campbell, Ebsworthy, and Holker (2002), students given training to attend away from negative words had reduced emotional response to a stress induction compared to students trained to attend to negative probes. This indicates that attentional bias can have a causal impact on emotional response.

In summary both semantic (words) and visual (faces) dot probe detection research provides the strongest experimental evidence for an automatic, preconscious hypervigilance for threat. Hypervigilance for threat is more likely when conscious elaborative processing is restricted (shorter exposures with reduced awareness), when threat stimuli match the current concerns or worries of the patient, and when threat intensity is moderate to severe. In addition facilitated attention to threat may be enhanced by an impaired disengagement from highly threatening stimuli in anxious individuals (e.g., Koster et al., 2006). Attentional avoidance of threat clearly plays an important role in defining perceptual bias in anxiety but it may be less prominent in high trait anxiety (Mogg et al., 2004). Finally, attentional bias is probably not unique to anxiety, with depression, for example, characterized by an attentional bias for negative information (e.g., Gotlib, Krasnoperova, et al., 2004; Mathews et al., 1996).

Stimulus Identification Tasks

Stimulus identification paradigms involve a search for threatening or nonthreatening words within a matrix of random words or measurement of latency to identify words presented at participants' threshold of awareness. In a number of studies panic patients had enhanced identification of threat stimuli (Lundh et al., 1999; Pauli et al., 1997; see Lim & Kim, 2005, for negative findings) and social phobia individuals had facilitated identification of angry faces (Gilboa-Schechtman, Foa, & Amir, 1999). However, studies of generalized anxiety have been more complicated, with some showing facilitated detection of threat (Mathews & MacLeod, 1986; Foa & McNally, 1986) and others indicating that the problem might be increased distraction by threatening stimuli (Mathews, May, Mogg, & Eysenck, 1990; Rinck, Becker, Kellerman, & Roth, 2003).

Summary

There is strong empirical support for the first hypothesis of the cognitive model. Despite some inconsistencies across studies, there is still substantial evidence from a variety of experimental methodologies that anxiety is characterized by a hypervigilance for threatening stimuli and that this attentional bias is absent in low anxiety states. However, it is also clear that a number of qualifications must be added to this statement. Attentional threat bias is more evident in the immediate or early stages of processing when conscious awareness is reduced, when threat stimuli match the specific anxiety-relevant concerns of the individual, and when threat intensity has reached a moderate to high level. Figure 3.2 provides a schematic illustration of how exposure duration, meaning, and threat value determine the role of selective attentional processing for threat in anxiety (see Mogg & Bradley, 1998, 2004, for further elaboration).

Hypervigilance for threat will be absent when mildly threatening and impersonal stimuli (e.g., general threat words) are presented at long exposure intervals. At the other extreme, all individuals will exhibit heighten vigilance when stimuli are extremely threatening, highly personal, and preconscious or automatic. That is, anyone will attend to stimuli evaluated as posing a significant threat. However, it is the moderately threatening, personally specific stimuli presented at brief, preconscious exposure intervals that will result in the exaggerated attentional threat bias that characterizes the anxiety disorders. Moderately threatening stimuli are considered threatening by vulnerable individuals but nonthreatening to those with low anxiety (Mogg & Bradley, 1998). However, selective attention to threat (i.e., facilitation effects) must be understood as an interplay with avoidant (i.e., inhibitory) attentional processes, which in turn depends

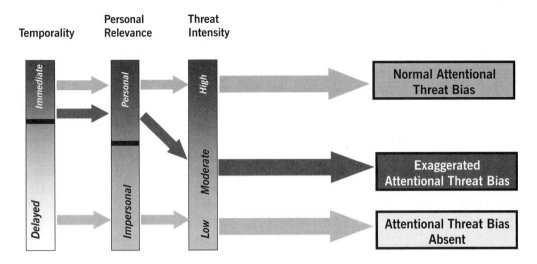

FIGURE 3.2. Schematic representation of threat gradient for attentional bias.

on an evaluation of stimulus threat value (Mathews & Mackintosh, 1998). An apparent hypervigilance for threat may be due to any combination of facilitated threat detection, impaired threat disengagement, or subsequent avoidance of threat cues with prolonged exposure. The following clinical implication can be drawn from this research.

Clinician Guideline 3.1

Clinically anxious and vulnerable individuals automatically orient toward threat without conscious awareness of this tendency. Some form of attentional training might help counter this orienting bias.

Hypothesis 2. Diminished Attentional Processing of Safety

Anxious individuals will exhibit an automatic attentional shift away from safety cues that are incongruent with their dominant threat concerns, whereas nonanxious individuals will show an automatic attentional shift toward safety cues.

The selective attentional bias for threat reflects a narrowing of attention that accompanies emotional arousal (Barlow, 2002). "Narrowing of attention" is based on Easter-brook's (1959) proposal that increased emotional arousal will cause a reduction in the range of cues utilized (processed) by an organism. From an information-processing perspective, this means the higher the anxiety level, the more one's attention will become narrowly focused on a restricted range of mood-congruent stimuli, thereby causing a reduction in the scope of stimulus processing (Barlow, 2002; Wells & Matthews, 1994; see also Mathews & Mackintosh, 1998). In the present context this means that highly anxious individuals should exhibit the greatest amount of attentional narrowing for threat-relevant stimuli, with little attentional resources remaining to process information that is mood-incongruent, such as cues of nonthreat or safety. We predict that information signifying safety or absence of threat would be a stimulus category most likely to be ignored in anxiety states because it is highly incongruent with this intense focus on a narrow band of threatening information.

Two questions are relevant for this second hypothesis. First, do highly anxious individuals exhibit significantly reduced processing of relevant safety information? Second, do nonanxious individuals show an enhanced processing bias for safety cues? Two other issues that are related but less central to this hypothesis are whether nonanxious individuals automatically shift their attention away from threat and whether highly anxious individuals eventually avoid threatening cues in an effort to intentionally compensate or suppress the earlier automatic hypervigilance for threat and danger (Mathews & Mackintosh, 1998; Mogg & Bradley, 2004; Wells & Matthews, 1994).

High Anxiety: Reduced Safety Signal Processing

As noted in Chapter 2 inhibited processing of safety information is an important faulty information-processing characteristic of anxiety. Diminished processing of safety might be a cognitive factor that underlies the propensity of anxious individuals to engage in safety-seeking behavior, an important factor in the persistence of anxiety (i.e., Rachman, 1984a; Salkovskis, 1996a, 1996b; Salkovskis, Clark, Hackmann, Wells, & Gelder, 1999). This is because avoidance and other safety behaviors (e.g., holding on to objects, venturing out only when accompanied, having immediate access to medication, reassurance seeking, checking) deprive individuals of opportunities to disconfirm their catastrophic beliefs. For example, a person with panic disorder who will only go to a store with a close family member fails to learn that she will not have a heart attack from chest pain (i.e., the catastrophic fear belief) even though she may feel intense anxiety when alone in the store. The catastrophic belief, then, persists despite the nonoccurrence of heart attacks because the person engages in safety-seeking behavior (avoids stores or takes a friend) that averts the dreaded outcome and reduces anxiety, but it also prevents the person from learning that the belief is groundless (Salkovskis, Clark, & Gelder, 1996).

Research has shown a link between safety-seeking behavior, catastrophic beliefs, and persistent anxiety. A questionnaire study of panic disorder (Salkovskis et al., 1996) found evidence of the predicted associations between threat beliefs and actual safety-seeking behavior when individuals were questioned about their responses during their most panicky or anxious episodes. In addition, brief treatment analogue studies have shown that decreases in safety-seeking behavior lead to greater reductions in catastrophic beliefs and anxiety (Salkovskis et al., 1999; Sloan & Tech, 2002; Wells et al., 1995). If anxious individuals exhibit less rapid and efficient processing of safety information, this would leave them with a narrowed intense focus on the threatening aspects of a situation. This hypervigilance for threat combined with diminished processing of mood-incongruent safety cues might promote more extreme and effortful attempts to reestablish a sense of security through safety-seeking behavior (see Figure 3.3 for proposed relationships).

Only a few studies have investigated information processing of safety cues in anxiety. Mansell and D. M. Clark (1999) found that socially anxious individuals exposed to a social-threat manipulation (give a short speech) recalled significantly fewer positive public self-referent trait adjectives and Amir, Beard, and Prezeworski (2005) reported

	Early Processing		*Later Processing*
HIGH ANXIETY	Heightened Attention to Threat	X	Delayed Threat Disengagement
	Diminished Attention to Safety		Inadequate Safety Cue Processing
			↓
			Increased Safety-Seeking Behavior
LOW ANXIETY	Reduced Attention to Threat	X	Low Threat Engagement
	Enhanced Attention to Safety		Appropriate Safety Cue Processing
			↓
			Safety-Seeking Behavior Absent

FIGURE 3.3. Proposed relation of threat and safety processing biases in high and low anxiety.

that individuals with generalized social phobia had difficulty learning nonthreat interpretations of ambiguous social information. Also, a psychophysiological study found that combat veterans with PTSD were less expressive to emotionally positive standard pictorial stimuli (i.e., lower zygomatic facial EMG response) after viewing a 10-minute trauma videotape (Litz, Orsillo, Kaloupek, & Weathers, 2000; see Miller & Litz, 2004, for failure to replicate). These findings suggest that diminished processing of nonthreat or safety information may be evident in anxiety but this may only occur at the later stage of strategic processing (see Derryberry & Reed, 2002). Also, the provision of safety cues may have difficulty overriding the strong information-processing bias for threat (i.e., Hayward, Ahmad, & Wardle, 1994) and there is even evidence that individuals with panic may show a recognition bias for "safe" facial expressions (Lundh, Thulin, Czyzykow, & Öst, 1998).

At this point too few studies have investigated the processing of safety cues in anxiety and so the empirical status of Hypothesis 2 cannot be determined. Clearly, studies are needed that directly compare the automatic and strategic processing of threat-relevant and safety-relevant information in clinically anxious and nonanxious controls. In addition it would be important to establish a relationship between diminished safety cue processing as a mediator of safety-seeking behavior.

Low Anxiety: Enhanced Safety Signal Processing

Two outcomes are possible when investigating safety signal processing in the absence of anxiety. It is possible that attention is drawn toward positive stimuli or safety cues so that a positivity bias is evident in nonanxious states. An alternative outcome is that no attentional bias occurs in low anxiety so that an evenhanded processing of threatening and safety cues prevails.

At this point we know very little about the processing of safety-relevant information in low anxiety states. In the original dot probe experiment MacLeod et al. (1986) found that the nonanxious control group tended to shift their attention away from threat words (see also Mogg & Bradley, 2002). However, this effect has not been replicated in most subsequent studies (e.g., Mogg, Mathews, & Eysenck, 1992; Mogg, Bradley, et al., 2004; Mogg et al., 2000). On the other hand, MacLeod and Rutherford (1992) found that low trait-anxious students evidenced a significant reduction in color-naming interference for threat words as their state anxiety level increased in a high stress condition. Based on a color perception task, Mogg et al. (1992, Experiment 3) found that low state anxiety individuals attended more often to manic than to neutral words. However, in most studies the nonanxious group shows little differential result across stimuli, suggesting an evenhanded attention to threat and nonthreat cues. Although the key research is missing, Figure 3.3 illustrates a possible interaction between attentional processing of threat and safety in high and low anxiety, and how these combined effects might contribute to safety-seeking behavior in highly anxious individuals.

Threat Avoidance: An Empirical Perspective

As previously mentioned, there is emerging evidence that specific fears may be characterized by an initial vigilance for threat (at brief exposures), followed by an attentional avoidance of threat at longer intervals, whereas high trait anxiety simply shows the initial orientation toward threat (Amir, Foa, & Coles, 1998a; Mogg, Bradley, et al., 2004; Vassilopoulos, 2005). However, others have reported a vigilance-avoidance pattern of attentional bias for high trait anxiety (Rohner, 2002) and increased distraction for threat (Fox, 1994; Rinck et al., 2003). Thus questions remain about the relation between an initial orientation to threat and subsequent disengagement followed by sustained attention away from threatening cues. It is evident that threat hypervigilance can be countered through treatment interventions, by intentional suppression efforts, or by creating a state of low anxiety (Mogg & Bradley, 2004). However, it is unknown how this disengagement from threat might influence the processing of safety cues.

Summary

Empirical support for Hypothesis 2 is meager at this time because of the dearth of relevant studies. There is some preliminary evidence that highly anxious individuals may have diminished processing of nonthreat or safety information but this processing bias may be evident only at the strategic and not at the automatic processing level. The relationship between reduced safety cue processing and the occurrence of safety-seeking behavior has not been investigated and little is known about safety signal processing in low anxiety. Finally, mixed findings have been reported in studies on threat disengagement or avoidance, and there has been no research on its relation to safety cue processing.

Clinician Guideline 3.2

Diminished safety signal processing suggests that deliberate attentional training for safety cues may be a useful component of anxiety treatment.

Hypothesis 3. Exaggerated Threat Appraisals

Anxiety is characterized by an automatic evaluative process that exaggerates the threatening valence of relevant stimuli in comparison to the actual threat valence of the stimuli. Nonanxious individuals will automatically evaluate relevant stimuli in a less threatening manner that approximates the actual threat level of the situation.

There is now considerable evidence that an automatic threat appraisal process is involved in the preattentive threat bias in anxiety. Mathews and Mackintosh (1998) proposed that the representation of potential threat is dependent on activation of a *threat evaluation system* (TES). The TES represents the threat value of a previously encountered stimulus and is computed automatically at an early stage of information processing. During heightened anxiety, the output from the TES increases so that a lower threshold of stimulus intensity is required for threat valuation. Thus Mathews and Mackintosh argue that a hypervigilant attentional threat bias occurs in response to a prior preconscious automatic threat appraisal. Mogg and Bradley (1998, 1999a, 2004) also proposed that threat stimulus evaluation is a critical part of the automatic information processing that occurs in anxiety (see also the self-regulatory executive function model proposed by Wells, 2000). Recent theoretical accounts of fear and anxiety derived from a conditioning perspective propose that information is first analyzed by feature detectors and a preconscious "significance evaluation system" that results in a quick judgment of the fear relevance of stimuli (Öhman, 2000). Thus our contention that automatic threat appraisal is a critical component of primal threat mode activation is entirely consistent with other cognitive and behavioral models of fear and anxiety.

Implicit memory tasks offer an excellent experimental paradigm for investigating the presence of automatic threat evaluation in anxiety. These tasks involve memory retrieval in which some previously encoded information causes enhanced performance on a subsequent task even though the individual has no awareness or recollection of the relation between the prior experience and the task at hand (Schacter, 1990; Sternberg, 1996). In other words, previous exposure to a stimulus passively facilitates subsequent processing of the same stimuli and this "priming effect" is thought to reflect the degree of integrative processing that occurs during stimulus encoding (MacLeod & McLaughlin, 1995). Implicit memory more likely reflects automatic information processing, whereas explicit memory, a deliberate and effortful retrieval of stored information, maps more closely onto controlled, strategic processes (Williams et al., 1997).

Word Stem Completion

Implicit memory was first investigated with the word completion task. In this task individuals are presented with a list of anxiety-relevant (e.g., *disease, attack, fatal*) and neutral (e.g., *inflated, daily, storing*) words. After a filler task, individuals are given a set of word fragments, such as the first three letters of a word, and are asked to complete the fragment with the first word that comes to mind. A tendency to complete the word fragment with a less common word that was included in a previously presented word list would be an example of implicit memory. In the following example a threat-priming effect would be evident by completing the word fragment with a previously presented threat word rather than with a more common neutral word.

Encoded List	Word Fragment	Possible Response
coronary	cor_____	coronary vs. corn
attack	att_____	attack vs. attend
fatal	fat_____	fatal vs. father

Studies employing word stem completion have produced mixed results that can only be interpreted as weak evidence of implicit memory in anxiety. In some studies clinically anxious patients or high trait-anxious individuals have generated more threat word completions, which suggests an implicit memory for threat (e.g., Cloitre, Shear, Cancienne, & Zeitlin, 1994; Eysenck & Byrne, 1994; Mathews, Mogg, May, & Eysenck, 1989; Richards & French, 1991). However, other studies have failed to find an implicit threat bias (e.g., Baños, Medina, & Pascual, 2001; Lundh & Öst, 1997; Rapee, McCallum, Melville, Ravenscroft, & Rodney, 1994). McNally (1995) considers word stem completion a poor test of implicit memory in anxiety because it is strongly affected by the physical attributes of words rather than by their meaning.

Lexical Decision Tasks

In lexical decision tasks individuals are shown a list of mixed-valence words in which some may be anxiety-relevant, some depression-relevant, and others neutral. After a filler task individuals are shown a second list of words that will contain some of the "old" words, some "new" words, and also some nonword distractors (e.g., *eupine, mard, fledge*). Participants are told to indicate as quickly as possible whether the stimulus is a "word" or a "nonword." Quicker lexical decision for previously presented words suggests an implicit memory priming effect. In anxiety we would predict quicker lexical decision for previously presented threat than nonthreat words. In this experimental paradigm priming effects can be investigated subliminally or supraliminally depending on whether the first exposure occurs above or below the threshold of awareness.

In two lexical decision experiments, Bradley and colleagues (Bradley, Mogg, & Williams, 1994, 1995) failed to find evidence of an anxiety-congruent implicit memory bias in either subliminal or supraliminal priming conditions (see also Foa, Amir, Gershuny, Molnar, & Kozak, 1997, for negative results). Amir and colleagues utilized a more sensitive measure of automatic encoding of the meaning of information by requiring perceptual rather than word judgments to more complex stimuli. In two studies socially anxious individuals exhibited a significant auditory or visual preferential rating for previously presented threat stimuli that was interpreted as indicating an implicit memory-priming effect for social threat stimuli (Amir, Bower, Briks, & Freshman, 2003; Amir, Foa, & Coles, 2000). However, Rinck and Becker (2005) failed to find an implicit memory bias for socially threatening words in an anagram task (i.e., identify the word from scrambled letters). Thus findings from standard lexical decision experiments or more recent perceptually oriented priming studies have not been particularly supportive of implicit (automatic) threat evaluation in anxiety.

Primed Stimulus Identification Tasks

A number of studies have investigated implicit memory bias by determining if anxious individuals show more accurate detection of briefly presented threatening words (stimuli) as a result of prior exposure to threat and nonthreat stimuli. MacLeod and McLaughlin (1995) found an implicit memory bias for threat in GAD patients compared to nonanxious controls based on a tachistoscopic word identification task. The GAD group exhibited better detection of old threat than nonthreat words, whereas nonanxious controls had better identification on nonthreat than threat stimuli. However, others have failed to find speeded detection of previously presented threat versus nonthreat words in panic disorder or PTSD (Lim & Kim, 2005; Lundh et al., 1999; McNally & Amir, 1996). There is little evidence, then, for an implicit memory bias for threat from stimulus identification priming studies.

Other Tests of Automatic Threat Evaluation

Amir et al. (1998a) employed a homograph paradigm to investigate activation and inhibition of threat-relevant information in individuals with generalized social phobia (GSP) and healthy controls. Individuals read short sentences that were followed by a single word that either did or did not fit the meaning of the sentence. Individuals had to decide whether or not the cue word matched the meaning of the sentence. As predicted, only the GSP group showed a slower response to cue words that followed homographs with a possible social threat meaning. This effect was only present at short sentence priming intervals, which suggests that GSP individuals were able to suppress or inhibit an automatic evaluation of the sentence's threat meaning when more effortful processing was allowed.

Employing a memory task called *release of proactive interference* (RPI) that taps into the semantic organization of memory, Heinrichs and Hofmann (2004) failed to find the predicted memory effects of socially threatening information for high socially anxious students. In fact, the opposite effect was found with the low social anxiety group demonstrating a RPI effect for socially threatening words. In a study involving analysis of eye movement to angry, happy, and neutral faces, Rohner (2004) was able to show that individuals learned to avert their attention away from angry faces. In this experiment, then, anxiety was related to an implicit memory for threat avoidance.

Finally, an experimental paradigm called the Implicit Association Test (IAT) has been used to examine automatic memory-based associations between two concepts (Greenwald, McGhee, & Schwartz, 1998). It is considered an index of implicit attitudes because it is relatively uninfluenced by conscious controlled processes (Teachman & Woody, 2004). In a study involving individuals highly fearful of snakes or spiders, Teachman, Gregg, and Woody (2001) found significant differences in implicit negative associations for snake versus spider attitudes across several semantic categories that matched individuals' fear concerns (Teachman & Woody, 2003; see de Jong, van den Hout, Rietbrock, & Huijding, 2003, for negative findings of implicit associations for spider cues in a group with high fear of spiders). Moreover, fear-related implicit associations were shown to change over the course of a three-session group exposure treatment for phobias (Teachman & Woody, 2003).

Two studies have compared high and low socially anxious individuals on the IAT. Tanner, Stopa, and de Houwer (2006) found that both high and low socially anxious groups had positive implicit self-esteem as indicated by their reaction times to IAT word classification. However, implicit self-esteem was significantly less positive in the high social anxiety group, suggesting that a self-favoring effect was weaker in those with high self-reported social anxiety. De Jong (2002) also concluded that high socially anxious individuals have a weaker self-favoring bias, but his results suggested this was due to significantly higher esteem associations for others. Although only a few IAT studies have been published to date, they do provide some tentative support for automatic threat association in anxiety. However, most of the studies relied on analogue samples and so it is possible that stronger results would be found in clinical samples (Tanner et al., 2006).

Summary

Despite consensus across various models of anxiety that some level of automatic evaluation of threat must be present in anxious states, it has been difficult to demonstrate this effect experimentally. The few studies that are relevant to Hypothesis 3 have produced inconsistent findings. Coles and Heimberg (2002) concluded from their review that there is modest support for implicit memory biases in all the anxiety disorders. It may be that the results would be more supportive if priming manipulations were more sensitive to the semantic meaning of stimuli as opposed to its perceptual properties. It is also apparent that evidence for automatic threat bias will vary depending on the experimental cognitive task employed. Some of the early results using the IAT suggest that implicit associations for threat may characterize anxiety, but the results are still too preliminary.

Clinician Guideline 3.3

The presence of automatic threat evaluation in anxiety indicates that deliberate identification, tracking and questioning of the initial threat evaluation might be helpful in diminishing the impact of automatic threat appraisals.

CONSEQUENCE OF THREAT MODE ACTIVATION

Hypothesis 4. Threat-Biased Cognitive Errors

Highly anxious individuals will commit more cognitive errors while processing particular threatening stimuli, which will enhance the salience of threat information and diminish the salience of incongruent safety information. The reverse pattern will be evident in nonanxious states where a cognitive processing bias for nonthreat or safety cues is present.

Hypothesis 4 refers to the cognitive effects of fear activation that involve preconscious hypervigilance of threat, the automatic generation of threat meaning, and diminished access to safety cues. This automatic selectivity for threat will lead to further biasing in effortful or strategic processing. We predict that threat mode activation will lead to:

1. Overestimation of the probability, severity, and proximity of relevant threat cues.
2. Underestimation of the presence and effectiveness of relevant safety cues.
3. The commission of cognitive processing errors such as minimization, magnification, selective abstraction, and catastrophizing.

Biased Threat Estimations

One of the most consistent findings in cognitive research on anxiety is that anxious individuals tend to overestimate the probability that they will encounter situations that provoke their specific anxiety state. In an early study Butler and Mathews (1983) gave clinically anxious individuals, depressed individuals, and nonclinical controls 10 ambiguous situations. The anxious group generated significantly more threatening interpretations and rated these negative threatening events as significantly more probable and severe (i.e., subjective cost) than nonclinical controls but not the depressed group. This finding was later replicated with high trait-anxious students (Butler & Mathews, 1987). Biased estimates of threat probability have been found in subsequent research in which social phobics overestimate the probability of experiencing negative social events (Foa, Franklin, Perry, & Herbert, 1996; Lucock & Salkovskis, 1988), claustrophobics exaggerate the likelihood they will encounter closed spaces (Öst & Csatlos, 2000), individuals with panic disorder interpret arousal-related scenarios and negative physical outcomes more probable and costly (McNally & Foa, 1987; Uren, Szabó, & Lovibond, 2004), and worriers generate higher subjective probabilities for future negative events (e.g., MacLeod, Williams, & Bekerian, 1991). In this latter study increased access to reasons why the negative event would happen and reduced access to why it would not happen (i.e., safety features) predicted probability judgments.

Cognitive bias should be most evident during fear activation. The positive correlation between heightened probability or severity (i.e., costly) estimates of threat and intensity of anxious symptoms is consistent with this prediction (e.g., Foa et al., 1996; Lucock & Salkovskis, 1988; Muris & van der Heiden, 2006; Öst & Csatlos, 2000; Woods, Frost, & Steketee, 2002). Moreover, causal relations between anxiety and threat perception have been found in fear provocation experiments. In various studies anxious and phobic individuals predict that they will experience more fear and panic attacks than actually happens when exposed to the fear situation (e.g., Rachman, Levitt, & Lopatka, 1988b; Rachman & Lopatka, 1986; Rachman, Lopatka, & Levitt, 1988). This tendency to overestimate the likelihood of threat has also been found in the worry concerns of chronic worriers (Vasey & Borkovec, 1992) and in the exaggerated negative appraisals of social performance generated by socially anxious individuals (Mellings & Alden, 2000; Stopa & Clark, 1993). However, with repeated experience, individuals show a decrease in their overpredictions of fear so that their estimates more closely match their actual fear level.

Maladaptive Looming Effect

Along with exaggerated estimates of threat probability and severity, inaccurate appraisals of the proximity of danger are also an aspect of biased cognitive processing in anxiety. Riskind and Williams (2006) emphasize that "mental representations of dynamically intensifying danger and rapidly rising risk" (pp. 178–179), termed *looming maladaptive style*, are a key component of threat appraisal in anxiety. According to Riskind and colleagues, a critical feature of any threatening stimulus is the perception of the threat as moving and intensifying in relation to the self in terms of physical or temporal proximity of real events but also in terms of the mental rehearsal of the potential time course of future events (Riskind, 1997; Riskind, Williams, Gessner, Chrosniak, & Cortina,

2000). Exaggerated threat in anxiety must be understood in terms of this dynamic danger content involving qualities such as the velocity (directional speed), accelerating momentum (rate of increase), and direction (coming toward the person) of threat (Riskind, 1997; Riskind & Williams, 1999, 2005, 2006). The looming vulnerability model, then, maintains that anxiety occurs when threat is appraised as rapidly approaching or developing such as an approaching snake, a deadline, an illness, or a social failure (Riskind, 1997). It is considered a key feature of the danger schema activated in anxiety and so is a specific construct that is applicable to all anxiety states from simple phobias to more abstract phenomena like worry and GAD (Riskind & Williams, 1999).

Riskind and Williams (2006) review an emerging research literature that supports the role of perceived intensifying danger and rapidly rising risk (i.e., looming) in predicting other features of anxious phenomenology. Experimental studies indicate that moving fear stimuli (e.g., videotape of tarantulas) elicit more fear and threat-related cognitions than stationary fear or neutral stimuli (Dorfan & Woody, 2006; Riskind, Kelly, Harman, Moore, & Gaines, 1992) and phobic anxiety is associated with a greater tendency to perceive a fear stimulus (e.g., spider) as changing or moving rapidly toward one's self (e.g., Riskind et al., 1992; Riskind, Moore, & Bowley, 1995; Riskind & Maddux, 1993). In addition, the Looming Maladaptive Style Questionnaire (LMSQ), which assesses a tendency to generate mental scenarios that involve movement toward some dreaded outcome, is uniquely associated with several features of anxious phenomenology (Riskind et al., 2000) and may be a latent common factor that underlies OCD, PTSD, GAD, social phobia, and specific phobias (Williams, Shahar, Riskind, & Joiner, 2005). Overall these findings are consistent with the observation that anxious individuals misjudge the impending nature of threatening stimuli, leading them to the erroneous conclusion that danger is closer or more immediate than is actually true. Riskind's research indicates this heightened sensitivity to the kinetic qualities of danger is an important aspect of biased threat appraisals in anxiety.

Cognitive Errors

Surprisingly little research has investigated the relevance of depressive cognitive errors (e.g., dichotomous thinking, overgeneralization, selective abstraction) for anxiety. In a study of thought content individuals with GAD generated more imperatives ("have to/ should") and catastrophizing words than dysphoric and nonanxious students, and all participants generated more cognitive errors during worry than during a neutral condition (Molina, Borkovec, Peasley, & Person, 1998). Despite a paucity of research, it is likely that anxious individuals do exhibit many of the same cognitive errors found in depression, especially when dealing with information relevant to their fear concerns. However, research is needed to determine the role of inferential cognitive errors in the anxiety disorders.

Summary

We began our review of Hypothesis 4 with three predictions concerning the role of cognitive errors in fear activation. Unfortunately, only one of these predictions has been tested empirically. The empirical evidence is consistent in showing that anxious individuals exaggerate the likelihood and probably the severity of negative situations related to their anxious concerns. This cognitive bias for threat estimation appears relevant to most of the anxiety disorders, although it is still debatable whether it is specific only to anxiety. The research on looming cognitive style clearly indicates that overestimating the proximity or impending nature of danger is a critical aspect of biased threat evaluation that potentiates the anxious state.

It is likely that highly anxious individuals generate the same types of cognitive errors that we see in depression. Catastrophizing is well known in panic disorder, but it is likely that dichotomous thinking, selective abstraction, magnification/minimization, overgeneralization, and other forms of rigid and absolutistic thinking are prominent in all the anxiety disorders. Research is needed to determine whether some of these cognitive errors are specific to anxiety-relevant concerns and what role they play in the persistence of fear activation. It would also be helpful to move beyond static paper-and-pencil measures of cognitive errors to "online assessment" of thought content during fear provocation.

At this time we have no information on the role of cognitive errors in the diminished processing of safety cues that is considered an important feature of fear activation. We assume that if cognitive processing errors can lead to an overestimation of threat, then this same cognitive processing style might lead to an underestimation of safety. This latter proposition, however, must await empirical investigation.

Clinician Guideline 3.4

Repeated experiences with situations involving varying levels of impending threat that disconfirm anxious individuals' exaggerated threat expectancies are critical in modifying the erroneous thinking style that contributes to the persistence of the anxious state.

Hypothesis 5. Negative Interpretation of Anxiety

Highly anxious individuals will generate more negative and threatening interpretations of their subjective anxious feelings and symptoms than individuals experiencing low levels of anxiety.

In the cognitive model (see Figure 2.1) increased autonomic or physiological arousal is another prominent feature of threat mode activation. Hypothesis 5, however, refers to the cognitive processes associated with physiological arousal. It is proposed that highly anxious individuals will perceive their heightened arousal, anxious feelings, and other somatic symptoms of anxiety as more threatening and unacceptable than low anxious individuals. It is also expected that this "fear of fear" (Chambless & Gracely, 1989) will be more evident during highly anxious states and will motivate individuals to terminate the fear program.

Beck et al. (1985, 2005) identified another aspect of this negative interpretation of anxiety, *"emotional reasoning,"* in which the state of feeling anxious is itself interpreted as evidence that danger must be present. Later Arntz, Rauer, and van den Hout (1995) referred to this as *"ex-consequentia reasoning"* which involves the fallacious proposition "If I feel anxious, there must be danger" (p. 917). They found that spider phobic, panic, social phobic, and other anxiety disorder patients but not nonclinical controls were significantly influenced in their danger ratings of hypothetical anxiety scripts by the presence of anxiety response information.

It is proposed that different aspects of the subjective experience of anxiety will be perceived as threatening depending on the nature of the anxiety disorder. In some cases it will be the physiological symptoms that are considered most unacceptable, whereas in other disorders it is cognitive phenomena (i.e., worry or unwanted intrusive thoughts) or even the heightened sense of general anxiousness that is perceived as most disturbing. Whatever the actual focus, it is the state of being anxious that is considered threatening and intolerable to the person. Table 3.1 presents the specific negative interpretations of anxiety associated with each of the anxiety disorders discussed in this volume.

Empirical Evidence

Negative interpretation of physiological arousal is a central process in the cognitive model of panic disorder (see Chapter 8 for further discussion). Questionnaire studies indicate that individuals with panic disorder are more likely to negatively (even catastrophically) misinterpret bodily sensations associated with anxiety and to report more distress when experiencing these symptoms than nonclinical individuals or those with other types of anxiety disorders (e.g., D. M. Clark et al., 1997; Harvey, Richards, Dziadosz, & Swindell, 1993; Hochn-Saric, McLeod, Funderburk, & Kowalski, 2004; Kamieniecki, Wade, & Tsourtos, 1997; McNally & Foa, 1987; Rapee, Ancis, & Barlow, 1988). Also, experimental research indicates that panic patients are more likely to feel anxious or even to panic when they focus on induced or naturally occurring bodily sensations (Antony, Ledley, Liss, & Swinson, 2006; Pauli, Marquardt, Hartl, Nutzinger, Hölzl, & Strain, 1991; Rachman, Lopatka, & Levitt, 1988; Rachman, Levitt, & Lopatka, 1988; Hochn-Saric et al., 2004). Together these studies provide a strong empirical basis that a heightened misinterpretation of physiological arousal is a key process in panic.

For individuals with GAD a focus on the more cognitive symptoms of anxiety will characterize their negative interpretation of anxiousness. Adrian Wells first noted that "worry about worry" (i.e., metaworry) is a prominent feature of GAD that distinguishes high worriers from those who are nonworriers (Wells, 1997; Wells & Butler, 1997;

TABLE 3.1. Specific Negative Interpretations of Anxiety Associated with Each of the Anxiety Disorders

Anxiety disorder	Focus of negative interpretation of anxiety
Panic disorder	Physiological arousal, specific bodily sensations
Generalized anxiety disorder	Subjective experience of worry ("worry about worry")
Social phobia	Somatic and behavioral indicators of being anxious in social settings
Obsessive–compulsive disorder	Anxious feeling associated with certain unwanted intrusive thoughts, images, or impulses
Posttraumatic stress disorder	Specific physiological and emotional arousal symptoms associated with trauma-related mental intrusions

Wells & Mathews, 1994). Metaworry involves a subjective negative appraisal of the significance, increased incidence, and perceived difficulties associated with the uncontrollability of worry (Wells & Mathews, 1994). Evidence that GAD is associated with heightened metaworry would support Hypothesis 5 and indicate that in generalized anxiety a negative interpretation of the act of worrying (e.g., "If I don't stop worrying, I'll end up an emotional wreck") contributes to an intensification and persistence of the anxious state. In fact, various studies have shown that GAD patients were distinguished from patients with other anxiety disorders (especially social phobia) by heightened scores on metaworry (Wells & Carter, 2001) and there is a strong relationship between metaworry and increased tendency to experience pathological worry (Wells & Carter, 1999; Wells & Papageorgiou, 1998a; see also Rassin, Merchelback, Muris, & Spaan, 1999). An early study by Ingram (1990) found that generalized anxiety and depression were characterized by a heightened focus on one's thoughts, sensations, and feelings as indicated by Fenigstein, Scheier, and Buss's (1975) Self-Consciousness Scale (SCS). These studies are consistent with Hypothesis 5, indicating that an increased focus on the negative characteristics of worry will exacerbate the general anxiety state.

In social phobia negative interpretation of anxious symptoms in social situations because of a concern that anxiety will be perceived negatively by others is a central feature of the disorder (see D. M. Clark & Wells, 1995; Wells & Clark, 1997). Various studies have found that social phobia is characterized by negative appraisal of anxiety-related interoceptive cues that leads to erroneous inferences about how one appears to others and subsequently to heightened subjective anxiety (for review, see D. M. Clark, 1999; Bögels & Mansell, 2004). Elevated self-focused attention has been found in social anxiety (e.g., Daly, Vangelisti, & Lawrence, 1989; Hackman, Surawy, & Clark, 1998; Mellings & Alden, 2000). Moreover, a specific focus on anxious symptoms (e.g., blushing) intensifies anxiety in high social anxiety but not in low social anxiety (Bögels & Lamers, 2002; see Bögels, Rijsemus, & De Jong, 2002, for contrary findings).

Experimental research has also supported the cognitive model. Mansell and D. M. Clark (1999) found a significant association in high but not low social anxiety between perception of bodily sensations and ratings of how anxious individuals thought they appeared to others. Mauss, Wilhelm, and Gross (2004) compared high and low socially anxious students before, during, and after a 3-minute impromptu speech and found that the high social anxiety group perceived a greater level of physiological arousal, felt more anxious, and exhibited more anxious behavior than the low anxious group even though there were no significant group differences in actual physiological activation. Moreover, self-reported anxiety correlated with perceived but not actual physiological activation for the total sample. These findings are consistent with Hypothesis 5. Social phobia is characterized by a heightened focus on anxious symptoms that clearly intensifies the anxious state.

In cognitive accounts of OCD the central problem is the faulty appraisal of unwanted intrusive thoughts, images, or impulses of dirt, contamination, doubt, sex, causing injury to others, and the like (D. A. Clark, 2004; Salkovskis, 1989, 1999; Rachman, 1997, 1998, 2003). Thus obsessional thinking develops when an unwanted intrusive thought, image, or impulse is misinterpreted as representing a significant potential threat to one's self or others and the person perceives a heightened sense of personal responsibility to prevent this anticipated threat. Rachman (1998) suggested that "emotional reasoning" could play an important role in the faulty appraisal of obsessional intrusions. Any anxiety associated with an intrusion could be misinterpreted as confirming the significance and potential dangerousness of the thought. This would be an example of "ex-consequentia reasoning" (Arntz et al., 1995) contributing to the faulty appraisal and escalation of the intrusion (e.g., "If I feel anxious by the thought of being dirty and potentially contaminating others, then I must be in danger of infecting others.").

There is a strong association between the subjective anxiousness or emotional distress of an intrusive thought, and its frequency, uncontrollability, and obsessionality (e.g., Freeston, Ladouceur, Thibodeau, & Gagnon, 1992; Parkinson & Rachman, 1981a; Purdon & Clark, 1993, 1994b; Salkovskis & Harrison, 1984). Moreover, individuals with OCD rate their obsessions and other unwanted intrusions as more anxiety-provoking than do nonobsessional controls (Calamari & Janeck, 1997; Janeck & Calamari, 1999; Rachman & de Silva, 1978). In a diary study involving 28 patients with OCD the individual's most upsetting obsession was rated as more frequent and more meaningful in terms of importance and control of thought than the least upsetting obsessions (Rowa, Purdon, Summerfeldt, & Antony, 2005). These findings are consistent with the view that OCD is characterized by a heightened sensitivity to certain OCD-related mental intrusions that may in part be due to the anxiety-eliciting properties of the obsession. However, research is needed that specifically investigates whether OCD is characterized by a misinterpretation of anxious feelings associated with obsessional intrusions and that this, in turn, contributes to a heightened state of general anxiousness.

Negative interpretation of anxious symptoms associated with trauma-related intrusions is a key process emphasized in cognitive theories of PTSD (Brewin & Holmes, 2003; Ehlers & Clark, 2000; Wells, 2000). Many studies have now shown that negative interpretation of initial PTSD symptoms plays a causal role in the persistence of PTSD (see review by Brewin & Holmes, 2003). In addition, negative appraisal of unwanted trauma-relevant intrusive thoughts or images is predictive of the severity and persistence of PTSD (Halligan, Michael, Clark, & Ehlers, 2003; Steil & Ehlers, 2000; Mayou, Bryant, & Ehlers, 2001). These findings, then, are entirely consistent with Hypothesis 5, indicating that negative and threatening interpretations of trauma-related anxious symptoms contribute significantly to the persistence of PTSD.

Summary

This brief review of the empirical research on enhanced negativity bias in the interpretation of anxious symptoms indicates strong empirical support for Hypothesis 5. Research spanning all five anxiety disorders found evidence that enhanced negative interpretation of anxiety or "fear of fear" was a contributor to the persistence of anxiety (see also chapter 4 on the related concept of anxiety sensitivity). Panic disorder is characterized by threat misinterpretations of the physical symptoms of anxiety, GAD by metaworry, social phobia by heightened self-focused attention on internal states of anxiousness, OCD by the anxiety-arousing properties of mental intrusions, and PTSD by physiological arousal elicited by trauma-related internal and external triggers. In each case a tendency to perceive anxiety itself in a threatening manner contributed to the persistence of the unwanted emotional state.

Clinician Guideline 3.5

The idiosyncratic meaning of anxious symptoms (i.e., the significance of heightened anxiousness) must be assessed and treated with cognitive restructuring as part of the intervention for reducing primal threat mode activation.

Hypothesis 6. Elevated Disorder-Specific Threat Cognitions

Anxiety will be characterized by an elevated frequency, intensity, and duration of negative automatic thoughts and images of selective threat and danger in comparison to nonanxious states or other types of negative affect. Furthermore, each of the anxiety disorders is characterized by a particular thought content relevant to its specific threat concerns.

One of the conscious phenomenal manifestations of primal threat mode activation is the frequent and repeated intrusion into conscious awareness of automatic thoughts and images related to the specific fear concerns of the individual. There is, in fact, a very large empirical literature that has demonstrated a preponderance of harm, threat, and danger cognitions and images in panic disorder (Argyle, 1988; McNally, Hornig, & Donnell, 1995; Ottaviani & Beck, 1987); GAD (Beck, Laude, & Bohnert, 1974; Hibbert, 1984); social phobia (Beidel, Turner, & Dancu, 1985; Hackmann et al., 1998; Turner, Beidel, & Larkin, 1986); and OCD (Calamari & Janeck, 1997; Janeck & Calamari, 1999; Rachman & de Silva, 1978; Rowa et al., 2005); as well as posttrauma-relevant threatening intrusions in PTSD (Dunmore, Clark, & Ehlers, 1999; Mayou et al., 2001; Qin et al., 2003; Steil & Ehlers, 2000). This "softer version" of Hypothesis 6, then, has been well documented in the empirical literature.

The more controversial aspect of Hypothesis 6 is the "strong version" predicting that each of the anxiety disorders will show a specific cognitive profile, and that this profile will distinguish anxiety from other negative emotional states. Table 3.2 presents the automatic thought content that characterizes each of the anxiety disorders.

There are two aspects to the "specificity" question in this hypothesis. First, to what extent is anxiety distinguishable from depression, with the former characterized by thoughts of harm and danger whereas the latter is distinguished by thoughts of loss and failure? And second, is there a specific cognitive profile that characterizes each of the anxiety disorder subtypes?

Cognitive Specificity: Distinguishing Anxiety from Depression

The content-specificity hypothesis states that "each psychological disorder has a distinct cognitive profile that is evident in the content and orientation of the negative cognitions and processing bias associated with the disorder" (Clark et al., 1999, p. 115). The content or orientation of the automatic thoughts and processing bias that characterizes anxiety states focuses on the possibility of future physical or psychological threat/danger and the sense of increased personal vulnerability or lack of safety. In depression the predominant cognitive theme concerns past personal loss or deprivation. In fact, global hopelessness as well as hopelessness about specific life problems is significantly greater in major depression than in GAD (Beck, Wenzel, Riskind, Brown, & Steer, 2006). The

TABLE 3.2. Types of Automatic Thoughts and Images That Characterize Specific Anxiety Disorders

Anxiety disorder	Thematic content of automatic thought/image
Panic with/without agoraphobic avoidance	… of physical catastrophe (e.g., fainting, heart attack, dying, going crazy)
Generalized anxiety disorder	… of possible future loss and failure in valued life domains as well as fear of losing control or inability to cope
Social phobia	… of negative evaluation by others, humiliation, poor social performance
Obsessive–compulsive disorder	… of losing mental or behavioral control that results in serious harm to self or others.
Posttraumatic stress disorder	… of past trauma and its sequelae

cognitive model, then, asserts that anxiety and depression can be distinguished by the content (and temporal orientation) of the negative automatic thoughts and interpretations generated by the individual.

In our own studies future-oriented threat-related cognitions distinguished panic and GAD from major depression/dysthymia (Clark, Beck, & Beck, 1994) and threat-related cognitions showed a closer, more specific relation with an anxiety than a depression symptom dimension (Clark, Beck, & Stewart, 1990; Clark, Steer, Beck, & Snow, 1996). These findings have been supported in other studies, although anxious cognitions appear to have a greater degree of nonspecificity than depressive cognitions (e.g., Beck, Brown, Steer, Eidelson, & Riskind, 1987; Ingram, Kendall, Smith, Donnell, & Ronan, 1987; Jolly & Dykman, 1994; Jolly & Kramer, 1994; Jolly, Dyck, Kramer, & Wherry, 1994; Schniering & Rapee, 2004). In a meta-analysis of 13 studies, R. Beck and Perkins (2001) found only partial support for the content-specificity hypothesis. Anxious and depressive cognition measures were significantly correlated with both their corresponding and noncorresponding mood/symptom measures and the cognition measures showed an average correlation of .66 with each other. Yet, quantitative comparisons did reveal that the depressive cognition measures had significantly higher correlations with depression than with anxious symptoms, but the anxious cognitions were equally correlated with depression and anxiety. The authors concluded that threat-related cognitions may not have the same degree of specificity as depressive cognitions (R. Beck & Perkins, 2001; see similar conclusion reached in review by Clark et al., 1999), although certain clinical populations or levels of symptom severity may show more or less specificity (Clark et al., 1996; Ambrose & Rholes, 1993).

The apparent lack of specificity for anxious cognitions may reflect a greater degree of heterogeneity for anxious than depressive cognitions. R. Beck and Perkins (2001) suggest two possibilities for the lack of specificity with anxious cognitions. Is it possible that a subset of anxious thought can be identified that is specific to particular anxiety disorders, whereas other types of anxious thinking may be more generally related to anxiety and depression? Or depressive cognitions may show greater specificity because they are related to low positive affect, which is a specific mood–personality construct of depression, and anxious cognition is less specific because it is the cognitive face of high negative affect, which is a mood–personality dimension common to all emotional disorders.

There is evidence that specificity may only apply to a subset of anxious cognitions. Jolly and Dykman (1994) reported that some threat cognitions were more related to a general negativity factor, whereas other cognitions related to physical or health-related threat were more specific to anxiety. In other research anxious overconcern (i.e., worry) emerged as a common feature of all anxiety disorders, whereas negative evaluation of others or social threat may evidence more subtype-specificity (Becker, Namour, Zayfert, & Hegel, 2001; Mizes, Landolf-Fritsche, & Grossman-McKee, 1987). Finally, Riskind (1997) has argued that looming vulnerability, the perception of threat movement, may offer better precision in distinguishing anxiety from depression because it incorporates time and rate of change in its conceptualization of threat appraisal. Although still tentative, it appears that only certain types of threat-related cognitions such as concerns about physical symptoms, health, social evaluation, and impending danger are specific to anxiety, whereas anxious apprehension or worry may be more evident in both anxiety and depression.

Cognitive Specificity in Anxiety Disorder Subtypes

Less research has investigated whether a specific cognitive content is associated with the anxiety disorder subtypes. In two studies R. Beck and colleagues found that worry was common to anxiety and depression and a strong predictor of negative affect, whereas hopelessness was predictive of low positive affect and panic-related cognitions were clearly specific to anxiety states (R. Beck, Benedict, & Winkler, 2003; R. Beck et al., 2001). In a confirmatory factor analysis of self-reported anxious and depressive self-statements, self-statements reflecting depression/hopelessness and self-statements reflecting anxiety/uncertainty about the future had large and significant loadings on a general negativity factor (Safren et al., 2000).

One of the most direct tests of cognitive content-specificity among anxiety disorder subtypes was reported by Woody, Taylor, McLean, and Koch (1998). They found that patients with panic disorder scored significantly higher on a measure of threat-related cognitions that were unique to panic (i.e., the UBC Cognitions Inventory—Panic subscale) compared to patients with major depression. However, the two groups did not differ on the Cognitions Checklist—Anxiety subscale, which the authors claim assesses more general conceptions of anxious cognitions.

Summary

Over the years numerous studies have shown that automatic thoughts and images of threat, danger, and harm occur with greater frequency and intensity in the anxiety disorders when fear is activated. Consequently there is ample evidence supporting the basic assertion of Hypothesis 6. Whether thoughts of threat and danger are a specific marker of anxiety has been more equivocal, and whether each anxiety disorder has its own unique cognitive content that distinguishes it from other emotional states has not been subjected to adequate empirical investigation. However, a number of tentative conclusions can be drawn about cognitive content-specificity in anxiety. It is likely that only some forms of anxious thought will show the level of specificity predicted by Hypothesis

6. Specificity is more likely when researchers focus on thought content that characterizes each of the disorder subtypes (see Table 3.2) rather than more general forms of apprehensive thought. Moreover, cognitive content-specificity may be more apparent at higher levels of symptom severity or in clinical groups that present with greater diagnostic homogeneity (e.g., pure anxiety disorder groups). Failure to find specificity in the anxiety disorders could reflect the inadequacies of the measures employed, especially if self-report questionnaires are used that underrepresent the more specific forms of cognition associated with the anxiety subtypes. Also, the high rate of comorbidity between anxiety and depression has complicated efforts to investigate level of specificity in pathognomonic processes. Cognitive specificity research would be advanced if investigators compared "pure" (single-diagnosis) anxiety and depression groups using specialized instruments of negative thought content. Until then, much remains unknown about the parameters of cognitive content-specificity in anxiety.

Clinician Guideline 3.6

Clinicians should use thought records, diaries, and other self-monitoring forms to obtain a "real-time" assessment of the automatic thought and image content that intrudes into conscious awareness during fear activation. Specific themes of threat and danger will provide valuable diagnostic and assessment information for constructing a case formulation of the anxiety disorder.

Hypothesis 7. Ineffective Defensive Strategies

Highly anxious individuals will exhibit less effective immediate defensive strategies for diminishing anxiety and securing a sense of safety relative to individuals experiencing low levels of anxiety. In addition, highly anxious individuals will evaluate their defensive abilities in threatening situations as less effective than nonanxious individuals.

Hypothesis 7 focuses on the final consequence of threat mode activation (see Figure 2.1). It is proposed that fear activation involves an automatic defensive response that is aimed at immediate reduction or avoidance of fear and the reinstatement of safety. This rapid response system is not an effortful intentional coping response but instead a fundamental biologically based adaptational system that is triggered when the organism encounters a potentially life-threatening situation (Öhman & Mineka, 2001). The adaptational value of fear is partly due to its ability to trigger an immediate defensive response.

Fear has evolved to deal with situations involving physical danger that are potentially life-threatening and so primitive alarm reactions may be effective for external dangers. However, they are less useful, even counterproductive, for the more abstract, protracted, and internally oriented threats that characterize the anxiety disorders. Beck et al. (1985, 2005) proposed that two automatic behavioral defensive systems can be triggered by threat. The first is an active, energic system involving mobilization (e.g., fight, flight) in response to danger. The second is a more passive, anergic system that involves a stereotypic immobility response (e.g., fainting). Craske (2003) presented a threat immi-

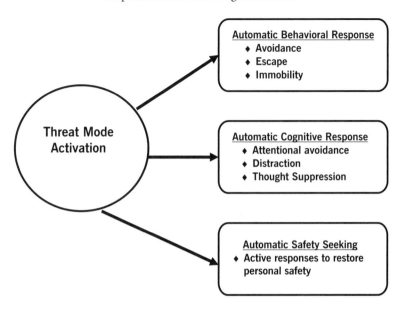

FIGURE 3.4. The automatic defensive response system associated with threat mode activation.

nence model in which increased proximity and detection of a threat is associated with a corresponding state of autonomic arousal in preparation for fight or flight.

Figure 3.4 summarizes the behavioral, cognitive, and safety-seeking processes involved in the automatic defensive reaction elicited by threat mode activation.

Behavioral Escape and Avoidance

Escape and avoidance behavior is so prominent in anxiety states that it is included as one of the cardinal DSM-IV diagnostic features of social phobia, PTSD, specific phobia, and panic disorder (APA, 2000). Furthermore, attempts to ignore, suppress, or neutralize obsessions in OCD and the ineffective control of worry in GAD can be considered examples of escape responses in these disorders. Escape and avoidance responses are so closely associated with subjective fear that their occurrence is taken as an important marker of fear expression (Barlow, 2002).

Behavioral, biological, and emotion theories of fear are almost universal in their agreement that an automatic escape and avoidance response is part of fear activation (Barlow, 2002). Various defensive reactions such as withdrawal (flight, escape, avoidance), attentive (freezing) or tonic (unresponsive) immobility, aggressive defense, and deflection of attack (appeasement or submission) are associated with fear arousal in all animals including humans as a means of protection against danger (Marks, 1987). Active avoidance of fear stimuli, which has been demonstrated in numerous animal and human aversive conditioning experiments, is known to have reinforcing effects because it is associated with the avoidance of punishment (Gray, 1987; Seligman & Johnston, 1973). Avoidance learning, then, is resistant to extinction because it terminates exposure to punishment (the aversive stimulus) and engenders a sense of control over the situation, the latter of which augments fear reduction (for review and discussion, see Mineka, 1979, 2004). It is not surprising that escape and avoidance responding has played a prominent role in learning theories of fear acquisition and persistence (for further discussion, see Barlow, 2002; Craske, 2003; Öhman & Mineka, 2001; LeDoux, 1996; Marks, 1987).

Phenomenological studies of the anxiety disorders have found that some form of immediate escape and avoidance is evident in most anxiety states. Escape and avoidance is more prevalent in high levels of state and trait anxiety (Genest, Bowen, Dudley, & Keegan, 1990). Most individuals with panic disorder (i.e., 90%) evidence at least mild to moderate levels of agoraphobic avoidance (Brown & Barlow, 2002; Craske & Barlow, 1988). In social phobia individuals are more likely to engage in subtle avoidance behaviors like not giving eye contact or looking away while in social evaluative situations (Beidel et al., 1985; Bögels & Mansell, 2004; Wells et al., 1995), whereas emotional numbing, avoidance of trauma-related cues, or foreshortened future are active and passive avoidance responses in PTSD that reflect attempts to reduce the aversiveness of reexperiencing the trauma (e.g., Feeny & Foa, 2006; Wilson, 2004). Between 75 and 91% of individuals with OCD have both obsessions and compulsions, the latter being an active avoidance or escape response (Akhtar, Wig, Varma, Peershad, & Verma, 1975; Foa & Kozak, 1995). For the vast majority of anxious patients, behavioral avoidance plays an important role in their daily experience of this negative emotional state.

Cognitive Avoidance: An Automatic Defensive Reaction

Various cognitive processes have been identified as part of the automatic avoidance response to threat. Attentional shift away from threat stimuli, distraction, thought suppression, and the initiation of worry are all protective cognitive processes that are aimed at terminating or preventing exposure to threat (Craske, 2003). Ironically, these immediate responses may actually increase accessibility to the very schemas that represent threat (Wells & Matthews, 2006). Moreover, all of these processes involve a mix of automatic and more conscious, effortful processing. In this section we consider evidence for an automatic cognitive avoidance, whereas the more elaborative aspects of distraction, worry, and thought suppression will be discussed as deliberate avoidant coping strategies under Hypothesis 10.

An automatic avoidance of threat has been more consistently demonstrated in specific and social phobias than in GAD and the other anxiety disorders (see reviews by Bögels & Mansell, 2004; Mogg & Bradley, 2004; e.g., experiment by Mogg, Bradley, Miles, & Dixon, 2004). As a result it is still unknown whether an automatic attentional avoidance of threat is a universal feature of all high anxiety states.

If a delayed automatic attentional avoidance of threat does emerge more consistently across the anxiety disorders, then this process could be a key element in triggering the more conscious, strategic cognitive avoidance responses like distraction, thought suppression, and worry (see also Mathews & Mackintosh, 1998, for similar view). Borkovec and colleagues present compelling evidence that worry functions as a cognitive avoidance reaction to threatening information (Borkovec, 1994; Borkovec, Alcaine, & Behar, 2004; see also Mathews, 1990) that is instigated by the automatic attentional biases for threat. Although worry is predominantly a conscious effortful coping strategy with an avoidant function, the initiation of the worry process may be a product of automatic vigilance for threat.

Automatic Safety Seeking

Safety-seeking behavior is an important class of escape and avoidance behavior that is evident in the persistence of agoraphobia (Rachman, 1984a), panic disorder (D. M. Clark, 1997; Salkovskis, 1996a), social phobia (Rapee & Heimberg, 1997; Wells & Clark, 1997), and PTSD (Ehlers & Clark, 2000). Various studies have shown that increased use of safety-seeking behaviors is related to the persistence of anxiety and avoidance (e.g., Dunmore et al., 1999; Dunmore, Clark, & Ehlers, 2001; Salkovskis et al., 1999; Sloan & Telch, 2002; Wells et al., 1995). White and Barlow (2002) reported that 74% of their patients with panic disorder with agoraphobia engaged in one or more safety behaviors such as carrying a medication bottle, food/drink, bags, bracelets, or other objects. In another study individuals with social phobia exhibited more safety behavior that was associated with increased anxiety and that mediated actual deficits in social performance (Stangier, Heidenreich, & Schermelleh-Engel, 2006).

Cognitive models of specific anxiety disorders and the few studies that have been conducted on safety seeking suggest that this form of response may be important in the pathogenesis of anxiety. However, this research is of limited relevance to Hypothesis 7 because it focuses on safety seeking as a deliberate avoidant coping strategy. Whether there are more immediate automatic aspects of safety seeking that would make it part of the immediate defense response is unknown at this time.

Summary

There is overwhelming clinical and laboratory evidence for a fairly automatic escape and avoidance response in high anxiety, and this responding is part of a characteristic automatic defensive pattern aimed at protecting the organism against threat and danger. What is less well known is whether the elimination of escape and avoidance responses is necessary for the successful treatment of anxiety states. Much less is known about the more automatic features of cognitive avoidance and safety-seeking behaviors. The research that has been published has examined these topics in terms of conscious deliberate coping strategies aimed at the reduction of anxiety. Thus more research is needed that directly compares the automatic defensive response of high and low anxious individuals in terms of its immediate impact on anxiety level and perceived effectiveness as a direct test of Hypothesis 7. Until this research has been conducted, the empirical status of the cognitive and safety-seeking aspects of Hypothesis 7 is unknown.

Clinician Guideline 3.7

Relatively automatic and idiosyncratic cognitive, behavioral, and safety-seeking defensive responses must be identified and targeted for change. A broad perspective on avoidance, one that recognizes its cognitive and safety-seeking characteristics as part of an automatic rapid response system to threat, is essential.

SECONDARY ELABORATIVE REAPPRAISAL: THE STATE OF ANXIOUSNESS

Hypothesis 8. Facilitated Threat Elaboration

A selective threat bias will be evident in explicit and elaborated cognitive processes such that in anxiety memory retrieval, outcome expectancies, and inferences to ambiguous stimuli will show a preponderance of threat-related themes relative to nonanxious individuals.

As discussed in Chapter 2, the cognitive model of anxiety postulates that a secondary, compensatory stage of information processing occurs in response to threat mode activation (i.e., the immediate fear response). Whereas the earliest moments of anxiety are dominated by automatic processes that characterize primal threat mode activation, the later secondary phase primarily involves deliberate and effortful processing that reflects a conscious strategic approach to anxiety reduction.

The secondary elaborative phase plays a primary role in the persistence of anxiety. In fact, most cognitive-behavioral interventions of anxiety focus on change at this elaborative phase. The modification of effortful cognitive processing can lead to a significant reduction even in the more automatic aspects of fear activation. In his review Mansell (2000) presented clinical and experimental evidence that conscious interpretations can have a significant positive or negative impact on the automatic processes involved in anxiety. Psychological intervention that effectively reduces anxious symptoms has been shown to also lessen automatic attentional bias for threat (see MacLeod, Campbell, Rutherford, & Wilson, 2004). Nevertheless, we consider conscious effortful information processing that involves making judgments, generating expectancies, evaluating or appraising information, reasoning and decision making, and explicit memory retrieval important aspects of the threat-biased cognitive architecture of anxiety. As evident from the review below, there has been much debate in the research literature on the role of elaborative, strategic processing in anxiety.

Threat-Biased Interpretations

A variety of experimental tasks have been employed to determine if anxious individuals exhibit a greater tendency to make biased threat-related judgments than nonanxious individuals. In some studies threat and nonthreat words were presented but evidence for a clear preference for threat was mixed (e.g., Gotlib et al., 2004; Greenberg & Alloy, 1989). More consistent findings emerged from emotional priming experiments in which participants are shown positive and negative trait adjectives preceded by a positive or negative sentence prime. In these studies GAD and panic patients exhibited a preferential response to primed threat stimuli (e.g., D. M. Clark et al., 1988; Dalgleish, Cameron, Power, & Bond, 1995).

Biased judgment is more accurately investigated with experimental paradigms that present threatening and nonthreatening ambiguous stimuli, with the prediction that anxious individuals will endorse the more threatening interpretation. Ambiguous tasks are more sensitive to evaluation biases because they allow for the possibility of generating alternative interpretations that vary in their aversiveness (MacLeod, 1999). One experimental paradigm used to investigate interpretation bias involves auditory presentation of homophones, which are words with identical pronunciation but distinct spelling, and threatening or nonthreatening meaning (e.g., *die/dye*; *weak/week*; *flu/flew*). Individuals are asked to write down the word they heard presented. In an early study Mathews, Richards, and Eysenck (1989) found that anxious patients generated signifi-cantly more threatening spellings than nonanxious patients. This finding has been rep-licated in other studies (e.g., Mogg, Bradley, Miller, et al., 1994, Experiments 2 and 3).

One could argue that the presentation of ambiguous sentences and other forms of text comprehension might provide a more accurate representation of the complex concerns we find in the anxiety disorders than single word stimuli. In these studies anxiety disorder patients are more likely to generate or endorse threatening rather than nonthreatening interpretations of the sentences (e.g., Amir, Foa, & Coles, 1998b; D. M. Clark et al., 1997; Eysenck, Mogg, May, Richards, & Mathews, 1991; Harvey et al., 1993; Stopa & Clark, 2000; Voncken, Bögels, & de Vries, 2003). On the other hand, Constans, Penn, Ilen, and Hope (1999) found that non-socially anxious individuals had a positive interpretation bias for ambiguous social information whereas socially anxious individuals were more even-handed in their interpretations (see also Hirsch & Mathews, 1997). Brendle and Wenzel (2004) found that socially anxious students had particularly pronounced negative interpretation bias to self-relevant positive unambiguous passages and reduced positive interpretation of the same passages after 48 hours. Thus it may be that both enhanced threat interpretation and reduced postivity bias operate differently, especially in social phobia, but both are important in characterizing the interpretation bias in anxiety.

One problem with homophones and ambiguous (or unambiguous) passages is that the threatening productions of the anxious may reflect a response bias (i.e., tendency to emit a particular response) rather than an interpretation bias (i.e., tendency to encode or interpret stimuli in a certain threatening manner; see MacLeod, 1999). Macleod and Cohen (1993) used a text comprehension task to show that only the high trait-anxious students had quicker comprehension latency for ambiguous sentences that were fol-lowed by a threatening continuation sentence. This priming effect indicates that the high but not the low trait-anxious students were more inclined to impose a threatening meaning on the ambiguous sentences. A more recent study of homograph pairs (i.e., a word with two different meanings; e.g., *bank* could mean a financial institution or side of a river) suggests that when threat meanings are primed in generalized social phobia, this activated interpretative bias may persist longer than it does in nonsocially anxious individuals (Amir et al., 2005). Furthermore, recent studies employing inter-pretative bias training suggest a possible causal relation between threat interpretations and anxiety. Nonanxious individuals trained to make negative or threat interpretations to ambiguous sentences experienced subsequent increases in state anxiety or anxiety reactivity (Mathews & Mackintosh, 2000; Salemink, van den Hout, & Kindt, 2007a; Wilson, MacLeod, Mathews, & Rutherford, 2006). The training effect, however, may be more pronounced for positive interpretations (e.g., Mathews, Ridgeway, Cook, & Yiend, 2007; Salemink et al., 2007a), with some studies even finding weak or insig-nificant effects of negative interpretative training on anxiety levels (Salemink, van den Hout, & Kindt, 2007b).

In summary there is considerable evidence that the anxiety disorders are character-ized by a conscious, strategic interpretation bias for threat that is particularly evident when processing ambiguous information that is relevant to the specific anxiety concerns of the individual. The fact that this effect has been found in priming studies indicates that it can not simply be dismissed as response bias. Interpretative biases have been demonstrated in panic disorder for body sensation information and in social phobia for ambiguous social scenarios (see Hirsch & Clark, 2004). In addition, the interpretative bias training studies provide evidence of a possible causal role in anxiety (see also Chapter 4). Although much remains to be understood about the specificity of the interpretative bias, we believe the findings are sufficiently well advanced to conclude that it plays a contributory role in anxiety and so warrants a "strongly supported" designation.

Threat-Related Expectancies

If anxiety is characterized by a threat bias in elaborative processing, then anxious individuals should be more likely to hold heightened expectations for future threat or danger that are relevant to their anxious concerns. MacLeod and Byrne (1996) reported that anxious students anticipated significantly more negative personal future experiences than nonanxious controls. In a 6-month follow-up of New York City workers after the 9/11 terrorist attacks, individuals who reported more PTSD symptoms also appraised the threat of future terrorist attacks more likely (Piotrkowiski & Brannen, 2002).

Research on covariation bias indicates that heightened expectations of negative experiences can bias perceptions of environmental contingencies (MacLeod, 1999). In this experimental paradigm, individuals are presented fear-relevant or neutral slides that are randomly associated with a mild shock (aversive response), a tone (neutral response), or nothing. Participants are asked to pay attention to the stimulus–response associations and determine whether or not there was a particular relationship between type of stimulus and response. Tomarken, Mineka, and Cook (1989) found that high fearful women consistently overestimated the percentage of times that the fear slides were associated with an electric shock, which reflects a processing bias for threat. This overestimation of threat as indicated by exaggerated judgments of fear stimuli and shock associations was replicated in spider-phobic individuals (de Jong et al., 1995), although prior fear may have a greater effect on future covariation expectancies rather than post hoc estimates of past covariation (de Jong & Merckelbach, 2000). Covariation bias for threat has also been demonstrated in panic-prone individuals exposed to slides of emergency situations (Pauli, Montoya, & Martz, 1996) and, more recently, in generalized social phobia when estimating the contingency between negative outcomes and ambiguous social events (Hermann, Ofer, & Flor, 2004; see Garner, Mogg, & Bradley, 2006, for contrary results). Although it is unclear whether the covariation bias is as prominent in the anxiety disorders as it is in specific phobic states, it is evident that negative expectancies can bias judgments of contingencies that characterize anxiety-relevant situations.

Explicit Memory Bias

Information-processing research has also investigated whether anxiety is characterized by a biased recall of threat-congruent information. If threat-relevant schemas are activated in anxiety, one would expect increased access to schema-congruent memories. However, evidence that anxious individuals exhibit a mnemonic advantage for threat-relevant information has not been compelling (Mathews & MacLeod, 1994; MacLeod, 1999). Williams et al. (1997) concluded that biased implicit memory for threat is more often found in anxiety, whereas a negative bias in explicit memory is more likely found in depression. In addition, MacLeod (1999) concluded that anxiety vulnerability is characterized by implicit but not explicit memory bias for threat.

Presence of an explicit memory bias for threat is indicative of bias at the strategic, elaborative phase of information processing. Contrary to earlier assertions, Coles and Heimberg (2002) concluded in their review that explicit memory biases for threat-relevant information is evident in panic disorder and, to a lesser extent, in PTSD and OCD. However, explicit memory bias is less apparent in social phobia and GAD.

The self-referent encoding task (SRET) has been used most often to assess explicit memory bias in anxiety and depression. Individuals are shown a list of positive, negative (or threatening), and neutral self-relevant words and asked to indicate which words are self-descriptive. After the endorsement task, individuals are given an incidental recall exercise in which they write down as many words as they can remember. Based on this experimental paradigm or various modifications, a negative or threat recall bias has been found for social phobia (Gotlib et al., 2004); panic disorder (Becker, Rinck, & Margraf, 1994; Cloitre et al., 1994; Lim & Kim, 2005; Nunn, Stevenson, & Whalan, 1984); PTSD (Vrana, Roodman, & Beckham, 1995); and GAD or high trait anxiety (Mogg & Mathews, 1990). However, other studies have failed to find a negative cued or free recall (or recognition) bias for GAD or high trait anxiety (Bradley, Mogg, & Williams, 1995; MacLeod & McLaughlin, 1995; Mathews, Mogg, et al., 1989; Mogg et al., 1987, 1989; Richards & French, 1991); social phobia (Cloitre, Cancienne, Heimberg, Holt, & Liebowitz, 1995; Lundh & Öst, 1997; Rapee et al., 1994, Experiments 1 and 2; Rinck & Becker, 2005); OCD (Foa, Amir, Gershuny, et al., 1997); and even panic disorder (Baños et al., 2001).

Coles and Heimberg (2002) noted that explicit memory bias for threat was more apparent when conceptual or "deep" processing of information was required at the encoding stage, when individuals did not have to produce the stimuli they fear at the retrieval stage, when recall rather than recognition is tested, and when externally valid experiences are used that relate directly to the fear concerns of the individual. To this end, some researchers have investigated memory for threatening experiences by exposing individuals to imagined or real-life situations. Most of these studies involved socially anxious individuals who were exposed to hypothetical or actual social encounters and then assessed for encoding and retrieval of various elements of the experience. In the majority of cases the high socially anxious group did not show an explicit threat recall bias (e.g., Brendle & Wenzel, 2004; Rapee et al., 1994, Experiment 3; Stopa & Clark, 1993; Wenzel, Finstrom, Jordan, & Brendle, 2005; Wenzel & Holt, 2002). Radomsky and Rachman (1999) found evidence for enhanced recall of prior contact with perceived contamination objects (see also Radomsky, Rachman, & Hammond, 2001), but this effect was not replicated in a later study of OCD patients with washing compulsions (Ceschi, van der Linden, Dunker, Perroud, & Brédart, 2003).

A sufficient number of studies have found evidence of an explicit memory bias for threat, especially when recall rather than recognition is assessed, to conclude that this body of research provides a modest level of empirical support for Hypothesis 8. It would appear that the conscious elaborative processing involved in the encoding and retrieval of information may be biased toward threat in anxiety. However, an explicit memory bias for threat has been most apparent in panic disorder and least evident in GAD and social phobia. In fact, most studies have been unable to find evidence of an explicit memory bias for threat in social phobia even with information-processing manipulations that map closely to real-life social experiences. Too few memory studies have been conducted in OCD or PTSD to allow any conclusions to be drawn, although Muller and Roberts (2005) recently concluded in their review that OCD is characterized by a positive memory bias for threatening stimuli. Overall research on explicit memory bias provides only modest support for Hypothesis 8.

Autobiographical Memory

If anxiety is characterized by threat-biased elaborative processing, then we would expect anxious individuals to exhibit an elevated tendency to recall past personal experiences of threat or danger. Selective retrieval of autobiographical memories has been demonstrated most clearly in depression where a negative mood-congruency effect has been found across numerous studies (for review, see D. A. Clark et al., 1999; Williams et al., 1997). In the typical autobiographical study, individuals are asked to report the first memory that comes to mind in response to neutral or valenced cue words. The autobiographical memory task has good ecological validity because it assesses individuals' personal memories and experiences, although biased recall could be caused by a greater number of past threatening experiences in the lives of anxious individuals (MacLeod, 1999). Thus retrieval differences may not reflect memory differences as much as differences in life experiences.

Only a few studies have investigated autobiographical memory in anxiety. Rapee et al. (1994, Experiment 4) failed to find any differences between socially anxious and nonanxious groups in number of positive or negative memories recalled to social or neutral stimulus words, although Burke and Mathews (1992) produced more positive results indicative of an autobiographical memory bias in GAD. Mayo (1989) found that high trait anxiety was associated with recall of fewer happy and more unhappy personal memories. Wenzel, Jackson, and Holt (2002) reported that individuals with social phobia recalled more personal memories involving negative affect in response to social threat cues but this effect was weak, accounting for only 10% of their social threat-cued memories. Although only a few studies of autobiographical memory in anxiety have been published, it may emerge that this memory bias may be specific to certain anxiety disorders such as GAD but not to others like social phobia.

Summary

Overall there is considerable empirical support for Hypothesis 8, that anxiety is characterized by facilitation of threat at the elaborative, strategic stage of information processing. The strongest research support is from the interpretative bias research. The most frequent finding is biased threat-related judgments in high anxiety. This is most apparent when ambiguous information is presented that is specific to the fear concerns of the individual (e.g., body sensations for panic disorder and negative social evaluation for social phobia). There is some indication that the interpretation bias in anxiety is persistent, focuses mainly on the severity of threat, and has a causal impact on anxiety. Questions still remain on whether the interpretation bias primarily involves the exaggeration of threat or the diminution of a positivity bias that characterizes nonanxious states.

There is some evidence that a conscious strategic processing of threat is evident in the form of heightened negative expectancies. Anxious individuals may be more likely to expect that negative or threatening future events will happen to them, although more research is needed to establish this finding. Experiments on the covariation bias indicate that fear-related expectancies in phobic states can result in biased perceptions of environmental contingencies (MacLeod, 1999). Whether covariation biases also operate in the anxiety disorders requires further research. However, at this stage there is at least some experimental support for the view that anxiety involves a biased expectancy for future negative or threatening personal events.

Finally, the considerable research literature on explicit memory bias in anxiety has established that a biased retrieval of threat-relevant information is evident in panic disorder but not in social phobia or GAD. Too few memory studies have been conducted on individuals with OCD or PTSD to allow firm conclusions. In addition anxious individuals may have a tendency to recall personally threatening memories and this could contribute to other elaborative processes such as anxious rumination and postevent processing (see Hirsch & Clark, 2004). However, evidence for selective autobiographical memory for threat is very tentative at the present time.

Clinician Guideline 3.8

Considerable empirical evidence supports therapeutic interventions that seek to change the conscious strategic information processing that is the basis of an exaggerated reappraisal of threat. Modify intentional threat evaluations, expectancies, and memory retrieval to establish a more balanced reappraisal of immediate threat that can have a positive impact on the automatic processes of fear activation.

Hypothesis 9. Inhibited Safety Elaboration

Explicit and controlled cognitive processes in anxiety will be characterized by an inhibitory bias for safety information relevant to selective threats such that memory retrieval, outcome expectancies, and judgments of ambiguous stimuli will evidence fewer themes of safety in comparison to nonanxious individuals.

If anxious individuals have a bias for consciously and effortfully processing threat-relevant information, is it not possible that these same strategic processes might be biased against safety-related cues? Unfortunately, very little experimental research has addressed this possibility. Even though a number of attentional deployment studies have shown that anxious individuals exhibit attentional avoidance of threat stimuli at longer presentation intervals (see discussion under Hypotheses 1 and 2), there is practically no research on whether anxious persons show a more deliberate inhibition of safety information processing. Other researchers, such as D. M. Clark (1999), have emphasized that safety behaviors play an important role in the persistence of anxiety, but they fail to consider whether highly anxious individuals might actively inhibit the processing of safety material.

In a series of experiments Hirsch and Mathews (1997) investigated the emotional inferences that high and low anxious individuals made when primed with ambiguous sentences after they read about and imaged being interviewed. The main difference between groups occurred with the nonanxious group, who showed a quicker latency to make positive inferences after a positive prime. The high anxiety group failed to show this positivity bias in their online inferences. The authors concluded that biased judgments in anxiety may be better characterized in terms of an absence of a protective positive bias that characterizes healthy individuals (see also Hirsch & Mathews, 2000). If we extend this deficit inferential processing of positive information to include safety material, then these results might suggest that nonanxious individuals have a propensity to elaborate safety-relevant information whereas individuals with social anxiety may lack such a deliberate, strategic processing bias.

Self-report measures can also be used to assess whether anxious individuals are less likely to deliberately process safety or corrective information. Researchers at the Center for Cognitive Therapy in Philadelphia developed a 16-item questionnaire called the Attentional Fixation Questionnaire (AFQ) to assess whether individuals with panic disorder fixate on distressing physical symptoms and ignore corrective information during panic attacks (Beck, 1988; Wenzel, Sharp, Sokol, & Beck, 2005). A number of the AFQ items deal with safety issues such as "I am able to focus on the facts," "I can distract myself," "I can think of a variety of solutions," or "I remember others' advice and apply it." Fifty-five patients with panic disorder completed the questionnaire at four time intervals: pretreatment, 4 weeks, 8 weeks, and termination. Patients who continued to have problems with panic attacks scored higher on the AFQ than individuals with panic disorder who no longer had panic attacks, and treatment improvement was associated with large pre–posttreatment differences on the ATQ. While only suggestive, these results are consistent with Beck's (1988) contention that during a panic attack individuals are less able to consciously process safety or corrective information.

Summary

At this point it is unknown whether the interpretation threat bias in anxiety also affects the processing of safety cues. We might expect that safety information would not be encoded as deeply if the information-processing apparatus is oriented toward threat. However, to date there is only suggestive evidence for inhibited or diminished elaborative processing of safety information in anxiety, with a present lack of critical research on this issue.

Clinician Guideline 3.9

Treatment of anxiety might benefit from training that improves deliberate and effortful processing of safety and corrective information during periods of anticipatory and acute anxiety.

Hypothesis 10. Detrimental Cognitive Compensatory Strategies

In high anxiety states worry has a greater adverse effect by enhancing threat salience whereas worry in low anxiety states is more likely to be associated with positive effects such as the initiation of effective problem solving. In addition, other cognitive strategies aimed at reducing threatening thoughts, such as thought suppression, distraction, and thought replacement, are more likely to exhibit paradoxical effects (i.e., rebound, increased negative affect, less perceived control) in high than low anxiety states.

Worry: A Maladaptive Coping Strategy

As a product of threat mode activation worry has a deleterious impact on the persistence of anxiety by enhancing the perceived likelihood and severity of threat as well as one's personal sense of vulnerability or ability to cope. Worry, then, has a dual function both as a "downstream" consequence of automatic threat processes and a "feedback" contributor to the persistence of anxiety. This leads to three specific predictions about worry in the anxiety disorders:

- Highly anxious individuals will have more excessive, exaggerated, and uncontrolled worry than those with low anxiety.

- Worry in high anxiety will have a more negative consequence, resulting in greater threat reappraisal and increased subjective anxiety.

- The worry process in low anxiety is characterized by more adaptive and effective problem solving, whereas worry in high anxiety is counterproductive.

EXCESSIVE, UNCONTROLLABLE WORRY

Considerable evidence indicates that worry is a prominent feature of all the anxiety disorders and when it occurs in these clinical states, it is much more excessive, exaggerated, and uncontrollable than the worry reported by nonclinical individuals. In a recent review of cognitive specificity of the anxiety disorders, it was concluded that pathological worry is not only evident in GAD but in other anxiety disorders as well, such as panic disorder and OCD (Starcevic & Berle, 2006). Worry is a prominent feature of symptom constructs considered common across the anxiety disorders such as anxious apprehension (Barlow, 2002), negative affect (Barlow, 2000; Watson & Clark, 1984), and trait anxiety (Spielberger, 1985). Although most studies find that worry is significantly more frequent, severe, and uncontrollable in GAD (Chelminski & Zimmerman, 2003; Dupuy et al., 2001; Hoyer, Becker, & Roth, 2001), nevertheless elevated levels are also present in panic disorder, OCD, social phobia, PTSD, and even depression as well as subsyndromal states of high anxiety (Chelminski & Zimmerman, 2003; Gladstone et al., 2005; Wetherell, Roux, & Gatz, 2003). Naturally, the actual content of worry will vary, with social phobia associated with social evaluative concerns, panic with the occurrence of panic attacks or some dreaded physical consequence, PTSD with past trauma or the negative impact of the disorder, and OCD with a variety of obsessional fears. Moreover, the worry in GAD may be distinguished by concerns about minor daily matters, remote future events, or illness/health/injury (Craske, Rapee, Jackel, & Barlow, 1989; Dugas, Freeston, et al., 1998; Hoyer et al., 2001). Overall, though, the research clearly indicates that excessive and maladaptive worry is commonly associated with states of high anxiety.

NEGATIVE EFFECTS OF PATHOLOGICAL WORRY

Anxious individuals worry in order to avoid unpleasant somatic anxiety or other nega-tive emotions, as well as a problem-solving strategy that seeks to avoid or at least pre-pare for anticipated future negative events (Borkovec et al., 2004; Wells, 2004). In his cognitive model of GAD, Wells (1999, 2004) emphasized that positive beliefs about the perceived benefits of worry are an important factor in the persistence of worry and the anxious state. However, worry is a problematic coping strategy that ultimately contrib-utes to an escalation in anxiety by intensifying perceived threat. For clinically anxious individuals, excessive worry will contribute to a reappraisal of the threat as even more dangerous and imminent, and their coping resources as less than adequate for the antici-pated event. Worry, then, causes an intensification of anxiety through its negative effect on emotional responding, cognition, and ineffective problem solving.

Wells (1999) argued that the worry process is problematic because (1) it involves the generation of numerous negative scenarios that cause a greater sense of threat and personal vulnerability, (2) it heightens sensitivity to threat-related information, (3) it increases the occurrence of unwanted intrusive thoughts, and (4) it leads to a misattribu-tion of the cause for the nonoccurrence of a catastrophe, thereby strengthening positive beliefs about worry (e.g., "I won't do well on an exam unless I worry").

There is considerable evidence that worry leads to an increase in subjective anxiety. Both cross-sectional and longitudinal studies indicate that increased worry is associ-ated with elevations in both anxiety and depression (Constans, 2001; Segerstrom, Tsao, Alden, & Craske, 2000). The close association between repeated anxious thoughts or worry and subjective negative emotion has been found in daily dairy studies (Papageor-giou & Wells, 1999) as well as in laboratory-based research in which nonclinical indi-viduals are assigned to an instructed worry condition (e.g., Andrews & Borkovec, 1988; Borkovec & Hu, 1990; York, Borkovec, Vasey, & Stern, 1987).

Another negative consequence of worry is an increase in unwanted negative intru-sive thoughts. In a number of studies worry-prone individuals who engaged in a worry induction condition later reported an increase in unwanted anxious and depressive intrusive thoughts (Borkovec, Robinson, et al., 1983; York et al., 1987). Pruzinsky and Borkovec (1990) found that self-labeled worriers had significantly more negative thought intrusions than nonworriers even without a worry induction manipulation, and Ruscio and Borkovec (2004) reported that GAD worriers had greater difficulty controlling neg-ative thought intrusions after a worry induction than did non-GAD worriers, although the negative intrusions caused by worry were short-lived. A causal relation between worry and unwanted intrusive thoughts has also been demonstrated after exposure to a stressful stimulus in which instructions to worry after viewing a film resulted in a greater number of unwanted film intrusions (see Butler, Wells, & Dewick, 1995; Wells & Papageorgiou, 1995).

PATHOLOGICAL WORRY, AVOIDANCE, AND PROBLEM SOLVING

The persistence of worry is a paradox. On the one hand, it is an aversive state associated with elevated anxiety and distress, and yet we are drawn to it in times of anxiousness. One explanation is that worry persists because of the nonoccurrence of that which we dread (Borkovec, 1994; Borkovec et al., 2004). Moreover, it is maintained by the belief that it helps in preparation for anticipated future negative outcomes (Borkovec & Roemer, 1995). Wells (1994b, 1997) has argued persuasively that positive beliefs about worry's effectiveness in threat reduction contribute to its persistence. However, the effectiveness of worry is immediately undermined by the fact that most of the things that people worry about never happen (Borkovec et al., 2004). Under these conditions a powerful negative reinforcement schedule is set in place in which positive beliefs about the effectiveness of worry for avoiding or preventing bad events become strengthened by the nonoccurrence of adverse events. So we worry not to gain any particular advantage but instead to prevent or avoid anticipated adversity.

Even though worry may be a superfluous cognitive activity, its negative effect is further compounded by evidence that its very occurrence thwarts effective problem solving. Measures of worry are negatively correlated with certain aspects of social problem-solving measures in both clinical and nonclinical samples (Dugas, Letarte, Rhéaume, Freeston, & Ladouceur, 1995; Dugas, Merchand, & Ladouceur, 2005). Chronic worry is unrelated to social problem-solving ability but more directly associated with lower problem-solving confidence, less perceived control, and reduced motivation to engage in problem solving (Davey, 1994; Davey, Hampton, Farrell, & Davidson, 1992; Dugas et al., 1995). In sum, this research suggests that although pathological worry may not be characterized by social problem-solving deficits, it probably interferes in the person's ability to implement effective solutions (Davey, 1994). In contrast, worry phenomena in nonclinical populations may be associated with more effective implementation of problem-solving responses (Davey et al., 1992; Langlois, Freeston, & Ladouceur, 2000b).

EXCESSIVE WORRY AND THE THREAT INTERPRETATION BIAS

A final negative consequence of worry is that it causes one to reappraise a fear stimulus in a more threatening manner. In a study of self-reported worriers and nonworriers in elementary school-aged children, Suarez and Bell-Dolan (2001) found that worriers generated more threatening interpretations to hypothetical ambiguous and threatening situations than children not prone to worry. Constans (2001) also found that worry-proneness 6 weeks before an exam was associated with increased estimated risk of failing the exam. These findings, then, are consistent with our proposition that worry will contribute to a reappraisal of threat as a more severe and probable occurrence.

Negative Impact of Safety Seeking

Even though various aspects of safety-seeking have been discussed previously, it can also be viewed as a maladaptive compensatory coping strategy. More extensive reliance on safety-seeking behavior has been linked to the persistence of anxiety and threat-related beliefs (see section on Hypothesis 2). Furthermore, there is some evidence of a weaker automatic processing of safety information and a later attentional avoidance of threat. If more direct experimentation upholds the notion that automatic processing of safety information is less efficient in high anxiety states, then this could help explain why the anxious person has to expend more elaborative resources in the pursuit of safety.

Anxious individuals are more likely to utilize safety-seeking behaviors as a means of coping with anxiety than nonanxious individuals (see section on Hypothesis 2). In the short term safety-oriented coping may result in some immediate relief of anxiety but in the long term it actually sustains threatening interpretations by preventing their disconfirmation (Salkovskis, 1996b). In this way, extensive reliance on safety seeking will contribute to the persistence of anxiety. The importance of safety seeking as a maladaptive strategic coping response that contributes to the pathogenesis of anxiety has been recognized as an important process in most of the specific anxiety disorders such as GAD (Woody & Rachman, 1994), panic disorder (D. M. Clark, 1999), social phobia (D. M. Clark & Wells, 1995), and PTSD (Ehlers & Clark, 2000). Like worry, then, extensive use of safety seeking is a detrimental coping strategy that contributes to the persistence of anxiety.

Thought and Emotion Suppression

The deliberate suppression of unwanted thoughts and emotions are two other coping strategies that may contribute to the persistence of anxiety. Wegner and his colleagues were the first to demonstrate that the deliberate suppression of even neutral cognitions, such as the thought of a white bear, will cause a paradoxical rebound in the frequency of the target thought once suppression efforts cease (Wegner, Schneider, Carter, & White, 1987). In the typical thought suppression experiment, individuals are randomly assigned to one of three conditions: a short interval (e.g., 5 minutes) in which they can think anything except a target thought (suppression condition), an express condition (purposefully think the target thought), or monitor-only condition (think any thoughts including the target thought). This is followed by a second interval of equal length in which all participants are given an express or monitor-only condition. In both intervals participants indicate whenever the target thought intrudes into conscious awareness. Evidence of postsuppression rebound is apparent when the suppression group reports a higher rate of target intrusions during the subsequent express or monitor-only period than the group that initially expressed or monitored their thoughts. The rebound phenomenon is attributed to the lingering effects of intentional thought suppression that becomes most apparent when mental control is relaxed (Wenzlaff & Wegner, 2000). The relevance of this research for emotional disorders is obvious (for critical reviews, see Abramowitz, Tolin, & Street, 2001; D. A. Clark, 2004; Purdon, 1999; Purdon & Clark, 2000; Rassin, Merckelbach, & Muris, 2000; Wegner, 1994; Wenzlaff & Wegner, 2000). If unwanted thoughts actually accelerate as a result of prior intentional suppression efforts, then deliberate mental control of distressing thoughts would be a maladaptive cognitive coping strategy that contributes toward higher rates of threatening and disturbing cognition seen in anxiety states. In this case thought suppression would be a major contributor to the persistence of anxiety. However, two issues must be addressed. First, how often do anxious individuals rely on deliberate thought suppression as a coping strategy? And second, when anxious individuals suppress their unwanted threatening and worrisome thoughts, is there a resurgence in anxious thinking and emotion?

PREVALENCE OF THOUGHT SUPPRESSION

The tendency to utilize thought suppression has been measured by self-report questionnaires like the White Bear Suppression Inventory (WBSI; Wegner & Zanakos, 1994). The WBSI is a 15-item questionnaire that assesses individual differences in the tendency to engage in deliberate mental control of unwanted thoughts. Positive correlations have been reported between the WBSI and various self-report measures of anxiety as well as measures of obsessionality (e.g., Rassin & Diepstraten, 2003; Wegner & Zanakos, 1994). Moreover, scores on the WBSI are significantly elevated in all the anxiety disorders but then decline in response to effective treatment (Rassin, Diepstraten, Merckelbach, & Muris, 2001). A factor analytic study of the WBSI, however, found that an unwanted intrusive thoughts rather than thought suppression factor correlated with anxiety and OCD symptoms (Höping & de Jong-Meyer, 2003). Nevertheless, other clinical studies have indicated that thought suppression is evident in the anxiety disorders. Harvey and Bryant (1998a) found that survivors of motor vehicle accidents with acute stress disorder (ASD) had higher ratings of natural thought suppression than survivors without ASD. A study of women who experienced a pregnancy loss revealed that a tendency to engage in thought suppression predicted PTSD symptoms at 1 month and 4 months postloss (Engelhard, van den Hout, Kindt, Arntz, & Schouten, 2003). Overall these findings indicate that thought suppression is a coping strategy that is very often employed by those who are suffering from anxiety.

NEGATIVE EFFECTS OF THOUGHT SUPPRESSION

It appears that individuals with an anxiety disorder are as effective as nonclinical or low anxious individuals in suppressing anxious target thoughts, at least in the short term (Harvey & Bryant, 1999; Purdon, Rowa, & Antony, 2005; Shipherd & Beck, 1999), although there are other studies that indicate less efficient suppression by diagnostically anxious individuals (Harvey & Bryant, 1998a; Janeck & Calamari, 1999; Tolin, Abramowitz, Przeworski, & Foa, 2002a). Moreover, the experimental evidence is inconsistent in whether suppression of anxious thoughts such as worries, obsessional intrusive thoughts, or trauma-related intrusions is more likely to result in postsuppression rebound. Some studies have reported rebound effects with anxious and obsessional target thoughts (Davies & Clark, 1998a; Harvey & Bryant, 1998a, 1999; Koster, Rassin, Crombez, & Näring, 2003; Shipherd & Beck, 1999), whereas others have generally failed to find any rebound suppression effects (Belloch, Morillo, & Giménez, 2004a; Gaskell, Wells, & Calam, 2001; Hardy & Brewin, 2005; Janeck & Calamari, 1999; Kelly & Kahn, 1994; Muris, Merckelbach, van den Hout, & de Jong, 1992; Purdon, 2001; Purdon & Clark, 2001; Purdon et al., 2005; Roemer & Borkovec, 1994; Rutledge, Hollenberg, & Hancock, 1993, Experiment 1). Generally, it appears that postsuppression rebound of anxious thoughts is no more or less likely in clinically anxious samples than in nonclinical individuals (see Shipherd & Beck, 1999, for contrary findings).

Even though an immediate postsuppression resurgence of unwanted thought intrusions has not been consistently supported, there is evidence that suppression of anxious thoughts may have other negative effects that are important to the persistence of anxiety. First, it appears that over a longer time period, such as a 4- or 7-day interval, previous suppression of anxious targets will result in a significant resurgence of unwanted thoughts (Geraerts, Merckelbach, Jelicic, & Smeets, 2006; Trinder & Salkovskis, 1994). Abramowitz et al. (2001) suggested that individuals can successfully suppress unwanted thoughts over short time periods, but as time progresses and individuals relax their control efforts, a resurgence of target thought frequency is more likely. Second, suppression does appear to have a direct negative effect on mood, causing anxious and depressive symptoms to intensify (Gaskell et al., 2001; Koster et al., 2003; Purdon & Clark, 2001; Roemer & Borkovec, 1994; Markowitz & Borton, 2002; Trinder & Salkovskis, 1994). Third, more recent studies have found that suppression of anxious or obsessional intrusions can sustain or even alter one's negative appraisal of their reoccurring target intrusions and in this way contribute to an escalation in anxious mood (Kelly & Kahn, 1994; Purdon, 2001; Purdon et al., 2005; Tolin, Abramowitz, Hamlin, Foa, & Synodi, 2002b). Finally, it is clear that certain parameters can accelerate the negative effects of suppression and/or reduce its immediate effectiveness such as the imposition of a cognitive load (see Wenzlaff & Wegner, 2000, for review) or presence of a dysphoric mood state (Conway, Howell, & Giannopoulos, 1991; Howell & Conway, 1992; Wenzlaff, Wegner, & Roper, 1988). Moreover, some researchers have suggested that individual difference variables might influence the effects of suppression (Geraerts et al., 2006; Renaud & McConnell, 2002). For example, highly obsessional individuals may be more likely to experience persisting negative effects of suppression than individuals low in obsessionality (Hardy & Brewin, 2005; Smári, Birgisdóttir, & Brynjólfsdóttir, 1995; for contrary findings, see Rutledge, 1998; Rutledge, Hancock, & Rutledge, 1996).

The nature of intentional thought suppression and its role in psychopathology is currently the subject of intense empirical investigation. It is obvious that the process is complex and initial views that suppression causes a postsuppression rebound in unwanted thought frequency that reinforces persistent emotional disturbance is overly simplified. At the same time, the research is sufficiently clear that suppression of anxious thoughts, especially worry, trauma-related intrusions, and obsessions, is not a healthy coping strategy for reducing distressing thoughts and anxiety. For example, in one study individuals with panic disorder who experienced a 15-minute CO_2 challenge were randomly assigned to either accept or suppress any emotions or thoughts during the challenge test (Levitt, Brown, Orsillo, & Barlow, 2004). Analyses revealed that the acceptance group reported less subjective anxiety and less avoidance in response to the 5.5% CO_2 challenge than the suppress group, although no differences were evident on subjective panic symptoms or physiological arousal. At this point it is probably safe to conclude that the intentional and effortful suppression of anxious thoughts is not a coping strategy that should be encouraged in the management of anxiety. Rather, the expression and acceptance of distressing thoughts and images no doubt has therapeutic benefits that we are only beginning to understand.

SUPPRESSION OF EMOTION

There has been increasing interest in the role that emotion regulation or stress reactivity might play in specific types of psychopathology as well as psychological well-being more generally (e.g., S. J. Bradley, 2000). One type of emotion regulation that is of particular relevance to the anxiety disorders is *emotion inhibition*. Gross and Levenson (1997) defined emotion inhibition as an active, effortful recruitment of inhibitory processes that serve to suppress or prevent ongoing positive or negative emotion-expressive behavior. In their study of 180 undergraduate women shown amusing, neutral, and sad film clips suppression of positive or negative emotion was associated with enhanced sympathetic activation of the cardiovascular system, reduced somatic reactivity, and a modest decline in self-rated positive emotion.

Researchers have begun to investigate emotion inhibition and its related construct of *experiential avoidance* in the anxiety disorders. The latter refers to an excessively negative evaluation of unwanted thoughts, feelings, and sensations as well as to an unwillingness to experience these private events, thereby resulting in deliberate efforts to control or escape from them (Hayes, Strosahl, Wilson, et al., 2004b). In a study comparing Vietnam combat veterans with and without PTSD, those with PTSD reported more frequent and intense withholding of positive and negative emotions and this tendency to suppress emotions was specifically associated with PTSD symptomatology (Roemer, Litz, Orsillo, & Wagner, 2001; see also Levitt et al., 2004, for panic disorder). Experiential avoidance is significantly correlated with a number of anxiety-relevant features like anxiety sensitivity, fear of bodily sensations and suffocation, and trait anxiety, and it prospectively predicted daily social anxiety and emotional distress over a 3-week period (Kashdan, Barrios, Forsyth, & Steger, 2006). Although these findings are preliminary, it would appear that the suppression of emotion may join the suppression of unwanted thoughts as a maladaptive coping strategy that inadvertently fuels distressing emotional states like anxiety.

Clinician Guideline 3.10

Anxious individuals rely on certain deliberate and effortful coping strategies as an immediate compensation for their highly aversive subjective state. Unfortunately, any immediate relief from anxiety due to worry, avoidance, safety-seeking behaviors, or cognitive/experiential suppression is temporary. Indeed, these strategies actually play a prominent role in the longer term persistence of anxiety states. Thus effective intervention must redress the detrimental impact that these maladaptive effortful coping strategies have on anxiety.

SUMMARY AND CONCLUSION

A review of the research literature relevant to the cognitive model of anxiety (see Figure 2.1) indicates there is mounting empirical support for the role of automatic cognitive processes in immediate fear activation. This is most evident for Hypothesis 1, where there is consistent experimental data indicating that fear is characterized by an automatic, preconscious attentional threat bias for moderately intense personal threat stimuli presented at very brief exposure intervals. Very little research has been conducted on the possibility of an automatic attentional processing against safety information (i.e., Hypothesis 2), although there is moderate research support for an automatic threat evaluation process in high anxiety states (i.e., Hypothesis 3).

Hypotheses 4 to 7 focus on various cognitive, behavioral, and emotional consequences elicited by immediate threat mode activation. There is considerable evidence that anxious individuals overestimate the probability, proximity, and, to a lesser extent, the severity of threat-relevant information (i.e., Hypothesis 4). There is consistent empirical evidence that highly anxious individuals misinterpret their anxious symptoms in a negative or threatening manner (i.e., Hypothesis 5) and that automatic negative thoughts and images of threat, danger, and personal vulnerability or helplessness characterize anxiety states (i.e., Hypothesis 6). However, research on cognitive content-specificity was much less consistent in demonstrating that threatening thought content is specific to anxiety. It may be that cognitive specificity would be more apparent if researchers focused on disorder-specific cognitions rather than on general forms of apprehensive thought.

Hypothesis 7, which proposes that an automatic defensive response is elicited by immediate threat mode activation, has mixed support. Although there is a well-established behavioral literature demonstrating the prominence of behavioral escape as an automatic defensive response in anxiety, there has been little research on an automatic cognitive avoidance and safety-seeking defensive response.

The final three hypotheses reviewed in this chapter deal with the secondary, elaborative phase of anxiety. This component of the anxiety program will be of greatest interest to practitioners because the processes involved in the elaboration of anxiety have a direct impact on its persistence. This is also the phase that is specifically targeted in cognitive therapy of anxiety. Empirical support for Hypothesis 8 was strong, with numerous studies demonstrating that anxious individuals exhibit a deliberate threat interpretation bias for ambiguous stimuli, which is indicative of a conscious, strategic threat-processing bias. However, it is unknown whether diminished elaborative processing of safety information occurs in anxiety (i.e., Hypothesis 9) because there is practically no research on the topic. Empirical evidence for maladaptive cognitive coping strategies in anxiety is very strong (i.e., Hypothesis 10), with numerous studies demonstrating the detrimental effects of worry, excessive safety-seeking behavior, thought suppression, and, more recently, experiential avoidance. This research clearly highlights the importance of targeting these response strategies when offering cognitive therapy for anxiety.

Our extensive review of the extant empirical research clearly supports a cognitive basis to anxiety. Specific cognitive structures, processes, and products are critical to the activation and persistence of anxiety. Although this research provides a basis for advocating a cognitive approach to the treatment of anxiety, it does not address the question of etiology. In the next chapter we consider whether there might be a causal role for cognition in the etiology of anxiety.

Chapter 4

Vulnerability to Anxiety

We walk in circles so limited by our own anxieties that we can no longer distinguish between true and false, between the gangster's whim and the purest ideal.
——INGRID BERGMAN (Swedish-born actress, 1915–1982)

People who have suffered years from an anxiety disorder are often perplexed about the origins of their disorder. Clients will frequently ask "Why me?," "How come I developed this problem with anxiety?", "Did I inherit this condition, do I have some kind of imbalance in my brain chemistry?," "Did I do something to bring this on myself?" "Is there a flaw in my personality or some weakness in my psychological makeup?" Unfortunately, clinicians facing questions about the etiology of anxiety have great difficulty providing satisfactory answers given that our knowledge of vulnerability to anxiety is relatively limited (McNally, 2001).

Even though research on vulnerability has lagged behind our knowledge of the psychopathology and treatment of anxiety, most would agree that susceptibility to developing an anxiety disorder varies greatly within the general population. This is well illustrated in the following case examples. Cynthia, a 29-year-old factory worker, who described herself as being highly anxious, worrisome, and lacking self-confidence since early childhood, developed moderately severe doubt and checking compulsions after leaving high school and assuming the increased responsibilities of work and living independently. Andy, a 41-year-old accountant, presented with a first onset of severe panic disorder and agoraphobic avoidance after promotion to a highly stressful, performance-driven managerial position that led to the onset of various physical symptoms, such as chest pressure and pain, heart palpitations, numbness, sweating, lightheadedness, and stomach tightness. He had a comorbid health anxiety that intensified after receiving treatment for hiatus hernia, high cholesterol, and acid reflux. Ann Marie, a 35-year-old government office worker, suffered from long-standing social phobia that remained untreated until she experienced her first full-blown panic attack after a promotion that caused a significant increase in her work stress. Ann Marie stated that she had always been a generally anxious and worrisome person since high school, but currently found social interactions the most threatening for her.

In each of these case illustrations the emergence of an anxiety disorder occurred within the context of predisposing factors and precipitating circumstances. Frequently individuals with anxiety disorders report a predisposition toward high anxiety, nervousness or worry, as well as precipitating events that escalate their daily stress. Since predisposing biological or psychological characteristics and environmental factors are both involved in the etiology of clinical anxiety, diathesis–stress models are frequently proposed to account for individual differences in risk for anxiety (Story, Zucker, & Craske, 2004). In many cases major life events, traumas, or ongoing adversities are involved in anxiety; in others, the precipitants are not so dramatic, and fall within the realm of normal life events (e.g., increased work stress, an uncertain medical test, an embarrassing experience). These differences in clinical presentations have led researchers to search for vulnerability and risk factors that might predict whether a person develops an anxiety disorder.

In this chapter we present the cognitive model of *vulnerability* to anxiety. We begin by defining some of the key concepts employed in etiological models of disorder. This is followed by an overview of the role that heritability, neurophysiology, personality, and life events may play in the origins of anxiety disorders. We then present the cognitive vulnerability model of anxiety that was first articulated in Beck et al. (1985). The chapter concludes with a discussion of the empirical support for the last two hypotheses of the cognitive model, elevated personal vulnerability and enduring threat-related beliefs, that pertain directly to the issue of etiology.

VULNERABILITY: DEFINITIONS AND CARDINAL FEATURES

Although often used interchangeably, the terms "vulnerability" and "risk" have very distinct meanings (see Ingram, Miranda, & Segal, 1998; Ingram & Price, 2001). *Risk* is a descriptive or statistical term referring to any variable whose association with a disorder increases its likelihood of occurrence (e.g., gender, poverty, relationship status) without informing about actual causal mechanisms. *Vulnerability*, on the other hand, is a risk factor that has causal status with the disorder in question. Vulnerability can be defined as an endogenous, stable characteristic that remains latent until activated by a precipitating event. This activation can lead to the occurrence of the defining symptoms of a disorder (Ingram & Price, 2001). Knowledge of vulnerability factors has treatment implications because it will elucidate the actual mechanisms of etiology (Ingram et al., 1998). However, vulnerability does not directly lead to disorder onset but instead is mediated by the occurrence of precipitating events.

Vulnerability factors are internal, stable, and latent or unobservable until activated by a precipitating event (Ingram et al., 1998; Ingram & Price, 2001). This private, unobservable nature of vulnerability in asymptomatic individuals has presented special challenges for researchers in search of reliable and valid methods for detecting vulnerability (Ingram & Price, 2001). Moreover, vulnerability constructs must have high sensitivity (i.e., must be present in disordered individuals), a moderate level of specificity (i.e., more prevalent in the target disorder than in controls), and be distinct from the precipitating life event (Ingram et al., 1998). In Beck's cognitive model vulnerability constructs are neither necessary nor sufficient but rather contributory causes of psychopathology that may interact or combine with other etiological pathways that are present at the genetic, biological, and developmental levels (see Abramson, Alloy, & Metalsky, 1988; D. A. Clark et al., 1999).

The cognitive model of anxiety presented in Chapter 2 (see Figure 2.1) describes the proximal cognitive structures and processes involved in the persistence of anxiety, whereas this chapter focuses on distal cognitive variables that are predispositions for anxiety. These distal cognitive vulnerability factors are *moderators* (i.e., they affect the direction and/or strength of association between stress and symptom onset), whereas more proximal cognitive variables are *mediators* (i.e., they account for the relationship between vulnerability, stress, and disorder onset) (see Baron & Kenny, 1986; Riskind & Alloy, 2006). In the cognitive model multiple distal vulnerabilities are present at the biological, cognitive, and developmental levels so that some individuals may have multiple vulnerabilities. These *compound vulnerabilities* might be associated with even higher risk for disorder onset, a more severe symptom presentation, or comorbid emotional conditions (Riskind & Alloy, 2006).

BIOLOGICAL DETERMINANTS

Individual differences in genetics, neurophysiology, and temperament will interact with a predisposing cognitive vulnerability to heighten or reduce one's anxiety-proneness in response to life adversity or threat. Barlow (2002) convincingly argued for a generalized biological vulnerability to anxiety disorders, in which heritability, a nonspecific vulnerability factor, accounts for 30–40% of variability across all anxiety disorders. This genetic vulnerability is most likely expressed through elevations in broad personality traits or temperaments like neuroticism, trait anxiety, or negative affectivity. Chronic arousal, prepotent neuroanatomical structures (e.g., amygdala, locus coeruleus, BNST, right prefrontal cortex), and neurotransmitter abnormalities in serotonin, GABA, and CRH are other biological vulnerabilities to anxiety that have etiological significance, in part by interacting in a synergistic fashion with cognitive vulnerability (see Chapter 1 for further discussion).

PERSONALITY VULNERABILITY

Neuroticism and Negative Affectivity

Eysenck and Eysenck (1975) described neuroticism (N) as a predisposition toward emotionality in which the highly neurotic individual is overly emotional, anxious, worrisome, moody, and has a tendency to overreact strongly to a range of stimuli. High N and low E (extraversion) individuals—or introverted individuals—were considered more likely to develop anxiety because they have an overreactive limbic system that causes them to more easily acquire conditioned emotional responses to arousing stimuli. Although there is strong empirical support for high N in the pathogenesis of anxiety (e.g., see review by Watson & Clark, 1984), empirical evidence for other characteristics of N, such as its neurophysiological basis, have not been as well supported (Eysenck, 1992).

Watson and Clark (1984) proposed a mood–dispositional dimension called *negative affectivity* (NA). NA reflects a "pervasive individual difference in negative emotionality and self-concept" (p. 465), with high NA individuals more likely to experience elevated levels of negative emotions including subjective feelings of nervousness, tension, and worry, as well as a tendency to have poor self-esteem and to dwell on past mistakes, frustrations, and threats (Watson & Clark, 1984). Research within the Big Five personality tradition have subsumed the notion of N and NA under the higher order, superordinate personality construct of "negative emotionality" (e.g., Watson, Clark, & Harkness, 1994).

There is a large correlational and factor analytic research showing an association between negative emotionality and anxiety in clinical and nonclinical samples (i.e., Longley, Watson, Noyes, & Yoder, 2006). Higher emotionality is evident in all the anxiety disorders as well as in depression (e.g., Bienvenu et al., 2004; Cox, Enns, Walker, Kjernisted, & Pidlubny, 2001; Trull & Sher, 1994; Watson, Clark, & Carey, 1988) and it predicts future anxious symptoms (Gershuny & Sher, 1998; Levenson, Aldwin, Bossé, & Spiro, 1988). Thus high NA or emotionality is a broad, nonspecific distal vulnerability factor for anxiety and its disorders that constitutes a temperamental characteristic of proneness to nervousness, tension, and worry with roots in genetic and early childhood experiences (i.e., Barlow, 2002).

Trait Anxiety

Another personality construct so closely related to negative emotionality (i.e., N or NA) that the two are considered almost synonymous is *trait anxiety* (Eysenck, 1992). Spielberger, the strongest proponent for distinguishing between state and trait anxiety, defined *state anxiety* as "a transitory emotional state or condition of the human organism that is characterized by subjective, consciously perceived feelings of tension, apprehension and heightened autonomic nervous system activity. A-States vary in intensity and fluctuate over time" (Spielberger, Gorsuch, & Lushene, 1970, p. 3).

Trait anxiety, on the other hand, is considered to be "relatively stable individual differences in anxiety proneness" (Spielberger et al., 1970, p. 3). Individuals with high trait anxiety are more likely to respond to situations of perceived threat with elevations in state anxiety and evaluate a greater range of stimuli as threatening, have a lower anxiety activation threshold, and feel more intense anxious states (Rachman, 2004; Spielberger, 1985). Although there is substantial evidence that Spielberger's State-Trait Anxiety Inventory is highly relevant for stress and anxiety (Roemer, 2001), high trait anxiety is a problematic vulnerability construct because (1) its temporal stability has not been consistently supported, (2) its unidimensional structure has been challenged, (3) it is too highly correlated with state anxiety, (4) it may lack specificity for anxiety, and (5) it embodies a vague idea of vulnerability that is closely aligned with Freud's concept of neurotic anxiety (Eysenck, 1992; Rachman, 2004; Reiss, 1997; Roemer, 2001). For these reasons researchers have looked elsewhere for more specific personality predictors of anxiety disorders.

Anxiety Sensitivity

In recent years anxiety sensitivity, a fear of or sensitivity to experiencing anxiety, has emerged as a more promising personality vulnerability construct that takes a more cognitive perspective with greater specificity to anxiety and its disorders. *Anxiety sensitivity* (AS) is the fear of anxiety-related bodily sensations based on enduring beliefs that negative physical, social, or psychological consequences might result from these anxious symptoms (Reiss, 1991; Reiss & McNally, 1985; Taylor, 1995a; Taylor & Cox, 1998). For example, a person with high AS might interpret chest pain as sign of an imminent heart attack and so feel highly anxious when experiencing this bodily sensation, whereas a person with low AS might interpret the chest pain as muscle tension due to physical exertion and so experience no anxiety with the bodily sensation.

A propensity to feel anxious about certain bodily symptoms is present in high AS because individuals believe anxiety and its physical symptoms can lead to serious consequences like heart attacks, mental illness, or intolerable anxiety (Reiss, 1991). Thus AS is a personality variable that amplifies fear when anxiety sensations and behaviors are experienced (Reiss, 1997). In this way it is thought to play both an etiological and a maintaining role in all the anxiety disorders, but particularly panic disorder and agoraphobia (Reiss, 1991; Taylor & Cox, 1998).

Psychometric Validation

The 16-item Anxiety Sensitivity Index (ASI) is the primary measure for assessing individual differences in AS (Reiss, Peterson, Gursky, & McNally, 1986; Reiss & McNally, 1985). Despite considerable debate over its factorial structure, it now appears that the ASI is a hierarchical multidimensional construct with two or three correlated lower order factors (i.e., Fears of Mental Catastrophe vs. Fears of Cardiopulmonary Sensations or Physical Concerns, Mental Incapacitation, and Social Concerns about Being Anxious) linked to a higher order general factor of AS (Mohlman & Zinbarg, 2000; Schmidt & Joiner, 2002; Zinbarg, Barlow, & Brown, 1997). There is also controversy over which dimensions best describe AS. Based on a 36-item ASI-R, only two correlated factors were replicated across data sets drawn from six countries: Fear of Somatic Symptoms and Social-Cognitive Concerns (Zolensky et al., 2003).

The most recent revision of the ASI, the 18-item ASI-3, may provide the best assessment of the three AS dimensions; physical, cognitive, and social concerns (Taylor, Zvolensky, et al., 2007). The ASI-3 subscales had improved internal consistency and good criterion-related validity, although the three subscales were very highly correlated (r's > .83). Nevertheless, findings across the various versions of the ASI indicate that subscales rather than a total score should be utilized to indicate level of AS.

The ASI measures have good internal consistency, test–retest reliability, and strong convergent validity with other measures of anxiety (Mohlman & Zinbarg, 2000; Reiss et al., 1986; Taylor & Cox, 1998; Zvolensky et al., 2003). Moreover, the AS lower order dimensions are generally consistent across various countries (Bernstein et al., 2006; Zvolensky et al., 2003), although there is some evidence that high AS scores may decrease over time even in the absence of a specific intervention (Gardenswartz & Craske, 2001; Maltby, 2001; Maltby, Mayers, Allen, & Tolin, 2005). There has been considerable debate on whether AS is distinct from trait anxiety (for discussion, see Lilienfeld, 1996; Lilienfeld, Jacob, & Turner, 1989; McNally, 1994). The current view is that AS is a distinct lower order construct hierarchically linked to the broader personality disposition of trait anxiety (Reiss, 1997; Taylor, 1995a).

Experimental Validation

If AS amplifies fear reactions, then high AS should lead to more intense anxiety in response to a wider range of stimuli (Reiss & McNally, 1985; see Taylor, 2000). This should be particularly evident in biological challenges that provoke panic attacks under controlled laboratory conditions or other experimental manipulations that elicit the physical symptoms of anxiety (McNally, 1996). In fact, there is now considerable empirical evidence that baseline AS predicts postchallenge anxiety symptoms and panic attacks in people with or without diagnosable panic disorder (for reviews, see McNally, 2002; Zvolensky, Schmidt, Bernstein, & Keough, 2006). High AS predicts fearful response and panic symptoms to carbon dioxide (CO_2) inhalation (e.g., Rapee, Brown, Antony, & Barlow, 1992; Rassovsky, Kushner, Schwarze, & Wangensteen, 2000; Schmidt & Mallott, 2006), hyperventilation (Carter, Suchday, & Gore, 2001; Holloway & McNally, 1987; McNally & Eke, 1996; Rapee & Medoro, 1994), and caffeine ingestion (Telch, Silverman, & Schmidt, 1996). Although ASI Physical Concerns may be the only AS dimension that predicts fear response to a physical challenge (Brown, Smits, Powers, & Telch, 2003; Carter et al., 2001; Zvolensky, Feldner, Eifert, & Stewart, 2001), these experimental findings support the predictive validity of the ASI and its special relevance to panic-spectrum psychopathology (Zvolensky et al., 2006).

Diagnostic Specificity

If AS is a specific cognitive-personality vulnerability factor for anxiety, then it should be significantly more elevated in anxiety, especially panic disorder, than in other clinical and nonclinical samples (McNally, 1994, 1996). Individuals with panic disorder or agoraphobia score on average two standard deviations above the normative mean on the ASI (McNally, 1994, 1996; Reiss, 1991; Taylor, 1995a, 2000) and anxiety disorder samples (except simple phobias) score significantly higher than depression or nonclinical comparisons (Taylor & Cox, 1998; Taylor, Koch, & McNally, 1992). Within the anxiety disorders, persons with panic disorder and agoraphobia score significantly higher than the other anxiety disorders, with PTSD, GAD, OCD, and social phobia scoring significantly higher than nonclinical comparison groups (Deacon & Abramowitz, 2006a; Taylor, Koch, & McNally, 1992a). At the symptomatic level ASI has a specific association with self-report of panic attacks in nonclinical child and adult populations (e.g., Calamari et al., 2001; Cox, Endler, Norton, & Swinson, 1991; Longley et al., 2006), although some studies have found AS relates to depressive symptoms as well (Reardon & Williams, 2007).

The ASI subscales appear to have differential specificity for anxiety and panic. ASI Physical Concerns is the only dimension specific to panic disorder whereas Social Concerns may be more relevant to social phobia (e.g., Deacon & Abramowitz, 2006a; Zinbarg et al., 1997) and Cognitive Dyscontrol may be related to depression (Cox et al., 2001; Rector, Szacun-Shimizu, & Leybman, 2007). However, caution must be exercised when using the ASI to screen for anxiety or panic. Hoyer and colleagues examined the predictive accuracy of the ASI, BAI, and several other anxiety measures in a large epidemiological sample of 1,877 young women in Dresden, Germany (Hoyer, Becker, Neumer, Soeder, & Margraf, 2002). None of the measures alone were able to accurately screen for anxiety disorders, although better predictive accuracy occurred when a specific anxiety disorder was targeted by more specific symptom questionnaires (e.g., screening for agoraphobia with the Mobility Inventory). Clearly, then, it would be incorrect to assume the presence or absence of panic solely on the basis of an individual's ASI score.

Prospective Studies

The best empirical evidence that AS is a cognitive personality vulnerability factor for panic disorder comes from longitudinal studies. Maller and Reiss (1992) reported that ASI scores predicted frequency and intensity of panic attacks 3 years later. In two separate samples of U.S. Air Force cadets assessed before and after a stressful 5 weeks of basic cadet training, the ASI predicted spontaneous panic attacks that occurred in 6% of the cadets during the 5-week period (Schmidt, Lerew, & Jackson, 1997, 1999). Additional analyses revealed that AS uniquely predicted changes in anxious symptoms (i.e., BAI scores) when controlling for the close association between anxiety and depression. Unexpectedly, analysis of the ASI subfactors revealed that it was ASI Mental rather than Physical Concerns that predicted the spontaneous panic attacks and changes in BAI scores.

In a 4-year community-based longitudinal study, adolescents classified as stable high or escalating ASI scorers were significantly more likely to experience a panic attack than low stable scorers (Weens, Hayward, Killen, & Taylor, 2002). However, there was little evidence that experiencing panic led to subsequent increases in AS (see Schmidt, Lerew, & Joiner, 2000, for contrary findings). Plehn and Peterson (2002) conducted an 11-year mailed follow-up survey with first year undergraduates initially assessed for AS and trait anxiety. After controlling for history of panic symptoms, only Time 1 ASI was a significant predictor of panic symptoms and panic attacks over an 11-year time interval. Surprisingly, trait anxiety, not AS, was the only significant predictor of panic disorder. In a retrospective cross-sectional study ASI Physical Concerns and exposure to aversive life circumstances predicted panic attacks and agoraphobic avoidance in the past week (Zvolensky, Kotov, Antipova, & Schmidt, 2005). Together these findings indicate that high AS constitutes a significant cognitive-personality predisposition for panic attacks. However, it is unclear which of the ASI subfactors is the most potent predictor of panic and whether having panic causes a "scarring effect" on AS (i.e., leads to subsequent increase in AS). McNally (2002) also reminds us that the amount of variance accounted for by AS is modest, suggesting that other factors are clearly important in the etiological of panic.

Treatment Effects

There is considerable evidence that AS is responsive to interventions (for reviews, see McNally, 2002; Zvolensky et al., 2006). For example, a primary preventive program that targeted AS produced significant reductions in AS that translated into lower subjective fear response to a biological challenge and a significant decrease in Axis I psychopathology over a 2-year follow-up period (Schmidt, Eggleston, et al., 2007). Thus targeting AS in cognitive therapy should produce immediate and long-term benefits in anxiety reduction.

Anxiety Sensitivity and the Cognitive Model

Empirical evidence that AS is a specific predisposing factor for anxiety, especially panic, fits with the cognitive vulnerability model of anxiety. AS is a cognitive construct that describes individual differences in the propensity to misinterpret the bodily sensations of anxiety in a threatening manner. It is a specific cognitive vulnerability construct that may have relevance beyond panic to the extent that negative interpretation of subjective anxiety and its symptoms is a consequence of automatic threat mode activation (see Chapter 2). In Chapter 3 we discussed empirical evidence that emotional reasoning or a tendency to interpret anxious symptoms in a negative or threatening manner is an important cognitive phenomenon in anxiety. We expect that individuals high in AS will more likely engage in emotional reasoning and other forms of biased interpretation of their anxious symptoms than individuals low in AS.

Based in part on correlational analyses between the ASI and the Fear Survey Schedule (see Taylor, 1995a), Rachman (2004) concluded that AS along with illness/injury sensitivity and fear of negative evaluation are distinct lower order traits that are nested hierarchically in the broader construct of trait anxiety. All three of these constructs are cognitive in nature since they focus on a tendency to misinterpret physical or social information in a negative or threatening manner. They describe specific cognitive-personality vulnerabilities for panic and social-evaluative anxiety states. And yet, even though there is strong empirical support that AS is a vulnerability factor in anxiety, its ability to account for only modest variance indicates that other cognitive-personality factors must be involved in the pathogenesis of anxiety disorder.

Clinician Guideline 4.1

Include the ASI or ASI-3 in the pretreatment assessment battery to evaluate the client's propensity to misinterpret physical, cognitive, and social symptoms in an anxious or fearful manner.

Diminished Personal Control

It has been suggested that the greatest human fear is of losing control, leading many researchers to consider impaired control a key feature of stress, anxiety, depression, and other aspects of psychological distress (Mineka & Kihlstrom, 1978; Shapiro, Schwartz, & Astin, 1996). In his account of the origins of anxious apprehension, Barlow (2002) posited that a generalized psychological vulnerability interacts with a generalized biological vulnerability and particular learning experiences in the development of specific anxiety disorders. *Psychological vulnerability* was defined as "a chronic inability to cope with unpredictable uncontrollable negative events, and this sense of uncontrollability is associated with negatively valenced emotional responding" (Barlow, 2002, p. 254). Earlier Chorpita and Barlow (1998) defined *control* as "the ability to personally influence events and outcomes in one's environment, principally those related to positive or negative reinforcement" (p. 5).

In anxiety uncertainty that one possesses the required level of control over an anticipated aversive outcome is an enduring characteristic (Alloy et al., 1990). This diminished sense of personal control is an individual difference variable that may be acquired through childhood experiences of stifled independence, limited exploration, and high parental protection. As a result of repeated experiences of uncontrollable or unpredictable events throughout early and middle childhood, the individual develops low perceived control over life circumstances and perhaps increased neurobiological activity in the behavioral inhibition system (Barlow, 2002; Chorpita & Barlow, 1998). According to Barlow, these beliefs of low personal control constitute a personality diathesis that interacts with negative or aversive life events to trigger anxiety or depression.

It has been long recognized that a decrease in perceived control is associated with anxiety and that lower control over a threatening event can increase estimates of the probability of danger and personal vulnerability (Chorpita & Barlow, 1998). Beck et al. (1985, 2005) recognized that fear of losing control is a prominent cognitive feature found in many anxiety states. Barlow and colleagues (Barlow, 2002; Chorpita & Barlow, 1998) note that the perception that threatening events occur in an unexpected, unpredictable fashion is part of a diminished sense of personal control over aversive events. However, there is a lack of direct support for a specific association between chronic diminished control and anxiety (see Barlow, 2002; Chorpita & Barlow, 1998). In fact there has been a long research tradition in locus of control, learned helplessness, life event appraisals, and attributional style that recognizes a role for perceived control in depression (e.g., Abramson, Metalsky, & Alloy, 1989; Alloy, Abramson, Safford, & Gibb, 2006; Hammen, 1988). Alloy et al. (1990), for example, stated that a generalized tendency to perceive negative events as uncontrollable is a distal contributory cause of depression.

Alloy and colleagues further proposed a helplessness–hopelessness theory that identifies certain key cognitive processes that underlie the high comorbidity between anxiety and depression (Alloy et al., 1990). According to the theory, anxiety is experienced when individuals expect to be helpless in controlling important future events but are uncertain about their helplessness, whereas this anxiety turns to hopelessness and depression when the future negative outcomes become certain. Unfortunately, research on the role of a cognitive style of diminished control for negative outcomes in anxiety, and its probable connection to depression, is limited (Chorpita & Barlow, 1998). This state of affairs is partly due to the lack of sensitive measures of perceived uncontrollability of threat. To rectify this situation, the 30-item Anxiety Control Questionnaire (ACQ) was developed to assess perceived control over anxiety-related symptoms, emotional reactions, and external problems and threats (Rapee, Craske, Brown, & Barlow, 1996). The ACQ has good internal consistency, 1-month test–retest reliability, and moderate correlations with anxiety and depression symptom measures (see also Zebb & Moore, 1999).

There is fairly consistent empirical evidence of a close association between anxiety and diminished sense of control over outcomes. In a panic disorder study agoraphobic avoidance was greatest in those who had high anxiety sensitivity and low ACQ perception of control (White, Brown, Somers, & Barlow, 2006). Likewise Hofman (2005) found that anxiety in social phobia persists because individuals have low perceived control over emotions and bodily sensations when exposed to social threat (see also McLaren & Crowe, 2003; Rapee, 1997, for similar findings).

Despite evidence of an association between diminished sense of control over potentially threatening outcomes and anxiety, there is a significant body of research from the attributional style literature showing that reduced perceived control over past negative events may have an even stronger relation to depression than to anxiety. A negative or pessimistic attributional style refers to the belief that the cause of past loss and failure can be attributed to internal, global, and stable or enduring personal deficiencies (Abramson, Seligman, & Teasdale, 1978). A negative attributional style can be viewed as a diminished sense of past control. There is now considerable evidence that negative attributional style is a cognitive-personality vulnerability for depression (for reviews, see Alloy et al., 2006; Sweeney, Anderson, & Bailey, 1986; e.g., Hankin, Abramson, & Siler, 2001; Metalsky, Halberstadt, & Abramson, 1987). However, studies that have examined the specificity of the negative attributional style reveal that it is also apparent in anxiety, though to a lesser degree, (e.g., Heimberg et al., 1989; Johnson & Miller, 1990; Luten, Ralph, & Mineka, 1997).

Perceived reduction in control over potentially threatening outcomes appears to be an important factor in the anxiety disorders, especially if there is elevated uncertainty about the threat (Alloy et al., 1990; Moulding & Kyrios, 2006). However, the necessary longitudinal research has not been conducted to determine whether there is an enduring belief in diminished personal control over threat that is a distal contributory factor to anxiety. Nevertheless, there is sufficient evidence to conclude that low perceived control is a contributor to anxiety, although it is probably a nonspecific cognitive-personality factor found in both depression and anxiety.

Clinician Guideline 4.2

Include assessment of perceived control over threat in the case formulation. Two aspects of control are important to assess in anxiety: (1) clients' perceived control over emotional responses, especially symptoms of anxiety; and (2) clients' evaluations of their ability to manage anticipated threats related to their primary threat concerns. The ACQ can be helpful when assessing perceived control of anxiety.

LIFE EVENT PRECIPITANTS OF ANXIETY

Diathesis–stress models have been proposed for anxiety that explain disorder onset in terms of an interaction between negative life events and a preexisting vulnerability diathesis (e.g., Barlow, 2002; Chorpita & Barlow, 1998). A life event, situation, or circumstance that is evaluated as a potential threat to one's survival or vital interests can activate an underlying vulnerability that will lead to a state of anxiety. This underlying diathesis can involve personality predispositions like high negative emotionality, trait anxiety, anxiety sensitivity, and a chronic sense of diminished control, as well as more specific cognitive vulnerabilities such as hypervalent threat schemas and heightened sense of personal weakness and ineffectiveness (see discussion below).

There is evidence that an excess of negative life events is associated with the anxiety disorders. In a large population-based twin study, the occurrence of high-threat life events was associated with a significant increase in risk of developing a pure generalized anxiety episode (e.g., Kendler, Hettema, Butera, Gardner, & Prescott, 2003). In a retrospective study of life adversity and onset of psychiatric disorders in over 1,800 community-based young adults, individuals who averaged over six major life events or potentially traumatic experiences and an accumulating exposure to lifetime adversity had increased risk of depressive or anxious episodes (Turner & Lloyd, 2004). Stressful or adverse life experiences have been shown to frequently precede and/or exacerbate the onset of OCD (i.e., Cromer, Schmidt, & Murphy, 2007), social phobia, panic disorder, GAD, and, of course, PTSD (for reviews, see Clark, 2004; Craske, 2003; Ledley, Fresco, & Heimberg, 2006; Taylor, 2000, 2006). However, one must keep in mind that many individuals develop an anxiety disorder without experiencing a major negative life event, and most people who experience life adversities never develop an anxiety disorder (McNally, Malcarne, & Hansdottir, 2001).

Although there is consistent evidence that life events play an etiological role in anxiety, it is also apparent that their contribution may be less prominent in anxiety than they are in depression. For instance, Kendler, Myers, and Prescott (2002) did not find evidence to support a diathesis–stress model for the acquisition of phobias (see also Brown, Harris, & Eales, 1996). Thus threatening life events and other experiences of life trauma and adversity are significant contributors in the pathogenesis of anxiety, but much remains to be learned about the exact nature of these proximal contributors and how they interact with the cognitive-personality vulnerability factors for anxiety.

Clinician Guideline 4.3

Given the prominence of threat-oriented stressful events, adversity, and traumatic experiences in anxiety disorders, include a life history in the assessment. The cognitive case formulation should include appraisals of control, perceived vulnerability, and expected outcomes associated with these experiences.

THE COGNITIVE VULNERABILITY MODEL

In their original account of the cognitive model of anxiety Beck et al. (1985, 2005) defined *vulnerability* as "a person's perception of himself as subject to internal or external dangers over which his control is lacking or is insufficient to afford him a sense of safety. In clinical syndromes, the sense of vulnerability is magnified by certain dysfunctional cognitive processes" (Beck et al., 1985, pp. 67–68). In this formulation vulnerability to anxiety is conceptualized as a predisposition to misinterpret potentially threatening or novel situations as dangerous and devoid of safety, leaving the individual in a state of perceived helplessness. In the anxiety disorders only certain types of threat will activate this underlying cognitive vulnerability. Once activated in a particular situation, the cognitive-affective program described in Chapter 2 (see Figure 2.1) maintains the individual in a heightened state of anxiety.

Beck et al. (1985, 2005) focused on two main characteristics of cognitive vulnerability. The first is an enduring tendency to misinterpret certain types of threatening or novel situations as dangerous. The second is a predisposition to perceive one's self as incompetent, weak, or lacking the personal resources to deal with certain types of threatening or stressful situations. In the current formulation of the cognitive model, the first feature of cognitive vulnerability is captured by Hypothesis 12, enduring threat-related beliefs, and the second falls under Hypothesis 11, elevated personal vulnerability. Both aspects of vulnerability must be present for an individual to be cognitively predisposed to anxiety. Furthermore, we would expect cognitive vulnerability to exhibit a high degree of selectivity within a diathesis–stress framework, so that it would only surface when the vulnerable person anticipates encountering specific types of potentially threatening situations. Thus an enduring tendency to misinterpret certain types of potential threat and one's ability to manage this threat would remain dormant until activated by relevant trauma or other forms of perceived stress. Once activated, the threat schemas would dominate the information-processing system whenever a relevant threat-related cue is encountered.

Like other anxiety researchers, we believe a cognitive vulnerability for anxiety develops through repeated experiences of neglect, abandonment, humiliation, and even trauma that can occur during childhood and adolescence (see Barlow, 2002; Chorpita & Barlow, 1998; Craske, 2003). Certain parenting practices such as overprotection, restriction of independence and autonomy, preoccupation with potential danger, and encouraging escape and avoidance in response to anxiety could all contribute to the development of a cognitive vulnerability to anxiety. Although there is some empirical evidence that supports this conjecture, much of it is based on retrospective assessment of childhood experiences (McNally et al., 2001). Large community-based longitudinal studies that begin in childhood are needed in order to determine the developmental antecedents of cognitive vulnerability to anxiety.

The present account of cognitive vulnerability is consistent with the proposals of other cognitive-behavioral researchers. M. W. Eysenck (1992), for example, proposed a hypervigilance theory of anxiety in which individuals with high trait anxiety have an attentional system that is oriented toward threat detection when they are in potentially threatening situations or in a state of high anxiety. Craske (2003) suggested that both negative affectivity and a threat-based style of emotional regulation (i.e., a response to arousal and distress characterized by avoidance and danger-laden expectations) are vulnerability factors for anxiety. Rachman (2004) noted that people may be primed to detect threat cues and overlook or minimize safety information. Mathews and MacLeod (2002) argued that attentional and interpretative biases for threat constitute a vulnerability to anxiety. And Wells (2000) proposed that enduring metacognitive beliefs (i.e., beliefs about one's thoughts) about worry, judgments of cognitive confidence, and the importance of monitoring one's thought processes constitutes a vulnerability for emotional disorders.

Our focus on the cognitive basis of vulnerability to anxiety must be understood within the context of other etiological factors such as biological and developmental determinants, NA, trait anxiety, anxiety sensitivity, diminished personal control, and the like. This broader view of vulnerability is represented in Figure 4.1.

Prepotent threat schemas and perceived personal vulnerability or weakness are more specific cognitive constructs that directly reflect the slightly broader constructs of high anxiety sensitivity, diminished personal control, and sensitivity to negative evaluation, which in turn are related to broad traits of negative emotionality and high trait anxiety. In this way vulnerability to anxiety disorders involves the interaction of multiple pathways emanating from constitutional, developmental, environmental, personality, and information-processing domains. Based on this framework for vulnerability, we turn to consider the empirical evidence for the two main components of the model: an enduring sense of personal vulnerability and the presence of hypervalent threat schemas.

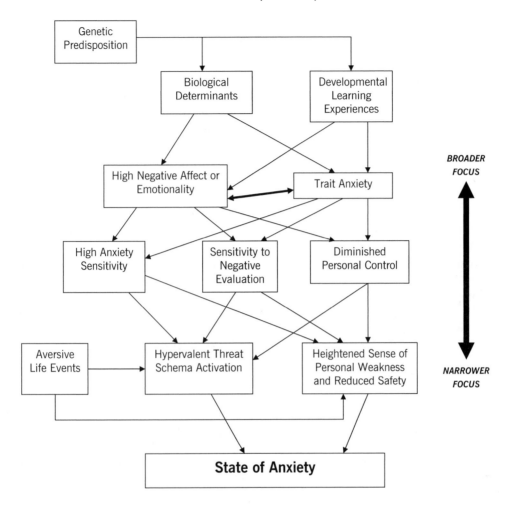

FIGURE 4.1. Cognitive vulnerability model of anxiety.

Hypothesis 11. Heightened Sense of Personal Vulnerability

Highly anxious individuals will exhibit lower self-confidence and greater perceived helplessness in situations relevant to their selective threats compared to nonanxious individuals.

Beck et al. (1985, 2005) considered diminished self-confidence and self-doubt an important aspect of cognitive vulnerability to anxiety. For the person who suffers from anxiety a self-confidence set is replaced by a vulnerability perspective. When in a vulnerability mode, individuals evaluate their own abilities and competence as inadequate for dealing with a perceived threat. As a result, they become tentative or withdraw from a situation in a self-protective manner. When a confident attitude is adopted, the individual focuses on the positives in a situation, minimizes the dangers, and may even assume a greater sense of personal control than when low self-confidence prevails (Beck et al., 1985, 2005). Adopting a confident mode increases the probability of success in a threatening situation, whereas dominance of the vulnerability mode is more likely to lead to failure and reinforce individuals' belief in their incompetence because it is associated with self-questioning, uncertainty, and a weak or tentative response in a challenging situation. Bandura's (1991) concept of low perceived self-efficacy, as well as uncontrollability and unpredictability, are distal vulnerability factors in anxiety proposed by other researchers (e.g., Chorpita & Barlow, 1998; Schmidt & Woolaway-Bickel, 2006) that are consistent with the cognitive vulnerability concept of diminished self-confidence for selective types of perceived threats.

There are three assumptions about the nature of low self-esteem in anxiety. First, the lack of self-confidence is highly specific to the anxious concerns of the individual. Unlike depression, where we find a generalized negative view of the self, the lower self-worth in anxiety is only evident in situations relevant to the person's anxious concerns. For example, a client with a specific phobia about swallowing was discouraged and disheartened about his ability to eat in the presence of others and yet felt very competent when performing in front of hundreds as an amateur comedian. Second, lack of self-confidence will be a significant determinant of self-protective responses in anxious situations such as escape and avoidance, and deficit performance in dealing with the situation. And third, lack of self-confidence in responding to certain types of perceived threat arises from early childhood and other learning experiences and so acts as a vulnerability factor for the later development of an anxiety disorder.

Empirical Evidence

The first criterion of vulnerability is sensitivity to the disorder in question. Anxious individuals should exhibit less self-confidence in dealing with threatening situations relevant to their anxiety state than nonanxious individuals. Like depression, presence of anxiety disorders is characterized by a significant lowering of self-esteem (e.g., Ingham, Kreitman, Miller, Sashidharan, & Surtees, 1986). In fact a connection between low self-esteem and anxiety has figured prominently in psychological theories and research on social anxiety, in particular. Various studies have shown that low self-esteem or dysfunctional beliefs about the self are related to heightened social anxiety or shyness (de Jong, 2002; Jones, Briggs, & Smith, 1986; Kocovski & Endler, 2000; Tanner et al., 2006; Wilson & Rapee, 2006). However, there are a number of qualifications that must be made about the nature of low self-esteem in social anxiety.

First, most of the research evidence indicates that the lack of self-confidence in social phobia is specific to social situations involving the perception of evaluation from others rather than a global low self-esteem. In fact social threat is often needed to prime low self-worth in socially anxious samples (e.g., O'Banion & Arkowitz, 1977; Rapee & Lim, 1992; Stopa & Clark, 1993). Second, it is not clear whether the lack of self-confidence in social anxiety reflects an elevation in negative self-evaluation or a reduction in positive self-evaluation. Mansell and Clark (1999) found that a high social anxiety group recalled fewer positive trait adjectives but not more negative adjectives than a low social anxiety group after giving a 2-minute videotaped speech (see de Jong, 2002; Tanner et al., 2006, for similar findings). Thus the primary problem in social anxiety may be a reduction in positive self-evaluation in social situations rather than an elevation in negative self-view. Third, it is still unclear which aspects of low self-esteem may be most important in social phobia. Wilson and Rapee (2006), for example, found that it was certainty of self-concept that was reduced in social phobia, whereas Mansell and Clark (1999) found that socially anxious individuals had reduced positivity recall for public but not private self-referent trait adjectives. Finally, differences in self-esteem may depend on whether automatic (i.e., implicit) or more effortful (i.e., explicit) processes are assessed. Implicit Association Test (IAT) studies suggest that the problem of low self-esteem in anxiety may be reflected in more controlled, effortful processes rather than an underlying, automatic evaluative bias (see de Jong, 2002; Tanner et al., 2006).

Although considerably less is known about the role of low self-esteem in other anxiety disorders, there is some preliminary research that is noteworthy. Ehntholt, Salkovskis, and Rimes (1999) found that both OCD and non-OCD anxious groups had significantly lower self-worth and generalized self-esteem than a nonclinical control group but concluded that low generalized self-esteem may be a consequence of anxiety rather than a predisposing factor. Wu, Clark, and Watson (2006) found that OCD patients were distinguished by a very low self-image based on profile analysis of the SNAP-2 and low self-esteem has been implicated in the development of PTSD symptoms (Piotrkowski & Brannen, 2002). Doron and Kyrios (2005) proposed that a restricted self-concept may constitute an underlying vulnerability for OCD. Thus there is increasing interest among researchers on the role that low self-esteem and other selfhood concepts might play in the pathogenesis of the anxiety disorders.

Summary

Although there is empirical evidence that low self-esteem characterizes the anxiety disorders, it is not clear whether this is a cause or a consequence of the disorder. Research on self-esteem vulnerability in anxiety has lagged far behind the empirical literature on low self-esteem in depression. Two types of studies are critical to progress beyond mere speculation. First, longitudinal studies are needed to determine if low self-worth is indeed a predisposing contributor to an anxiety disorder. These types of studies are practically nonexistent in the anxiety literature. And second, experimental research is needed to determine if variations in self-esteem have a corresponding causal effect on anxious symptoms. Causal effects must be demonstrated if low self-confidence in dealing with threat is a true cognitive vulnerability for anxiety.

If low self-worth is a cognitive vulnerability for anxiety, the preliminary findings suggest it is highly specific to threatening content perceived relevant to an individual's primary anxious concerns. In addition the lack of self-confidence is most likely evident at the secondary phase of anxiety where effortful, controlled processes predominant (see Figure 2.1). However, a conclusion on the empirical support for Hypothesis 11 must wait until further research has been completed.

Clinician Guideline 4.4

When assessing self-worth issues in anxiety, the clinician should evaluate the client's level of self-confidence in dealing with situations that exemplify the individual's primary anxious concerns.

Hypothesis 12: Enduring Threat-Related Beliefs

Individuals vulnerable to anxiety can be distinguished from nonvulnerable persons by preexisting maladaptive schemas (i.e., beliefs) about particular threats or dangers and associated personal vulnerability that remain inactive until triggered by relevant life experiences or stressors.

The cognitive model of anxiety (see Chapter 2) considers automatic activation of the primal threat mode a central process in the experience of anxiety. Threat mode activation sets in motion the symptoms that constitute a state of anxiety. Moreover, the dysfunctional beliefs or schemas that comprise the primal threat model are personal and quite idiosyncratic to each individual. They are primarily learned through various positive or negative experiences of threat or danger that occurred to self or significant others. As such they are enduring representations of threat, which in the anxiety disorders are often excessive, biased and maladaptive. These dysfunctional threat-related schemas will result in exaggerated appraisals of the probability and severity of threat, underestimate personal coping ability, and minimize the presence of safety (Beck et al., 1985, 2005).

In the cognitive model threat-relevant schemas constitute the core cognitive vulnerability for anxiety. The threat schemas of the anxiously vulnerable person are not only qualitatively different from those of the nonvulnerable person in terms of containing misinformation and bias about particular threats, but they are also "prepotent" in that a broader range of less intense stimuli will activate the schemas. For example, most people feel some anxiety before giving a public address that reflects activation of beliefs such "It is important that I do a good job" and "I expect the audience will be receptive." However, the person vulnerable to social anxiety might feel intense anxiety when asked a question in a work-related meeting because of activation of schemas like "I can't speak-up, people will notice that my voice is trembly," "They'll think there is something wrong with me," "They'll assume I must have an anxiety problem—a mental illness." In comparison to the nonvulnerable person, the individual with social anxiety has more extreme, exaggerated schemas that lead to an exaggerated appraisal of the danger. Also notice that a much less threatening situation triggers the threat schemas of the socially anxious person. In this way the schematic representations of threat in the vulnerable person are prepotent or hypervalent, leading to more frequent and intense activation. Unlike the nonvulnerable person, activation of certain threat schemas in the vulnerable person will tend to capture much of the information-processing resources so that the more constructive schemas become relatively inaccessible to the person.

Empirical Evidence

Is there any evidence that threat-relevant beliefs or schemas constitute an enduring cognitive predisposition for clinical anxiety states? We have already reviewed a considerable amount of empirical evidence that is consistent with a schema-based cognitive vulnerability to anxiety. In the previous chapter numerous studies by MacLeod, Mogg, Bradley, Mathews, and others found that nonclinical individuals with high trait anxiety had an attentional processing bias for threat, especially under conditions of stress (see reviews by Mathews & MacLeod, 1994, 2002, 2005; Mogg & Bradley, 1998). The conclusion reached by Mathews and MacLeod (2002) is that high trait-anxious individuals have a cognitive vulnerability to anxiety in the form of a lower threshold for switching from an avoidance to a vigilant information-processing mode.

A second source of supportive evidence for a schematic vulnerability to anxiety comes from the anxiety sensitivity and diminished control studies reviewed in this chapter. Although it would be inaccurate to describe the ASI as a beliefs measure, it does assess appraisals that are based on a variety of preexisting beliefs about physical sensations and anxiety. For example, the ASI item "It scares me when I become short of breath" would be based on a preexisting belief such as "I am putting myself at severe risk of being unable to breath when I feel short of breath." If high ASI scores predict elevated likelihood of subsequent anxiety, we can generalize from these findings to the beliefs that underlie ASI appraisals as supportive evidence that these beliefs constitute vulnerability for anxiety. The same generalization can be made from the research on diminished control and negative attributional style in anxiety. Certain preexisting beliefs about lack of control over anticipated threats will underlie control perceptions, making these beliefs an important element in the proposal that diminished sense of personal control is a vulnerability factor in anxiety. To summarize, the notion of preexisting dysfunctional beliefs that predispose to anxiety is a common feature of many cognitive theories of anxiety disorders (e.g., D. A. Clark, 2004; Ehlers & Clark, 2000; Wells, 2000; Wells & Clark, 1997).

DYSFUNCTIONAL ANXIETY BELIEFS

In order to investigate the role of dysfunctional beliefs in the etiology of anxiety, specific belief measures are needed that directly assess threat schema content. Unfortunately, research in this area is not as well developed as the experimental studies on attentional bias or the brief prospective diathesis–stress studies found in depression. Nevertheless, we are beginning to see more research on the role of threat-relevant schemas and beliefs in clinical anxiety.

In recent years there has been considerable research on the belief structure of OCD. An international group of researchers called the Obsessive Compulsive Cognitions Working Group (OCCWG) proposed six belief domains as constituting a cognitive vulnerability to OCD: inflated responsibility, overcontrol of thoughts, overimportance of thoughts, overestimated threat, perfectionism, and intolerance of uncertainty (OCCWG, 1997). Definitions of these belief domains can be found in Table 11.3.

An 87-item self-report questionnaire, the Obsessive Beliefs Questionnaire (OBQ), was developed to assess the six OCD belief domains. Later factor analysis indicated it could be reduced to 44 items that assessed three belief dimensions: responsibility/threat estimation, perfectionism/intolerance of uncertainty, and importance/control of thoughts (OCCWG, 2005). Two large-scale multisite clinical studies based on the 87-item OBQ revealed that OCD patients scored significantly higher than other nonobsessional anxious and nonclinical comparison groups on OBQ Control of Thoughts, Importance of Thoughts, and Responsibility subscales, in particular, and the six OBQ belief scales correlated better with self-reported OCD measures than with the BAI or BDI (OCCWG, 2001, 2003; see Steketee, Frost, & Cohen, 1998, for similar results). However, the six OBQ subscales are highly intercorrelated and they have strong correlations with other non-OCD measures like the Penn State Worry Questionnaire. At present the OBQ is probably the best measure of OCD beliefs, although certain weaknesses are apparent in its construct validity.

It is also becoming increasing clear that only certain belief domains like responsibility, importance, and control of thoughts may be specific to OCD whereas other domains like threat overestimation and perfectionism are common across the anxiety disorders. Although there has been some inconsistency across studies, beliefs about the importance of thoughts and need to control thoughts have tended to differentiate OCD patients from other anxiety groups, with responsibility and overestimated threat sometimes showing specificity but perfectionism and intolerance of uncertainty more often emerging as nonspecific across the anxiety disorders (e.g., Anholt et al., 2006; Clark, Purdon, & Wang, 2003; Sica et al., 2004; Tolin, Worhunsky, & Maltby, 2006; see Emmelkamp & Aardema, 1999, for contrary results). Moreover, some beliefs may be particularly relevant for certain OCD subtypes such as importance/control of thoughts for pure obsessions, or perfectionism/intolerance of uncertainty for OCD checking (Calarami et al., 2006; Julien, O'Connor, Aardema, & Todorov, 2006). Also, cluster analytic studies with the OBQ suggest that not all patients with OCD will necessarily endorse these OCD beliefs, leading some researchers to question whether dysfunctional beliefs plays a role in all OCD cases (Calamari et al., 2006; Taylor et al., 2006).

Recently there has been an attempt to determine whether preexisting dysfunctional beliefs might prospectively predict an escalation in OC symptoms. Eighty-five parents who were expecting their first child were administered the OBQ-44 and other measures of anxious and obsessional symptoms prenatally and then 3 months postpartum (Abramowitz, Khandker, Nelson, Deacon, & Rygwall, 2006). Most of the mothers and fathers reported distressing intrusive thoughts about their newborns at the follow-up assessment, and regression analyses revealed that OBQ Total Scores predicted an increase in postpartum OC symptoms as determined by the Yale–Brown Obsessive Compulsive Scale and the Obsessive–Compulsive Inventory—Revised. In a 6-week prospective study involving 377 undergraduates, Coles and Horng (2006) found that OBQ-44 Total Scores predicted an increase in OC symptoms as measured by the Obsessive Compulsive Inventory Total Score but the interaction between beliefs and negative life events failed to reach significance. However, in a second study Coles and colleagues failed to entirely replicate this finding (Coles, Pietrefesa, Schofield, & Cook, 2007), with OBQ-44 showing only a trend toward significance and no interaction with negative life events.

Researchers have examined the types of dysfunctional beliefs found in other anxiety disorders. Preexisting maladaptive beliefs about worry and its consequences are evident in chronic worry and GAD (Cartwright-Hatton & Wells, 1997; Dugas et al., 2005; Dugas, Gagnon, Ladouceur, & Freeston, 1998; Wells & Cartwright-Hatton, 2004; Ruscio & Borkovec, 2004; Wells & Papageorgiou, 1998a). Wenzel, Sharp, Brown, Greenberg, and Beck (2006) found that beliefs relevant to panic such as the anticipation of anxiety, concern about physical and emotional catastrophes, and self-deprecation were more closely associated with anxiety and panic symptoms than with self-reported depression. Individuals with social anxiety may endorse a number of early maladaptive schemas as indicated by elevated scores on the Young Schema Questionnaire subscales of Emotional Deprivation, Guilt/Failure, Social Undesirability/Defectiveness, Dependence, and the like (Pinto-Gouveia, Castilho, Galhardo, & Cunha, 2006). Overall there is some indication that enduring maladaptive beliefs about threat and vulnerability characterize the anxiety disorders, but this research is still in its infancy and many fundamental questions about the nature of schematic vulnerability in anxiety have not been addressed.

INDUCED THREAT INTERPRETATION BIAS

It is now well established that a tendency to endorse threatening interpretations of ambiguous information is an important feature of the selective processing bias for threat that characterizes anxiety (Mathews, 2006). However, demonstrating that threat-processing bias, and its underlying schematic threat activation by extension, has causal influence is more difficult because most of the research has been correlational or involved cross-sectional research designs. Mathews and MacLeod (2002) note that evidence of differential bias in anxious and nonanxious groups, reduction of threat bias with treatment, or differential activation of bias in high and low trait anxious individuals after a stressful event can not rule out a noncausal explanation such as the influence of a third unidentified variable. Thus research showing that experimental manipulation of interpretative bias through deliberate training conditions has a considerable impact on emotion is strong empirical evidence for causality in evaluative processing of threat. Furthermore, this research is important for cognitive vulnerability because it provides evidence for a basic precondition of vulnerability: that biased information processing has a causal effect on emotion.

The basic aim of induction procedures is to train volunteers to engage in selective processing of new anxiety-relevant information and assess changes in subsequent anxiety. Two effects are necessary to demonstrate. First, that training in differential processing bias has been successful and generalizes to the processing of new information. And second, an increase or decrease in threat-processing bias results in changes in level of anxiety. A third question often addressed is whether there are individual differences in susceptibility to threat-bias training that might suggest heightened vulnerability to anxiety.

MacLeod and colleagues conducted a series of experiments on induced attentional bias for threat in student volunteers. In the typical experiment individuals were randomly assigned to an attentional threat training condition or the avoidance of threat in favor of emotionally neutral cues (Mathews & MacLeod, 2002). In a series of unpublished pilot experiments (see discussion in Mathews & MacLeod, 2002), MacLeod and colleagues adapted the dot probe detection paradigm so that participants were randomly assigned to 576 training trials in which the dot always appeared in the location of threatening or neutral words. Analysis of 128 test trials revealed a significant training effect in which participants trained to detect threat words were significantly faster at probe detection after a threat word and slower to detect probes after a neutral word. This training effect was replicated in another pilot experiment using happy and angry faces.

In their first major published study, MacLeod et al. (2002) reported on two studies involving experimental manipulation of attentional bias. In the first experiment 64 nonvulnerable students (trait anxiety scores in the middle range) were randomly assigned to an "attend negative" training condition or an "attend neutral" condition. Training involved 576 trials in which 50% of the word pair presentations were at a short exposure interval (i.e., 20 milliseconds) and the other 50% were at a longer exposure duration (i.e., 480 milliseconds). Ninety-six test trials were distributed throughout the training trials. Thus half of the participants were trained to attend to the negative information and the other half were trained to attend away from negative stimuli (attend to neutral words). After the dot probe training all participants completed a stressful anagram task. Analysis revealed that students in the negative training condition exhibited faster dot probe detection to negative words in the test trails, whereas participants trained to attend away from negative words exhibited a speeding effect to dot probes following the neutral words. However, this training effect was only evident at the longer exposure trials, indicating that differential bias was not preconscious. Furthermore, attentional training had no immediate effect on mood, although after the anagram stress students trained to attend away from negative information showed significantly lower elevations in negative mood. The authors concluded that *attentional threat avoidance training* may reduce vulnerability for negative emotional response to stress.

In a second replication study all training trials were conducted at a longer exposure interval and emotional reactivity to stress was assessed before and after attentional training (MacLeod et al., 2002). Analysis revealed that a differential training effect was again achieved and that attentional training away from negative stimuli resulted in no negative emotional response to the anagram stressor, whereas the group that had negative attentional training showed a pronounced negative emotional response to the stressor. These differential effects were due to training because at baseline the groups did not differ in showing elevations in negative mood to a preinduction baseline anagram task. The authors concluded that attentional training modified the degree of emotional response to a subsequent stressor. Thus the training had its greatest impact not on mood directly but rather on affecting emotional vulnerability to stress.

Of greatest relevance to Hypothesis 12 are a series of published studies on interpretative bias training. Grey and Mathews (2000) first investigated whether interpretative bias for threat could be trained in volunteers with normal trait anxiety scores. Individuals were randomly assigned to a threatening or a nonthreatening homograph training condition in which volunteers were trained to complete a word fragment with a threatening or nonthreatening homograph. In the first experiment, Grey and Mathews (2000) found that threat training resulted in faster response for generating threat solutions on 20 critical test items, and the biasing effect of threat training was found to generalize to a lexical decision task in two further experiments. In a final study that included an untrained control group, individuals exposed to homograph threat training showed faster lexical decision for threat than the baseline group. These studies, then, demonstrated that an interpretative threat bias for ambiguous stimuli can be trained in nonvulnerable individuals.

Mathews and Mackintosh (2000) conducted five experiments in which interpretative bias training involved making a negative (threatening) or positive (nonthreatening) interpretation to a short description of an ambiguous social situation. Sixty-four descriptions were presented with each one followed by a word fragment that matched a threatening or nonthreatening interpretation. In the first experiment, volunteers randomly assigned to interpretative threat training were faster at completing negative probe word fragments and gave higher recognition ratings to threatening interpretations of the ambiguous descriptions. Furthermore, there was a direct effect on mood, with the threat group reporting an increase in anxiety after training, although this mood effect was not replicated in the second experiment. In the fourth experiment interpretative threat training did result in an increase in state anxiety but its effects were shown to dissipate rather rapidly. The final experiment demonstrated that induced bias for threat will lead to an increase in anxiety only when it is activated by generating personally threatening meanings. The authors conclude that their results provide direct experimental evidence that activation of threat interpretation bias plays a causal role in anxiety.

In a more recent study Wilson et al. (2006) used the homograph interpretative bias induction of Grey and Mathews (2000) and randomly assigned 48 nonanxious students to a threat or nonthreat training condition. Analysis revealed the expected differential interpretation bias with training but no direct effect on depressed or anxious mood. However, interpretation bias did have a significant impact on emotional reactivity to four stressful video clips with the threat-trained group showing an elevation in state anxiety in response to the stressor. The authors concluded that threat interpretation bias can make "a causal contribution to anxiety reactivity" (Wilson et al., 2006, p. 109).

Yiend, Mackintosh, and Mathews (2005) used the text-based ambiguous social scenarios from Mathews and Mackintosh (2000) to demonstrate that the induction of a threat interpretation bias can endure over at least 24 hours but, like previous studies, there was no significant direct effect on state anxiety. In another study Mackintosh, Mathews, Yiend, Ridgeway, and Cook (2006) again found that induced interpretation bias endured over a 24-hour time period and survived changes in environmental context between training and testing. This enduring effect of induction training was replicated in a second experiment using text-based scenarios involving potential physical threat. Furthermore, individuals with the negative interpretation training showed the largest increases in state anxiety after viewing stressful accident video clips a day after training. However, a replication study of Mathews and Mackintosh (2000) failed to find that the effects of interpretative bias training generalized to indices of interpretative processing that differed from the training task, although they did find that negatively trained individuals had significant increases in state anxiety (Salemink et al., 2007a). A second experiment, however, produced negative results, with positive and negative interpretative bias training having no significant effect on state anxiety or emotional reactivity to stress (Salemink et al., 2007b). Together these results indicate that interpretative training effects can endure over time and across differing environmental and possibly stimulus contexts, and that changes in emotional reactivity due to training may also have some measure of durability.

In a special issue of the *Journal of Abnormal Psychology* a series of studies based on cognitive bias training demonstrated that significant therapeutic benefits could be achieved from directly training anxious individuals to generate benign or positive interpretations to emotionally ambiguous material, or to selectively attend to nonthreatening stimuli; the procedures were labeled *cognitive bias modification* (for a discussion see MacLeod, Koster & Fox, 2009). Four studies are of particular relevance in demonstrating the causal status of threat bias. In the first study nonclinical students who were trained over several days to selectively avoid emotionally negative or threatening words using a home-based dot probe program had significantly lower trait anxiety scores and weakened stress reactivity to a naturalistic stressor encountered 48 hours after training than a no-train control group (MacLeod & Bridle, 2009).

In a second study high worriers trained to access benign meanings to threat-related homographs and emotionally ambiguous scenarios had significantly fewer negative thought intrusions and less anxiety during a focused breathing task than the no-training control group (Hirsch, Hayes, & Mathews, 2009). In two final studies involving attentional training using a dot probe task, individuals with GAD trained to selectively attend to neutral words had a significant decrease in attentional threat bias and anxiety symptoms (Amir, Beard, Burns, & Bomyea, 2009), and in a second similar study socially anxious participants trained to disengage from negative social cues also reported significantly greater reductions in social anxiety and trait anxiety than the no-training control group (Schmidt, Richey, Buckner, & Timpano, 2009). Together these studies indicate that cognitive bias training may be effective in reducing anxiety, which provides further support for a causal basis to threat bias in anxiety.

Summary

There is relatively little research on cognitive vulnerability to anxiety that has employed self-report questionnaires of dysfunctional beliefs about threat, except for some studies reporting inconsistent findings on enduring beliefs in OCD. However, more recent experimental studies employing different training protocols have demonstrated that a threat interpretation bias can be created in nonanxious individual that may be similar to the selective processing bias for threat that characterizes anxiety. Evidence of some durability over time and transfer of induced processing style to novel stimuli and changes in environmental context suggests that these training effects may be quite robust. However, the causal effects of induced threat interpretation bias on anxiety are not simple. It is apparent that training effects on anxiety are most likely when the induced bias is activated when individuals are required to generate personally threatening meanings (Mathews & Mackintosh, 2000) or, possibly when interpretation bias activates personally threatening imagery (Hirsch, Clark, & Mathews, 2006). Moreover, the mood-congruency effects of induced interpretation bias are most notable with exposure to a stressor. Thus the evidence to date indicates that threat interpretation bias plays a causal role in modifying vulnerability to emotional reactivity. However, this research is still in its infancy and many fundamental questions remain unanswered.

Training in positive interpretation bias may prove to be an effective treatment for clinical anxiety states. Studies on cognitive bias modification have demonstrated significant reductions in anxious symptoms. Mathews et al. (2007) found that training in positive interpretation bias reduced trait anxiety scores. Furthermore, use of imagery during interpretation training might improve training effects as indicated by reductions in state anxiety and increases in positive affect (Holmes, Mathews, Dalgleish, & Mackintosh, 2006; see also Holmes, Arntz, & Smucker, 2007). The current findings, then, are most promising and are our strongest experimental evidence to date that schematic threat activation in the form of interpretative threat bias plays a significant contributory role in anxious reactivity to stress. Moreover, there may be significant therapeutic benefits in reversing the preexisting cognitive bias by training vulnerable individuals to make positive interpretations of ambiguous threat stimuli.

Clinician Guideline 4.5

Deliberate and sustained training in generating positive, nonthreatening interpretations of personally meaningful situations relevant to the client's primary anxious concerns can counter the hypervalent schematic threat activation that characterizes vulnerability to anxiety.

SUMMARY AND CONCLUSION

In this chapter we discussed a number of constructs that have been proposed in the etiology of anxiety disorders. Although various genetic, biological, developmental, and environmental factors have been implicated in the onset of anxiety, it is our contention that individuals can also possess cognitive vulnerability for anxiety. As depicted in Figure 4.1, the cognitive model recognizes that genetic predisposition, biological determinants, childhood experiences, and aversive life events all play a significant role in the etiology of an anxiety disorder. At the same time, however, general cognitive-personality factors interact with more specific enduring cognitive structures as contributory pathways to the expression of anxiety.

At the more general level the cognitive model recognizes that certain personality characteristics such as high negative emotionality or elevated trait anxiety are nonspecific vulnerability factors in anxiety. There is now considerable empirical evidence that nonclinical high trait-anxious individuals exhibit a propensity for a threat-related information-processing bias that is similar to that seen in the anxiety disorders, especially when induced by training or activated by a stressor (e.g., see review by MacLeod et al., 2004). High NA has been implicated in the etiology of both anxiety and depression. However, it is at the more specific level that we see contributory factors that have even more relevance for anxiety. An extensive literature now exists on the etiological role of anxiety sensitivity and while perceived uncontrollability is clearly involved in the pathogenesis of anxiety, it is doubtful its influence is limited to the anxiety disorders.

The remainder of the chapter discussed evidence for the final two hypotheses of the cognitive model. There is emerging evidence that enduring beliefs or schemas about threat and personal vulnerability are predisposing factors to anxiety. Although research on a cognitive vulnerability model of anxiety is still in its infancy, considerable progress has been made in the last few years in demonstrating the causal status of an information-processing bias for threat in anxiety. We are only beginning to see how this cognitive vulnerability research might lead to better treatments for the anxiety disorders.

PART II

COGNITIVE THERAPY OF ANXIETY
Assessment and Intervention Strategies

The reformulated generic cognitive model of anxiety presented in Part I provides a framework for assessment and case formulation as well as for cognitive and behavioral approaches to intervention that are common across the anxiety disorders. In this sense cognitive therapy is transdiagnostic, targeting maladaptive cognitive structures and processes that are common across the various subtypes of anxiety. The chapters in this part of the book provide detailed, step-by-step instructions for basic cognitive assessment and treatment approaches that are relevant to all forms of anxious symptom presentation. Chapter 5 discusses standardized measures for assessing general anxiety as well as a framework and case illustration for developing a cognitive case formulation for anxiety. Chapter 6 explains how to implement cognitive intervention strategies like education, self-monitoring, cognitive restructuring, and generating alternatives to modify the exaggerated threat and vulnerability appraisals and beliefs in anxiety disorders. Chapter 7 focuses on the critical role played by behavioral interventions such as exposure, response prevention, and directed behavioral change in cognitive therapy for anxiety disorders. Together these chapters provide basic instruction in how to implement core cognitive and behavioral intervention strategies that provide the scaffolding for the disorder-specific cognitive therapy discussed in Part III.

Cognitive Assessment and Case Formulation

> Our Age of Anxiety is, in great part, the result of trying to do today's jobs with yesterday's tools.
> —MARSHALL MCLUHAN (Canadian academic and author, 1911–1980)

Sharon is a 52-year-old single woman who worked as an information technology consultant for a large advertising firm. She had been employed with this firm for 10 years, and her job involved daily contact with a large number of employees who requested her assistance whenever they experienced problems with their computers. Thus her job required many daily one-to-one interactions with individuals at their workstations dealing with their computer and network problems as well as meetings with senior managers whenever there were questions about information technology.

Sharon decided to finally seek treatment for what she described as a "life-long struggle with anxiety." She indicated that her main problem was heightened anxiety whenever she engaged in social interaction with work colleagues. She reported only mild anxiety outside the work setting and so never before considered treatment until 6 months ago when she experienced a significant increase in her work setting anxiety level. She declined pharmacotherapy from her family physician and instead agreed to see a psychologist for psychotherapy. Before offering Sharon a course of cognitive therapy, there were a number of questions about her anxiety that needed to be addressed. What was the nature of her anxiety disorder and what were her primary anxiety symptoms? What external or internal cues triggered her anxiety? What were her automatic anxious thoughts and exaggerated appraisals of threat and personal vulnerability? Was she highly intolerant of anxiety and hypervigilant for certain symptoms of anxiety? How did she try to cope with her heightened anxiety? Were worry and avoidance prominent responses to anxiety? How did she interpret her failure to control anxiety? These are a few of the questions that were addressed during Sharon's assessment sessions that led to an individualized cognitive case formulation that is presented at the end of this chapter.

Assessment and case formulation stand as a bridge between cognitive theory and treatment. Since its earliest inception cognitive therapy has emphasized the importance of theory-guided assessment as the foundation for effective psychotherapy. In the first published cognitive therapy manual, Beck, Rush, Shaw, and Emery (1979) emphasized that diagnostic formulation, establishing treatment goals, educating the client into the cognitive model, and selecting target symptoms were critical elements in treatment for depression.

The tools of assessment and case formulation that are now available to the cognitive therapist are much more precise than those available in the early years of cognitive therapy. For example J. S. Beck (1995, 2005) developed a more detailed and refined cognitive case conceptualization scheme that can be applied to the anxiety disorders. She argues for the importance of conceptualization as a guide for focusing therapy on the critical problems and processes that underlie a psychological disturbance. Often treatment failure in difficult cases can be traced to a misguided or incomplete case conceptualization (J. S. Beck, 2005). Persons and colleagues (Persons, 1989; Persons & Davidson, 2001) provided one of the most comprehensive models for case formulation, emphasizing its individualized, theory-driven, and hypothesis-generating nature. Cognitive-behavioral treatment protocols for specific anxiety disorders like panic (S. Taylor, 2000), social phobia (Elting & Hope, 1995), GAD (Turk, Heimberg, & Mennin, 2004; Wells, 1997) and OCD (D. A. Clark, 2004) again emphasize the important role played by cognitive assessment and case formulation.

In this chapter we present a case formulation scheme for anxiety based on the cognitive model (see Figure 2.1). A general framework for cognitive case conceptualization is described that can be applied to all anxiety disorders. Precise applications of this case conceptualization scheme will be considered within the disorder-specific chapters. The first section of the chapter reviews diagnostic and general anxiety symptom measures that are an important assessment tool in cognitive therapy of anxiety. This will be followed by a discussion of the assessment of immediate fear activation (Phase I) and its sequelae. A third section focuses on assessment of secondary, elaborative processes that lead to a reappraisal of threat and personal vulnerability. The chapter concludes with a case illustration of cognitive formulation of anxiety and a consideration of difficulties that can arise at this stage of treatment.

DIAGNOSTIC AND SYMPTOM ASSESSMENT

The first two or three contact sessions should focus on assessment that leads to a preliminary case formulation. Figure 5.1 illustrates a three-pronged approach to assessment that will be present during the initial phase of cognitive therapy for anxiety.

Diagnostic Interviews

The diagnostic interview has always played an important role in cognitive therapy. Beck et al. (1979) argued that a complete diagnostic evaluation is essential for establishing symptom targets and treatment planning. Although clinicians are divided on the importance of differential diagnosis in psychotherapy, there is no debate that critical clinical

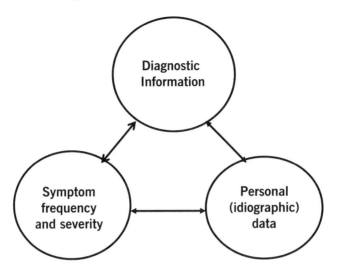

FIGURE 5.1. Three aspects of assessment for anxiety.

information is obtained in the course of conducting a diagnostic interview. A diagnostic interview is important to case conceptualization and treatment planning because:

- It provides detailed information on the presenting symptom typology, frequency, and severity.
- Key cognitive processes in the anxiety disorders are often assessed.
- Situational triggers and coping strategies, especially avoidance responses, are evaluated.
- Level of distress and impact on daily functioning is determined.
- Precipitating factors, symptom development, and course are delineated.
- Competing symptoms and other psychological processes that might complicate treatment are identified.

Two key questions must be settled before conducting a diagnostic assessment in cognitive therapy. Is it really necessary to spend the extra time doing a structured or semistructured clinical interview, or would a traditional unstructured interview suffice? Which is the best structured diagnostic for the anxiety disorders? Experts agree that structured or semistructured interviews must be used to establish diagnostic status in clinical research (Antony & Rowa, 2005). This is because structured interviews are significantly more accurate in determining a valid diagnosis than unstructured clinical interviews (Miller, Dasher, Collins, Griffiths, & Brown, 2001), and they have greater interrater reliability (Miller, 2001). Miller (2002) determined that the diagnostic imprecision of traditional unstructured clinical interviews was in large part due to incomplete data collection. Because semistructured interviews force the clinician to assess all key diagnostic symptoms, this error in data collection is overcome.

Despite the diagnostic superiority of semistructured interviews, they are rarely used in clinical practice (Antony & Rowa, 2005). This is because semistructured interviews can take upwards of 2 hours to administer, they require some degree of training, and the published booklets can be quite costly. Nevertheless, we believe that the wealth of information obtained from an interview like the Anxiety Disorders Interview Schedule for DSM-IV (ADIS-IV) or the Structured Clinical Interview for DSM-IV Axis I Disorders (SCID-IV) justifies the investment in clinical resources (see Miller, 2002, for cost–benefit analysis).

Although a fairly wide selection of interviews is available to the clinician, the ADIS-IV (Brown, Di Nardo, & Barlow, 1994) and SCID-IV (First, Spitzer, Gibbon, & Williams, 1997) have become the most widely used interviews in North America. Both are clinician-administered, semistructured interviews designed to make a differential diagnosis based on DSM-IV-TR criteria (APA, 2000). The SCID for Axis I has a published clinician version (SCID-CV) that covers the DSM-IV-TR diagnoses most commonly seen in clinical practice, whereas the unpublished research version (SCID-RV) is much longer and includes numerous diagnostic subtypes and course specifiers (First et al., 1997). Summerfeldt and Antony (2002) concluded that the SCID is superior in its breadth of diagnostic coverage and there is evidence of good interrater reliability for many of the most common diagnostic disorders (Williams et al., 1992; Riskind, Beck, Berchick, Brown, & Steer, 1987). However the SCID-CV provides only a brief symptom screener for certain anxiety disorders like specific phobia, GAD, social phobia, and agoraphobia without a history of panic disorder while failing to assess past history of other disorders. In order to obtain an accurate diagnosis of specific anxiety disorders, the SCID-CV must be supplemented with additional symptom questions from the SCID-RV. The addition of dimensional severity ratings on situational triggers is also recommended in order to provide important clinical data on the specific anxiety disorders (Summerfeldt & Antony, 2002).

The best diagnostic interview for the anxiety disorders is the ADIS-IV. Although the ADIS-IV has current and lifetime versions available for adults, the current version will be of most relevance in clinical practice. It includes sections on each of the anxiety disorders as well as highly comorbid conditions (e.g., mood disorders, hypochondriasis, alcohol/drug abuse or dependence). In each of the anxiety disorder sections, severity and distress ratings are obtained on specific symptoms, and the Hamilton Rating Scale of Anxiety (HRSA; Hamilton, 1959) and Hamilton Rating Scale of Depression (HRSD; Hamilton, 1960) are included so that the scales can be administered during the interview. Although the ADIS-IV covers all the key diagnostic criteria for the anxiety disorders, it goes well beyond DSM-IV-TR by providing information on psychopathological phenomena that are targeted in interventions for anxiety (e.g., partial symptom expression, avoidance, situational triggers, and apprehension).

The ADIS-IV has high interrater reliability for the DSM-IV-TR anxiety and mood disorders (see review by Summerfeldt & Antony, 2002). Brown and Barlow (2002) reported that the ADIS-IV current or lifetimes versions had good to excellent interrater agreement for principal diagnoses based on a clinical sample of 362 outpatients (see also Brown, Di Nardo, Lehman, & Campbell, 2001). Kappas for two independent interviews conducted within a 2-week interval ranged from .67 for GAD to .86 for specific phobia. The most common source of disagreement among the interviewers involved whether a case met threshold criteria for a particular anxiety disorder as well as information variance across interviews (i.e., patients giving different information to the interviewers). Summerfeldt and Antony (2002) noted that although the ADIS-IV provides more detailed information and dimensional ratings of anxious symptoms, it is more time-consuming and assesses a narrower range of disorders. The ADIS-IV can be purchased from Oxford University Press/Graywind Publications.

Clinician Guideline 5.1

Administer the ADIS-IV current version prior to implementing a course of cognitive therapy for anxiety. The ADIS-IV provides a precise diagnosis and crucial symptom data for the five anxiety disorders discussed in this volume.

Symptom Measures

A number of standardized self-report questionnaires and clinician rating scales are available to assess the frequency and severity of anxious symptoms. Here we focus on broadly based, general measures of anxiety with disorder-specific measures covered in later chapters. Standardized measures of general anxiety symptoms are useful because they provide:

- A broad overview or screening of various anxious symptoms.
- A measure of symptom severity that is important for evaluating treatment effectiveness.
- Access to normative data so that the relative severity of an anxiety state can be determined.
- Opportunity for repeated administration over the course of treatment so that progress can be charted and symptom clusters identified that have been unresponsive to treatment.

Over the years a variety of general anxiety measures have been developed. The following section presents a few measures that we believe are most relevant for cognitive therapy of anxiety. A more comprehensive review of anxiety measures is provided in an edited book by Antony, Orsillo, and Roemer (2001).

Beck Anxiety Inventory

The Beck Anxiety Inventory (BAI; Beck & Steer, 1990) is a 21-item questionnaire that assesses the severity of anxious symptoms on a 0 ("not at all") to 3 ("severely, I could barely stand it") scale. According to the manual (Beck & Steer, 1990), the normal range for the BAI Total Score is 0–9, mild anxiety is 10–18, moderate severity is 19–29, and severe anxiety ranges from 30 to 63. Psychometric studies indicate that the BAI has high internal consistency (alpha = .92) and a 1-week test–retest reliability of .75 (Beck, Epstein, Brown, & Steer, 1988; Steer, Ranieri, Beck, & Clark, 1993). The BAI Total Score correlates moderately with other anxious symptom measures like the Hamilton Rating Scale of Anxiety—Revised, State–Trait Anxiety Inventory, and weekly diary ratings of anxiety, and patients with anxiety disorders score significantly higher than those with other psychiatric diagnoses (Beck et al., 1988; Creamer, Foran, & Bell, 1995; Fydrich, Dowdall, & Chambless, 1992; Steer et al., 1993). As reported in the manual

(Beck & Steer, 1990), the BAI Total Score means and standard deviations for various diagnostic groups are as follows: panic disorder with agoraphobia (M = 27.27, SD = 13.11), social phobia (M = 17.77, SD = 11.64), OCD (M = 21.69, SD = 12.42), GAD (M = 18.83, SD = 9.08), and primary depressive disorder (M = 17.80, SD = 12.20).[1] Factor analyses indicate that the questionnaire is multidimensional with either a two or a four factor structure (e.g., Creamer et al., 1995; Hewitt & Norton, 1993; Steer et al., 1993). However, only one-quarter of the items assess the subjective or more cognitive aspects of anxiety (e.g., fear of the worst, unable to relax, terrified, nervous, scared) with the remainder assessing the physiological hyperarousal symptoms of anxiety. Thus the BAI is a good measure of the physical aspects of anxiety (especially panic disorder) and it is sensitive to treatment effects, although like most anxiety measures it correlates highly with self-report depression instruments (e.g., D. A. Clark, Steer, & Beck, 1994). The BAI is available from Pearson Assessment at *pearsonassess.com*.

Hamilton Rating Scale of Anxiety

The Hamilton Rating Scale of Anxiety (HRSA; Guy, 1976; Hamilton, 1959) is a 14-item clinician rating scale that assesses the severity of predominantly biological and behavioral symptoms of anxiety. Each symptom is rated on a severity scale from 0 ("not present") to 4 ("very severe/incapacitating") with symptomatic descriptions for each item. A cut-off score of 14 on the HRSA Total Scale differentiates individuals with an anxiety disorder from those with no current diagnosis (Kobak, Reynolds, & Greist, 1993). The HRSA Total Score has good internal consistency, interrater reliability, and 1-week test–retest reliability, and it has strong convergent and discriminant validity as well as sensitivity to treatment (Maier, Buller, Philipp, & Heuser, 1988; Moras, Di Nardo, & Barlow, 1992; see review by Roemer, 2001). However, the majority of individuals with major depression score above the cut-off score so the instrument does not accurately discriminate anxiety from depression (Kobak et al., 1993). Given that some training is required for the HRSA, the measure could be reserved for cases where a self-assessment of anxiety might be highly inaccurate (i.e., individuals who minimize or exaggerate their anxiety). A copy of the HRSA can be found in Appendix B of Antony et al. (2001) or in the appendix of the ADIS-IV.

Depression Anxiety Stress Scale

The Depression Anxiety Stress Scale (DASS; Lovibond & Lovibond, 1995a, 1995b) is a 42-item questionnaire with 14 items each assessing the severity of anxiety, depression, and stress. The anxiety subscale assesses autonomic arousal, skeletal musculature, situational, and subjective aspects of anxiety. For the DASS Anxiety Scale, 0–7 represents the normal range, 8–9 is mild anxiety, 10–14 is moderate, 15–19 is severe, and 20+ is extremely severe (see Lovibond & Lovibond, 1995b). The subscale has good internal consistency, temporal reliability, and convergent validity (Antony, Bieling, Cox, Enns, & Swinson, 1998a; Brown, Chorpita, Korotitsch, & Barlow, 1997;

---

[1] The BAI Total Score mean for the primary depressive disorder group (major depression, dysthymia, and adjustment disorder with depressed mood) was derived from an intake data set (N = 293) from the Center for Cognitive Therapy, University of Pennsylvania Medical School, that was available to the first author.

Lovibond & Lovibond, 1995a). For example, DASS Anxiety correlates .81 with the BAI and DASS Depression correlates .74 with the BDI in student samples (Lovibond & Lovibond, 1995b). In addition, individuals with panic disorder score significantly higher on DASS Anxiety than patients with major depression but those with OCD, social phobia, GAD, and simple phobia do not score higher than the major depression group (Antony, Bieling, et al., 1998; Brown et al., 1997). A shorter 21-item version of the DASS was developed by Antony, Bieling, and colleagues (1998) and has psychometric characteristics comparable to the original 42-item DASS. Although DASS Anxiety and Depression are moderately correlated (r's ~ .45) in clinical samples and DASS Anxiety has a predominant emphasis on autonomic arousal and fear (Antony, Bieling, et al., 1998; Brown et al., 1997), it is a promising measure. The DASS-42 is available in Appendix B of Antony et al. (2001) or it can be downloaded directly from *www.psy.unsw.edu.au/dass*. The manual and scoring template can be ordered from the same website.

State–Trait Anxiety Inventory

The State–Trait Anxiety Inventory (STAI—Form Y; Spielberger, Gorsuch, Lushene, Vagg, & Jacobs, 1983) consists of two 20-item scales with one scale assessing state anxiety ("how you feel *right* now, that is, *at this moment*") and the other measuring trait anxiety ("how you *generally* feel"). With its emphasis on current state, the STAI State scale has greater clinical relevance for tracking the effectiveness of cognitive therapy. Although the STAI has good reliability and convergent validity with other anxiety measures, its ability to distinguish anxiety from depression has been questioned (Roemer, 2001). For this reason we believe there are other anxiety symptom measures that provide a clearer assessment for the cognitive therapist. The STAI—Form Y can be purchased from Consulting Psychologists Press, Inc.

Cognitions Checklist

The Cognitions Checklist (CCL; Beck, Brown, Steer, Eidelson, & Riskind, 1987) comprises a 12-item anxiety subscale (CCL-A) and a 14-item depression subscale (CCL-D) that assesses the frequency of negative self-referent anxious and depressive thoughts along a 5-point scale ranging from 0 ("never") to 4 ("always"). The content of CCL-A revolves around themes of uncertainty and an orientation toward the future (Beck et al., 1987), with the majority of items (71%) focused on anxious thinking about physical or health-related concerns. Both subscales have good internal consistency, and factor analyses reveal the expected loadings of CCL items on separate anxiety and depression dimensions, especially in clinical samples (Beck et al., 1987; Steer, Beck, Clark, & Beck, 1994). Although CCL-A and CCL-D are moderately correlated, each subscale is more highly correlated with its congruent than incongruent symptom state (Beck et al., 1987; D. A. Clark et al., 1996; Steer et al., 1994). In clinical practice the CCL-A provides an estimate of the frequency of anxious thoughts, especially the physical or health concerns of most relevance to panic disorder. Individuals with anxiety disorders typically score in the midteens or higher on CCLA (Steer et al., 1994). A copy of the CCL can be obtained from the Center for Cognitive Therapy, Department of Psychiatry, University of Pennsylvania Medical School, Philadelphia, PA.

Penn State Worry Questionnaire

The Penn State Worry Questionnaire (PSWQ; Meyer, Miller, Metzger, & Borkovec, 1990) is a 16-item trait measure that assesses the propensity to worry as well as the intensity of worry experiences without reference to specific worry topics (Molina & Borkovec, 1994). The items are rated on a 5-point Likert scale from 1 ("not at all typical") to 5 ("very typical"), with items 1, 3, 8, 10, and 11 reverse scored. Although there is some debate over the factorial structure of the PSWQ (Brown, 2003; Fresco, Heimberg, Mennin, & Turk, 2002), only the Total Score is normally interpreted. The PSWQ has high internal consistency, test–retest reliability, and correlates with other self-report worry measures but it does have lower convergence with measures of general anxiety (Brown, Antony, & Barlow, 1992; Davey, 1993; Meyer et al., 1990; Molina & Borkovec, 1994). Group comparisons indicate that individuals with GAD score highest on the PSWQ, followed by other anxiety disorder groups and major depression who have similar elevated scores that are significantly higher than nonclinical controls (Brown et al., 1992; Chelminski & Zimmerman, 2003). A PSWQ cutoff score of 45 can be used to identify pathological worry or GAD in a treatment-seeking population (Behar, Alcaine, Zuellig, & Borkovec, 2003), although a higher cutoff score (62 or even 65) is needed to differentiate GAD from other anxiety disorders and possibly even depression (e.g., Fresco, Mennin, Heimberg, & Turk, 2003). Given that worry is prominent in most anxiety disorders (and depression), we suggest the PSWQ be included when assessing general anxiety. A copy of the PSWQ can be found in Molina and Borkovec (1994) or Appendix B of Antony et al. (2001).

Daily Mood Rating

In clinical practice daily idiographic ratings of general anxiety level can be a very useful metric for tracking fluctuations in subjective anxiety. For example, Craske and Barlow (2006) suggest that individuals complete a Daily Mood Record in which overall anxiety, maximum anxiety, overall physical tension, and preoccupation with worry are rated on a 0 (none) to 100 (extreme) scale at the end of each day. This can be augmented with single ratings on more specific symptom dimensions that may be more indicative of the person's particular anxiety disorder such as ratings on average worry about having a panic attack in panic disorder or mean daily social evaluative anxiety in social phobia. It is important that the cognitive therapist also assess changes in general anxiety as part of an evaluation of treatment effectiveness and for identifying situations that trigger anxiety. These data can be useful for suggesting issues that need to be addressed in therapy. We have found a 0 to 100 single scale most helpful in capturing the day-to-day changes in general anxiety (see Figure 5.2).

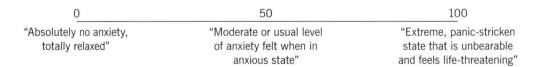

FIGURE 5.2. Daily mood rating scale.

This rating scale has been incorporated into a daily situation record form (see Appendix 5.1) that can be used to assess daily fluctuations in general anxiety.

Beck Depression Inventory–II

The Beck Depression Inventory–II (BDI-II; Beck, Steer, & Brown, 1996) is a 21-item questionnaire that assesses the severity of cognitive-affective, behavioral, and somatic symptoms of depression over a 2-week interval. The BDI-II is the third and latest revision of the original BDI that was published by Beck, Ward, Mendelson, Mock, and Erbaugh (1961). The second revision of the BDI (Beck & Steer, 1993) has been used widely in depression research and so most of the psychometric information has been generated on that measure. However, the BDI and BDI-II are highly correlated ($r = .93$; Dozois, Dobson, & Ahnberg, 1998), so the psychometric findings on the BDI are relevant for BDI-II. Although the BDI appears to be mulifactorial, the Total Score is most often used in clinical practice and research (Beck, Steer, & Garbin, 1988). There is extensive research demonstrating the internal reliability and the convergent and discriminant validity of the BDI (see Beck et al., 1988, for review; Tanaka-Matsumi & Kameoka, 1986). Individuals with major depression score significantly higher ($M = 26.52$, $SD = 12.15$) than those with anxiety disorders ($M = 19.38$; $SD = 11.46$; see Beck et al., 1996). The cut-off scores for the BDI-II are 0–13 nondepressed, 14–19 mildly depressed or dysphoric, 20–28 moderately depressed, and 29–63 severely depressed (Beck et al., 1996; see also Dozois et al., 1998). Given the high co-occurrence of depressive symptoms and disorder in those with high anxiety, it is recommended that the BDI-II be included in the standard assessment battery for anxiety. The BDI-II is available from Pearson Assessment at *pearsonassess.com*.

Clinician Guideline 5.2

To assess severity of general anxiety symptoms, administer the BAI, CCL, PSWQ, and daily ratings of average anxiety level. If desired, DASS Anxiety can be included and the HRSA can be used when clients over- or underreport their level of anxiety. The BDI-II should be added to assess level of comorbid depressive symptoms. A complete assessment will also include measures of specific anxiety disorders that are reviewed in subsequent chapters.

FEAR ACTIVATION: ASSESSMENT AND FORMULATION

Based on the cognitive model (see Figure 2.1) in this section we focus on assessment tools that provide critical information needed to develop a case formulation of the immediate fear response and its consequences. Experimental research on the immediate fear response uses information-processing tasks and psychophysiological measures that are not readily available to the therapist. However, the practitioner can use self-report, interview, and behavioral observation methods that rely on conscious, effortful processing in a manner that offers valuable information on a person's immediate fear response.

One of the most basic propositions of cognitive therapy is that schematic content, which is inaccessible to direct observation or detection, can be inferred from conscious, verbal report of one's thoughts, images, daydreams, ruminations, evaluations, and the like. Beck (1967) stated: "The schemas pattern the stream of associations and ruminations as well as the cognitive responses to external stimuli. Hence, the notion of schemas is utilized to account for the repetitive themes in free associations, daydreams, ruminations, and dreams, as well as in the immediate reactions to environmental events" (p. 283). If schemas direct conscious thought, then the differential activation and content of schemas can be inferred from verbal content (see also Kendall & Ingram, 1989). Furthermore, there is a direct link between automatic and elaborative processes as indicated by evidence that changes in conscious appraisal or meaning can modify automatic threat biases (see Mansell, 2000) and that an automatic attentional bias can be induced through an attentional training program that involves both brief and long processing intervals (e.g., Matthews & MacLeod, 2002; MacLeod et al., 2002). Together these considerations lead to the following proposition: *that the nature and function of automatic threat schema activation during the initial fear response can be determined from the cognitive, behavioral, and physiological products of this activation.*

Three primary questions must be addressed in any case formulation of the immediate fear response (Phase I).

- What situations, cues, or experiences trigger the immediate fear response?
- What is the core schematic threat or danger to self?
- What is the immediate inhibitory or defensive response to this threat?

Although standardized questionnaire and interview data can be helpful in building a case formulation, the most critical information will be obtained from idiographic measures. These are self-monitoring forms, rating scales, and diary records that allow the person to collect critical information when experiencing anxiety. They are tailored to the particular needs and circumstance of each client so that process-oriented, "online" data gathering is available that contributes to a more accurate case conceptualization.

Behavioral observation is another assessment approach that can provide important clinical information on immediate fear response. Some anxiety states like social phobia, OCD, and PTSD can be quite easily elicited in the therapy session by introducing relevant triggers of anxiety. Other anxiety disorders like panic and GAD require more ingenuity in order to trigger an immediate fear response. Often the therapist accompanies the client to particular external situations in order to observe an anxious state. In either case, direct observation of a fear response provides opportunity to gather detailed information on the nature, severity, and functional characteristics of the immediate fear response. We believe it is important for the therapist to have at least one opportunity to observe a client's acute anxiety state in order to develop an accurate case formulation and a sensitive individually tailored treatment plan.

Clinician Guideline 5.3

Daily self-monitoring and direct behavioral observation are important assessment strategies that should be a regular feature of any assessment and case formulation of anxiety. Both strategies are critical for determining the nature of immediate fear activation.

Situational Analysis

A cognitive case conceptualization of anxiety must begin with a thorough assessment of the situations, experiences, and cues that trigger anxiety. The cognitive therapist could begin at the most general level by asking about the problems or difficulties that led to a decision to seek treatment. With the anxiety disorders, the development of a Problem List (see Persons & Davidson, 2001) will inevitably lead into a discussion of the situations that trigger anxiety. Three types of situations should be assessed (see also Antony & Rowa, 2005). Table 5.1 presents a number of clinical questions that can be asked in the assessment interview.

Environmental Triggers

Information on the external or internal cues, situations, or experiences that trigger a state of fear or anxiety is a critical part of an evidence-based assessment strategy for the anxiety disorders (Antony & Rowa, 2005). It is important that the cognitive therapist obtain a comprehensive list of anxiety-provoking situations with sufficient detail to fully understand the specific cues that trigger an anxious response. In practically all cases, objects, events, or situations in the external environment can be identified that trigger anxiety. Examples of anxiety-eliciting situations include a variety of social settings or interactions in social phobia, in GAD daily events involving some degree of uncertainty or possibility of negative outcome (e.g., going on a trip, scheduling an appointment, paying bills), or in OCD situations that elicit fear of contamination or doubt would be prominent (e.g., washroom, sitting on park bench). Since a comprehensive knowledge of anxiety-eliciting situations is critical to case formulation, treatment planning, and later exposure interventions, the therapist should complete a broad list of triggering situations that range from the mild to most severe anxiety-arousing triggers.

The cognitive therapist can obtain initial information on environmental triggers from the clinical interview by asking specific questions about the types of situations that elicit anxiety (see Table 5.1). However, most anxious clients have selective and inaccurate recall of their anxiety-provoking situations so daily self-recording forms should be assigned in the early phase of treatment. Appendix 5.2 provides a Situational Analysis Form that can be used to collect key information on provoking situations. In some cases where there has been a long history of avoidance or where the client's self-report may be unreliable, it may be necessary to interview a spouse, close friend, or family member to obtain more complete information on provoking situations. The therapist could accompany the client to particular situations or set a homework assignment that involved exposure to a situation in question in order to assess its anxiety-eliciting properties. However, this might be too threatening for many anxious individuals, especially in the early phase of treatment.

Interoceptive Triggers

Most anxious individuals have a heightened awareness and responsiveness to the bodily sensations that characterize physiological hyperarousal in anxiety. Physiological sensations such as increased heart rate, feeling warm, lightheadedness, weakness, tension, and the like can themselves become triggers for elevated anxiousness. Thus it is impor-

TABLE 5.1. Interview Questions for Assessing Different Types of Situational Triggers in Anxiety

Type of situational triggers	Clinical questions
External situations, settings, objects	• "Have you noticed whether there are certain situations or experiences that are most likely to cause you to become anxious?"
	• "Are there some situations that cause only mild anxiety or occasionally cause you to be anxious and other situations that cause more extreme levels of anxiety?"
	• "Can you tell me about the last time you were in each of these situations and felt anxious." [Therapist probes for a full account of anxiety-provoking situations by obtaining examples from client's immediate past.]
	• "Have you noticed whether there is anything about a situation that might make the anxiety worse?"
	• "Is there anything about a situation that might ease your anxiety?"
	• "How often do you experience these situations in your daily life?"
	• "Do you try to avoid the situation? How much does this interfere in your daily life?"
Interoceptive (physical) cues	• "When you are in an anxious situation, have you noticed any changes in how you feel physically?" [Therapist could mention a few of the most common signs of hyperarousal if client needs prompting.]
	• "Have you noticed whether any of these physical sensations occur before you start feeling anxious?"
	• "How often do you get these physical sensations when you're anxious? Are some always present whereas others are only present occasionally?"
	• "Which of the physical sensations is felt most strongly when you are anxious? Which of the sensations do you notice first when you're anxious?"
	• "Have you noticed whether you feel more anxious once you are aware of a physical sensation?" [e.g., client might feel more anxious about sudden increases in heart rate.]
	• "Have you ever had the physical sensation (e.g., chest pain) occur unexpectedly when you were not anxious? Can you recall an example of when this happened? How did you feel after noticing the sensation?"
	• "Do you take special precautions to ensure that you don't experience a particular physical sensation?" [e.g., client might avoid time pressures because wants to maintain state of calm and avoid feeling tense.]
Cognitive cues	• "Have you ever had a thought, image, or impulse about something quite weird, unexpected, even disturbing, suddenly pop into your mind?" [Therapist might have to give examples or provide client with a list of common unwanted intrusions to prompt self-report of intrusions.]
	• "When you are entering an anxious situation [therapist states specific situations], do you recall having any sudden thoughts or images pop into your mind?"
	• "Do any of these unexpected intrusive thoughts involve things that are totally out of your character or that would cause you considerable embarrassment or dreaded consequences?"
	• "How upset do these thoughts make you feel?"
	• "Have you ever felt concerned that something might be wrong with you or that something bad could happen because of the intrusive thought, image, or impulse?"

tant to determine if there are any particular bodily sensations that make clients feel more anxious. Although interoceptive cues to anxiety are particularly evident in panic, they will be present in all of the anxiety disorders (Antony & Rowa, 2005). For example, a person with social phobia might become even more anxious in a social setting if she begins to feel warm because this is interpreted as a sign of increased anxiety that might be noticed by others.

The therapist should include questions in the clinical interview about interoceptive cues (see Table 5.1), but many clients have even less insight into the presence of physical triggers to anxiety than they do to external cues. A self-monitoring checklist of physical sensations, such as the form in Appendix 5.3, can be assigned as homework in order to gather more accurate information on interoceptive triggers. An interoceptive exposure test is another useful strategy for assessing the physical triggers of anxiety. Taylor (2000) describes a number of exercises that can be used in the therapy session to induce physical sensations. For example, the client can be asked to breathe through a straw or jog on the spot to induce chest tightness, to tense muscles to induce trembling/shaking, or to face a heater to feel bodily sensations of warmth. Although the intentional induction of such sensations can not be equated with the spontaneous occurrence of these sensations *in vivo*, they give the therapist an opportunity to directly observe the client's reaction to the sensations.

Cognitive Triggers

Unwanted and disturbing intrusive thoughts, images, or impulses are an example of a cognition that can trigger anxiety. Practically everyone experiences unwanted mental intrusions and they are commonly found in all the anxiety disorders. First described by Rachman (1981) within the context of OCD, unwanted intrusive thoughts, images, or impulses are "any distinct, identifiable cognitive event that is unwanted, unintended, and recurrent. It interrupts the flow of thought, interferes in task performance, is associated with negative affect, and is difficult to control" (Clark & Rhyno, 2005, p. 4). Some examples of common intrusions are "unprovoked doubt about locking the door when I know I did," "touching something gross and dirty that is lying on the street," "saying an insulting or embarrassing remark for no apparent reason," "blurting out an obscenity in a public meeting," "swerving your car into oncoming traffic," and the like. Unwanted intrusions are very common in OCD as obsessions and in PTSD as sudden recollections of a past trauma. However, they can also occur in GAD as a negative consequence of excessive worry (Wells, 2005a) or as unwanted cognitions in the presleep phase of individuals suffering from insomnia (Harvey, 2005). Unwanted intrusions often involve the theme of losing control that leads to a dreaded negative consequence.

It is important that the cognitive therapist inquire about unwanted intrusive thoughts. Table 5.1 lists some possible questions for assessing this clinical phenomenon. With the exception of OCD or PTSD, individuals are often not very aware of their intrusive thoughts. A list of common unwanted intrusions can be used and clients asked if they ever had any of these thoughts, images, or impulses (lists can be found in D. A. Clark, 2004; Rachman & de Silva, 1978; Steketee & Barlow, 2002). Since most intrusions are provoked by external cues, clients can be asked to be especially vigilant for mental intrusions when in situations that typify their anxious concerns.

Elements of a Complete Situational Analysis

A thorough situational analysis should consist of the following elements:

- Detailed description of multiple situations or triggers
- Intensity of associated anxiety
- Frequency and duration of exposure to situation/trigger
- Presence of escape, avoidance responses
- Specific eliciting cues

A *detailed description* of each situation or trigger is needed. Subtle changes in context can alter the intensity of anxiety. For example, a patient with panic disorder might report little anxiety driving to work on a very familiar route. However, vary the route by one new street, and anxiety level might change dramatically. The proximity of a safety signal will also influence anxiety (e.g., presence of a trusted friend or distance from a medical facility). It may be that a particular situation (e.g., interacting with work colleagues) needs to be broken down into finer gradients in order to understand its anxiety-eliciting properties. The cognitive therapist should have enough detail about each anxiety-provoking situation or trigger so that accurate exposure assignments can be constructed.

It is important to know the *intensity of anxiety* felt in each situation since the therapist should have a range of situations or triggers that elicit mild to severe anxiety states. Some clients require considerable practice using the 0–100 rating scale to gauge their anxiety level, especially if they tend to engage in dichotomous thinking (e.g., they feel intensely anxious or not anxious at all). These ratings, however, are needed to develop an effective treatment plan.

The therapist must determine *how often* the person experiences an anxiety-provoking situation and *the duration* of his or her exposure to the situation. Anxiety-provoking situations that occur regularly in the person's daily life will be more helpful for treatment than rare or exceptional occasions. For example, daily social interactions with work colleagues that trigger anxiety in someone with social phobia will be much more important to treatment than a situation such as giving a speech that may rarely occur in the person's life. Also, does the provoking situation involve brief or prolonged exposure when the person encounters the circumstance? Again anxiety-provoking situations that involve longer exposure intervals (e.g., using a public washroom) will be more useful in treatment planning than triggers involving brief exposure (e.g., touching a public telephone as you walk by it).

The cognitive therapist should also obtain information on the extent that each situation is associated with *escape or avoidance*. Clients should be asked if they always try to avoid the situation or escape from the situation as quickly as possible. At this assessment stage the therapist should have a good understanding of how well the client tolerates anxiety in each provoking situation. If the situation is avoided on some occasions but not others, what determines the presence or absence of avoidance? Does this depend on the person's mood state or some subtle characteristic of the situation? Information on escape and avoidance will be critical in planning an exposure hierarchy.

Finally, the cognitive therapist should determine whether there are *specific cues or stimuli in a situation* that are first noticed by the anxious individual. For example, when a person with fear of contamination first enters a public area, what is first noticed that elicits some concern, the speck of dirt on the floor or the fact that a stranger just brushed past him? For a socially anxious individual, does he first notice that his throat feels dry or that his hand seems to be shaking? A person with PTSD might avoid a particular route to work because of anxiety but it is really the fact that driving past a particular ethnic store along the route triggers flashbacks that is the crux of the problem. In addition it is important to determine whether the person is hypervigilant for these subtle and specific anxiety-provoking cues. It is likely that a self-monitoring homework assignment will be needed in order to identify the salient attentional features of anxiety-provoking situations.

Clinician Guideline 5.4

A complete situational analysis should include detailed information on a wide range of anxiety-provoking external and internal situations or stimuli, with a specific focus on the intensity of anxiety, frequency, and duration of situational exposure, extent of escape/avoidance, and presence of eliciting cues.

The First Apprehensive Thoughts or Images

One of the main consequences of threat schema activation during the immediate fear response phase is the production of automatic threat-oriented thoughts and images (see Figure 2.1). These threat-oriented automatic thoughts and images occur at the earliest point in anxiety generation and provide a window into the schematic content that is the basis of the anxiety disorder.

In the context of assessment the cognitive therapist can refer to these initial threat-oriented automatic thoughts as *the first apprehensive thoughts*. They are defined as *brief, sudden, and completely automatic thoughts or images that something bad or unpleasant is about to happen, or at least could happen, to persons or their valued resources.* In panic disorder these first apprehensive thoughts might refer to the dangers posed by a perceived physical sensation, in social phobia it might be the thought of drawing the attention of others, in OCD it might be of some catastrophe for others as a result of one's action or inaction, in PTSD it could be a sense of losing control and increased personal vulnerability, and in GAD it could be the occurrence of some serious negative life event. Notice that the first apprehensive thoughts always reflect some important aspect of the person's primary anxious concerns. In fact the situational analysis will provide the therapist some clues as to first apprehensive thoughts because of the types of situations that provoke anxiety.

Discovering the client's first apprehensive thoughts presents special challenges for assessment. Often these thoughts are so rapid and transient that the person only experiences them as a sudden feeling of fear or apprehension. The actual automatic thought content is lost because it is quickly replaced by more elaborative, reasoned reappraisal of the situation. So, when the therapist questions clients about their first apprehensive thoughts, what is recalled and reported are the more deliberate reappraisal thoughts that occur in the second phase of anxiety. Clients interviewed when not feeling anxious may dismiss the first apprehensive thoughts as too exaggerated and unrealistic, and so deny they ever occurred during an anxious episode.

So how can the cognitive therapist gain access to this fleeting cognitive content? It is important to introduce the topic of first apprehensive thoughts in a collaborative, exploratory manner. A description of the first apprehensive thoughts should be provided and the client should be warned that it is often difficult to identify these thoughts in the anxiety cycle. Explain that when entering an anxious situation, most people are so focused on how they feel and the details of the situation, that their first apprehensive thoughts are often lost to them. The following example can be used to introduce clients to the concept of *the first apprehensive thoughts*.

"Imagine for a moment that you are walking down a deserted street or country road by yourself and it is getting dark. Suddenly you hear a noise behind you. You immediately stiffen, your heart beats quickly, and you quicken your pace. Why this sudden surge of adrenalin? No doubt you instantly interpret the noise as a danger-ous possibility: 'Could someone be approaching from behind who could cause me harm?' You turn around and there is no one there. Quickly you think to yourself 'No one is there, it must have been the wind, a squirrel, or my imagination.' It is this secondary thought, this reevaluation of the situation, that sticks in your mind. If later I asked you about your walk, you would remember a momentary twinge of fear and the later realization that 'nothing was there.' That first apprehensive thought that triggered the fear 'Is there an attacker behind me?' is lost to recall, instead replaced by your reasoned response to the situation.

"In the last couple of sessions you have described a number of situations that cause you considerable anxiety. In these situations you would have had some initial apprehensive thoughts or images that fueled your fear or anxiety. It may be that now you can't remember what they are because you don't feel threatened at the moment and you are not in an anxiety-provoking situation. However, it is impor-tant to our treatment that we discover the first apprehensive thoughts. We want to know what 'kick-starts' the anxiety. Together, by carefully going over each situa-tion and collecting some further information, we may discover the types of appre-hensive thoughts or images that define your anxious experiences."

The first assessment strategy for identifying the initial apprehensive thoughts is the *clinical interview*. Although individuals often don't remember their initial automatic anxious thoughts, a few specific, well-phrased questions can provide some initial clues to these thoughts. Here are some examples of clinical questions:

- "You indicated that in situation X you feel intensely anxious. For you what would be the worst thing that could happen in this situation? What would be the worst possible outcome? Try to think about the worst consequence without considering whether or not you think it is likely to happen."
- "Is there anything specific about the situation or about how you are feeling that concerns you? What is not quite right for you? What is different from your nor-mal self?"
- "How could the situation change so you feel less concern, less uneasy?"
- "What do you tell yourself to ease your anxiety, to reassure yourself that every-thing will be fine?"

It is important that the first apprehensive thought be recorded in the person's own words and not reflect the therapist's own suggestions. The therapist might probe for a certain type of thought content, but its actual expression should reflect the idiosyncratic concerns of the client. This will ensure that the apprehensive thought content is highly relevant to the specific anxious concerns of the client.

It is also important to remember that even in the same anxiety-provoking situation, people will differ in the focus of their apprehension and so it is important for the therapist to discover each client's unique anxious apprehension. As an example, a client reports intense anxiety about going to a meeting with work colleagues. The first apprehensive thought could be any of the following possibilities:

- "What if I'm asked a question in the meeting that I can't answer? Everyone will think I'm incompetent." (performance evaluation cognition)
- "What if I have to say something and everyone stares at me? This makes me so nervous." (social evaluation cognition)
- "What if my voice trembles when I speak? Everyone will know that I am nervous and wonder what's wrong with me." (social phobia cognition)
- "What if I have a panic attack in the meeting?" (panic disorder cognition)
- "What if I accidentally blurt out an insulting remark?" (OCD cognition)
- "What if I'm not supposed to be at this meeting and everyone wonders why I am there?" (interpersonal acceptance cognition)
- "What if I feel nauseated in the meeting and have to run out and vomit?" (cognition about specific fear of vomiting)
- "I never really know what to say in these meetings and how to chit-chat with others; I really hate this." (social skills deficit cognition)

As can be seen from this example, there are a large number of possible apprehensive thoughts triggered by any anxiety-provoking situation. The purpose of the cognitive assessment is to identify the anxious thought content that is unique to each client.

Self-monitoring homework tasks must be assigned in order to obtain more immediate and accurate assessment of the first apprehensive thoughts or images. The "immediate anxious thoughts" column of the Situational Analysis Form (Appendix 5.2) can be used as an initial attempt to collect self-monitoring data on the first apprehensive thought. Clients must be encouraged to focus on "what is the worst that could happen in this situation" without considering whether it is probable, realistic, or rational. They should be encouraged to write down the automatic threat thoughts while they are in the anxious situation. They can ask themselves "What is so bad about this situation?", "What am I thinking is the worst that could happen?," or "What could harm me in this situation?". If a more detailed self-monitoring form is needed, the Apprehensive Thoughts Self-Monitoring Form can be used (see Appendix 5.4).

Imagery or role plays can be used in the therapy session to determine individuals' apprehensive cognitions in anxious situations. In fact anxious patients often have conscious fantasies or images of physical or psychosocial harm that can elicit intense subjective feelings of anxiety (Beck et al., 1974). It is important, then, that the therapist determine whether the initial apprehension may take the form of an intrusive image such as reliving a traumatic event. Whatever the case, the client can be asked to imagine a recent anxiety-provoking situation or the therapist and client could role-play the situation in order to elicit automatic anxious thoughts or images. Throughout, the therapist probes for a client's anxious appraisals of the situation and her ability to cope. Naturally the effectiveness of this assessment approach depends on the client's imaginative ability or capacity to engage in role playing.

Induction exercises can also be used to elicit apprehensive thoughts. For example, various physiological hyperarousal symptoms can be induced and clients encouraged to verbalize their "stream of thoughts" as they experience these symptoms. A situation could be created in the therapy session or stimuli introduced to elicit anxiety and clients could again be asked to verbalize their emerging thoughts. For example, someone with fear of contamination could be given a dirty cloth to touch and then report on his anxious thoughts.

Finally, the most effective procedure for eliciting the first apprehensive thoughts is to accompany the client into a *naturalistic anxiety-provoking situation*. Although the presence of the therapist might have a safety cue effect, careful probing of clients' stream of consciousness should reveal their first apprehensive thoughts. Even generating an expectation of exposure to an anxiety-provoking situation might be sufficient to elicit these primary automatic anxious thoughts.

Clinician Guideline 5.5

Obtain an accurate assessment of the client's first apprehensive thoughts in a variety of anxiety-provoking situations to determine the underlying threat schema responsible for the anxious state.

Perceived Autonomic Arousal

Individuals are usually very aware of the physical symptoms of anxiety and so can quite readily report these symptoms in the clinical interview. They should be asked for examples of recent anxiety episodes and the physical symptoms experienced at these times. Rather than have clients report on the typical anxiety attack, it is better for them to report on specific incidents of anxiety and the exact physical symptoms experienced during these episodes. Some variation in the physical symptoms of anxiety can be expected across different anxiety episodes.

The practitioner will be relying mainly on clients' self-report of their physiological responses since use of psychophysiological laboratory-based or ambulatory equipment for monitoring purposes is rarely feasible in the clinical setting. Self-monitoring forms should be used for clients to collect "online" data of their physiological responses when anxious. In most cases the Physical Sensation Self-Monitoring Form (Appendix 5.3) can be given as a homework assignment and will provide the needed information on the client's autonomic arousal profile. In certain cases where physiological arousal plays a particularly important role in the persistence of anxiety (i.e., panic disorder, hypochondriasis), an expanded checklist of bodily sensations can be administered (see Appendix 5.5).

Three questions must be addressed when assessing subjective physiological hyperarousal in the immediate fear response phase. First, what is the typical physiological response profile when the person is in a state of heightened anxiety? It is important to determine whether the client typically experiences the same physiological symptoms in a variety of anxiety-provoking situations. Which bodily sensations are most intense? Which arousal symptoms are experienced first? How long do they persist? Does the person do anything to achieve relief from the hyperarousal?

A second question concerns how the state of physiological hyperarousal is interpreted. Are there certain bodily sensations that are the primary focus of attention? What is the client's concern or fears about that sensation? Identifying the exaggerated threat appraisal of a particular body sensation is another important source of information on the core threat schemas that are driving the anxiety. Table 5.2 presents the exaggerated threat appraisals and schemas that may be associated with a number of physiological hyperarousal symptoms.

A final question when assessing physiological arousal is their role in the persistence of anxiety. Catastrophic misinterpretation of physical symptoms plays a key role in panic disorder (D. M. Clark, 1986a) and hypochondriasis (Salkovskis & Bass, 1997) but may be less prominent in OCD or GAD. In anxiety disorders where misinterpretation of physical symptoms is a prominent concern, treatment will focus on "decatastrophizing" these exaggerated appraisals. Thus case formulations for anxiety must take into account the nature, interpretation, and function of physiological hyperarousal during the phase of immediate fear.

Clinician Guideline 5.6

The nature, function, and interpretation of physiological hyperarousal and other bodily sensations must be determined as part of any case formulation for anxiety.

TABLE 5.2. **Exaggerated Threat Appraisals and Schemas That May Be Associated with Common Physical Symptoms of Anxiety**

Physical sensation	Exaggerated faulty appraisal	Threat-oriented schema
Difficulty breathing, shortness of breath	"I can't breath properly, I feel like I'm not getting enough air."	Risk of slow, agonizing death by suffocation
Chest tightness, pain, heart palpitations	"Maybe I am having a heart attack."	Death from sudden cardiac arrest
Restless, agitated	"I am losing control; I can't stand this feeling of anxiety."	Risk of going crazy, embarrassing myself, being overwhelmed with unending anxiety, etc.
Dizzy, lightheaded, faint	"I might be losing consciousness."	Might never regain consciousness; cause embarrassment by fainting in public
Nausea	"I might be sick to my stomach; vomit."	Suffocate from vomiting; embarrassment from being sick in public setting

Note. Based on Taylor (2000).

Immediate Inhibitory Responses

Immediate, defensive responses such as escape, avoidance, freezing, or fainting (Beck et al., 1985, 2005) are part of an automatic inhibitory strategy to reduce fear. An important part of any cognitive assessment of anxiety is to identify these fear-inhibiting responses and yet their detection can be difficult because they are so automatic, with the individual having little conscious awareness of their presence. However, it is important to determine the presence of these responses because they should be targeted for change given their capacity to reinforce the anxious state and undermine treatment effectiveness. As an example, a number of years ago one of us treated a woman with driving fear after having been rear-ended in a motor vehicle accident. Upon assessment it was discovered that while in traffic she anxiously kept her eye on the rearview mirror, checking to ensure that the car behind her was not too close. This checking behavior was done quite automatically as a defensive response. However, it meant that she was not attending as closely as she should to the traffic in front of her, thus increasing the likelihood of another accident.

Once again a detailed clinical interview, self-monitoring, and behavioral observation during heightened anxiety are the primary assessment approaches for identifying immediate defensive behaviors. There are a number of subtle defensive reactions that the clinician should be aware could occur as an immediate inhibitory response.

- *Avoids eye contact* to threatening stimulus (e.g., socially anxious person fails to make eye contact when conversing with others).
- *Cognitive avoidance* in which attention is shifted away from a disturbing thought or image (e.g., in PTSD a trauma-related intrusion might trigger a state of dissociation).
- *Immediate escape (flight) behavior* (e.g., a person with fear of contamination quickens her pace as she walks past a park bench where homeless people sit).
- *Behavioral avoidance* (e.g., a person with mild agoraphobia automatically chooses a less crowded store aisle).
- *Reassurance seeking* (e.g., a person keeps reciting the phrase "There is nothing to fear").
- *Compulsive response* (e.g., a person automatically pulls the car door handle repeatedly to make sure it is locked).
- *Defensive physiological reflex response* (e.g., a person anxious about swallowing food starts to gag when attempting to swallow; a person with driving fear stiffens body or is generally tense whenever he is a passenger in a car).
- *Tonic immobility (freezing)* (e.g., during a brutal assault a person may feel paralyzed, feeling like she is unable to move [see Barlow, 2002]).
- *Fainting* (e.g., a person experiences a sudden drop in heart rate and blood pressure at the sight of human blood or mutilated bodies).
- *Automatic safety behaviors* (e.g., a person automatically clutches an object to avoid falling or losing balance).

Given the automatic, rapid nature of these defensive responses, it is likely that some form of behavioral observation will be necessary to accurately assess their presence. It would be preferable if the cognitive therapist accompanied the client into anxious situations and then noted any inhibitory responses. Alternatively, a friend, family member, or spouse could be given the above list of defensive responses and asked to note whether any of these responses were observed when accompanying the client in anxious situations.

Clinician Guideline 5.7

Uncover automatic cognitive and behavioral inhibitory responses through behavioral observation to identify reactions that could later undermine the effectiveness of exposure.

Cognitive Processing Errors

Cognitive processing during the immediate fear response tends to be highly selective, with attention narrowly focused on the source of threat and one's ability (or inability) to deal with this threat. As a result certain unintended errors will be evident in the client's evaluation of the threat that will not be readily apparent to the individual. These cognitive errors can be determined from the automatic anxious thoughts and behaviors that are elicited in anxiety-provoking situations. Appendix 5.6 provides a list of the common cognitive errors seen in anxiety disorders, followed by a self-monitoring form that clients can use to become more aware of their anxious processing biases. This should be introduced after the client has been taught how to identify the first apprehensive thought. Teaching clients how to identify their cognitive errors will not only provide information for the case formulation but it is a useful cognitive intervention strategy (see Chapter 6).

Many anxious clients have difficulty identifying the cognitive errors in their anxious thinking. It may take a number of sessions before the client can capture examples of his own thinking biases. In the meantime the therapist can use the form in Appendix 5.6 to identify some of the thinking errors that are apparent from the clinical interview and self-monitoring of anxious thoughts. This can be incorporated in the case formulation until more accurate data are available from clients' own recording of their thinking errors.

Clinician Guideline 5.8

Use Appendix 5.6, Common Errors and Biases in Anxiety, to train clients to identify the automatic cognitive errors that occur whenever their anxiety is provoked by certain internal or external triggers.

SECONDARY REAPPRAISAL: ASSESSMENT AND FORMULATION

Anxiety is always the result of a two-stage process involving the initial activation of threat followed by a slower, more reflective processing of the threat in light of one's coping resources. For this reason the cognitive therapist also assesses secondary elaborative processing, focusing on two questions that must be addressed in the case conceptualization.

1. How does the individual's more elaborative reappraisal of the situation lead to an increase in anxiety?
2. How effective is the individual's reflective reappraisal in reducing or terminating the anxiety program?

Assessment of secondary reappraisal is not as difficult as assessment of the immediate fear response because these processes are less automatic and so more amenable to conscious awareness. Individuals tend to have more insight into these slower, more deliberate processes that are responsible for the persistence of anxiety. Because cognitive therapy tends to focus on this secondary level, an accurate assessment of elaborative processes is critical to the success of the intervention. In this section we examine five domains of secondary processing that should be included in the assessment.

Evaluation of Coping Abilities

Reliance on maladaptive coping strategies and failure to adopt healthier responses to threat are considered key factors in failed emotional processing in general and the persistence of anxiety in particular (e.g., Beck et al., 1985, 2005; Wells, 2000). One of the most common distinctions in the coping literature is between strategies that focus on emotion regulation versus those that focus directly on life problems. Lazarus and Folkman (1984) originally defined emotion-focused coping as "directed at regulating emotional response to the problem" (p. 150) and problem-focused coping as "directed at managing or altering the problem causing the distress" (p. 150). There is now a large body of research indicating that certain aspects of emotion-focused coping (e.g., rumination) are related to the persistence of negative emotional states, whereas problem-focused coping is associated with reduction in negative affect and the promotion of positive emotion and well-being (e.g., Carver, Scheier, & Weintraub, 1989; see reviews by Fields & Prinz, 1997; Folkman & Moskowitz, 2004; for discussion of positive aspects of emotion expression, see Austenfeld & Stanton, 2004).

In the present context this distinction between an emotion- and a problem-focused approach is useful in understanding the persistence of anxiety. Coping responses that focus on "how can I make myself feel less anxious" are more self-defeating (i.e., lead to persistence of unwanted anxiousness), whereas coping that is more problem-oriented (i.e., "I have a real life problem that I must address") is more likely to lead to a reduction in anxiety.

The cognitive therapist should keep this distinction in mind when assessing the coping responses of anxious clients. To what extent is the client's coping repertoire dominated by emotion-focused versus problem-oriented strategies? In addition three other questions on coping must be addressed in the assessment:

1. How often does an individual use various maladaptive and adaptive coping responses when feeling anxious?
2. What is the client's perception on the effectiveness of the coping strategies in reducing anxiety?
3. Does the client perceive that an increase or persistence of anxiety is associated with the coping response?

Appendix 5.7 provides a checklist of 34 behavioral and emotional coping responses that pertain to anxiety. We suggest the therapist go over the checklist as part of the clinical interview since most clients should be quite aware of their coping responses when anxious. Also most anxious individuals probably have not considered the perceived effectiveness of their coping and its effects on the intensity and duration of anxiety. Therefore some probing and questioning may be necessary in order to obtain this information.

From this assessment one should be able to specify in the case formulation which maladaptive coping strategies are frequently associated with anxiety and their perceived effectiveness, the relative effectiveness of any adaptive strategies that the client already employs, and the overall level of confidence or helplessness felt in dealing with anxiety. This will also provide the therapist with clues about behavioral changes that may be targeted in treatment. However, it is also likely that this checklist assessment must be complemented with questions about coping responses that may be unique to the specific anxiety disorders. Also many of the strategies listed in Appenditx 5.7 could be stress management responses. Therefore it is important that clients be asked to focus on activities employed directly in response to their anxiety and not activities they use to relieve general stress, improve mood state, or enhance their overall sense of well-being.

Clinician Guideline 5.9

Use Appendix 5.7, Behavioral Responses to Anxiety Checklist, to assess how often various behavioral and emotional coping strategies are used to control anxiety. Highlight the role of these strategies in the persistence of anxiety in the case conceptualization.

Deliberate Safety-Seeking Behavior

White and Barlow (2002) define safety behaviors as "those actions that a patient engages in to help him or her feel more secure or protected" (p. 343). The focus of safety behaviors is to feel secure, safe, which has the obvious benefit of reducing feelings of anxiety (see Chapter 3, Hypotheses 2 and 7, for further discussion).

It is important to clearly identify in the case formulation the main safety-seeking responses whether they are more automatic and habitual in nature or more consciously mediated, deliberate coping responses. By this point in the assessment much of this information has already been collected from individuals' self-monitoring of their responses in anxious situations (i.e., Situational Analysis Form, Apprehensive Thoughts Self-Monitoring Form) or from the previous evaluation of coping strategies (i.e., Behavioral Responses to Anxiety Checklist). The cognitive therapist can go back over these forms and select out responses that often occur when the person is anxious. For each response the following questions should be asked to assess the safety-seeking function of the response:

- "I notice from your form that you often do X [state actual response] when you feel anxious. To what extent do you feel safer or more secure after you have done this? [e.g., How much safer do you feel going to the mall with a friend versus going to the mall alone?]"

- "What would happen to your anxiety if you did not engage in this safety activity? [e.g., What would happen to your anxiety if you didn't carry your medication with you?]"
- "How important is this activity to your way of dealing with or managing your anxiety? Is it something you do deliberately or is it more automatic, like a habit that you are hardly aware of doing?"

Once the client's primary safety-seeking responses have been identified, it is important to also specify the cognitions and physical sensations associated with safety seeking (i.e., Salkovskis, Clark, et al., 1999). This might be quite obvious from the cognitive-behavioral responses recorded on the self-monitoring forms or on occasion the cognitive therapist might have to assess more specifically. The following fictitious clinical excerpt illustrates the type of inquiry that could be used to identify safety-seeking cognitions.

THERAPIST: I notice from the checklist that you indicated you always carry your Ativan with you at all times. Could you tell me why this is so important for you?

CLIENT: Well, I just feel better knowing that I have the medication if I ever need it. I haven't used the Ativan in months but knowing that it is there makes me feel better.

THERAPIST: What would happen if you forgot to take the medication bottle with you?

CLIENT: I know that I would feel a lot more anxious if I realized I didn't have it. The Ativan is so effective in relieving my anxiety. If I have it with me, I know that I could always take a pill if the anxiety gets too severe. Even though I haven't used the medication in months, just knowing that the anxiety can't get out of hand because I could always take an Ativan seems to help.

THERAPIST: Is there anything you feel or experience when in an anxious situation that is somehow better just knowing you have the medication?

CLIENT: Well as you know I get really afraid of having another panic attack when I notice that I'm becoming more anxious. The worst thing is feeling like I am losing control. Knowing that I could take an Ativan and be calmer and in control within a few minutes makes me feel a lot better; it makes me feel more confident.

A number of cognitions are evidently associated with this client's medication-related safety-seeking behavior. She believes just having access to the medication gives her more confidence and makes her feel safer, more secure. More importantly, there is a direct functional relationship between the catastrophic thought "of losing control" and being able to take the medication. This belief that the medication is an important source of regaining control and thwarting overwhelming anxiety will become a target in treatment. If the cognitive basis of safety seeking cannot be determined by interview or review of the self-monitoring forms, direct observation of the client's anxiety either by accompanying the person into an anxious situation or conducting an anxiety-induction exercise in the session might be necessary. In all anxiety cases identifying the primary safety-seeking behaviors and their cognitive basis is an important part of the case formulation for anxiety.

Clinician Guideline 5.10

Identify the primary intentional safety-seeking behaviors by reviewing the client's Behavioral Responses to Anxiety Checklist (Appendix 5.7) and determine the functional significance and cognitive basis of the responses. Also reconsider the safety-seeking function that may be associated with the more automatic, inhibitory reactions noted in Guideline 5.7. This should result in a clear specification of the subtle, more automatic and more conscious, deliberate safety-seeking behaviors that characterize the client's anxiety.

Constructive Mode

An important part of the secondary phase of anxiety is the activation of a more constructive, problem-oriented approach to the threatening situation. It must be recognized that all treatment-seeking individuals will have some capacity to respond to their anxiety in a more constructive manner. It is important to identify these strengths in the case formulation so this can be incorporated into the treatment plan. What behavioral responses to anxiety does the client already exhibit that indicates a more constructive approach? Is the person able to engage in adaptive problem-solving? Are there any cognitive strategies that lead to a reduction in the perceived level of threat? It is useful to assess the constructive mode when the person is in a nonanxious state. How do they perceive threat and their personal vulnerability when not anxious? How well can they bring this more realistic, adaptive perspective to bear when they are anxious? How difficult is it to believe the constructive perspective when anxious?

Very often individuals who seek cognitive therapy for anxiety have had previous treatment or read cognitively oriented self-help books on anxiety. Thus it is very likely that some constructive response to their anxiety is already present. Table 5.3 presents various types of constructive responses to anxiety and sample clinical questions that can be used to assess constructive mode activation when anxious.

Assessment of clients' "spontaneous" use of various constructive approaches to anxiety is important for two reasons. First, it provides some indication of the clients' strengths around which a treatment plan can be formulated. And second, it may be that a particular constructive approach has not been employed effectively and so the client has negative expectations about its success. It would be important for the therapist to know this before assigning this strategy as homework. In sum, assessment of constructive mode activation is an important part of the case formulation.

Clinician Guideline 5.11

Identify adaptive coping strategies that are present in the client's repertoire and the extent to which these responses are utilized during periods of anxiety. Evaluation of the constructive mode should also include an assessment of the client's ability to engage in a more realistic appraisal of his or her anxious concerns when not anxious and whether this more realistic perspective is available during anxious episodes.

TABLE 5.3. Examples of Constructive Responses to Anxiety That Should Be Assessed as Part of the Case Conceptualization

Constructive response	Clinical questions
Spontaneous exposure	• How often does the client deliberately expose himself to anxiety-provoking situations? • How intense and for how long is the anxiety tolerated before escape occurs? • Does exposure occur on a regular basis? Are safety cues present or absent? • What is the client's evaluation of the exposure experience? Is it seen as reducing her anxiety or exacerbating it?
Self-initiated response prevention	• How often does the client inhibit responses that are intended to reduce anxiety (e.g., a compulsive ritual in OCD)? • How hard is it to resist the urge to engage in the anxiety-reduction activity? • Does resistance occur on a regular basis? • How is the attempt to resist the anxiety-reducing activity evaluated? Is the resistance viewed as making the anxiety worse or better?
Relaxation response	• How often does the client engage in progressive muscle relaxation, controlled breathing, or meditation in response to anxiety? • What is the client's evaluation of the effectiveness of these strategies in managing anxiety? • Is there any evidence that the client is using relaxation as an escape strategy because of a fear of being anxious? To what extent is relaxation an adaptive or maladaptive response strategy for anxiety?
Problem-solving ability	• Does the client take a problem-solving approach to the source of anxiety? (e.g., a student worried about exam failure works on improving study skills) • What is the perceived effect of these problem-solving attempts on anxiety level? • Are there any weaknesses to the problem-solving strategy that may undermine its positive effect on anxiety?
Realistic threat reappraisal	• Does the client engage in any questioning or reappraisal of his initial threat appraisal, and if so, how effective is this questioning? • Can he practice evidence gathering where he seeks out contrary information that the threat is not as great as initially thought? • Does he ever turn to some form of empirical hypothesis testing where he seeks out experiences to determine if his fears are realistic or exaggerated?
Reappraisal of personal vulnerability	• Does the client engage in any form of evidence gathering about her ability to cope with the threat? • Can she recall past experiences of successful coping as a means of readjusting her initial sense of personal vulnerability? • Does she deliberately engage in anxiety-provoking activities to test-out her vulnerability?

Cognitive Coping and the Role of Worry

Excessive Worry

We previously argued that worry in highly anxious individuals is an important contributor to the persistence of anxiety because of domination of threat mode activation (Beck & Clark, 1997; see Chapter 2). It is a detrimental cognitive coping strategy (see Chapter 3, Hypothesis 10) that is evident in most of the anxiety disorders, especially GAD. Thus it is important that the nature, extent, and function of worry be assessed when developing a case formulation for anxiety.

The first question to address is whether the client worries when anxious and, if so, what is the worry content, its frequency, and its persistence. The therapist can expect worry content to broadly fit within the main anxious concerns of the client. For example, in panic disorder the worry is about disturbing bodily sensations, whereas in social phobia worry about performance in social settings and the evaluation of others are dominant.

Appendix 5.8 presents the Worry Self-Monitoring Form A that can be used to assess any worry content associated with anxious episodes. This can be given as a homework assignment or the cognitive therapist could complete the form in the therapy session based on anxious situations identified on the Situational Analysis Form or the Apprehensive Thoughts Self-Monitoring Form. The purpose of the Worry Self-Monitoring Form A is to collect qualitative information on any worry themes that may play an important role in the persistence of the worry. This worry content will provide useful information for cognitive interventions the therapist will employ later in treatment. It is also important to determine how often the client worries when anxious and the duration of the worry episode. Worry that is frequent and lasts for 1–2 hours has a very different treatment implication from the occasional bout of worry that is dismissed within a few minutes.

In Chapter 3 we discussed a number of negative consequences associated with worry that may account for its pathological effects on anxiety (e.g., heightened sensitivity to threat information, increased sense of personal vulnerability, an increase in unwanted intrusive thoughts, an escalation in negative emotions, cognitive/emotional avoidance, and ineffective problem solving). However, most individuals will not have sufficient insight into the negative effects of worry to allow collection of this information from a homework assignment. Instead the therapist could use the worry episodes recorded on the Worry Self-Monitoring Form A as the basis for questioning that explores the negative consequences of worry. The following is a therapy excerpt based on a client with social phobia who was anxious about interrupting his supervisor to ask an important question:

THERAPIST: John, I notice from the Worry Self-Monitoring Form that you were particularly anxious on Friday about having to go to your supervisor's office to ask an important question about a project you were trying to finish. You rated your anxiety as 80/100 and the first apprehensive thought was "he is going to be so angry that I am interrupting him with such a stupid question."

JOHN: Yeah, I was really upset about this situation. These kinds of things really bother me. I find I get so anxious.

THERAPIST: It appears that you spent approximately a half hour worrying about this before you went and then you were worried most of the day afterward that your supervisor was angry with you for interrupting him. You've written that before you asked the question you were worried mainly about his angry reaction (i.e., would he be abrupt with me), whether you would be able to make yourself clearly understood, and whether you would understand your supervisor's response. Afterward you kept replaying the conversation in your mind to determine whether you sounded stupid or not. Furthermore, you worried about your supervisor's opinion of you and whether this would reflect negatively on your year-end performance evaluation. You've also written that you were worried that others overheard the conversation in your supervisors' office and were thinking that you were "so pathetic" (using your expression).

JOHN: I find I worry a lot about how I come across to other people and the negative effects of my "bumbling" conversations with others.

THERAPIST: John, in this situation did you notice any changes in your anxiety level while you were worrying before or after the interaction with your boss?

JOHN: Not sure what you mean.

THERAPIST: Did you notice any increases or decreases in your anxious feelings while you were worrying?

JOHN: Oh, I definitely felt more anxious. Before the interaction I tried to convince myself everything would be okay but all I could think about was his anger, and afterward I again tried to reassure myself that everything would be fine but the more I thought about it the more convinced I became that he thinks I'm incompetent.

THERAPIST: So one of the negative effects of worry is that it makes you more anxious rather than less anxious. Do you think worrying about talking to your boss made you more effective when you actually went and asked him the question?

JOHN: No, I don't think worrying about it gave me more confidence or improved the conversation. All I could think about was getting it over and dealing with the negative consequences later.

THERAPIST: You've mentioned a couple of other ways that worry may have a negative effect. It sounds like it makes you think about avoiding or escaping as quickly as possible. Also it doesn't sound like worry helps you cope with situations or problems more effectively. Did you notice anything else about your thinking when you were worrying?

JOHN: Not sure what you mean.

THERAPIST: Did you notice whether a lot of upsetting thoughts kept popping into your mind even though you didn't want them?

JOHN: Oh, yes. I kept seeing an image of my supervisor's angry face, I could hear him shouting at me, and I kept having the thought "He thinks I'm such an idiot."

THERAPIST: From your description, John, it sounds like worry has a number of negative effects on your anxiety. It is associated with an increase in anxious feelings; it may interfere with your ability to deal with situations; it intensifies the urge to escape or avoid the anxiety; and it increases unwanted distressing thoughts and images. This is not unusual in anxiety. Our research on worry indicates that it has far-reaching negative effects that can contribute to the persistence of anxiety. Would you like to make worry reduction an important goal in your anxiety treatment plan?

JOHN: Yeah, I definitely think I need to learn how to get a handle on my worry.

Other Cognitive Coping Strategies

In Chapter 3 (see Hypothesis 10) attempts to deliberately suppress unwanted thoughts and feelings were considered compensatory coping strategies that may contribute to the persistence of anxiety. In addition the intentional suppression of emotional expression may have adverse effects on negative emotion, although far fewer studies have investigated this possibility. An assessment of intentional thought suppression and emotional inhibition should be included in the case formulation. Appendix 5.9 presents a cognitive coping checklist that includes emotion inhibition along with a number of other intentional thought control strategies that may exacerbate the anxious state.

The Cognitive Responses to Anxiety Checklist (Appendix 5.9) can be assigned as a homework exercise. However, most anxious clients are probably not aware of their thought control strategies because these responses can become quite habitual over time. Thus some training and education will be required to teach clients how they may engage in maladaptive thought control strategies that only make anxious thoughts more salient. One might be able to review a recent anxious episode and use the checklist to determine which of the 10 strategies occurred and to what extent they contributed to anxiety reduction. Alternatively, a state of anxiety could be induced in the therapy session (or observed in a naturalistic setting) and clients could be asked whether they use any of the checklist strategies to control their anxious thoughts or worries.

Another way to highlight the nature of thought control in clients' experience of anxiety is to conduct a modified thought suppression experiment. This is illustrated in the following example.

THERAPIST: Lorraine, I would like to take a closer look at your anxiety about having a panic attack. You've indicated that often you feel your chest tighten and your first apprehensive thoughts are "I must be getting anxious. I really need to calm down. If I don't I could have another of those terrible panic attacks."

LORRAINE: Yes, that is exactly how I feel. I really hate those feelings and would do anything to get rid of them.

THERAPIST: Okay, what I would like to do is a little exercise with you right here in the office. First, I would like to see if you could focus on your anxious thoughts right now. Maybe you could bring these thoughts to your mind by tightening your chest muscles or imagining you are in a recent anxious situation. It doesn't matter how you do it, but I would like you to think about feeling anxious and the possibility of having a panic attack.

LORRAINE: I'm not sure I want to do this. I'm afraid I could trigger a panic attack. Already I'm beginning to feel anxious.

THERAPIST: I understand your concern. We can stop the exercise at any time. I simply want you to bring the anxious thoughts to your full attention. If you are beginning to feel anxious, then maybe you can focus on these anxious thoughts right now even without tightening your chest muscles.

LORRAINE: Oh, I have no trouble thinking about my anxiety right now and the possibility of a panic attack.

THERAPIST: Okay, Lorraine, please close your eyes and focus your attention on thoughts of being anxious right now. Think about how you are feeling and the last time you had a panic attack. I am going to ask you to hold that thought for 30 seconds.... [pause] Now stop thinking about your anxiety. I am going to give you another 30 seconds to stop thinking about your anxiety and the possibility of panic. You can do this anyway you choose.... Okay, stop [pause]. Were you able to stop yourself from thinking about your anxiety and the possibility of a panic attack?

LORRAINE: This is really hard. I tried not to have the thoughts but it was almost impossible. I think it was too short. I needed more time to get rid of my anxious thoughts.

THERAPIST: It is true that I gave you only half a minute. However, many people find the exercise even more frustrating if I drag it out longer. The important point is whether or not you were able to stop the anxious thinking.

LORRAINE: Not really. I seemed to be getting more and more anxious the harder I tried to get the thoughts out of my mind.

THERAPIST: You've just made an important point. The harder you try "not to think about the anxiety, the more you think about it." I have here a checklist of various strategies people use to change their anxious thinking. [Therapist passes Lorraine a copy of the Cognitive Responses to Anxiety Checklist.] Could you look through this checklist and tell me whether you just used any of these strategies in your attempt to not think about the anxiety.

LORRAINE: Well, I tried to deliberately not think about the anxiety (item #1), and I kept telling myself it is stupid to be anxious because I'm sitting here in your office (#6), and I tried to convince myself that I couldn't possibly have a panic attack right now (item #3). None of this seemed to work very well, though.

THERAPIST: From this exercise we've discovered a couple of things. First, you've reported that the harder you try to control your anxious thoughts, the worse they get. And second, you've reported a number of different mental control strategies you used to try and get rid of anxious thoughts. I realize that you've just done a "simulation" because in real life your anxious thoughts and feelings would be a lot more intense than they were while you were sitting in this office. I wonder how often you might automatically try to control your anxious thoughts whenever you feel anxious using the same strategies you reported just now. And I wonder what effect this might have on your anxiety. I wonder if it makes your anxiety worse or better. Would you like to find out?

LORRAINE: Sure, I think that would be a good idea.

THERAPIST: Okay, before our next session, could you take a copy of the Cognitive Responses to Anxiety Checklist that we just used and see if you could capture some times when you were anxious. Try to focus on your attempts to control the anxious thinking. Which of these thought control strategies did you use and how effective were they? Under the "how often" category, just check whether you used the strategy or not. You don't have to capture all your anxious moments, just one or two a day. It should take only a few minutes each day to fill out the form. Do you think that is doable?

LORRAINE: Yeah, I should be able to do this in the next week. I'm still having lots of anxiety.

Clinician's Guidelines 5.12

Assessment of the nature, frequency, and function of worry and other cognitive control responses is an important aspect of the case formulation of the persistence of anxiety. The Worry Self-Monitoring Form A (Appendix 5.8) can be used to obtain clinical information on worry, and the Cognitive Responses to Anxiety Checklist (Appendix 5.9) is available to assess deliberate thought control strategies.

Threat Reappraisal

This final aspect of case conceptualization is a culmination of all the assessment activities that have been described previously. As clients consciously and deliberately reflect back on their anxiety when in a safe and relaxed context, what is their evaluation of the threat and their ability to cope? Appendix 5.10, the Anxious Reappraisal Form, can be used to explore with clients their threat and vulnerability cognitions when feeling anxious and then their evaluation of the threat and personal vulnerability when calm, not anxious. One would expect that when anxious the thinking should be biased toward exaggerated threat and underestimated ability to cope, whereas during periods of no anxiety the person's threat evaluation would be more realistic and self-confidence elevated.

The Anxious Appraisal Form should be used as a clinical resource in the therapy session to help the therapist explore and then record the client's anxious and nonanxious appraisals rather than assigned as a homework exercise. The cognitive therapist should point out the differences between the client's thinking when anxious and not anxious. It should be emphasized that the client is capable of thinking in a more realistic fashion about her anxious concerns when in a calm and relaxed state. This means that the goal of therapy is to help clients learn to generalize their more realistic thinking about the threat and their ability to cope to their most difficult anxious moments. In this way the information obtained on the Anxious Reappraisal Form can be used to define one of the primary treatment goals of cognitive therapy for anxiety.

Clinician Guideline 5.13

Use the Anxious Reappraisal Form (Appendix 5.10) to assess clients' ability to generate a more realistic reappraisal of threat and personal vulnerability during periods of no anxiety. This can be used to highlight the biased, exaggerated nature of their thinking when anxious. Shifting to the more realistic appraisal that is evident in low anxiety should be a stated goal of treatment.

CASE FORMULATION OF ANXIETY: A CASE ILLUSTRATION

Cognitive Case Formulation

We conclude this chapter with a case illustration to demonstrate how the clinician can utilize the theory-driven assessment perspective described in this chapter to arrive at an overall cognitive case conceptualization of anxiety. Although we have described a very detailed cognitive approach to assessment and case formulation, it should be obvious from the following case presentation that much of the critical information can be obtained from the clinical interview, self-monitoring forms, observation of anxiety within the session, and standardized diagnostic interview and questionnaire measures. Thus it is reasonable to expect that an initial cognitive case conceptualization can be developed within the first two to three sessions, which will then be frequently revised and elaborated throughout the treatment process. In fact it is this changing, evolving nature that is the heart of case conceptualization (Persons, 1989).

A diagram of the cognitive case conceptualization of anxiety that is available in Appendix 5.11 can be used to summarize the assessment information and derive an individualized case formulation. Although there are many components to case formulation, the clinician is never expected to have a "finalized formulation" before initiating treatment. Certain core elements of the conceptualization should be apparent after the initial assessment and prior to treatment such as the situational triggers, first apprehensive (automatic anxious) thoughts, physiological hyperarousal, defensive (i.e., safety-seeking) responses, primary worry content (if relevant), and coping strategies. These aspects of the formulation will be revised and other components completed during subsequent treatment sessions. An individualized case formulation, then, evolves over the course of therapy.

Cognitive Case Conceptualization

We return to the clinical case presented at the beginning of this chapter. Sharon sought treatment for a long-standing problem with persistent anxiety that manifested itself mainly while interacting with work colleagues in her employment setting.

Diagnostic and Symptom Assessment

Sharon was administered the ADIS-IV as well as the general anxiety measures discussed in this chapter. Based on the ADIS-IV her primary axis I disorder was social phobia. Panic disorder without agoraphobic avoidance was a secondary axis I diagnosis. She also met criteria for a past major depression, single episode. The depression spontaneously remitted after 2 months and occurred in response to the death of a pet. She also reported a subclinical fear of heights and worry, but the latter was clearly related to her social anxieties at work. She obtained the following scores on the questionnaire battery; Beck Anxiety Inventory Total = 6, Beck Depression Inventory–II Total = 12, Hamilton Anxiety Rating Scale = 10, Cognitions Checklist—Depression = 15 and Cognitions Checklist—Anxiety = 7, and Penn State Worry Total = 64. Sharon also completed the Social Phobia and Anxiety Inventory (SPAI; Turner, Beidel, & Dancu, 1996) and obtained a Difference Score of 105.9, which is consistent with untreated generalized social phobia. Thus the psychometric data suggest only mild anxiety symptoms that are more cognitive than physiological in nature. The Penn State Worry score is elevated, but this is due to the client's worry about her social interactions at work. The BDI-II and CCL-D suggest the presence of some depressive symptoms. A pretreatment average daily anxiety level of 21/100 again confirmed a rather low level of anxiety.

The diagnostic assessment clearly indicated that the social phobia should be the primary focus of treatment. Although she met diagnostic criteria for panic disorder, the initial onset was 15 months ago, with the last full-blown panic attack occurring 1 year ago. In total she experienced four full-blown panic attacks and a number of limited symptom attacks, with many of the later occurring in social contexts at work. However, Sharon reported only minimal, brief periods of concern about the panic attacks that lasted only 3–4 days after a full-blown episode. Sharon also indicated that the panic attacks had limited interference in her daily functioning. Thus it was concluded that treatment of panic attacks that were not related to her social anxiety was not warranted at this time.

Assessment of Immediate Fear Response

Sharon listed a number of situations that trigger her anxiety at work. These include speaking up or interacting in a small group meeting, talking to persons in authority like her supervisor, one-to-one interaction with work colleagues over their computer problems, and initiating phone calls at work. These activities were associated with moderate to severe anxiety and a moderate level of avoidance. Given that her job primarily involves consultation with others, Sharon was frequently confronted with these anxiety-provoking situations on a daily basis. Other social activities that triggered considerable anxiety and avoidance were going to parties and being assertive, especially refusing unreasonable requests. Sharon completed a Situational Analysis Form as part of a homework assignment and reported a number of anxious episodes focused on small meetings and one-to-one interaction at work. The only cognitive trigger to anxiety was the anticipatory thought "I must speak to my supervisor about this problem." It was decided to target her anxiety in small meetings and one-to-one interaction with work colleagues since these represented the main triggers to her anxiety.

Two main automatic apprehensive thoughts became apparent from Sharon's self-monitoring homework assignments and subsequent interview sessions. When anticipating or first encountering a social situation at work, Sharon would think "I hope I am able to perform okay" and "I hope my face doesn't turn red." The only physiological sensations she reported when anxious was feeling warm and her face turning red (i.e., blushing). Blushing was a major concern for Sharon. She interpreted this as a sign that she was anxious, losing concentration, and would be less able to speak clearly and sensibly to others. She was also concerned that people would notice that her face was red and wonder what was wrong with her.

As a result of these anxious cognitions and the negative interpretations of blushing, Sharon exhibited a number of automatic defensive responses. Behaviorally she would say as little as possible in meetings (i.e., avoidance) and would speak very rapidly when she was forced to interact with others (i.e., escape response). She avoided eye contact in her social interactions. She also was hypervigilant about feeling warm and would often touch her face or check in a mirror to determine if she was visibly red. Her main automatic cognitive defense was to reassure herself that everything was okay and to try to relax. In sum her primary automatic defensive response to ensure safety was to say as little as possible in social situations, to avoid eye contact, and to locate herself in a setting so as to draw as little attention as possible.

A number of cognitive errors were evident in Sharon's anxious thinking about social situations. Catastrophizing was apparent in her belief that having a red face was highly abnormal and something that others would also interpret as a sign of abnormality. She was also convinced that once her face turned red, it meant she was anxious and would lose her concentration. This would result in poor performance, which others would evaluate as social incompetence. Tunnel vision was another cognitive error since Sharon would often become preoccupied with her face and whether she was feeling warm in social settings. She also engaged in emotional reasoning in that feeling uncomfortable in social settings meant that she was in greater danger of not functioning well and more likely to draw the attention of others. Finally, she tended to think of anxiety from an all-or-nothing perspective with certain situations associated with social threat and so intolerable, whereas other situations were entirely safe (e.g., working alone in her office).

Assessment of Secondary Reappraisal

Sharon exhibited a number of deliberate coping strategies in response to her social anxiety. She would try to physically relax in social situations by engaging in deep, controlled breathing, she tried to answer questions via e-mail in order to avoid face-to-face interaction with work colleagues, she would procrastinate about such things as asking her supervisor for clarification on an issue, and she was quiet and withdrawn in meetings, saying as little as possible. She also tried to suppress her feelings to hide any sense of discomfort. The intentional use of alternative means of communication with others (e.g., e-mail) had a prominent safety-seeking function. These strategies were all somewhat effective in reducing her social anxiety. Sharon was concerned that if she changed her approach to social anxiety if might make her work life more stressful.

Worry played a secondary role in Sharon's social anxiety. She worried on a daily basis about the possible social interactions she might encounter, whether she would experience a lot of anxiety throughout the day, and whether she would be socially incompetent as a result. She also worried outside the work setting that the extra stress and anxiety she was feeling at work might have a negative effect on her health and well-being. Sharon's cognitive coping strategies to control her anxiety were quite limited other than the use of reassurance and rationalization that everything will be fine and self-instructions to control her anxiousness. She concluded she was generally ineffective in controlling the anxiety and that the best strategy was to minimize social contact as much as possible. Interestingly, this perspective on social threat and vulnerability was evident even when she was not anxious and alone.

Treatment Goals

Based on our cognitive case conceptualization, the following goals were developed in Sharon's treatment plan:

- Decatastrophize her misinterpretation and maladaptive beliefs about blushing and the consequent negative evaluation of others.
- Modify the belief that anxiousness in social settings must be controlled because it will lead to dire negative outcomes such as social incompetence (i.e., reappraise the probability and severity of threat).
- Reduce avoidance and increase exposure to socially anxious situations.
- Eliminate maladaptive defensive and coping strategies such as speaking too quickly when anxious, reliance on deep breathing, and self-rationalization focused on convincing herself there is no threat.
- Reduce the negative effects of worry about being anxious whenever social interaction is anticipated.
- Improve assertiveness and other verbal communication skills when interacting with authority figures such as a supervisor.

SUMMARY AND CONCLUSION

In this chapter we presented a cognitive case conceptualization perspective that is based on the cognitive model of anxiety (see Chapter 2). Although this framework will be applicable to all anxiety cases, it will require some modification for each of the specific anxiety disorders. Case formulation plays an important role in cognitive therapy for all psychological problems. For the anxiety disorders assessment begins with clinical diagnosis and administration of standardized questionnaires. It is important that presence of anxious and depressive symptoms be assessed. Utilizing interview methodology, self-monitoring forms, and direct observation, the clinician gathers information on the immediate or automatic cognitive, physiological, and behavioral responses that characterize the initial fear program. This is followed by assessment of more deliberate cognitive and behavioral coping strategies that are intended to terminate the anxious episode but instead inadvertently contribute to its long-term persistence. Particular attention is given to automatic and intentional responses that have a safety-seeking function. The assessment will culminate in a specification of the threat and personal vulnerability appraisals generated when the individual is an anxious and a nonanxious state. This detailed cognitive formulation should lead to the development of specific treatment goals that will guide the intervention process. A Quick Reference Summary is provided in Appendix 5.12 to assist the clinician in applying our cognitive perspective on assessment and case formulation in clinical practice.

Daily Anxiety Ratings and Situation Record

Name: _____ Date: _____

Instructions: Use the rating scale below to record a number from 0 to 100 that indicates the average level of anxiety you experienced during the day. In the far right column briefly describe any situations that you found particularly anxiety provoking on a particular day.

0	50	100
"Absolutely no anxiety, totally relaxed"	"Moderate or usual level of anxiety felt when in anxious state"	"Extreme, panic-stricken state that is unbearable and feels life-threatening"

Day of the Week/Date	Rating of Average Anxiety Level (0–100)	Provoking Situations (Note any situations that increased your anxiety during the day)
1. Sunday		
2. Monday		
3. Tuesday		
4. Wednesday		
5. Thursday		
6. Friday		
7. Saturday		

Situational Analysis Form

Name: _____   Date: _____

Directions: Please write down any situations that triggered an anxiety response. Very briefly describe the situation in column two and in the third column rate the intensity of anxiety (0–100) and its duration (number of minutes). In the fourth column note the most prominent anxious symptoms you experienced and in the fifth column record any immediate thoughts in the situation. In the final column please comment on your immediate response to the anxiety.

Date/Time	Situation	Anxiety Intensity (0–100) and Duration (min)	Primary Anxious Symptoms	Immediate Anxious Thoughts	Immediate Response to Feeling Anxious
1.					
2.					
3.					
4.					

Physical Sensation Self-Monitoring Form

Name: _____   Date: _____

Directions: Please write down any situations or experiences that caused an increase in your anxiety. Pay particular attention to whether you experienced any of the bodily sensations listed on this form while you were in that situation. Use the rating scales beside each sensation to indicate how you felt about the bodily reaction.

1. ***Briefly describe anxious situation***: _____

Record level of anxiety in situation (0–100 scale): _____

Checklist of physical sensations experienced in situation:

Physical Sensation	Intensity of Physical Sensation [Use 0–100 scale defined below]	Anxiousness about Physical Sensation [Use 0–100 scale defined below]
Chest tightness		
Elevated heart rate		
Trembling, shaking		
Difficulty breathing		
Muscle tension		
Nausea		
Lightheaded, faint, dizzy		
Weak, unsteady		
Feeling warm, sweaty		
Dry mouth		

(cont.)

2. ***Briefly describe anxious situation***: _____

Record level of anxiety in situation (0–100 scale): _____

Checklist of physical sensations experienced in situation:

Physical Sensation	Intensity of Physical Sensation [Use 0–100 scale defined below]	Anxiousness about Physical Sensation [Use 0–100 scale defined below]
Chest tightness		
Elevated heart rate		
Trembling, shaking		
Difficulty breathing		
Muscle tension		
Nausea		
Lightheaded, faint, dizzy		
Weak, unsteady		
Feeling warm, sweaty		
Dry mouth		

Rating Scale Instructions: *Intensity of Physical Sensations Scale,* 0 = barely felt the sensation; 50 = strong sense of the sensation; 100 = dominant, overwhelming feeling.

Anxiousness about Physical Sensations Scale, 0 = not at all anxious about having the sensation; 50 = considerable concern that I am having this sensation; 100 = feel intensely anxious, panicky that I am having this sensation.

Apprehensive Thoughts Self-Monitoring Form

Name: _____   Date: _____

Directions: Please write down any situations or experiences that caused an increase in your anxiety. After rating the level of anxiety experienced in the situation in the second column, write down your response to the questions posed in the next columns based on what you were thinking and feeling in the situation. Try to fill in this form while you are in the anxious situation or as soon afterward as possible.

Anxiety-Provoking Situation [Describe briefly in a few words and include date and time of day]	Average Anxiety Level [0–100 scale]	Worst Possible Outcome [What's the worst possible thing that could happen regardless of how unlikely or unrealistic?]	What's not right about the situation? [What's disconcerting about the situation or about how you feel or could behave? Or how could others behave toward you that would be upsetting?]	What would ease your anxiety? [How could the situation change to ease your anxiety? How could you change or others change to ease your anxiety?]
1.				
2.				

APPENDIX 5.5

Expanded Physical Sensations Checklist

Name: _____   Date: _____

Instructions: Below you will find a list of physical sensations that can be experienced during periods of high anxiety or during panic attacks. Please indicate the intensity of the physical sensation during a typical anxiety episode or panic attack. The checklist should be completed during the anxiety episode or as soon afterward as possible. *Also please circle the bodily reaction or sensation that you noticed first during the episode of anxiety.*

Physical Sensation	Absent	Slight	Moderate	Severe	Very Severe
Tense muscles					
Muscle pain					
Weakness					
Muscle twitches, spasms					
Numbness in hands, feet (or pins and needles sensation)					
Tingling in hands, feet					
Nausea					
Stomach cramps					
Indigestion					
Feeling of urgency to urinate					
Diarrhea					
Congested, buildup of mucus in throat or nose					
Dry mouth					

(cont.)

Physical Sensation	Absent	Slight	Moderate	Severe	Very Severe
Difficulty taking a deep breath, shortness of breath					
Throat feels constricted (like you could choke)					
Chest tightness					
Chest pain					
Heart pounding, palpitations					
Heart skipping a beat					
Trembling, shaky					
Feeling restless, fidgety					
Feelings of unreality					
Muscle twitches					
Dizziness					
Feeling lightheaded					
Feeling faint					
Unsteady, loss of balance					
Hot flushes or chills					
Sweating					
Other sensations (state):					

Common Errors and Biases in Anxiety

The following is a list of thinking errors that are common when people feel afraid or anxious. You may find that you make some of these errors when you feel anxious but it is unlikely that you make all of the errors every time you are anxious. Read through the list of errors with their definition and examples. Put a check mark beside the ones that are particularly relevant for you. You will notice the errors overlap because they all deal with different aspects of overestimating threat and underestimating safety when feeling anxious. After reading through this list, turn to page 170 where you will find a form that you can use to become more aware of your own thinking errors when anxious.

Thinking Error	Definition	Examples
Catastrophizing	Focusing on the worst possible outcome in an anxious situation.	• Thinking that chest tightness is sign of a heart attack • Assuming friends think your comment is stupid • Thinking you'll be fired for making a mistake in your report
Jumping to conclusions	Expecting that a dreaded outcome is extremely likely.	• Expecting that you will fail the exam when unsure of a question • Predicting that your mind will go blank during the speech • Predicting that you will be extremely anxious if you make the trip
Tunnel vision	Focusing only on possible threat-relevant information while ignoring evidence of safety.	• Notice that a person looks bored while you are speaking in a meeting • Notice a spot of urine on the floor of an otherwise very clean public washroom • Person with combat PTSD experiences flashback when seeing newsclip of a far-off regional conflict
Nearsightedness	Tendency to assume that threat is imminent (close at hand).	• An individual with OCD is convinced of possible contamination even coming within a few yards of a homeless person • Worry-prone individual is convinced he will be fired any day • Person with fear of vomiting is concerned she is about to become sick to her stomach because she has an "unsettled feeling"
Emotional reasoning	Assuming that the more intense the anxiety, the greater the actual threat.	• Flying must be dangerous because I feel so anxious when I fly • Person with panic assumes the likelihood of "losing control" is greater when feeling intense anxiety • Worry-prone individual is even more convinced something bad will happen because she feels anxious
All-or-nothing thinking	Threat and safety are viewed in rigid, absolute terms as either present or absent.	• Person with obsessional doubts is always concerned that the light switch is not completely off • Person with social anxiety is convinced his work colleagues will think that he is incompetent if he speaks up • Person who experienced past trauma is convinced she must avoid anything that reminds her of the past incident

(cont.)

Identifying Anxious Thinking Errors

Name: _____   Date: _____

Instructions: With the handout entitled "Common Errors and Biases in Anxiety" as your reference, use the form below to write down examples of your own thinking errors that occur when you feel anxious. Please focus on how you are thinking when you are in anxious situations or anticipating the situation. Also focus on your most immediate apprehensive thoughts rather than any secondary reconsideration of the situation.

Thinking Error	Examples of My Own Anxious Thinking Errors
Catastrophizing	
Jumping to conclusions	
Tunnel vision	
Nearsightedness	
Emotional reasoning	
All-or-nothing thinking	

Behavioral Responses to Anxiety Checklist

Name: _____   Date: _____

Instructions: You will find below a checklist of various ways that people tend to respond to anxiety. Please indicate how often you engage in each response *when you are anxious*, how effectively the strategy reduces or eliminates anxious feelings, and whether you think the strategy unintentionally leads to the persistence of your anxiety.

Scale Descriptions: How often do you engage in this response when you feel anxious? [0 = never, 50 = half of the time, 100 = all the time]; When you engage in this response, how effectively does it reduce your anxiety? [0 = not at all; 50 = moderately effective in reducing anxiety, 100 = completely eliminates my anxiety]; Based on your experience, to what extent do you think this response contributes to a persistence of your anxiety? [0 = does not contribute at all, 50 = makes a moderate contribution, 100 = is a very important factor in the persistence of my anxiety]

Behavioral and Emotional Responses	How Often [0–100 scale]	Effective in Reducing Anxiety [0–100 scale]	Increases Persistence of Anxiety [0–100]
1. Try to physically relax (e.g., muscle relaxation, controlled breathing, etc.)			
2. Avoid situations that trigger anxiety			
3. Leave situations whenever I feel anxious			
4. Take prescription medication			
5. Seek reassurance, support from spouse, family, or friends			
6. Engage in a compulsive ritual (e.g., check, wash, count)			
7. Distract myself with activities			
8. Suppress my feelings (i.e., hold in my feelings)			
9. Use alcohol, marijuana, or other street drugs			
10. Get very emotional, tearful			
11. Have an anger outburst			
12. Become physically aggressive			

(cont.)

Behavioral and Emotional Responses	How Often [0–100 scale]	Effective in Reducing Anxiety [0–100 scale]	Increases Persistence of Anxiety [0–100]
13. Speak or act more quickly in a hurried manner			
14. Become quiet, withdraw from others			
15. Seek medical/professional help (e.g., call therapist or GP; go to emergency)			
16. Use Internet to chat with friend or obtain information			
17. Reduce physical activity level			
18. Rest, take a nap			
19. Try to find solution to the problem causing me anxiety			
20. Pray, meditate in effort to reduce anxious feelings			
21. Have a smoke			
22. Have a cup of coffee			
23. Gamble			
24. Engage in pleasurable activity			
25. Eat comforting food (e.g., favorite junk food)			
26. Seek some place that makes me feel safe, not anxious			
27. Listen to relaxing music			
28. Watch TV or videos (DVDs)			
29. Do something that is relaxing (e.g., take a warm bath or shower, have a massage)			
30. Seek out a person who makes me feel safe, not anxious			
31. Do nothing, just let the anxiety "burn itself out"			
32. Engage in physical exercise (e.g., go to the gym, run)			
33. Read spiritual, religious, or meditative material (e.g., Bible, poetry, inspirational books)			
34. Go shopping (buy things)			

Worry Self-Monitoring Form A

Name: _____   Date: _____

Instructions: Using the form below, please record whether or not you have any worries associated with your anxiety. In the first column write down some occasions when you are feeling anxious, then rate the intensity of the anxiety on the 0–100 scale, and then try to capture your first apprehensive (anxious) thought in the situation. You can go back to the Apprehensive Thoughts Self-Monitoring Form if you need help identifying the apprehensive thought. In the final column write down anything that worried you about that situation as well as how long the worry lasted (number of minutes or hours).

Anxious Situation [Describe briefly and include date and time]	**Intensity of Anxiety** [0–100 scale]	**First Apprehensive (Anxious) Thought**	**Worry Content** [Is there anything that worries you about the situation or the effects of anxiety? Is there any negative consequence that worries you? How long did you worry?]
1.			
2.			
3.			
4.			
5.			

Cognitive Responses to Anxiety Checklist

Name: _____   Date: _____

Instructions: You will find below a checklist of various ways that people try to control their anxious and worrisome thoughts. Please indicate how often you engage in each response *when you are anxious* and how effective the strategy is in reducing or eliminating anxious thoughts.

Scale Descriptions: How often do you engage in this response when you feel anxious? [0 = never, 50 = half of the time, 100 = all the time]; When you engage in this cognitive strategy, how effectively does it reduce or eliminate the anxious thoughts? [0 = not at all; 50 = moderately effective in reducing anxiety, 100 = completely eliminates my anxiety]

Cognitive Control Response to Anxious Thinking	How Often Strategy is Used [0–100 scale]	Effectiveness in Reducing Anxious Thinking [0–100 scale]
1. Deliberately try not to think about what is making me anxious or worried.		
2. Tell myself that everything will be okay and will turn out fine.		
3. Try to rationalize the anxiety; look for reasons why my anxious concerns might be unrealistic.		
4. Try to distract myself by thinking about something else.		
5. Try to replace the anxious thought with a more positive or comforting thought.		
6. Make critical or negative remarks to myself about being anxious.		
7. Tell myself to simply "stop thinking" like this.		
8. Think a comforting phrase or prayer.		
9. Ruminate on the anxious thought or worry; I keep going over in my mind what happened in the past or what could happen in the future.		
10. When I start to feel anxious I try to suppress the feelings so I don't look nervous or upset.		

Anxious Reappraisal Form

Name: _____   Date: _____

Instructions: Please complete the form below to record your perspective when feeling anxious and when not feeling anxious. When you are anxious, describe the worst outcome that you fear most and rate its felt probability from 0 (not at all likely to happen) to 100 (absolutely expect it to happen). Then indicate how well you think you could cope with the anxiety and rate your level of confidence in yourself from 0 (no confidence) to 100 (absolute confidence). Next repeat the form when you are not feeling anxious. As you look back on those anxious situations, what is the expected outcome and what is your perceived ability to cope with your anxiety?

When Feeling Anxious		When Not Feeling Anxious	
Feared Outcome	*Ability to Cope with Anxiety*	*Expected Outcome*	*Ability to Cope with Anxiety*
[Describe worst outcome and rate its probability 0–100]	[Describe coping ability and confidence 0–100]	[Describe most likely outcome and rate its probability 0–100]	[Describe coping ability and confidence 0–100]

Diagram of Cognitive Case Conceptualization of Anxiety

Name: _____   Date of Initial Assessment Session: _____

A. CURRENT DIAGNOSTIC INFORMATION
[Based on ADIS or SCID; duration refers to length of current disorder]

Primary axis I diagnosis _____   Duration: _____

Secondary axis I diagnosis: _____   Duration: _____

Tertiary axis I diagnosis: _____   Duration: _____

Additional subclinical diagnoses: _____

Number of episodes of primary diagnosis: _____

B. SYMPTOM PROFILE

Beck Anxiety Inventory Total: _____   Beck Depression Inventory–II Total: _____

Cognitions Checklist—Anxiety: _____   Cognitions Checklist—Depression: _____

Hamilton Anxiety Rating Scale Total Score *(optional)*: _____

Penn State Worry Questionnaire Total: _____

Pretreatment Daily Anxiety Mean *(sum of ratings over week/7)*: _____

C. PROFILE OF IMMEDIATE FEAR RESPONSE

Situational Analysis

List Primary External Triggers

1. _____
2. _____
3. _____
4. _____
5. _____

List Primary Internal/Cognitive Triggers

1. _____
2. _____
3. _____
4. _____
5. _____

↓

First Apprehensive Thoughts/Images
List Core Automatic Anxious Thoughts/Images
[present during episodes of anxiety]

1. _____
2. _____
3. _____
4. _____

↓

(cont.)

Perceived Physiological Hyperarousal

List Primary Physical Sensations/Symptoms

1. _____
2. _____
3. _____
4. _____
5. _____

Misinterpretation of Sensation/Symptom

1. _____
2. _____
3. _____
4. _____
5. _____

↓

Automatic Inhibitory/Defensive Responses

List Primary Behavioral Defenses

1. _____
2. _____
3. _____
4. _____

List Primary Cognitive Defenses

1. _____
2. _____
3. _____
4. _____

Mark defenses with safety-seeking function with asterisk.

↓

Primary Cognitive Errors
[evident during anxious episodes]

Type of Cognitive Error

1. _____
2. _____
3. _____
4. _____
5. _____

Actual Example of Error from Client Assessment

1. _____
2. _____
3. _____
4. _____
5. _____

D. PROFILE OF SECONDARY REAPPRAISAL

Primary Behavioral and Emotional Coping Strategies

Briefly Describe the Coping Strategy

1. _____
2. _____
3. _____
4. _____
5. _____

Perceived Effect
in Reducing Anxiety

1. _____
2. _____
3. _____
4. _____
5. _____

Mark coping strategies with safety-seeking function with asterisk.

↓

(cont.)

Primary Worry Symptoms
Briefly describe the main worry content during anxious episodes

1. _____
2. _____
3. _____
4. _____
5. _____

↓

Principal Thought Control Strategies

Briefly Describe the Control Strategy

Perceived Effect
in Reducing Anxiety

1. _____
2. _____
3. _____
4. _____
5. _____

1. _____
2. _____
3. _____
4. _____
5. _____

Threat and Vulnerability Appraisal
When Anxious
[briefly summarize the client's perspective
on threat and vulnerability when anxious]

_____
_____
_____
_____
_____
_____
_____
_____
_____

Threat and Vulnerability Reappraisal
When Not Anxious
[briefly summarize the client's
perspective on threat and vulnerability
when not anxious]

_____
_____
_____
_____
_____
_____
_____
_____
_____

Chapter 5 Quick Reference Summary: Cognitive Assessment of Anxiety

I. Conduct Diagnostic Interview (ADIS-IV or SCID-IV)

II Assess Symptom Profile

Beck Anxiety Inventory (cutoff score 10+), Cognitions Checklist—Anxiety subscale ($M = 18.13$, $SD = 10.06$ for primary diagnosis of anxiety disorder),[*] Penn State Worry Questionnaire (cutoff score 45+), Anxiety Sensitivity Index ($M = 19.1$, $SD = 9.11$ for nonclinical; $M = 36.4$, $SD = 10.3$ for panic disorder)[+], BDI-II (cutoff score 14+), Daily Mood Rating (Appendix 6.1—Daily Anxiety Ratings and Situation Record); optional measures (HRSA, DASS, STAI)

III. Immediate Fear Activation Profile

1. *Situational Analysis* (assess environmental, interoceptive, and cognitive triggers; use Appendix 5.2—Situational Analysis Form; detailed description, rate intensity and duration of anxiety, escape/avoidance responses, specific triggering cues; begin with in session and then assign as self-monitoring)

2. *Assess First Apprehensive Thoughts* (give illustrative explanation on page 142; probe— "What's the worst that could happen?", "What concerns you about the situation?"; use Appendix 5.4—Apprehensive Thought Record to self-monitor; begin with in-session probing)

3. *Perceived Autonomic Arousal* (typical physiological responses and their interpretation; use Appendix 5.3—Physical Sensation Self-Monitoring Form or Appendix 5.5—Expanded Physical Sensations Checklist for self-monitoring; in session and self-monitor)

4. *Automatic Defensive Responses* (probe for automatic cognitive avoidance, reassurance seeking, compulsions, immediate fight/flight, avoids eye contact, fainting, automatic safety seeking, freezing, etc.; complete in session and observation)

5. *Cognitive Processing Errors* (give client list of common errors—Appendix 5.6, and use Identifying Anxious Thinking Errors to discover client's typical errors; complete in session)

IV. Secondary Elaborative Response Profile

1. *Evaluate Coping Responses* (assess behavioral and emotional coping responses when anxious; use Appendix 5.7—Behavioral Responses to Anxiety Checklist in session)

2. *Assess Safety-Seeking Function of Coping Responses* (identify responses used to instill sense of safety and its effects on anxiety; complete in session)

3. *Identify Constructive, Adaptive Approaches to Anxiety* (any evidence that client has healthy ways of coping with anxiety in other situations; complete in session)

4. *Assess Role of Worry* (use Appendix 5.8—Worry Self-Monitoring Form A to assess worry content; determine its effects on anxiety; complete in session)

5. *Identify Cognitive Coping Strategies* (use Appendix 5.9—Cognitive Responses to Anxiety Checklist to identify reliance and perceived effectiveness of maladaptive cognitive responses like thought suppression, reassurance seeking, thought stopping, etc.; complete in session)

6. *Obtain Description of Threat Reappraisal* (use Appendix 5.10—Anxious Reappraisal Form to obtain anxious and nonanxious appraisals; latter becomes goal of treatment; complete in session)

V. Complete Case Formulation (use Appendix 5.11—Diagram of Cognitive Case Conceptualization of Anxiety)

---

[*]Steer, R. A., Beck, A. T., Clark, D. A., & Beck, J. S. (1994). Psychometric properties of the Cognitions Checklist with psychiatric outpatients and university students. *Psychological Assessment*, 6, 67–70.

[+]Antony, M. M. (2001). Measures for panic disorder and agoraphobia. In: M. M. Antony, S. M. Orsillo, & L. Roemer (Eds.), *Practitioner's guide to empirically based measures of anxiety* (pp. 95–125). New York: Kluwer Academic/Plenum.

Cognitive Interventions for Anxiety

Courage is not the lack of fear but the ability to face it.
—LT. JOHN B. PUTNAM JR. (23-year-old
American airman killed in World War II)

Pierre is a 33-year-old married man with two preschool children who had a 15-year history of panic disorder and a single episode of major depression in remission. Past treatment was primarily pharmacotherapy that proved quite effective in reducing his depression but had less impact on his anxiety symptoms. Pierre was now interested in pursuing a course of CBT for anxiety and panic symptoms.

At intake Pierre met diagnostic criteria for panic disorder. He reported at least five full-blown panic attacks in the past month that included heart palpitations, sweating, nausea, shortness of breath, hot flushes, dizziness, and lightheadedness. Nausea was the initial physical sensation that often precipitated a panic attack. Pierre was fearful that the nausea would lead to vomiting. His greatest fear was losing control and vomiting in a public setting. As a result he was hypervigilant for any signs of nausea or abdominal discomfort. He discovered that social situations were more likely to trigger nausea and heightened levels of anxiety and so he tended to avoid these situations or leave as soon as he felt abdominal discomfort. Because of his apprehension about heightened anxiety and panic, Pierre developed limited agoraphobic symptoms in order to avoid the risk of panic.

The main cognitive basis to Pierre's anxiety was his belief that "feeling nausea or abdominal discomfort in a public setting could cause vomiting, or at least intense anxiety or panic." His catastrophic misinterpretation of nausea was not related to a fear of vomiting per se (i.e., he was not fearful of becoming ill), but rather that he would have a panic attack that would cause intense embarrassment from vomiting in public. He could only recall one incident in which he vomited in response to a severe panic attack. It appears that this incident may have been caused by a recent increase in his medication. More recently there was evidence that the anxiety may be generalizing to other situations such as flying, travel away from home, and sleep.

Pierre developed a number of coping strategies to minimize his anxiety. Although escape and avoidance were his dominant safety-seeking response style, he carefully monitored what he ate and drank, would sit at the back of a gathering and close to an aisle, and he always carried his clonazepam with him whenever he left home. Pierre's exaggerated appraisal of threat associated with nausea was not apparent in other areas of his life. He was an avid ice hockey player who continued to play goalie on a senior men's team. Thus he regularly put himself in harm's way, stopping pucks and often causing significant injury or pain to himself. This did not make him the least bit anxious. Instead it was feeling nausea or abdominal discomfort that was associated with appraisals of unacceptable threat and danger.

Therapy focused on Pierre's catastrophic misinterpretation of nausea. *In vivo* exposure was of limited value because Pierre was already forcing himself into anxious situations, although he would often leave whenever he became concerned with nausea. Interoceptive exposure was not utilized because of the difficulty in producing nausea sensations in a controlled setting. Instead therapy utilized mainly cognitive intervention strategies that targeted Pierre's faulty appraisal of nausea, dysfunctional belief that nausea will lead to panic and vomiting, and the belief that escape provided the most effective means of ensuring safety. Education into the cognitive therapy model of panic, evidence gathering, generating alternative interpretations, and empirical hypothesis testing were the primary cognitive intervention strategies employed. After eight sessions, Pierre reported a significant reduction in panic even with increased exposure to anxiety-provoking situations. Symptoms of general anxiety showed some improvement, although to a lesser degree. Therapy continued with a focus on other issues related to his general level of anxiousness and depressive symptoms such as low self-confidence and pessimism.

In this chapter we describe cognitive therapy for the maladaptive appraisals and beliefs that contribute to the persistence of anxiety. We begin with the purpose and main objectives that underlie cognitive interventions. This is followed by a discussion of how to educate the client into the cognitive model and teach skills in the identification of automatic anxious thoughts and appraisals. We then describe the use of cognitive restructuring to modify exaggerated threat and vulnerability appraisals as well as the need to eliminate intentional thought control responses. Empirical hypothesis testing is next described as the most potent cognitive intervention strategy for modifying anxious cognition. The chapter concludes with a brief consideration of some newer cognitive interventions such as attentional training, metacognitive intervention, imaginal reprocessing, mindfulness, and cognitive diffusion that appear promising adjuncts in cognitive therapy of anxiety.

MAIN OBJECTIVES OF COGNITIVE INTERVENTIONS

The cognitive treatment strategies outlined in this chapter are based on the cognitive model of anxiety described in Chapter 2 (see Figure 2.1). They are intended to target the anxious thoughts, appraisals, and beliefs highlighted in the assessment and case conceptualization (see Chapter 5). Cognitive interventions seek to shift the client's perspective from one of exaggerated danger and personal vulnerability to a perspective of minimal acceptable threat and perceived ability to cope. There are six main objectives of cognitive interventions for anxiety.

Shift Threat Focus

One of the first objectives of cognitive interventions is to shift the client's focus away from an internal or external situation or stimulus as the cause of fear and anxiety. Most individuals with an anxiety disorder enter therapy believing that the cause of their anxiousness is the situation that triggers their anxious episodes. For example, individuals with panic disorder believe they are anxious because they have chest pain that could result in a heart attack, whereas individuals with GAD believe the cause of their anxiety is the real possibility of negative life experiences in the near future. As a result of this belief, anxious individuals seek interventions that will alleviate what they consider the source of the anxiety. The person with panic disorder seeks to eliminate chest pain, thereby removing the possibility of a heart attack, whereas the person with social phobia may look for signs that he is not being negatively evaluated. One of the first tasks in cognitive therapy is to guide clients into an acknowledgment that the situational triggers and perceived possibilities of terrible outcomes is not the cause of their anxiety. This is accomplished through the cognitive restructuring and empirical hypothesis-testing interventions that are discussed below.

It is critical that the cognitive therapist avoid any attempt to verbally persuade anxious clients against their anxious threat. This warning against trying to verbally modify threat content was emphasized by Salkovskis (1985, 1989) for treatment of obsessions. Thus the therapist must not engage in verbal debates about the possibility of having a heart attack, suffocating, contaminating others with a deadly germ, making a mistake, being negatively evaluated in a social setting, being the victim of another assault, or experiencing some negative outcome in the future. After all, any clever arguments that can be concocted by the therapist will be immediately dismissed by the client because mistakes do happen, people can become the victim of disease by contamination, and even the occasional young person dies from a heart attack. The reality is that threat can never be eliminated entirely. At best such persuasive debates will only amount to reassurance that provides temporary relief from anxiety and at worst the client's outright dismissal of the effectiveness of cognitive therapy. Thus it is critical to the success of cognitive therapy that therapy avoids a direct focus on the client's threat content.

Clinician Guideline 6.1

Avoid any attempt to use logical persuasion to directly target primary threat content. Such attempts will undermine the effectiveness of cognitive therapy and result in the persistence of the anxious state.

Focus on Appraisals and Beliefs

The cognitive perspective views anxiety in terms of an information-processing system that exaggerates the probability and severity of threat, minimizes personal ability to cope, and fails to recognize aspects of safety (i.e., Rachman, 2006). An important objective in cognitive therapy, then, is to shift the client's focus from threat content to how they appraise or evaluate threat. For cognitive therapy to be effective, the client must accept the cognitive model (i.e., treatment rationale) that their anxiety arises from their faulty thoughts, beliefs, and appraisals of threat rather than from the threat content itself.

This approach to anxiety recognizes that individuals with an anxiety disorder often fail to adopt a rational, realistic appraisal of the dangers related to their anxious concerns, especially during anxious states. In fact anxious individuals often recognize that a danger is highly unlikely, or even impossible. However, the problem is that they will appraise even a remote danger (1/1,000,000,000) as an unacceptable risk. Thus the cognitive therapist must focus on the thoughts, appraisals, and beliefs about threat (e.g., feelings of nausea) and vulnerability rather than threat content per se. The following is a clinical vignette that illustrates how this shift in therapeutic orientation can be achieved with a person suffering from social phobia:

THERAPIST: Looking over your diary, I see that you were especially anxious in a meeting you had with work colleagues last week.

CLIENT: Yes, the anxiety was really intense. I was so scared someone would ask me a question.

THERAPIST: What would be so bad about that?

CLIENT: I'm afraid I would say something stupid and everyone would think I'm an idiot.

THERAPIST: What do you think was making you anxious about the meeting?

CLIENT: Well I was anxious because I could be asked a question and then I would say something stupid and everyone would think badly of me. [focus on threat content]

THERAPIST: It sounds like you certainly had anxious thoughts like "what if I'm asked a question" and "what if I say something stupid." Do you suppose other people who do not have social anxiety also have these same thoughts from time to time?

CLIENT: Well, I suppose they do but I feel so anxious and they don't.

THERAPIST: True, that is an important difference. But I wonder if this difference is caused by how you evaluate these thoughts when you have them and how a nonanxious person evaluates the thoughts when she has them about a work meeting.

CLIENT: I'm not sure I understand what you mean.

THERAPIST: When you think "I could be asked a question" and "I could say something stupid," how likely do you think this is and what do you think could be a consequence or outcome?

CLIENT: When I'm anxious I tend to be entirely convinced I'm going to say something stupid and that everyone will think I'm an idiot.

THERAPIST: So when you have these anxious thoughts you evaluate the probability that it will happen as very high ("you will say something stupid") and that terrible consequences will result ("everyone will think I'm an idiot"). Do you suppose this might be the source of your anxiety, that it is these appraisals of high probability and serious consequences that are making you anxious? [focus on appraisals of threat]

CLIENT: Well, I don't really know. I always thought that what made me anxious is that I tend to say stupid things when I'm around people.

THERAPIST: Let's see if we can find out more about this. For a homework assignment, do you have some close friends or family you could ask about whether they have ever had concerns about saying something stupid in a public setting? It would be interesting to find out how they appraise or think about these situations that results in not feeling anxious.

CLIENT: Yes, I could do that.

THERAPIST: Great! So let's see whether the way we appraise or think about situations (e.g., "I will probably say something stupid and everyone will think I'm an idiot") is an important cause of anxiety or not. If these appraisals are important, then we will want to change them as part of our treatment for social anxiety.

Clinician Guideline 6.2

A key element of cognitive therapy of anxiety is teaching clients that the source of persistent anxiety is their biased appraisals of threat. The success of other cognitive interventions depends on clients' acceptance of this cognitive or information-processing formulation of anxiety.

Modify Biased Threat, Vulnerability, and Safety Appraisals and Beliefs

In cognitive therapy of anxiety the main objective of cognitive interventions is to modify overestimated appraisals of threat and personal vulnerability related to the primary anxious concern as well as change the client's perspective on the safety aspects of the situation. Cognitive interventions tend to focus on four key elements of faulty cognition.

- *Probability estimates:* What is the perceived threat or danger? Is the client generating an exaggerated probability estimate of the threat or danger?
- *Severity estimates:* Is there a biased evaluation of the severity of the perceived outcome or consequence of the threat?
- *Vulnerability estimates:* What is the level of perceived personal vulnerability when in the anxious situation? To what extent are the client's perceived weaknesses exaggerated when anxious?
- *Safety estimates:* What safety information is being ignored or undervalued, resulting in a downgraded estimate of perceived safety in the anxious situation?

The faulty appraisals of threat and vulnerability are evident in the automatic apprehensive thoughts or images, misinterpretations of physiological arousal, cognitive errors, dysfunctional defenses and coping strategies, and primary worry symptoms identified in the case conceptualization (see Appendix 5.11). Table 6.1 illustrates typical appraisals that are associated with the anxiety disorders.

Once the biased appraisals have been well articulated in therapy, the goal of cognitive interventions is to arrive at a more balanced, realistic appraisal of the probability

TABLE 6.1 Illustrative Examples of Threat, Vulnerability, and Safety Appraisals Associated with the Anxiety Disorders

Anxiety disorders	Threat probability appraisals	Threat severity appraisals	Perceived vulnerability estimates	Biased safety estimates
Panic disorder	"I'm having difficulty breathing; I'm not getting enough air."	"What if I can't breathe and suffocate to death?"	"I can't handle this feeling of not being able to breathe; it is a terrifying experience."	"No one is around to help me. I'm so far from a hospital. I need more oxygen."
Generalized anxiety disorder	"I just know that I'm going to do poorly in the job interview."	"I'll make such a fool of myself; the interviewers will wonder why I ever applied for this job. I'll never find a good job."	"I never interview well. I become so anxious that I lose my concentration and end up rambling all over the place."	"Job interviewers are just looking for an excuse to reject you. Besides they have already made up their mind not to hire you before you start the interview."
Social phobia	"People are looking at me and notice that I'm shaky."	"They'll wonder what's wrong with me; does she have a mental illness?"	"I can't cope with these social situations; I get too anxious."	"I can't conceal my anxiety from others; how could anyone not see that I'm anxious."
Obsessive–compulsive disorder	"I have a terrible feeling that I didn't turn off the stove."	"If I did leave the stove burner on, it could start a fire."	"I am prone to making mistakes, being forgetful, and so could easily leave the burner on."	"I don't have an accurate memory of turning it completely off. I need to check and concentrate hard on whether the knob is completely off."
Posttraumatic stress disorder	"I have to avoid situations that remind me of the trauma because I will have intrusive recollections of what happened to me."	"I feel so helpless, alone, and frightened when I have these intrusive thoughts and memories of the ambush. It's almost as bad as when I was under fire."	"I've got to stop having these intrusive thoughts and flashbacks of the ambush. And yet I can't control them; they've taken over my life."	"The only time I can forget is when I'm drinking. There is no escape from the memories even when I'm asleep."

and severity of threat, the person's actual ability to cope with the situation, and whether it is more realistic to assume safety rather than danger. This latter perspective can only be achieved by helping clients abandon their maladaptive safety-seeking practices and focus on aspects of the anxious situation that denote safety. Interventions such as cognitive restructuring and empirical hypothesis testing are used to achieve this modification in anxious thoughts, beliefs, and appraisals.

A focus on the modification of threat appraisals has always been at the heart of cognitive therapy for anxiety (e.g., D. M. Clark, 1986b; Wells, 1997). Beck et al. (1985, 2005) state that cognitive restructuring teaches clients to replace questions about "why" they are feeling anxious with "how" they are making themselves feel anxious (i.e., appraisals of threat). Recent cognitive behavioral treatment manuals for the anxiety disorders have also emphasized the use of cognitive interventions to modify threat appraisals (e.g., Craske & Barlow, 2006; D. A. Clark, 2004; D. M. Clark, 1997; Rachman, 2003; Rygh & Sanderson, 2004; Taylor, 2006). In addition, evidence from the social experimental literature on emotion regulation indicates that cognitive reappraisal as a coping strategy is associated with greater positive emotion, less negative emotion, and better psychological health (John & Gross, 2004). Thus our emphasis on the reappraisal of threat and vulnerability has broad support in the psychotherapeutic and experimental literature.

Clinical Guideline 6.3

The primary focus of cognitive interventions is the modification of exaggerated estimates (appraisals) of the probability and severity of threat as well as evaluations of personal vulnerability and lack of safety.

Normalize Fear and Anxiety

Normalizing anxiety was first discussed by Beck et al. (1985) in their chapter on modifying the affective component of anxiety. At that time normalizing anxiety was highlighted as a way to help clients become less self-absorbed in their anxiety symptoms. There are three aspects of the normalization of anxiety that must be considered.

1. *Normalizing in relation to others.* The actual situations, thoughts, and sensations that are associated with anxiety should be normalized. Anxious individuals are often so focused on their own experience of anxiety that they fail to recognize that these phenomena are almost universal. For example, how often do people experience chest pain or breathlessness, a concern that they have made a bad impression on others, doubt over their actions or decisions, uncertainty about the possibility of some accident or future calamity, or recollections about some frightening experience? The therapist can ask clients to consider the "normality of threat" and possibly even collect survey data on whether nonanxious individuals ever experience the anxious threat. The purpose of this exercise is to shift individuals' focus away from threat content as the source of their anxiety to their appraisal of threat as the main contributor to their anxious state.

2. *Normalizing in relation to past experiences.* The therapist should explore clients' past experience with the situations, thoughts, or sensations that now trigger their anxiety. "Was there a time when having tightness in your chest didn't really bother you?" "Have you always been so concerned about what others think of you?" "Was there a time when concern about germs was not such a big deal in your life?" By inquiring about their past, clients will be remembering a time when they coped much better with the perceived threat. Again this shifts the focus from "I am an anxious person" to "What am I doing now that has made my anxiety so much worse?"

3. *Normalizing in relation to situations.* When assessing the situations that trigger anxiety, the cognitive therapist can also identify other situations that trigger the same thoughts or sensations but that do not lead to an anxious episode. For example, when working with panic disorder it is often helpful to inquire whether the client experiences physical sensations when exercising or engaging in vigorous activity but does not feel

anxious. In fact clients could be asked to exercise as a behavioral experiment to highlight their different appraisals of physical sensations (see discussion in next chapter). This type of normalization highlights the situational nature of anxiety and again emphasizes the client's ability to cope with anxiety-related triggers when they occur in nonanxious situations. It also reinforces the cognitive perspective that anxiety arises from appraisals rather than the actual stimuli that trigger anxiousness. (E.g., "When you are exercising and you feel tightness in your chest, you attribute this to physical exertion. You expect to feel tense while exercising. But when you feel spontaneous chest tightness, you attribute this to a possible impending heart attack. You tell yourself something is wrong, this shouldn't be happening. So when exercising you interpret chest tightness in a way that results in no anxiety, whereas when the chest tightness arises unexpectedly, you interpret the sensations in another way that leads to anxiousness, even panic.")

Normalizing fear and anxiety is an important objective in cognitive therapy of anxiety. It not only reinforces the focus on threat appraisals as the source of anxiety, but it produces a more optimistic attitude toward overcoming anxiety. Clients are reminded that very often they react to threat in a nonanxious, even courageous manner. As Rachman (2006) recently noted, "In specifiable circumstances virtually everyone, including patients suffering from anxiety disorders, can behave courageously" (p. 7). In cognitive therapy we remind clients that they often "turn off the fear program" in a variety of situations not related to their anxiety disorder. The goal of treatment, then, is to build on their own natural abilities to overcome fear and apply these resources to the anxiety disorder.

Clinician Guideline 6.4

Normalization of fear and anxiety, an important element of cognitive therapy, is achieved by emphasizing the universality of threat, the client's past experiences with anxious cues, and the situational or variable nature of anxious triggers.

Strengthen Personal Efficacy

In cognitive therapy therapeutic interventions do not focus only on modifying faulty threat appraisals but also on correcting erroneous beliefs about personal vulnerability and perceived inability to deal with one's anxious concerns. The cognitive therapist can construct the client's vulnerability perspective from the first apprehensive thoughts, automatic defensive responses, coping strategies, and worries identified in the cognitive case conceptualization. An important theme that runs throughout the course of treatment is "You're stronger than you think" when it comes to dealing with the anxious concerns. Building a greater sense of self-efficacy (i.e., Bandura, 1977, 1989) by structuring experiences and highlighting information that reinforces perceived control or mastery of the anxiety-related threat are critical elements in cognitive therapy of anxiety that will help clients override the threat-schema activation.

During cognitive restructuring and empirical hypothesis-testing exercises the cognitive therapist emphasizes the difference between an initial vulnerability estimate and the actual outcome related to an anxious situation. The goal is to teach clients how their initial thoughts and beliefs about vulnerability are a faulty representation of reality that makes them more anxious and contributes to avoidance and ineffective coping responses. The following clinical vignette illustrates how perceived vulnerability can be challenged with a client suffering from generalized anxiety.

CLIENT: I have been worried for a few days about my daughter's visit. I am so concerned that everything will go well. You know I haven't seen her for so long. When she left home a couple of years ago we had such a big argument. At that time she swore she would never come back home again.

THERAPIST: What's the worst that could happen when she visits?

CLIENT: Well, she could bring up the past and then we would get into a huge argument. She would then storm out of the house and never return.

THERAPIST: That would certainly be a terrible outcome for you. I know how much you really love your daughter.

CLIENT: Yeah, I've been trying to think how I can avoid an argument.

THERAPIST: And what have you come up with?

CLIENT: Basically nothing. Every time I try to visualize how it will go and what I will do if she brings up the past, all I can see is anger, shouting, and her slamming the door as she leaves the house. [low self-efficacy appraisals and beliefs]

THERAPIST: Sounds like you feel pretty helpless. When you are thinking like this what happens to your anxiety and worry?

CLIENT: I just end up feeling more anxious and worried about the visit.

THERAPIST: So one effect of thinking that you are incapable of handling this situation is that your anxiety and worry escalate. How do you think all of this will affect your interactions with your daughter?

CLIENT: I don't think it is helping me in any positive way. I end up feeling so scared and confused, probably I will end up blurting out something stupid when she is with me that will only make matters worse.

THERAPIST: Okay, let me summarize. You've described worries over your daughter's visit next weekend. One of the themes running through this worry is "I'm helpless to avoid a conflict" and this helplessness makes you feel even more anxious and less prepared for your daughter's visit. But I wonder if you are as helpless as you think. I wonder if you as poor at coping with confrontation or your daughter's anger as you think. I would like to suggest a couple of things. First, let's go over some of your past experiences with people who are angry or confrontational and see how you've managed. Are you as bad at dealing with these situations as you think? And second, let's take a problem-solving approach and write down, maybe even role-play, some strategies you might use with your daughter when she visits. [The therapeutic intervention seeks to contrast the client's predicted self-efficacy with actual outcomes in the past in order to highlight discrepancy and exaggeration of low perceived self-efficacy.]

CLIENT: This sounds like a good idea. I'm really worried about this visit.

Clinician Guideline 6.5

The therapist focuses on correcting low perceived self-efficacy for anxiety by pointing out how a discrepancy between predicted ability to cope and actual past outcomes contributes to anxiety. In addition the therapist adopts a problem-solving approach to expand the client's repertoire of adaptive coping resources and to foster positive experiences to enhance self-efficacy.

Adaptive Approach to Safety

In Chapter 3 we reviewed empirical research indicating that safety-seeking thoughts, beliefs, and behaviors are important contributors to anxiety. Consequently dealing with safety-seeking issues is an important theme in CT for anxiety. Three aspects of safety seeking should be considered in treatment.

Faulty Risk Appraisals

Salkovskis (1996a) noted that threat appraisal that leads to safety seeking is a balance between the perceived probability and severity of threat, on the one hand, and coping ability and perceived rescue factors, on the other. Kozak, Foa, and McCarthy (1988) commented that in OCD danger is assumed unless there is evidence for complete safety whereas the opposite viewpoint prevails in nonanxious states in which safety is assumed unless there is valid evidence of danger. The person with panic disorder may find heart rate increases too risky, or the person with OCD might be convinced that any observable dirt is a harbinger of disease and destruction. This strategy will confirm the patient's fear while disconfirming safety evidence is overlooked.

An important goal of cognitive therapy is to investigate with clients whether they hold faulty appraisals and assumptions about risk. What, then, constitutes "an acceptable level of risk"? "Can one eliminate all possibility of risk?" "What effect does this have on a person's life?" "Do nonanxious people live with risk"? "How successful have you been at eliminating all risk and at what cost to you?" These are questions that the cognitive therapist explores with clients when reviewing their self-monitoring diaries in an effort to correct maladaptive risk appraisal.

Enhance Safety-Seeking Processing

There are many aspects of anxious situations that signal safety rather than threat, but the anxious person often misses this information. When reviewing homework assignments, attention can be drawn to safety elements that the client may have ignored or minimized. Furthermore, anxious clients can be asked to intentionally record any safety information conveyed in an anxious situation. This safety information can be contrasted with threat information in order to generate a more realistic reappraisal of the magnitude of the risk associated with a particular situation. Throughout treatment the cognitive therapist must be vigilant for biases that minimize safety and maximize threat, thereby resulting in a threat-oriented information processing bias.

Dysfunctional Avoidance and Safety-Seeking Behavior

An important objective in cognitive therapy for anxiety is the identification and subsequent correction of avoidance and maladaptive safety-seeking behavior that contributes to the persistence of anxiety. As noted in the cognitive case conceptualization, these safety-seeking strategies can be cognitive or behavioral in nature. For example, clients with panic disorder might use controlled breathing whenever feeling breathless in order to avert a panic attack, or the person with social anxiety may avoid eye contact in social interactions.

Often safety-seeking responses have been built up over many years and may occur quite automatically. In such cases one can not expect the client to immediately cease the safety-seeking behavior. Instead the cognitive therapist should challenge the safety-seeking gradually, first working with the client to understand the role of such behavior in the persistence of anxiety. Once the client acknowledges its deleterious effects, then the maladaptive coping can be gradually phased out and substituted with more positive adaptive strategies. It is likely that this process may have to be repeated a number of times for anxious clients with multiple avoidant and safety-seeking responses.

Clinician Guideline 6.6

The clinician must address faulty risk appraisals, inhibited processing of safety cues, and maladaptive avoidant and safety-seeking responses throughout the course of cognitive therapy of anxiety disorders. Gradually phase out maladaptive safety-seeking responses and replace them with alternative, more adaptive strategies over an extended period of time.

COGNITIVE INTERVENTION STRATEGIES

In this section we present the actual therapeutic strategies that can be used to achieve the main objectives of cognitive therapy for anxiety. Naturally, these intervention strategies will be modified when used with the specific anxiety disorders discussed in the third part of this volume.

Educating the Client

Educating clients has always played a central role in cognitive therapy (Beck et al., 1979, 1985, 2005). Today it continues to be emphasized in practically every cognitive therapy and cognitive-behavioral treatment manual (e.g., J. S. Beck, 1995; D. A. Clark, 2004; D. M. Clark, 1997; Craske & Barlow, 2006; Rygh & Sanderson, 2004; Rachman, 1998, 2003, 2006; Taylor, 2006; Wells, 1997). The didactic component of treatment may not only improve treatment compliance but it can also directly contribute to the correction of faulty beliefs about fear and anxiety (Rachman, 2006).

There are three aspects of educating the client that are important in cognitive therapy for anxiety. First, individuals often have misconceptions about anxiety and so a discussion of fear and anxiety should be given with reference to the client's personal experiences. Second, a cognitive explanation for the persistence of anxiety should be

TABLE 6.2. Primary Elements of Educating the Client into the Cognitive Model and Treatment of Anxiety

Themes emphasized when educating the client

- Define anxiety and the role of fear
- The universal and adaptive nature of fear
- Cognitive explanation for inappropriate activation of the anxiety program
- Consequences of inappropriate activation of anxiety
- Escape, avoidance, and other attempts to control anxiety
- Treatment goal: turning off the anxiety program
- Treatment strategies used to deactivate the anxiety program
- The role of other approaches to anxiety reduction (e.g., medication, relaxation, herbal remedies)

provided in a manner that clients can readily understand and apply to their own situation. And third, the cognitive treatment rationale should be clarified so that clients will fully collaborate in the treatment process. In our experience clients who terminate therapy within the first three to four sessions often do so because they have not been educated into the cognitive model or they fail to accept this explanation for their anxiety. Either way, educating the client begins at the first session and will be an important therapeutic ingredient in the early sessions.

Table 6.2 presents the main themes that should be addressed when educating the client about the cognitive approach to anxiety. We briefly discuss how the therapist can communicate this information to clients in a comprehensible manner.

Defining Anxiety and Fear

Clients should be provided with an operational definition of what is meant by fear and anxiety from a cognitive perspective. Based on the definitions in Chapter 1, *fear can be described as perceived threat or danger to our safety or security.* Clients can be asked for examples of when they felt fearful and what the perceived danger was that characterized the fear (e.g., near accident, waiting for results of medical tests, threatened with violence or aggression). It should be pointed out that even thinking about or imaging worst-case scenarios can elicit fear. Again examples of imagined fears could be discussed. In the same way anxiety can be described *as a more complex, prolonged feeling of unease or apprehension involving feelings, thoughts, and behavior that occurs when our vital interests are threatened.* Whereas fear is usually momentary, anxiety can last for hours, maybe even days. Given the ubiquitous nature of computers and information technology in modern society, most people will readily understand if anxiety is described as analogous to *"a computer program that gets turned on, takes over the operating system, and won't quit until it is deactivated or turned off."* Throughout treatment, we find it useful to refer to "activating and deactivating the fear program" and the importance of "turning off the fear program" in order to eliminate anxiety. The therapist should be asking the client for personal examples of fear and anxiety in order to reinforce a full understanding of the concepts. This will ensure that client and therapist have a common language when talking about experiences of anxiety.

Adaptive Value of Fear

Most individuals suffering from an anxiety disorder have forgotten about the important role that fear plays in our survival. The therapist should discuss the universal nature of fear and its survival function. Clients can be asked about times when being afraid "saved their life" by mobilizing them to deal with a potential threat or danger. Beck et al. (1985, 2005) noted that it is often helpful to discuss with clients the "fight-or-flight" response that characterizes fear.

In the same way mild to moderate levels of subjective anxiety (nervousness) can be adaptive if it is not too intense or prolonged. Being nervous about an impending exam or job interview might motivate a person to be better prepared. Performers acknowledge that some degree of nervousness is both expected and beneficial before going on stage. Again the therapist can solicit past experiences from the client when anxiety was actually functional.

The reason for including a discussion on the positive function and adaptive value of fear and anxiety is to emphasize that these states are not abnormal. The problem in anxiety disorders is not the experience of fear or anxiety, but the fact that the fear program is inappropriately activated or turned on. Thus the goal of therapy is not to eliminate all anxiety but rather to reduce anxiety that is inappropriate or maladaptive. Another reason for emphasizing the survival value of fear is to normalize clients' anxiety so they view it as an exaggeration or misapplication of normal emotion. This should bolster a great sense of hope and optimism in treatment since they are not as different from "normal people" as they may have been thinking.

Cognitive Explanation for Inappropriate Activation of Anxiety

The preceding discussion on the normality of fear and anxiety will naturally lead into the issue of why the client's anxiety is so much more intense, persistent, and triggered by things that don't bother most people. This is the crux of the educational phase because it is critically important to the success of therapy that clients realize that their appraisals of threat are the primary determinants of their clinical anxiety. A copy of Figure 6.1 can be given to clients in order to facilitate an explanation of the cognitive model of anxiety.

Education into the cognitive model will occur after the assessment so the therapist can draw on the cognitive case conceptualization to obtain examples of the client's typical responses when anxious. The therapist should go through each step in Figure 6.1 and elicit from the client examples of typical situations, automatic thoughts, anxious symptoms, search for safety and avoidance, worry and preoccupation with anxiety and helplessness, and failed attempts to control anxiety. These experiences could be written down on Figure 6.1 as a record for the client on how the cognitive model explains inappropriate fear activation and the persistence of her clinical anxiety. Any questions or doubts concerning the applicability of the cognitive explanation for the client's anxiety should be addressed using the guided discovery in which the therapist questions the client in a manner that will encourage her to reevaluate her misgivings about the cognitive explanation (Beck et al., 1979). In most cases it is helpful to assign a homework assignment such as having the person fill in Figure 6.1 immediately after an anxiety episode. This will help consolidate a better understanding and acceptance of a cognitive explanation for the clinical anxiety state.

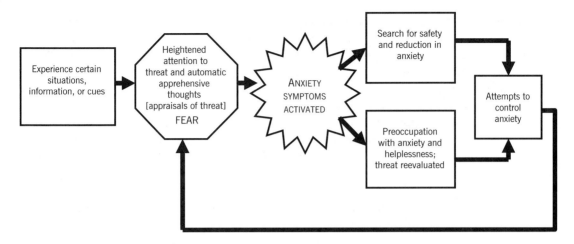

FIGURE 6.1. Diagram of the cognitive model of anxiety for use with clients.

Consequences of Inappropriate Anxiety

Most individuals with an anxiety disorder are all too familiar with the negative consequences of their anxiety. However, it is important to discuss consequences because having "fear of anxiety" is a prominent feature of clinical anxiety (Beck et al., 1985, 2005; D. M. Clark, 1986b). The therapist can explore with the client whether being "anxious about being anxious" might actually intensify the clinical disorder by making a person more sensitive or vigilant for any signs of anxiety (i.e., latter phase in Figure 6.1).

It is important to discuss how anxiety is manifested in the three major response systems; the physiological, the behavioral, and the cognitive. This should be discussed in reference to the clients' own experience of anxiety. Craske and Barlow (2006) provide a very helpful explanation of the three components of anxiety in their self-help book for worry called *Mastery of Your Anxiety and Worry*. They note that a better understanding of the physical, cognitive, and behavioral components of anxiety helps reduce the mystery and uncontrollability of anxiety and provides a framework for learning ways to reduce anxiety.

Some discussion of the broader consequences of having anxiety should be incorporated into educating the client. What effect does anxiety have in the client's daily life at work, home, and leisure? Are there restrictions or limitations imposed on what individuals can do or where they can go? The broader negative impact of anxiety needs to be emphasized in order to encourage client commitment to the therapeutic process by helping individuals think in terms of the costs and benefits of change. A consideration of the "personal burden of anxiety" can also help in the establishment of treatment goals.

The Role of Avoidance and Safety Seeking

It is useful to ask clients what they think is the most effective way to reduce anxiety. Although a variety of answers may be given, it should be emphasized that escape and avoidance (or completion of a compulsive ritual in OCD) ensure the quickest reduction in anxiety. The therapist and client can discuss a number of life-threatening examples where escape or avoidance actually ensures one's survival. Examples can also be given of animals (i.e., the client's pets) that automatically escape or avoid perceived danger. It should be emphasized that escape and avoidance are natural responses to perceived threat and danger.

A discussion of the natural, automatic character of escape and avoidance should lead into a consideration of their negative consequences and how escape and avoidance contribute to the persistence of anxiety. In their self-help book on panic entitled *10 Simple Solutions to Panic*, Antony and McCabe (2004) cite four disadvantages of escape/avoidance:

- It prevents learning that situations are safe, not dangerous or threatening (i.e., failure to disconfirm faulty appraisals and beliefs of threat).
- The subjective relief associated with escape/avoidance reinforces this behavior in future episodes of anxiety.
- Giving into escape/avoidance will increase a sense of guilt and disappointment in one's self and a loss of self-confidence.
- The immediate relief associated with escape/avoidance increases one's sensitivity to threat cues so that in the long term it will maintain or even increase fear and anxiety.

Throughout this discussion of the negative effects of escape/avoidance, the therapist should be soliciting personal examples and questioning the client on any perceived adverse consequences of continued escape/avoidance. By educating the client on the role of escape/avoidance in anxiety the therapist seeks to increase awareness that elimination of this control strategy is critical to the success of treatment. It will also lay the groundwork for introducing prolonged exposure to threat as the obvious remedy for this maladaptive defensive strategy (a fact that most individuals with anxiety are most reluctant to accept).

The therapist should also explore with clients any dysfunctional safety-seeking behaviors that may be used to alleviate anxious feelings. Do clients carry anxiolytic medications at all times just in case they are needed? Do they only venture into certain places when accompanied by a close friend or family member? Are there other more subtle forms of safety seeking such as holding onto railings when feeling dizzy or automatically sitting down when feeling weak? After examples of safety seeking are elicited, the therapist should discuss how this form of coping with anxiety might contribute to its persistence because:

- It prevents one from learning that his fears (i.e., perceived threats) are groundless (Salkovskis, 1996a).
- It creates a false sense of security (e.g., person with panic disorder develops maladaptive belief that having a friend close by somehow reduces the risk of heart palpitations and a heart attack).

Once again the purpose for educating clients about the role of safety-seeking responses is to increase their acceptance that reduction in this behavior is an important goal of treatment.

Treatment Goal

In keeping with our metaphor of fear as "a computer program," the therapist introduces the treatment rationale by explaining the goal of cognitive therapy in terms of "deactivating or turning off" the fear program by deliberately and intentionally engaging in activities that will "override" or "counter" fear and anxiety. The therapist should refer to Figure 6.1 and indicate that the fear program can be deactivated by intervening at all the different steps that contribute to the persistence of anxious symptoms. Clients could be asked to provide examples of their own success in deliberately overcoming an initial fear. It is also important to question the client about treatment expectations in order to elicit any misconceptions that could undermine the success of cognitive therapy.

There are a number of common faulty misconceptions about treatment that might need addressing. First, treatment can not permanently shut down fear. The goal is not to eliminate anxiety totally (if that was even possible) but to help clients develop effective ways to override the fear program when it is inappropriately activated. Second, the experience of anxiety will feel more natural, whereas efforts to reduce anxiety will seem much more difficult. This is because the former is an automatic response to perceived threat and the latter requires a much more deliberate, effortful response. This does not mean that intentional responses to anxiety are not powerful enough to deactivate fear and reduce anxiety. What it does mean is that repeated experiences with these effortful responses will be needed in order to improve their efficiency and effectiveness. And third, the objective of cognitive therapy is not to teach people more effective ways to "control their anxiety." Instead cognitive therapy focuses on helping individuals develop a more "accepting attitude" toward anxiety rather than a "combative (i.e., controlling) attitude." When thoughts like "I can't let these anxious feelings continue" are replaced with "I can allow myself to feel anxious because I know I'm exaggerating the threat and danger," then the intensity and persistence of anxiety are greatly diminished (Beck et al., 1985, 2005).

Treatment Strategies

Clients should be provided with a brief description and rationale for the intervention strategies that will be used to "turn off" the fear program and diminish their anxious feelings. The therapist should explain that a greater understanding of one's anxiety through education and the self-monitoring of anxious episodes are important interventions in cognitive therapy of anxiety. These components of treatment help counter the unexpected and unpredictable nature of anxiety.

The therapist explains that a second class of cognitive therapy interventions focuses directly on changing anxious thoughts and beliefs. This is accomplished by learning to critically question whether one's initial apprehensive thoughts are an accurate appraisal of the situation and then replacing these anxious interpretations with a more realistic way of thinking. Specific behavioral experiments are designed that will help the client develop a less anxious way of thinking. The therapist should emphasize that developing new ways of thinking about their anxious concerns is an important part of treatment because it directly targets the automatic apprehensive thoughts that give rise to anxious symptoms (refer to Figure 6.1).

A third category of cognitive therapy interventions deals with behavioral responses and coping strategies that may contribute to the persistence of anxiety. Escape, avoidance, safety-seeking behavior, and other cognitive or behavioral responses employed by clients in an effort to control their anxiety are targeted for change. Alternative ways of responding to anxiety are introduced and clients are encouraged to evaluate the utility of these approaches through use of behavioral exercises.

A final ingredient of cognitive therapy for anxiety involves graduated and repeated exposure to anxiety-provoking situations and a phasing out of escape, avoidance, safety seeking, or other forms of neutralizing responses (e.g., compulsive rituals in OCD). When introducing the concept of fear exposure, it must be realized that this can be terrifying to anxious individuals. Many anxious clients refuse to continue with treatment at the mere mention of exposure because they can not imagine dealing with the intense anxiety they expect to experience in highly fearful situations. To counter the client's negative expectations, the therapist should emphasize that exposure to fear situations is the most potent intervention for achieving lasting fear reduction. Exposure exercises will be introduced later in therapy in a very gradual fashion starting with experiences with a low to moderate level of anxiety in order to elicit core cognitions that underlie anxious feelings. All assignments will be discussed in a collaborative fashion with the client having the final say on what is expected at any point in therapy. The therapist should also reassure clients that an exposure task that seems too difficult can always be broken down or modified to reduce the level of anxiety. Finally, the therapist should explain the benefits of exposure to anxious situations. It reduces anxiety by providing evidence against threat-related "hot" cognitions and beliefs, it bolsters self-confidence, and it provides opportunity to practice more adaptive ways of coping with anxiety.

Other Approaches to Anxiety

Often clients will inquire whether medication, meditation, herbal remedies, and the like can be used while having a course of cognitive therapy for anxiety. However, these approaches are somewhat counterproductive to cognitive therapy because they all emphasize the short-term reduction and avoidance of anxious symptoms without concomitant change in cognition. For many individuals these interventions may have become an important part of their coping strategy for anxiety. Thus any withdrawal of these interventions should be done *gradually*, commensurate with a reduction in the client's anxiety level with progress through cognitive therapy. Naturally no change in medication should be recommended unless prescribed by the client's medical practitioner.

Methods of Educating the Client

Although a certain amount of verbal teaching is an evitable part of the educational process, it should not be the sole means of communicating the cognitive model and treatment rationale. The therapist should be asking clients about their personal experiences and using guided discovery to emphasize key aspects of the cognitive model that can be identified in these experiences. Clients are much more likely to accept the model if it has immediate relevance to their own experiences with anxiety.

The therapist can also assign self-monitoring homework to encourage the client to explore whether different aspects of the cognitive model are relevant to his anxiety. For example, a client with social phobia could be asked to experiment with the effects of giving eye contact versus avoiding eye contact in social interactions as a way of determining whether subtle forms of avoidance and safety seeking have an effect on her anxiety level. A client with OCD could be asked to try hard to suppress an anxious obsession on one day and then relinquish control efforts on an alternative day and record the effects of trying to control anxiety. A person with panic disorder could be asked to record the effects of thinking about a heart attack when his chest feels tight versus thinking that it is muscle strain. Notice that all of these assignments focus more on highlighting some aspect of the cognitive model in the client's experience of anxiety rather than directly modifying thoughts or behavior.

Bibliotherapy is an important method of educating the client into the cognitive model. We are currently in the process of writing a client workbook based on the present volume that will provide explanations and case examples useful for educating clients into the cognitive therapy perspective on anxiety. A number of other excellent self-help manuals have been published as well on cognitive therapy or CBT for anxiety disorders that can be given to clients as assigned reading. Appendix 6.1 presents a selected list of self-help manuals that are consistent with the cognitive model. Often clients are even more accepting of cognitive therapy after reading published accounts because it provides external validation that cognitive therapy is a well established and widely recognized treatment for anxiety.

Clinician Guideline 6.7

In the initial sessions of cognitive therapy, focus on educating the client into the cognitive model of anxiety and providing a rationale for treatment. Describe clinical anxiety as an automatic affective response to inappropriate fear activation that overtakes one's mental operating system. The goal of cognitive therapy is to deactivate, or "turn off," the fear program through deliberate and effortful changes in how we think and respond to anxiety. Educate clients into the cognitive model not by minilectures but by emphasizing its applicability to their personal experience of anxiety.

Self-Monitoring and the Identification of Anxious Thoughts

Teaching clients how to catch their anxious thoughts has been a central ingredient in cognitive therapy for anxiety since its inception (Beck et al., 1985). And yet this is one of the hardest skills for clients to master. The reason is that anxious thinking can be very difficult to recall when the person is in a nonanxious state. However, when individuals are highly anxious, they can be so overwhelmed with anxiety that any attempt to record anxious thinking is practically impossible. Moreover, it is during periods of intense anxiety that the person is most likely to exhibit the exaggerated estimates of threat probability and severity that are the core cognitive basis of anxiety (Rachman, 2006). Thus in cognitive therapy for anxiety considerable effort is focused on training in self-monitoring automatic anxious thoughts. Rachman (2006) also notes that it is important to identify the *current threat* that maintains anxiety. Daily diaries and self-monitoring of anxiety will play a critical role in identifying the perceived threat in everyday life.

There are two ways to introduce anxious clients to thought recording. First, have clients focus on writing down anxiety-provoking situations, rating their anxiety level, and noting any primary physical symptoms and any behavioral responses. These aspects of anxiety are often readily available to individuals, and will give them practice in tracking and dissecting their anxiety episodes. Second, it is important that the first introduction to anxious thinking be done in the therapy session (Beck et al., 1985). Since clients are often not anxious while in session, some form of mild anxiety induction exercise may be needed to elicit anxious thinking. For example, a panic induction exercise such as 2 minutes of overbreathing or spinning in a chair could be used to induce panic-like physical sensations. The client could be asked to verbalize any thoughts related to the exercise such as fear of heart attack, fainting, losing control, or the like. A person with PTSD could be asked to recall aspects of a past trauma and then verbalize his present thoughts about his recollected memories. A mild fear of contamination or doubt could be induced with someone suffering from OCD to elicit her appraisals about the threat. In each case the therapist would ask probing questions about the client's immediate thoughts. "What went through your mind as you were breathing harder and harder?," "What were your thoughts focused on?", "What were your main concerns?", "What was the worst that could happen?", "Did it feel like the worst outcome was likely to happen?", "Did you have any competing thoughts, such as maybe it wasn't so bad after all?"

Once the client has demonstrated some rudimentary skills at identifying his initial apprehensive (automatic) thoughts and appraisals in the therapy session, the therapist should assign a self-monitoring homework task. The Apprehensive Thoughts Self-Monitoring Form (Appendix 5.4) will be especially useful in this regard. Most clients need extended practice in self-monitoring their anxious thoughts between sessions. In fact self-monitoring of anxious thoughts and symptoms will continue throughout the course of treatment. Cognitive restructuring and empirical hypothesis testing can not be successfully employed until clients have become capable of identifying their automatic threat-related thinking.

It is important that the self-monitoring component of treatment increase the anxious person's awareness of two primary characteristics of anxious thinking:

- Overestimated probability appraisals—"Am I exaggerating the likelihood that some threat or danger will happen?"
- Exaggerated severity appraisals—"Am I overly focused on the worst possible outcome? Am I exaggerating the severity of a negative outcome?"

Sensitizing clients to their evaluations of threat is important in shifting their focus from threatening content (e.g., "What if the medical tests indicate cancer?") to how their appraisals contribute to anxiety (e.g., "Am I exaggerating the probability that the test will be positive and lead to the worst possible outcome?, If so, what effect is this having on my anxiety?"). Individuals will need repeated practice in identifying their initial apprehensive thoughts in order to improve their ability to catch the exaggerated threat appraisals. When reviewing self-monitoring homework, the cognitive therapist probes for exaggerated likelihood and severity of threat appraisals in order to reinforce the importance of this thinking in the persistence of anxiety.

Homework Compliance

Homework compliance is an important issue in cognitive therapy for anxiety and often it will be felt most keenly at the early phase of treatment when first assigning self-monitoring homework. Many clients do not like filling in forms or writing about their anxious thoughts and feelings. Even though there is mounting empirical evidence of an association between treatment improvement and homework compliance (Kazantzis, Deane, & Ronan, 2000), many clients still have great difficulty engaging in homework. This problem has been addressed in a number of recent volumes on cognitive therapy, and various suggestions have been offered for improving homework compliance (see J. S. Beck, 2005; Leahy, 2001; Kazantzis & L'Abate, 2006). In the present context the therapist should deal with any misconceptions or difficulties the client may have about homework. The importance of homework and learning to identify anxious thinking should be emphasized as an essential skill that must be acquired before utilizing the other cognitive and behavioral strategies for reducing anxiety. Homework should be assigned in a collaborative fashion with instructions written for client convenience. However, if an individual persists in refusing to engage in homework, termination of further treatment may be necessary.

There is one reason for homework noncompliance that may be specific to the anxiety disorders. Sometimes clients are reluctant to engage in any self-monitoring of their anxious thoughts and symptoms because they are concerned it will make the anxiety worse. For example, a 33-year-old man with abhorrent obsessions about pedophilic sex was afraid that writing down the occurrence and accompanying appraisals of the thoughts would not only make them more frequent and raise his anxiety level, but these thoughts were also a violation of his moral values. He was also concerned that drawing even more attention to the thoughts would erode what little control he had over the obsessions. In this example concerns about escalating anxiety, the repugnant and immoral nature of the obsessions, and fear of losing control all contributed to reluctance to engage in self-monitoring his anxious thoughts.

A number of steps can be taken to address this situation. First, it is important to make homework noncompliance a therapeutic issue. The faulty beliefs contributing to reluctance to self-monitor anxious thoughts should be identified and cognitive restructuring can be utilized to examine these beliefs and generate alternative interpretations. Possibly the homework assignment could be broken down into less threatening steps such as asking the client to experiment with self-monitoring thoughts on a certain day (or period within a day) and record the effects of the monitoring. This would be a direct behavioral test of the belief that "writing down my anxious thoughts will make me more anxious."

The cognitive therapist should spend time during the educational phase introducing the importance of homework and then periodically throughout treatment reminding the client of the role that homework plays in the success of cognitive therapy. The following is one way to explain homework to anxious clients:

"Homework assignments are a very important part of cognitive therapy. Approximately 10–15 minutes toward the end of each therapy session, I will suggest that we summarize the main issues we've dealt with in the session and then decide on a homework assignment. We will discuss the assignment together and make sure it is something that you agree is doable. I will write the assignment down so we are both clear on what needs to be done. From week to week I will also be giving you different types of forms on which to record the results of the assignment. The assignments will be short and not involve more than a few minutes out of your day.

At the beginning of each session I will review last week's homework with you. You can expect that each week we'll spend at least 10–15 minutes of the session reviewing the outcome of the homework and any problems you may have encountered. Do you have any questions at this point?

"You may be wondering, do I really have to do homework? I always hated homework in school. Besides I'm too busy for this sort of thing. You can think of cognitive therapy like 'mental exercise.' In any physical training program, you need to run, walk, or go to the gym three to five times a week in order to gain strength or lose weight. You wouldn't expect to meet your physical goals just by meeting with the trainer once a week. The same thing happens in cognitive therapy. You are developing a different mental approach to your anxiety that involves learning to respond to anxiety in ways that are not natural to you. You need lots of practice in using this alternative approach to override the automatic anxiety program. Switching off the anxiety program takes repeated practice and it won't happen just by meeting with the therapist once a week. The best way to overcome anxiety is through repeated practice in your daily life so that gradually the new way of responding becomes second nature to you. Just like in physical exercise, we've found in our research that cognitive therapy is most effective for people who do homework. Very often when clients do not benefit from treatment one of the main reasons is that they have not been doing homework. How do you feel about this aspect of therapy? Are you able to make a commitment to engage in homework at this time?"

Clinician Guideline 6.8

One of the first skills taught in cognitive therapy is the ability to identify and record the automatic apprehensive thoughts, images, and appraisals that characterize anxious episodes. In addition clients write down their observations of the physical and behavioral symptoms of anxiety. Self-monitoring anxious thoughts is a prerequisite skill for cognitive restructuring. It may be necessary to deal with homework noncompliance at this point in therapy.

Cognitive Restructuring

The goal of cognitive restructuring is to modify or literally "restructure" a person's anxious beliefs and appraisals about threat. It is an integral part of treatment for deactivating the anxiety program. The focus is on "current threat," that is, what is perceived as dangerous or threatening at this moment. Also the cognitive restructuring interventions are directed at the appraisals of threat rather than at threat content. The central question is "Am I exaggerating the probability and severity of threat and underestimating my ability to cope?" and not whether a threat could happen or not. For example, in panic disorder cognitive structuring would focus on whether the client is relying on exaggerated and biased appraisals of bodily sensations. The therapist would avoid any debate on whether or not the client could have a heart attack. The same is true for social phobia where the focus is on probability and severity appraisals of perceived negative evaluation from others and not on whether some people may be having negative thoughts about them. In this section we describe six cognitive intervention strategies: evidence gathering, cost–benefit analysis, decatastrophizing, identifying cognitive errors, generating alternatives, and empirical hypothesis testing.

Evidence Gathering

This intervention involves questioning clients on the evidence for and against their belief that a threat is highly probable and will lead to severe consequences. Evidence gathering is the sine qua non of cognitive restructuring (Beck et al., 1979, 1985, 2005) and has been variously labeled verbal disputation, logical persuasion, or verbal reattribution (Wells, 1997). After identifying a core anxious thought or belief and obtaining a belief rating on the thought, the therapist asks the following questions:

- "At the time when you are most anxious, what is happening that convinces you the threat is highly likely to occur? Is there any evidence to the contrary, that is, that the threat is not likely to occur?"
- "When you are feeling most anxious, what evidence is there that the outcome will be so serious? Is there any contradictory evidence that the outcome may not be as bad as you are thinking?"
- "What makes the evidence for your anxious thinking believable?"
- "Do you think you might be exaggerating the probability and severity of the outcome?"
- "Based on the evidence, what is a more realistic or likely estimate of the probability and severity of the worst that might happen?"

Appendix 6.2 provides an evidence-gathering form that can be used with clients. The therapist and client first write down the primary anxious thought or belief that characterizes an anxious episode. The client then provides probability and severity estimates based on how he feels during anxiety episodes. Using the Socratic form of questioning, the therapist probes for any evidence that supports such a high probability and severity estimate of outcome. Although Appendix 6.2 is limited to six entries, additional pages may be necessary to fully document the evidence supporting the anxious thought or belief. After writing down all the supporting evidence, the therapist then asks for evidence that suggests the probability and severity estimates may be exaggerated. Normally the therapist has to take more initiative in suggesting possible contradictory evidence because anxious individuals often have difficulty seeing their anxiety from this perspective. Once all the evidence against the anxious thought or belief has been recorded the client is asked to rerate the likelihood and severity of the outcome based solely on the evidence.

Individuals will sometimes protest, saying "Yes, but when I'm anxious it feels like the worst is going to happen even though I know it probably won't happen." The cognitive therapist should remind the client that "evidence gathering" is simply one approach out of many that can be used to deactivate anxiety. Whenever the client feels anxious, what has been learned from evidence gathering can be used to lower threat probability and severity appraisals to a more realistic level, thereby countering a major factor in the escalation of subjective anxiety. The following clinical example illustrates an evidence-gathering approach with a 27-year-old traveling salesperson who suffered from panic disorder and mild agoraphobic avoidance.

THERAPIST: Renée, I notice from your panic log that last Wednesday you were driving alone to a retail customer along a route that you don't normally take when you suddenly felt like you couldn't breathe. You indicated that you pulled the car to the side of the road and got out to get some fresh air. You wrote down a number of bodily sensations like a lump in your throat, feeling like you couldn't get enough air, grasping for breath, chest tightness, heart palpitations, dizziness, and general tension.

CLIENT: Yes, it was one of the worst panic attacks I've had in a long time. I just couldn't seem to breathe properly. The harder I tried the worse it got. I took sips of water to clear my throat but that didn't help.

THERAPIST: What were your afraid might be happening?

CLIENT: I was really afraid that I would suffocate. That's what it felt like. Here I was alone, in the middle of nowhere, and I couldn't breathe. It got so bad I wondered if I could actually suffocate to death.

THERAPIST: Okay, Renée, let's write that anxious thought—*"Thought that I would suffocate alone and die"*—here on this line using a form called "Testing Anxious Appraisals: Looking for Evidence" (Appendix 6.2). Now I would like you to think back to when you had the panic attack. When you were off to the side of the road, alone, and struggling to catch your breath, how likely was it that you were suffocating to death? In other words, based on how you were feeling, what did the probability that you were suffocating feel like to you from 0% (no chance it will happen) to 100% (certain it is happening).

CLIENT: Well, at the time it felt like a 90% probability that I was suffocating.

THERAPIST: And what about the severity of the outcome? How serious did it feel to you? Were you focused on the worst possible outcome like death by suffocation or something less serious like feeling the discomfort of panic? What rating would you use from 0 to 100 to indicate how serious the consequence seemed to you when you were panicky.

CLIENT: Oh, it was serious. All I could think about was suffocating to death by myself. I would give this a 100 rating.

THERAPIST: Okay, now let's look at the evidence, such as anything that was happening at the time, or past experiences, or information of any kind that would indicate that you were at high risk of experiencing a serious outcome like death by suffocation.

CLIENT: Well, one thing that makes me wonder if this suffocation feeling is serious is that it comes on me so suddenly, out of the blue. One minute I'm fine and then before I know it I can't breathe.

THERAPIST: Okay, let's put that down on the first line under evidence for the anxious thought: *"onset of suffocation feeling is rapid and unexpected."* Any other evidence that makes you think you're likely to suffocate to death?

CLIENT: The anxiety associated with this feeling is very intense, even panic. It's so bad I'm convinced something serious must be happening.

THERAPIST: Let's put that down under the second entry: *"feel intensely anxious, even panicky."* Anything else?

CLIENT: Well, the fact that I try to calm myself down by taking long, slow breaths and yet it doesn't help makes me convinced something is terribly wrong. If all of this was just bad nerves, shouldn't it go away when I breathe more slowly?

THERAPIST: Okay, a third piece of evidence for the anxious thinking is *"controlled breathing doesn't make the suffocation feelings disappear."* Is there anything else?

CLIENT: As I mentioned previously, I have very vivid memories of my uncle grasping for breath. He had a long battle with emphysema which in the final stage of the disease left him unable to breathe. It was a most horrifying way to die.

THERAPIST: So the fourth evidence for the anxious thought is *"memories of an uncle who eventually died from suffocation because of emphysema."* Is there any other evidence for your anxious thoughts about suffocation?

CLIENT: No, that pretty well covers it.

THERAPIST: Now let's look for evidence that does not support the view that you are at high risk of dying from suffocation. Can you think of any?

CLIENT: This is much harder to do. Huh.... I suppose one thing is that I haven't died yet. I mean I've had these suffocation feelings for months and yet I'm still here.

THERAPIST: Have you come close to death? For example, did you ever almost pass out, turn blue, or were paramedics ever called to provide you with oxygen?

CLIENT: No nothing like that. I've never had any tangible signs that I'm dying from suffocation.

THERAPIST: Let's write that down as evidence against your anxious thought on this first line in the right-hand column of the form: *"I've never experienced any tangible medical signs that I am dying from lack of oxygen."* Can you think of anything else?

CLIENT: Well, my family doctor has ordered various medical tests and I have seen specialists but they all say I am healthy. They say my respiration system is fine.

THERAPIST: So a second piece of evidence against the anxious thought is that *"I am physically very healthy as far as can be determined by medical science."* Is there any other evidence?

CLIENT: I can't think of any.

THERAPIST: Well, how hard is it to stop breathing? How long can you hold your breath? Let's try it. [Therapist times client on length of breath holding.]

CLIENT: That was really hard, even though I tried not to breathe, eventually I couldn't help myself. I had to breathe.

THERAPIST: Exactly, breathing is an automatic response. It is very difficult to stop breathing, even when you try your very best. Because breathing is such an automatic physiological response, people rarely just stop breathing spontaneously for no apparent reason. Have you ever heard of that happening to someone?

CLIENT: No, I haven't.

THERAPIST: So let's write that down as the third piece of evidence against your anxious suffocation thought: *"Breathing is such an automatic physiological response it is exceedingly rare to suddenly, unexpectedly stop breathing for no apparent reason."* Can you think of any other contrary evidence?

CLIENT: No, I'm stuck.

THERAPIST: Have you ever noticed whether there is anything you can do that reduces the suffocation feelings? For example, what happens to the feelings if you get distracted or are busy at work?

CLIENT: Well, on a couple of occasions when I started to get the feeling of not catching my breath and then I got real busy at work, I somehow forgot about it and the feelings went away.

THERAPIST: Okay, so maybe distraction can cause a reduction in suffocation feelings. Is there anything that seems to make the feelings worse?

CLIENT: My worst panic attacks have been when I'm driving alone in the car along a remote, unfamiliar highway. I seem to become really preoccupied with my physical state.

THERAPIST: Is there any chance, then, that focusing on breathing sensations makes the suffocation feelings worse?

CLIENT: It is possible.

THERAPIST: So let's write this down as the fourth evidence against the anxious thought: *"Suffocation feelings are worse when I focus on my breathing and least when I am distracted."* Does that sound like a condition that could lead to death? Do you suppose doctors warn people not to focus on their breathing because it might cause them to suffocate or if they have breathing problems, just distract themselves? Does this sound like a cure for emphysema?

CLIENT: No, obviously not. But I suppose it is consistent with anxiety as the cause of suffocation feelings. This is what my doctors have been telling me.

THERAPIST: Okay, so let's rerate your anxious thought *"I will suffocate alone and die."* Based on the evidence (and not on your feelings), what is the likelihood that you will die from suffocation?

CLIENT: Well, I suppose it is much less than 90% but it is certainly not zero. I'll say 20%.

THERAPIST: And based solely on the evidence, how serious is the likely outcome of your suffocation feelings?

CLIENT: Again, it's probably not 100% because death is highly unlikely. I guess the seriousness is about 60%.

THERAPIST: What this tells us is that you tend to overestimate the probability and severity of threat (*"I'll die from suffocation"*) when you are anxious. However, when you focus on the evidence (and not on your feelings) you realize the threat is much less severe. We know that making exaggerated threat estimates makes anxiety worse and when a person sees the threat more realistically, her anxiety declines. So, one way to reduce your anxiety is to correct your exaggerated anxious thoughts by reminding yourself of all the evidence against the thought and then rerating its probability and severity. After you do this a few times using Appendix 6.2 as a guide you'll become skilled at correcting your anxious thinking.

CLIENT: That sounds fine but when I'm really anxious I can't think straight.

THERAPIST: I understand but the more you practice correcting the anxious thoughts and appraisals, the more automatic the whole process becomes and the better you will get at using this technique to reduce your anxiety. Would you like to give this a try with a homework assignment?

CLIENT: Sure, let's give it a try.

[*Note:* If the client had difficulty utilizing evidence gathering in response to *in vivo* anxiety episodes, the therapist could have the client imagine panic situations and practice countering the anxiety with contradictory evidence.]

Clinician Guideline 6.9

Teach clients how to gather evidence for and against their appraisals of heightened probability and severity of threat related to their anxious concerns. Threat probability and severity estimates are recalculated solely on the basis of the evidence that is generated. Evidence gathering can be an effective method of challenging exaggerated anxious thinking by encouraging the anxious person to shift from affect-based appraisals (i.e., ex-consequentia reasoning: "I feel anxious, therefore I must be in danger") to evidence-based appraisals of a situation.

Cost–Benefit Analysis

In anxiety disorders cost–benefit analysis is a particularly versatile and effective intervention because individuals are already focused on the consequences of their thoughts and feelings. The therapist helps the client consider the question "What is the consequence, the advantages and disadvantages, of holding this particular belief or perspective in regards to my anxiety?" (see Leahy, 2003). Wells (1997) noted that cost–benefit analysis can also improve motivation for treatment. After identifying a core anxious thought, belief, or appraisal, the therapist can pose the following questions:

- "From your experience, what are the immediate and long-term consequences of embracing this anxious thought?"
- "Are there costs and benefits, or advantages and disadvantages to believing in the anxious thought?"
- "What immediate and long-term effect does this thinking have on your anxiety?"
- "If you had a different outlook on your anxiety, what would be the costs and benefits?"

The therapist can use the Cost–Benefit Form in Appendix 6.3 to conduct a cost–benefit analysis on an anxious thought or belief. The anxious thought is first recorded. Then, using guided discovery, the therapist explores the immediate and long-term advantages and disadvantages of accepting the anxious thought. Clients are asked to circle the consequences, both positive and negative, that are really important to them. Next an alternative way of thinking about the anxious situation is considered and the costs and benefits of this approach are written in the lower half of the form. Again the consequences of most significance to the client are circled. The objective of this exercise is to emphasize the heavy costs associated with anxious thinking and the immediate benefits of an alternative perspective. Homework assignments can be constructed to test out the consequences of anxious thinking and the benefits of an alternative approach. The therapist encourages clients to practice shifting their focus when anxious from the threat content to the question "Is this anxious thinking helpful or harmful?" The therapist emphasizes that repeatedly reminding oneself of the costs of anxious thinking is another effective way to weaken or deactivate the anxiety program. This intervention is particularly effective if clients fully realize that anxious thinking actually fuels their discomfort rather than helping them cope with or avert the perceived threat.

Jeremy suffered for years with GAD. One of his primary worries concerned finances despite having secure, well-paid employment. He always paid his bills, had enough money each month to contribute to his investment account, and had never even approached bankruptcy or financial hardship. And yet Jeremy continually worried that he was not putting enough into his investments and as a result he would not be prepared for the possibility of financial ruin. Using the Cost–Benefit Form, we identified Jeremy's anxious thought as *"I'm not saving enough money to prepare myself for the possibility of some future financial disaster"* (e.g., losing my job and having no income). Jeremy believed that his worry about saving money had a number of important advantages such as (1) it forced him to save more each month and so his investments were growing, (2) he watched his expenses much more closely, (3) he'll be better prepared to absorb a financial loss, (4) it ensures that he wouldn't lose the house or go bankrupt if he did lose his job, and (5) he feels better about himself when he is saving. Jeremy circled (1) and (3) as the most significant advantages of his worry.

Exploring the disadvantages of the worry proved more difficult but with therapist guidance the following list was generated: (1) the more he thinks about not saving enough, the more anxious and tense he feels; (2) once he starts to worry about saving enough, he can't seem to stop it, it completely takes over his mind; (3) he hasn't slept well because of worry over his savings; (4) there is little enjoyment in his life because he is constantly worried about finances; (5) he frequently deprives himself of little pleasures for fear of spending money; (6) he gets into severe arguments with his wife over saving and spending money and she has threatened to leave; (7) he feels distant and uninvolved with his children because of his preoccupation with finances; and (8) he spends long, frustrating hours each night monitoring his investments. Jeremy indicated that (1), (3), (6) and (7) were the most important costs associated with his worry over saving money.

At this point in therapy, Jeremy was still heavily invested in his financial worries. As a result he had difficulty generating an alternative perspective. Eventually, after considerable discussion, it was agreed that the following way of thinking could become a goal of treatment. *"I am saving enough money for temporary, moderate financial loss but there is little I can do to guarantee protection against a sustained period of total financial ruin."* We then discussed a number of advantages to this perspective on his finances: (1) less anxiety about saving because he no longer needs to amass a huge safety net of savings, (2) more tolerance for stock market fluctuations, (3) less need to monitor his investments, (4) more freedom to spend on everyday pleasures and comforts, and (5) fewer conflicts with spouse over finances because of less attempt to control expenditures. Both (1) and (5) were marked as significant advantages of the new perspective. In terms of disadvantages, Jeremy wondered (1) if he might end up with a smaller investment account because he is saving less money, and (2) he would be prepared for a narrower range of future financial losses. Overall, Jeremy agreed that the disadvantages of the anxious thoughts about saving and the advantages of adopting a more moderate view were clearly evident.

The therapist was able to use the cost–benefit analysis in future sessions by reminding Jeremy to think about "the consequences of anxious thinking about savings" and the benefits "of thinking about moderate savings." In particular, whenever Jeremy engaged in anxious worry about his finances, the therapist reminded him to "remember the cost–benefit form, and what you are doing to yourself by worrying about saving for the ultimate financial disaster." "Based on the cost–benefit analysis, how can you think about saving that will lead to less anxiety?" Again clients are reminded that repeatedly thinking in terms of cost–benefit analysis whenever they engage in anxious thinking is a useful tool for weakening the fear program and diminishing their anxiety.

Clinician Guideline 6.10

Cost–benefit analysis is a cognitive intervention that teaches clients to take a pragmatic approach by examining the immediate and long-term advantages and disadvantages of assuming exaggerated threat, or alternatively, of adopting a more realistic perspective. The therapist uses guided discovery and homework assignments to help clients achieve a full realization of the heavy costs associated with "assuming the worst" and the benefits derived from a more realistic alternative perspective. Clients can use this insight to counter their anxious thoughts and beliefs.

Decatastophizing

A third cognitive intervention that can be especially useful for most anxiety disorders involves having the client "hypothetically" confront his dreaded catastrophe or the worst that could happen. Beck et al. (1985, 2005) provided an extensive discussion of the use of decatastrophizing to modify exaggerated threat appraisals and beliefs. Craske and Barlow (2006) describe catastrophizing as "blowing things out of proportion" (p. 86) and decatastrophizing as "imaging the worst possible outcome and then objectively judging its severity" (p. 87). They note that catastrophizing involves thinking about outcomes that are entirely unlikely to happen, even impossible (e.g., "I could get a mental illness by coming in close proximity to a homeless person"), or exaggerating events that are highly unlikely (e.g., "People will notice I am nervous and think I am mentally unstable"), or jumping to an extreme conclusion from a minor event (e.g., "If I make a mistake on this form, it will be completely invalidated and I won't receive my long-term disability benefits").

Decatastrophization is an effective intervention when it is clear that catastrophic thinking is apparent in the client's threat and vulnerability appraisals. It is a particularly useful approach when dealing with the cognitive avoidance evident in pathological worry (Borkovec et al., 2004). Decatastrophizing confronts cognitive avoidance by encouraging the client to face the imagined catastrophe and its associated anxiety. This intervention also has a number of other therapeutic benefits such as realigning threat probability and severity estimates to a more realistic level, increasing a sense of self-efficacy for dealing with future negative outcomes, and enhancing information processing of safety and rescue features in future dreaded situations.

There are three components to decatastrophizing:

1. Preparation stage
2. Description of catastrophe ("What's the worst that could happen?"; "What would be so bad about that?")
3. Problem-solving stage

Timing is everything when using decatastrophizing. Given the level of anxiety and avoidance often associated with "thinking about the worst-case scenario," other cognitive and behavioral interventions should be employed as preparation for this form of "imaginal exposure." Later in the course of therapy, decatastrophizing could be introduced as a way of confronting "the fears in your own mind." The rationale and benefits of the intervention should be explained and the client's readiness to engage in decatastrophizing should be evaluated.

Assuming proper timing and preparation, the next step is to obtain a complete, detailed discussion of the worst-case scenario from the client. Probing questions such as "What's the worst that can happen" or "What's so bad about that" can be used. The downward arrow technique is often useful for arriving at the dreaded catastrophe. The client should be encouraged to describe all aspects of the feared catastrophe including its consequences to self and others ("How would your life change?"), its probability of occurrence, its severity, and the client's perceived inability to cope. The therapist should determine whether the client recognizes any safety or rescue features in the worst-case scenario. If possible, imaging the catastrophe is a more potent way to obtain the emotionally charged aspects of the worst possible outcome. Ratings on anxiety experienced while discussing or imagining the catastrophe should be obtained as a way of demonstrating the anxiety-inducing effects of catastrophizing. Having the client provide a written description of the catastrophe is an effective way to reduce possible cognitive avoidance that can occur when imagining or even discussing the "worst-case scenario." Also the therapist should determine the client's level of insight into the exaggerated or irrational nature of the catastrophizing and its effects on anxiety.

After a clear description of the worst-case scenario, a problem-solving approach to catastrophizing can be introduced as a way to counter this form of thinking. The evidence-gathering approach can be used to evaluate the likelihood of the worst-case scenario. A best possible outcome can also be developed as a way of framing the most extreme negative and positive outcome (Leahy, 2005). A more realistic, middle-of-the-road, negative outcome can be developed as an alternative to the catastrophe. Together the therapist and client can work out an action plan that would involve how to cope with the more realistic negative outcome. This action plan would be written out and the client encouraged to work on the plan whenever she started to catastrophize.

As an example, Josie had two to three severe panic attacks on a daily basis. She was hypervigilant about her pulse rate and became very anxious whenever she perceived that her heartbeat was too fast and possibly irregular. She engaged in catastrophic misinterpretation of her pulse rate, believing that she would have a life-threatening heart attack if her heart rate was too high. After a number of sessions involving education and less threatening interventions that focused on her misinterpretation of an accelerated heart rate, Josie agreed to engage in an imaginal exposure exercise in which she imagined an accelerated pulse rate that led to a severe heart attack in which she is lying on the ground grasping her chest, alone and dying. After an extensive evidence-gathering exercise in which the client and the therapist were able to examine evidence on whether the probability and severity of the catastrophic outcome was exaggerated or not, an alternative negative outcome was considered. Josie decided that a more likely very negative outcome might be chest tightness, a racing heart, followed by severe chest pain. She rushes to an emergency room and finds out she has had a mild heart attack. An action plan was then developed on how she would manage the rest of her life knowing that she has a heart condition. Josie was encouraged to work on the "mild heart attack" plan whenever she started to catastrophize. Notice that the purpose of this intervention was to reduce Josie's fear (and catastrophizing) about heart disease and to increase her perceived ability to cope if this situation ever occurred.

Clinician Guideline 6.11

Decatastrophizing involves the identification of the "worst-case scenario" associated with an anxious concern, the evaluation of the likelihood of this scenario, and then the construction of a more likely moderate distressing outcome. Problem solving is used to develop a plan for dealing with the more probable negative outcome.

Identifying Thinking Errors

Teaching anxious clients to become more aware of the cognitive errors they tend to make when feeling anxious is another useful strategy in the modification of faulty appraisals of anxiety. Highlighting the errors in one's thinking style reinforces the message to clients that threat perceptions are inaccurate when people are highly anxious. It encourages a more critical, questioning approach to one's anxious thinking. Thus it is important that clients understand the rationale for identifying and then correcting cognitive errors. The therapist could use the following explanation:

> "Although everyone engages in these erroneous thinking styles from time to time, these errors are particularly prominent when we are anxious. When we commit these errors in our thinking they tend to lead to more exaggerated and biased conclusions. For example, if I always focused only on the flaws or mistakes in a talk whenever I gave a public address (tunnel vision error), I would end up concluding that the talk was terrible and I was a dismal failure. The same thing happens when we commit these cognitive errors when we're feeling anxious. They lead us to exaggerated and false conclusions about the threat or danger in a situation and our inability to cope. So learning to identify these errors and correct them is an important intervention for reducing anxious thoughts and feelings."

Clients can be given a copy of Appendix 5.6 in order to familiarize themselves with the six forms of cognitive errors that are common in anxiety: catastrophizing, jumping to conclusions, tunnel vision, nearsightedness, emotional reasoning, and all-or-nothing thinking. Error identification should be introduced by first going over thought records produced in the session and discussing cognitive errors that are apparent in the client's anxious thinking. This can be followed with a homework assignment in which clients record examples of thinking errors taken from their everyday experiences (use Appendix 5.6). After this exercise the therapist encourages clients to incorporate error identification into a cognitive strategy utilized whenever they engage in anxious or worrisome thinking.

Taylor (2000) describes an inductive reasoning approach that can be very useful in countering the erroneous thinking style that leads to exaggerated threat appraisals. Through the use of Socratic questioning and a guided discovery approach, the therapist explores with the client how a particular situation or symptom can lead to a dreaded outcome. For example, a client could be asked how tightness in the chest could cause a heart attack, or how lying down prevents such heart attacks. A person with PTSD who becomes anxious when remembering a past trauma could be asked how such recollections increase the likelihood of present danger or a future trauma. Individuals with repugnant sexual obsessions could be asked to explain how such thoughts would lead to committing a sexual offense, or a person with social phobia could explain how a nervous feeling would lead to public humiliation. By engaging in this form of inductive questioning, the therapist is provided material that can be used to highlight the cognitive errors in anxious thinking that lead to faulty conclusions about threat and personal vulnerability.

Clinician Guideline 6.12

Clients learn to identify the cognitive errors and faulty inductive reasoning that characterizes an anxious thinking style. This intervention helps clients develop a more critical stance toward their automatic anxious thoughts.

Generating an Alternative Explanation

During periods of heightened anxiety, an individual's thinking is often extremely rigid and inflexible, with a narrow focus on the perceived threat or danger (Beck et al., 1985, 2005). Clients will often recognize that their anxious thinking is irrational but the strong emotional charge associated with the thoughts makes them difficult to ignore. Thus searching for alternative explanations for anxious situations can be extremely difficult. Repeated practice with the cognitive therapist coaching the client in generating alternative explanations to a variety of anxious situations will be necessary before this skill generalizes to naturalistic anxious situations that occur outside the therapy setting. It may be necessary to present the alternative as a tentative possibility that the client is encouraged to at least entertain as another way to understand a situation (Rouf, Fennell, Westbrook, Cooper, & Bennett-Levy, 2004). At the same time, learning to produce less anxious alternative interpretations is a critical component of cognitive therapy for anxiety because clients need credible explanations that replace their catastrophic interpretation.

The Alternative Interpretations Form in Appendix 6.4 can be used as a within-session therapeutic tool or a homework assignment for generating alternative explanations. Most clients will be able to produce the "most dreaded outcome" and the "most desired outcome" with little difficulty. The alternative, more realistic or probable outcome will require considerably more prompting and guidance from the therapist. A good alternative view should have the following characteristics:

1. Be clearly distinct from the catastrophic interpretation.
2. Have a better fit with the facts and reality of the situation.
3. Be amenable to empirical evaluation.

A client with OCD described as his primary obsession various disturbing sexual thoughts about being gay. Although he was embarrassed by his apparent homophobic reactions, nevertheless he continued to feel intensely anxious whenever situations triggered questioning thoughts about his sexual orientation. His catastrophic interpretation was "What if these frequent thoughts about being gay means that I am a latent homosexual. I will then have to divorce my wife and move in with a gay lover." His most desired outcome was "Never to have thoughts about being gay and have absolute certainty that I am 100% heterosexual." The more probable alternative explanation was "My frequent thoughts about being gay are not due to some latent homosexual orientation but rather to my overreaction to these thoughts because the thoughts represent a violation of my personal moral standards." Notice that the alternative interpretation is a polar opposite to the catastrophic explanation. Whereas the anxious view is "These thoughts may be caused by an unconscious homosexual orientation," the alternative explanation is "These thoughts are caused by a faulty response that stems from an extreme aversion to a homosexual orientation (i.e., homophobia)." Evidence gathering and empirical hypothesis testing are more effective when the alternative view and the catastrophic explanation are polar opposites. In this way the results from such exercises will be incontrovertible evidence for the alternative and against the catastrophic conclusion.

Table 6.3 presents examples of catastrophic interpretations, desired outcomes, and alternative explanations that may be found in specific anxiety disorders. The goal is to work with the client in generating credible alternative explanations that are subjected to empirical verification. With practice the client can learn to replace the catastrophic interpretation with the alternative explanation, thereby reducing the exaggerated threat appraisals and associated subjective anxiety.

Clinician Guideline 6.13

Remediation of anxious thinking requires the discovery of more realistic alternative interpretations that can replace exaggerated threat-related appraisals. The most effective alternatives for countering automatic anxious thoughts and beliefs are those that offer a more balanced, evidence-based perspective that is clearly distinct from the anxious schemas.

Empirical Hypothesis-Testing

One of the most important interventions for cognitive change is behavioral experimentation or empirical hypothesis testing. First introduced in the cognitive therapy manual

TABLE 6.3. Illustrations of Clients' Catastrophic, Most Desired, and Alternative Explanations That May Be Relevant for the Various Anxiety Disorders

Anxiety disorder	Catastrophic interpretation	Desired outcome	Alternative interpretation
Panic disorder (lightheaded, feelings of unreality)	"I'm losing control, contact with reality. Maybe I am going crazy and will have to be hospitalized."	"I want to always feel fully conscious and aware at any moment."	"Feelings of unreality and lightheadedness reflect normal variations in arousal level that can be affected by a variety of internal and external factors."
Social phobia (observes signs of increasing anxiety)	"Everyone will notice that I'm getting anxious and wonder what is wrong with me. I'll end up making a fool of myself."	"I want to always feel perfectly relaxed and confident in social settings."	"One can feel anxious and still perform competently in a social setting. Whether others observe my anxiety and draw negative conclusions can not be known."
Generalized anxiety disorder (worry about finishing minor daily tasks)	"I will be so worried about doing chores and errands that I'll be completely paralyzed and have to be re-hospitalized."	"I want full confidence and certainty that I will accomplish the daily goals that I set for myself."	"Worry will slow me down and reduce the amount that I can get done but it doesn't have to lead to complete paralysis and inactivity."
Obsessive–compulsive disorder (fear of mental contamination or morphing)	"If I get too close to people I feel are weird or different, I will lose my creative potential."	"I prefer to avoid all contact with people who are different and threaten my creativity."	"My creativity has been hampered by my OCD rather than by close proximity to people I perceive as undesirable."
Posttraumatic stress disorder (reaction to recurrent assault-related images)	"My inability to suppress these images means the PTSD is so bad I will never be able to function in life."	"I desire no unwanted recollections or memories of the brutal assault."	"Everyone who has been assaulted has to live with disturbing memories while minimizing their impact on daily living."

for depression (Beck et al., 1979), behavioral experiments are planned, structured experiences designed to provide the client with experiential data for and against threat and vulnerability appraisals or beliefs. The *Oxford Guide to Behavioural Experiments in Cognitive Therapy*, the most comprehensive clinical guide to behavioral experimentation, offered the following operational definition: "Behavioural experiments are planned experiential activities, based on experimentation or observation, which are undertaken by patients in or between cognitive therapy sessions" (Bennett-Levy et al., 2004, p. 8). They are derived from a cognitive formulation of anxiety, and their main purpose is to provide new information that can test the validity of dysfunctional beliefs, reinforce more adaptive beliefs, and verify the cognitive formulation. Based on conceptual considerations, clinical experience, and some empirical evidence, Bennett-Levy et al. (2004) make a compelling case for behavioral experimentation as the most powerful therapeutic strategy available to cognitive therapists for promoting cognitive, affective, and behavioral change.

In the anxiety disorders empirical hypothesis testing usually involves some form of exposure to a fear situation and a disconfirmatory manipulation that tests the validity of the anxious appraisal (D. M. Clark, 1986b; Wells, 1997). The most effective hypothesis-testing exercises are structured so that the outcome of the experiment can refute the anxious belief and supports the alternative interpretation. Given the overwhelming empirical evidence for the effectiveness of exposure in fear reduction (see discussion in Chapter 7), exposure-based hypothesis-testing exercises are a key intervention in cognitive therapy of anxiety. Behavioral experiments should be introduced early and continued throughout the course of treatment. Often they play a defining role in the modification of anxious thinking. In fact it is difficult to imagine an effective cognitive intervention for anxiety that does not include within- and between-session behavioral exercises. Behavioral exercises can take the form of fairly spontaneous within-session demonstrations such as asking the client to suppress thoughts of a white bear in order to illustrate the negative effects of intentional thought suppression. In the following section we discuss the critical steps in developing an effective empirical hypothesis-testing exercise. (See Rouf et al., 2004, for more detailed discussion of how to construct effective behavioral experiments.)

Step 1. The Rationale

Any empirical hypothesis-testing exercise should be derived from the primary issue of the therapy session and it should be consistent with the cognitive case formulation. The cognitive therapist introduces the exercise by providing a rationale. This can be illustrated in the following case example. Jodie was a 22-year-old university student who developed an incapacitating anxiety about attending large lecture-based classes. Her primary anxious thought was "Everyone in the class notices me and thinks that I don't belong in university." This led to escape (ie., leaving class early) and avoidance (i.e., skipping classes) behaviors that were jeopardizing her academic performance. In this situation the therapist introduced a behavioral experiment by stating:

> "So, Jodie, you are sitting in class and feeling very anxious. You have the thought 'everyone is probably looking at me and thinking she doesn't belong in university.' I wonder if we could come up with an experiment or some sort of exercise to test the accuracy of this thought. I could ask you to try and remember reasons why you think this interpretation might be true or false, but the most accurate way to find out is to collect information on site. The very best way to test out this anxious thought is to collect information on it while you are in the classroom. We all learn so much more from our own experiences than we do from listening to teachers or even therapists for that matter. In fact homework exercises such as this have been shown to be one of the most important ingredients for reducing anxiety. Not only does it give you an opportunity to test the anxious thinking, but it also provides an opportunity for you to directly work on the anxiety. Would you like to work together on constructing an exercise that would test out this anxious thought?"

Step 2. Statement of Threat Appraisal and Its Alternative

Assuming collaboration has been established with the client, the next step is to state the threat appraisal and its alternative. The Empirical Hypothesis-Testing Form in Appendix 6.5 can be used to formulate the behavioral experiment and collect the outcome data. A clear, specific statement of the threat interpretation (i.e., anxious thought or belief) targeted by the exercise is essential for an effective behavioral experiment. The therapist should record the anxious appraisal on the Empirical Hypothesis-Testing Form and ask clients to rate their belief in the statement on a 0–100 scale when they first begin the behavioral exercise. The therapist and client then come up with an alternative interpretation that is clearly distinct and more plausible than the anxious thought or belief (see previous section on generating alternatives). The alternative is recorded on the form and the client is asked to provide a belief rating at the conclusion of the behavioral experiment. The two belief ratings will provide an indication of whether the behavioral experiment has led to a shift in belief from a threat-related interpretation to the alternative perspective.

In our case illustration, Jodie's threat interpretation was "If I feel nervous in class everyone will notice me and think I don't belong in university." The alternative interpretation was "My nervous feelings are very evident to me but barely visible to my classmates. Besides they are too busy listening to the lecture, talking to the person beside them, sleeping, or daydreaming to take the time to notice me." Each of these statements was developed collaboratively during the therapy session for the behavioral experiment.

Step 3. Planning the Experiment

Devising a good behavioral experiment will probably take at least 10–15 minutes of therapy time. It is important to write out sufficient details of how the experiment should be conducted so it is clear to the client what is to be done at a certain time and in a particular location. The experiment must involve an activity that provides a clear test between the anxious and alternative interpretation. It is important that the exercise is planned out collaboratively with the client and there is agreement that the experiment is a relevant test of the anxious thought. There is little sense in pursuing an empirical hypothesis-testing exercise that the client doubts has relevance or has little intention of carrying out. Assuming a mutually agreed-upon relevant exercise, the therapist should write down specific instructions for completing the experiment in the left-hand column of the Empirical Hypothesis-Testing Form.

Rouf et al. (2004) discuss a number of considerations that should be taken into account when planning behavioral experiments. Make sure the purpose of the experiment is clear, that a time and place for the experiment has been identified, and that resources needed to carry out the exercise have been determined. Any anticipated problems should be worked out prior to assigning the exercise. The therapist can ask a client "What do you think might discourage or even prevent you from carrying out this exercise?" Problems such as insufficient time, limited opportunity, or heightened anticipatory anxiety must be addressed before assigning the exercise. It is important that something constructive is gained from the experiment regardless of the outcome (i.e., a win–win situation) and that the exercise is not too difficult or challenging for the client. Finally all doubts, fears, and other concerns expressed by the client must be addressed and any potential medical complications should be assessed by the client's physician.

In our case illustration, the following behavioral experiment was constructed. Jodie agreed to attend her next Chemistry 101 class on Wednesday at 9:00 A.M. She was asked to arrive at the lecture hall at 8:55 and to sit at least three seats in from the aisle in a middle row. Ten minutes into the lecture she agreed to write down anything she noticed in other students that indicated they were looking directly at her. Fifteen minutes into the lecture she would take three to four deep breaths and observe whether anyone noticed what she was doing. Twenty minutes into the lecture she would try to make her body shake ever so slightly for a few seconds and observe whether anyone noticed. The therapist and client practiced each of the elements of the experiment: how to record student reactions and what behavior would constitute a direct look, how to deep breath, and how to shake ever so slightly. Jodie agreed that this was a "doable exercise" and that it would be a good test of how much she is noticed in class.

Step 4. Hypothesis Statement

Under item 3 on the Empirical Hypothesis-Testing Form (Appendix 6.5), a specific hypothesis can be recorded that reflects the client's predicted outcome of the experiment. The hypothesis would directly reflect the anxious thought or belief stated in item 1. The therapist can ask, "Based on your anxious thought [state item #1 here], what do think will happen when you do this exercise? What outcome would make you feel more anxious?" In the present case Jodie wrote the following hypothesis on the form "Anything I do in class that is out of the ordinary such as arrive just before the beginning of the lecture, take deep breaths, or slightly shake will draw attention to myself. Once I notice people looking at me, I will feel intensely anxious." Notice that the hypothesis is derived from the anxious interpretation (i.e., "if I feel nervous in class everyone will notice me and think I don't belong in university") but it is a more specific application of the threat interpretation to the actual experiment.

Step 5. Record the Actual Experiment and Outcome

Clients should record how they conducted the experiment and its outcome as soon after completing the exercise as possible. A short description of what was done and its outcome can be written in the center and right columns on the Empirical Hypothesis-Testing Form. Often individuals do not conduct an experiment exactly as planned so a description of what was actually done is important in evaluating the success of the exercise. However, the actual outcome reported by the client is even more important when following up on the effects of the behavioral experiment. It is the client's perceived outcome that will provide the necessary information for determining whether the exercise had an effect on anxious thoughts and feelings. Thus the outcome recorded on the form becomes a main focus of therapy when reviewing the assigned homework.

Step 6. Consolidation Phase

The success of a behavioral experiment in large part depends on how effectively the therapist reviews the outcome of the exercise at the following session. Based on information recorded on the Empirical Hypothesis-Testing Form, the therapist uses a combination of active listening and probing questions to determine how the exercise was implemented and the client's evaluation of the outcome. Rouf et al. (2004) suggest that a number of issues should be explored including (1) the client's thoughts and feelings before, during, and after the experiment; (2) any changes in physical state; (3) evidence that any safety behaviors or other self-protective measures were utilized; (4) observations about how other people reacted to the client; (5) significant features of the environment; and (6) the outcome in terms of noticeable changes in the client's thoughts and feelings.

When discussing the experiment it is particularly important to evaluate the outcome in light of the previously stated hypothesis, or predicted outcome. Did the client experience as much anxiety as expected? Was her own response or the responses of others consistent with her prediction? Was the outcome more or less positive than expected? How similar was the actual outcome to the predicted outcome? If there was a discrepancy, what does this indicate about the relation between threat appraisals and anxiety? When reviewing the outcome of a behavioral experiment, the therapist is drawing the client's attention to the anxiety-provoking properties of heightened threat and vulnerability interpretations, and the anxiety-reducing effects of the alternative perspective. The goal is to reinforce the cognitive conceptualization of anxiety and to promote the idea that cognitive change is a critical component of anxiety reduction.

The overall purpose of the consolidation phase, then, is to arrive at the significance or personal meaning of the exercise for clients. Did the behavioral experiment provide a powerful demonstration of the cognitive conceptualization of anxiety? Did they learn something new about their thinking or way of coping with anxiety that might be responsible for its reduction? Did the exercise highlight how exaggerated threat and vulnerability appraisals can intensify subjective anxiety? What can the client take away from the experiment? This form of questioning will ensure that the behavioral experiment fits within the cognitive case conceptualization developed for the client. It will also help consolidate any therapy gains that have been made during the sessions. In fact the main purpose of behavioral experiments that are assigned as homework is to reinforce or consolidate what has been introduced in the cognitive therapy session by providing the client with personally relevant experiential evidence. It is this critical review of the experiment's outcome and its implications that enables empirical hypothesis-testing exercises to play a significant role in the therapeutic process.

Jodie reported at the following therapy session that she did the behavioral experiment and recorded a description of the experiment and its outcome on the Empirical Hypothesis-Testing Form. She noted that she arrived to the class at 8:55 and sat in the middle row. Ten minutes later she made a detailed observation of her peers and then 15 minutes into the lecture she took three to four deep breaths and observed possible reactions. However, she was unable to even slightly shake her body at the 20-minute mark because of fear someone would notice her odd behavior. In the outcome section of the form she wrote that only one or two students even glanced at her when she sat down in class or took the deep breaths. When the therapist reviewed this further, Jodie indicated she was actually quite surprised that her fellow students paid so little attention to her. She was also surprised that she actually experienced less anxiety than usual during the class. The therapist highlighted the discrepancy between the actual outcome ("Students pay little attention even when Jodie acted in a way that might draw some momentary attention") and Jodie's prediction ("If I do anything like breath differently it will draw attention to me and I'll get very anxious"). This experiment was a powerful demonstration for Jodie that thinking others are looking at her makes her more anxious than other people's actual momentary glances, and that testing out her anxious thoughts ("people are looking at me") with actual evidence ("people take much less notice of me than I think") will lead to a reduction in anxious feelings.

Step 7. Findings and Implications Summarized

A final step in empirical hypothesis testing is to summarize the findings and draw out their implications for developing a new approach to anxiety. This summary statement can be written on the Empirical Hypothesis-Testing Form and given to the client for future reference. For Jodie the classroom experiment was summarized in the following way:

> "People often have exaggerated threatening thoughts like 'everyone in the class is looking at me and thinking there is something wrong with me.' These thoughts are often biased and even untrue yet they cause considerable anxiety. When we put these thoughts to the test and realize they are not true, our level of anxiety will decrease substantially. So in the future, when you feel anxious, ask yourself 'Is my thinking accurate or am I exaggerating the threat or danger in this situation?' Test it out against reality. If there is little evidence to support the thinking, come up with an alternative view that you can act on."

Clinician Guideline 6.14

Empirical hypothesis testing is one of the most powerful clinical tools for changing anxious thoughts, feelings, and behavior. Exercises are designed to test the accuracy of anxious interpretations and reinforce the viability of alterative explanations. Effective behavioral experiments require careful planning and specification that are derived from the cognitive case formulation. Discussion of the outcome and its implications is an important component of this therapeutic intervention.

COGNITIVE STRATEGIES IN DEVELOPMENT: EXPANDING THE CLINICAL ARMAMENTARIUM

The cognitive therapy approach to anxiety disorders is an evolving psychotherapy that fosters new developments in therapeutic interventions that are derived from empirical research and clinical experience. There are four new cognitive procedures that have appeared in the clinical literature that may hold promise in the treatment of anxiety disorders. Unlike the standard cognitive interventions discussed in the previous section, these new interventions are still in the development phase and undergoing empirical investigation. Until more is known about their efficacy and incremental contribution to cognitive therapy, they should be utilized as auxiliary therapeutic strategies when conducting cognitive therapy for anxiety.

Attentional Training Technique

Wells (2000) introduced the attentional training technique (ATT) as a therapeutic procedure for modifying the perseverative nature of self-referent processing. Highly persistent, repetitive thought is often seen in the anxiety disorders in the form of worry, obsessions, or anxious rumination. The rationale behind ATT is to teach the anxious individual how to interrupt repetitive self-attentional processing that contributes to the persistence of the anxious state. Wells (2000) suggests that ATT may be effective in alleviating emotional distress (e.g., anxiety) by weakening self-focused attention, disrupting rumination and worry, increasing executive control over attention, and strengthening metacognitive processing.

According to Wells (2000), ATT consists of auditory attentional exercises in which clients are taught to selectively attend to neutral noises, rapidly switch their attention between different sounds, and divide their attention among diverse sounds. The entire procedure takes 10–15 minutes of therapy time and is practiced in a nonanxious state. First clients are provided a rationale for ATT. The main point communicated to the client is that ATT is a procedure for reducing self-focused attention which is known to intensify anxious thoughts and feelings. The therapist can use specific demonstrations to illustrate the negative effects of self-focused attention (e.g., have the client intensely focus on an anxious thought or image and note any changes in mood state). After ensuring that the rationale has been accepted, the therapist introduces a self-attention rating scale in which clients use a −3 to +3 bipolar scale to indicate the extent to which their attention is entirely focused on external stimuli (−3) to their attention is entirely self-focused (+3). These ratings are administered before and after the ATT practice session to ensure that the directed attention exercise resulted in a reduction in self-focused attention.

In the actual ATT procedure, the therapist instructs the client to focus on a dot on the wall. Seating behind the client, the therapist first instructs the client to attend fully and completely to her voice. Next the client is asked to attend to a tapping sound made by the therapist. Again the instructions are to shift one's attention so the client is fully and completely refocusing on the tapping sound and not letting any other sounds distract him from this task. Then the client is asked to attend to a third sound in the room such as a ticking clock. This procedure is then repeated for three different sounds in the near distance (i.e., just outside the room) and three sounds in the far distance (i.e., sounds that are outside in the street).

After clients have practiced focusing attention on different sounds, the therapist calls out the different sounds and they are asked to rapidly shift attention between the different sounds. This rapid shifting of attention is practiced for a few minutes. Finally, instructions are given to expand attention by trying to concentrate on all of the sounds simultaneously and to count the number of sounds heard at the same time. After completing the training procedure, the therapist obtains client feedback. It is emphasized that intentional direction of attention is difficult but with practice they will become more proficient. Homework is assigned consisting of 10–15 minutes of ATT practice twice a day. However, it is important to ensure that clients do not use ATT to avoid their anxious thoughts or to control anxious symptoms (Wells, 2000).

A variant of ATT that is probably even more applicable to the anxiety disorders is situational attentional refocusing (SAR). In SAR anxious clients are taught to shift attention from an internal focus to external information that may disconfirm the threat-related interpretation. Wells (2000) discusses the use of SAR in conjunction with exposure in which an individual with social phobia is taught how to shift attention to external information in the social situation which interrupts the deleterious self-focused attention that is often seen in social anxiety. For example, when an individual with social anxiety enters a feared social situation and becomes overly focused on herself (i.e., self-conscious) and how bad she feels, she is instructed to shift her focus of attention and observe the appearance and facial expressions of other people in the situation. Note whether these people really are looking at you (Wells, 2000). Although empirical support for the efficacy of ATT or SAR is still preliminary, findings from a series of single-case studies are promising (Papageorgiou & Wells, 1998; Wells & Papageorgiou, 1998b; Wells, White, & Carter, 1997).

Metacognitive Intervention

The ability to monitor and regulate our information-processing apparatus is a critical executive function that is important to human adaptation and survival. We not only evaluate external stimuli that impinge on our senses, but we also evaluate our own thoughts and beliefs. Flavell (1979) referred to this capacity to evaluate and regulate our thinking processes as *metacognition*, or "thinking about thinking." Metacognition is evident as a dynamic cognitive process in which we appraise the thoughts, images, and impulses that enter the stream of consciousness as well as more enduring beliefs or knowledge about cognition and its control. Wells (2000) defined *metacognition* as "any knowledge or cognitive process that is involved in the appraisal, monitoring or control of cognition" (p. 6).

An important function of metacognitive processes is the instigation of cognitive control strategies that could lead to the intensification or shift in internal monitoring (i.e., conscious awareness) toward or away from a particular thought (Wells, 2000). As evident from the review in Chapter 3, emotion has a significant biasing effect on information processing. It is conceivable that during anxious states, metacognitive beliefs about threat are activated and internal monitoring processes become biased toward detection and elaboration of threat-related thinking. Examples of threat-relevant metacognitive beliefs include "The more one thinks anxious thoughts, the more likely the feared outcome will happen," "I'll become completely overwhelmed with anxiety if I don't stop thinking this way," "If I think it is dangerous, the situation must be dangerous." In turn these beliefs could lead to activation of compensatory metacognitive control strategies, such as efforts to intentionally suppress anxious thoughts, which paradoxically cause an increase in the salience of the unwanted thoughts and persistence of the negative emotional state (Wells, 2000, 2009; Wells & Matthews, 2006).

The relevance of a metacognitive conceptualization is clearly evident in OCD and GAD where individuals engage in obvious appraisals of their unwanted distressing thoughts (i.e., obsessions, worry) and wage desperate attempts to control the mental intrusions (see D. A. Clark, 2004; Wells, 2000, 2009, for further discussion). However, metacognitive beliefs, appraisals, and control strategies are evident in most of the anxiety disorders and so it can be important to intervene at this level when offering cognitive therapy for anxiety. There are three aspects to cognitive therapy at the metacognitive level that must be considered.

Metacognitive Assessment

As a first step it is important to identify the primary metacognitive appraisals, beliefs, and control strategies that characterize the anxious state. Once the main automatic anxious thoughts have been identified, the therapist can probe for metacognitive processes in the following way.

- "When you have this anxious thought (e.g., 'I'm going to completely blow this job interview and never find decent work'), what makes this a significant or a threatening thought for you?"
- "Are you concerned about any negative consequences from having such thoughts?"
- "Why do you think you keep having these thoughts?"
- "Is it possible to get control over them? If so, which control strategies work and which ones don't work for you?"

Notice that this line of questioning focuses on how the individual appraises the experience of having anxious thoughts. In the present example, the client may indicate that he is concerned that having such anxious thoughts before the interview might make him even more anxious and more likely to perform poorly. A prominent metacognitive belief might be "Thinking you'll blow the interview makes it more likely you won't get the job" and "It's critical to get control of this thinking in order to have a good job interview." Once such metacognitive beliefs and appraisals have been identified, assessment should focus on the actual mental control strategies that an individual might employ to shift attention away from the anxious thinking.

Metacognitive Intervention

Having identified the key metacognitive appraisals and beliefs that characterize the anxious state, the cognitive therapist can employ standard cognitive restructuring strategies to modify this cognitive phenomenon. Strategies such as evidence gathering, cost–benefit analysis, decatastrophizing, and empirical hypothesis testing can be used to change metacognitive processes. The difference is not in the interventions but rather in what is targeted for change. In our previous discussion these cognitive strategies were used to directly modify the exaggerated threat and vulnerability appraisals that characterize anxious states. In the present discussion these same intervention strategies are used to modify "thinking about thinking," that is, the appraisals and beliefs about thought processes.

To illustrate, an anxious client believes "If I keep thinking I am going to have a car accident, I'm afraid this way of thinking will actually cause it to happen" (i.e., thought–action fusion). As a cognitive intervention the client could be asked to examine the evidence that motor vehicle accidents are caused by anxious thoughts. Inductive reasoning could be used to explore how a thought can lead to a physical catastrophe like a serious motor vehicle accident. A behavioral exercise could be set up in which the client observes the effects of such thoughts on her driving behavior or that of other motorists. A survey could be taken among friends, family, and work associates to determine how many people thought they would have an accident and then experienced a serious car accident. These cognitive interventions would focus on modifying the metacognitive appraisals of significance associated with the "accident premonition" so that the individual begins to interpret such thinking in a more benign fashion such as "the product of a highly cautious driver."

Metacognitive Control

An important part of intervention at the metacognitive level is a consideration of the actual thought control strategies used to deal with unwanted cognition. It is well known that certain control responses such as the intentional suppression of unwanted thoughts, rumination, self-critical or punishment responses, neutralization, reassurance seeking, and thought stopping are ineffective at best and counterproductive at worst (for review see D. A. Clark, 2004; Wells, 2000, 2009). The cognitive therapist should target any ineffective control responses used by the client. Cognitive restructuring and empirical hypothesis-testing exercises may be necessary in order to highlight the deleterious effect of cherished mental control responses. More adaptive approaches to mental control such as thought replacement, behavioral distraction, attentional training, or passive acceptance of the thought (e.g., mindfulness) can be introduced in a pragmatic fashion in order to empirically determine for the client the most effective mental control strategy to cope with unwanted anxious thoughts.

At this point we have no empirical data to indicate that cognitive therapy that incorporates a metacognitive perspective is more or less effective than a more standard cognitive therapy that focuses only on automatic anxious thoughts and beliefs. As will be seen in a later chapter, the CBT approach to OCD has a strong focus at the metacognitive level and a number of clinical trials have demonstrated its efficacy for OCD. Clinical experience would suggest that evidence of faulty metacognitive appraisals, beliefs, and control strategies in the persistence of a client's anxiety disorder would warrant a greater focus on these processes in therapy.

Imaginal Reprocessing and Expressive Writing

Although memories of past traumatic experiences are a prominent diagnostic feature of PTSD (DSM-IV-TR; American Psychiatric Association [APA], 2000), recollections of highly anxious experiences can play a key role in the persistence of any anxiety disorder. In fact threatening visual images of past experiences or anticipated possibilities in the future are common in all the anxiety disorders (Beck et al., 1985, 2005). These anxious fantasies or past recollections are often a biased and distorted representation of reality that can fuel an anxious state. For example, in panic disorder an individual might imagine a horrible death via suffocation, a person with social anxiety might remember a past experience of trying to speak up in a group of unfamiliar people, someone with OCD might recall a vivid memory of touching something quite disgusting and feeling a profound sense of contamination, or the individual with GAD might imagine her life after experiencing a financial disaster. In each of these cases the therapist should include imagery or memory modification as a therapeutic goal for treatment.

Modification of anxious memories or imagery begins with clients providing a full and detailed account of their memory or anxious fantasy. The therapist should elicit all relevant automatic thoughts, beliefs, and appraisals that constitute the biased threat interpretation of the memory or anticipated event. Descriptions of reliving approaches to traumatic memories in CBT for PTSD suggest a number of methods for enhancing clients' exposure to traumatic memories or anxious images and dealing with elevated anxiety levels (e.g., Foa & Rothbaum, 1998; Ehlers & Clark, 2000; Shipherd, Street, & Resick, 2006; Taylor, 2006). Extensive discussion and therapeutic questioning is an obvious initial step in exposure. This is followed by asking clients to write out a narrative of the traumatic memory or imagined catastrophe (for further discussion, see Chapter 12 on PTSD). This narrative should be as detailed as possible so it can be used as the basis of repeated exposure to the traumatic memory (i.e., reliving the experience).

Standard cognitive restructuring strategies are employed to modify faulty appraisals and beliefs associated with the memory or imagined catastrophe (Ehlers & Clark, 2000). The goal is to arrive at an alternative perspective toward the memory or anxious fantasy that is more adaptive and less anxiety-provoking. In addition, efforts should be made to construct a more balanced memory of the traumatic experience itself that is a closer approximation to reality. For individuals who are troubled by images of anticipated catastrophe, again a more realistic scenario can be developed. The client can be encouraged to practice replacing the maladaptive memory or fantasy with the more adaptive alternative. Behavioral exercises can be assigned that would strengthen the alternative memory or fantasy and weaken the traumatic recollection or anxious imagery. Given the extensive use of cognitive restructuring and construction of an alternative perspective, this form of imaginal intervention is better described as a "reprocessing intervention" (i.e., a reprocessing of the memory or anxious fantasy) rather than simply repeated exposure to an internal fear stimulus.

The contribution of memory or imagery reprocessing to the effectiveness of cognitive treatment for the anxiety disorders is unknown. Research that has focused specifically on the active ingredients of CBT for PTSD indicates that imaginal and situational exposure are critical components of the treatment's effectiveness (see review by Taylor, 2006). Moreover, Pennebaker (1993) found that thinking and talking about a traumatic event immediately after its occurrence is an important phase in the natural adaptation to traumatic events. More recently, Pennebaker and colleagues demonstrated that a relatively brief intervention in which individuals write on their deepest thoughts and feelings about an emotional upheaval produces positive emotional, behavioral, and health-related benefits including reductions in depressive symptoms for individuals who tend to suppress their thoughts (e.g., Gortner, Rude, & Pennebaker, 2006; see Pennebaker, 1997; Smyth, 1998). These findings, then, suggest that modification of highly distressing memories of past experiences or fantasies of future catastrophes is an important target for cognitive intervention when this phenomena plays a critical role in the maintenance of an individual's anxiety state.

Mindfulness, Acceptance, and Commitment

Segal, Williams, and Teasdale (2002) describe an eight-session group intervention for individuals who recovered from major depression aimed at reducing depressive relapse through training in mindfulness approaches that help individuals "decenter" from their negative thinking. Called mindfulness-based cognitive therapy (MBCT), the intent is to teach individuals a different way to become aware of and relate to their negative thinking. Rather than become engaged with their negative cognitions in an evaluative manner, individuals are taught to "decenter" from their thoughts, feelings, and bodily sensations. That is, negative thoughts are to be observed and described but not evaluated (Segal, Teasdale, & Williams, 2005). Group participants are taught to focus their awareness on their experience in the moment in a nonjudgmental manner. Eight-week

2-hour group sessions guide participants in exercises that increase moment-by-moment nonjudgmental awareness of bodily sensations, thoughts, and feelings. Daily homework in awareness exercises is a critical component of the treatment. The rationale behind mindfulness approaches is that a nonjudgmental "decentered" approach will counter the automatic patterns of cognitive-affective processing that can lead to depressive relapse (Segal et al., 2005).

Although clinical trials on the efficacy of MBCT are at a preliminary stage, there is evidence that the intervention can significantly reduce depressive relapse rates in those with three or more previous episodes of major depression compared with a treatment as usual condition (Ma & Teasdale, 2004; Teasdale et al., 2000). Furthermore, MCBT was most effective in preventing relapse/recurrence of episodes that were unrelated to negative life experiences. Since MBCT is an adaptation of Jon Kabat-Zinn's mindfulness meditation that has been used extensively at the University of Massachusetts for reduction of stress, pain, and anxiety, it has obvious relevance for treatment of anxiety disorders (see Germer, 2005; Kabat-Zinn, 1990, 2005; Kabat-Zinn et al., 1992). In a pilot study 14 patients with panic disorder and eight with GAD received an 8-week group meditation-based stress reduction and relaxation program (Kabat-Zinn et al., 1992). Twenty patients showed significant reduction in BAI and Hamilton Anxiety scores at posttreatment and a significant decrease in panic attacks. Although these preliminary findings are encouraging, full randomized controlled clinical trials will be needed before the full implication of mindfulness interventions for countering anxious cognition and reducing anxiety states is known.

Acceptance and commitment therapy (ACT), introduced by Dr. Steven Hayes, is a psychotherapeutic perspective linked to post-Skinnerian radical behaviorism that focuses on the context and function of psychological phenomena (i.e., cognition) rather than on its form and content (Hayes, 2004). ACT is based on an underlying philosophy of functional contextualism in which the function of phenomenon (e.g., a worrisome thought) is understood in terms of the whole organism interacting within a historical and situational context (Hayes, 2004; Hayes, Strosahl, & Wilson, 1999). The goal of functional contextualism is the prediction and influence of events that lead to psychological flexibility, that is, the ability to change or persist with functional behaviors that serve valued ends (Hayes, 2004). The following is a brief description of the six core therapeutic processes in ACT (for more detailed discussion, see Hayes, Follette, & Linehan, 2004; Hayes & Strosahl, 2004; Hayes, Strosahl, Buting, Twohig, & Wilson, 2004; Hayes et al., 1999).

- *Acceptance*—an openness to experience thoughts and feelings with nonjudgmental awareness; to embrace thoughts and feelings as they are rather than as events that must be controlled or changed. Clients learn through various experiential and mindfulness exercises to psychologically accept even their most intense thoughts, feelings, and bodily sensations.
- *Cognitive defusion*—refers to the process of objectifying thoughts so that thoughts are viewed as merely thoughts and no longer fused with the self or personal experience. A variety of techniques can be used to help clients defuse or separate themselves from the literal meaning of thoughts such as having clients repeatedly verbalize a difficult thought until it is merely heard without meaning or evaluation, or watch thoughts as external objects without use or involvement (Luoma & Hayes, 2003).

- *Self as context*—ACT focuses on helping clients release their attachment to an unhealthy conceptualized self and embrace a transcendent sense of self through a variety of mindfulness/meditation, experiential exercises, and metaphors (Hayes, Follette, et al., 2004).
- *Being present*—this refers to the promotion of an active, open, effective, and nonjudgmental awareness or contact with the present moment rather than fusion and avoidance which interfere with "being present in the moment."
- *Values*—clients are encouraged to select and clarify their fundamental life values which can be described as "chosen qualities of purposive action" (Hayes, Follette, et al., 2004). For example, clients can be asked what they would like to see written on their tombstone.
- *Committed action*—this involves choosing specific goals and then taking responsibility for behavioral changes, adapting and persisting with behavioral patterns that will lead to desired goals. Various intervention strategies such as psychoeducation, problem solving, behavioral homework, skills training, and exposure can be used to achieve committed action (Hayes, Follette, et al., 2004).

There are fundamental differences between ACT and cognitive therapy in their view of *cognition*. In cognitive therapy the term *cognition* refers to a thought process, whereas ACT considers it private behavior and so focuses on changing its function rather than its content (Hofmann & Asmundson, 2008). Furthermore, Hofmann and Asmundson (2008) note that the two approaches differ in their emotion regulation strategy, with cognitive therapy emphasizing change in the antecedents of emotion and ACT focusing on experiential avoidance or the response side of emotion regulation. This leads to fundamental differences in therapeutic approach, with ACT using mindfulness and other strategies to teach a nonevalutive, nonjudgmental approach to negative thoughts that encourage their acceptance and integration into a wide variety of actions (Luoma & Hayes, 2003). Of course, cognitive therapy emphasizes the evaluation and correction of negative thought content through cognitive and behavioral intervention strategies.

According to ACT, the main problem in the anxiety disorders is experiential avoidance, that is, an unwillingness to experience anxiety including its attendant thoughts, feelings, behaviors, and bodily sensations (Orsillo, Roemer, Lerner, & Tull, 2004). As a result, anxious individuals struggle against their anxiety, relying on ineffective and futile external and internal control strategies as well as escape and avoidance to alleviate the unacceptable anxiety. The goal of ACT is the reduction of experiential avoidance, which prevents the attainment of valued goals by teaching the anxious person experiential acceptance defined as "a willingness to experience internal events, such as thoughts, feelings, memories, and physiological reactions, in order to participate in experiences that are deemed important and meaningful (Orsillo et al., 2004, p. 76).

Orsillo and colleagues describe a 16-session individual ACT/mindfulness intervention for GAD that promotes experiential acceptance of anxiety through training in mindfulness, acceptance, cognitive defusion, meditation, relaxation, and self-monitoring. In addition an emphasis is placed on defining life values that have been impeded by experiential avoidance and commiting to behavioral changes that focus on valued activities so that the individual is behaving intentionally rather than reactively. In an open trial Roemer and Orsillo (2007) reported that ACT led to significant reductions on measures of GAD severity, worry, general anxiety, and stress symptoms that were maintained at

3-month follow-up. Twohig, Hayes, and Masuda (2006) utilized a multiple-baseline, across-participant research design involving eight weekly 1-hour sessions of ACT to demonstrate treatment effectiveness in four individuals with OCD. However, a recent meta-analysis of various "third wave" therapies, including ACT, concluded that their mean effect sizes were only moderate, the outcome studies lacked the methodological rigor seen in CBT, and so they fail to meet criteria for empirically supported treatments (Öst, 2008). It may be that a greater focus on training the anxious person to adopt a nonevaluative, benign acceptance and distancing perspective on anxious thinking has clinical utility in the treatment of the anxiety disorders, but this conclusion must await the results of more rigorous treatment outcome research.

Clinician Guideline 6.15

Attentional training may be used to interrupt heightened self-focused attention, whereas cognitive restructuring strategies can be redirected toward modification of faulty metacognitive processes and thought control strategies. Imaginal reprocessing and expressive writing may be helpful in modifying memories of past traumatic experiences or imagined future catastrophes, whereas mindfulness and cognitive diffusion derived from ACT may be used to teach clients a more detached, nonevaluative approach to anxious cognitions. Although promising, these approaches lack the strong clinical and empirical base of standard cognitive interventions for anxiety.

SUMMARY AND CONCLUSION

Modification of the exaggerated appraisals of threat, vulnerability, and safety seeking is the primary objective of cognitive therapy for anxiety disorders. This chapter presented the main cognitive strategies that comprise cognitive treatment protocols developed for the specific anxiety disorders. These strategies are entirely consistent with the cognitive model of anxiety (see Figure 2.1) and they target the aberrant cognitions identified in the case formulation.

The goal of any cognitive intervention is deactivation of the hypervalent threat schemas and heightened activation of more adaptive and realistic beliefs about threat and perceived ability to cope with one's anxious concerns. This is achieved by shifting the client's focus away from threat content and onto the faulty appraisals and beliefs that are the basis of the anxious state. Exaggerated appraisals of the probability and seriousness of threat are targeted as well as the heightened evaluations of personal vulnerability and need to seek safety. Cognitive interventions also seek to increase personal self-efficacy for dealing with anxiety by normalizing the fear response and fostering a more adaptive perspective on the balance between risk and safety.

A detailed description was provided on how to implement the main cognitive strategies that define this treatment approach to anxiety. Educating the client into the cognitive model of anxiety is an important first step in establishing therapeutic collaboration and compliance with treatment. Teaching self-monitoring skills in the identification of automatic anxious thoughts and appraisals, though critical to the success of cognitive therapy, can be especially difficult given the heightened emotional state and situational specificity of anxiety. However, once an awareness of exaggerated threat appraisals has been established, cognitive restructuring strategies such as evidence gathering, cost–benefit analysis, and decatastrophizing can be utilized to challenge anxious schemas.

Teaching the anxious individual to become much more aware of cognitive errors and faulty inductive reasoning during periods of intense anxiety helps foster a more critical attitude toward one's anxious thinking style. Formulating alternative perspectives on anxious situations and concerns that bear a closer approximation to reality offers a counterpoint to the exaggerated threat and vulnerability that characterizes anxiety. However, the most powerful tool in the cognitive therapist's armamentarium is the behavioral experiment or empirical hypothesis-testing exercise. Behavioral exercises provide clients with experiential data that refute threat and vulnerability schemas and support an alternative, adaptive perspective. A Quick Reference Summary is provided in Appendix 6.6 to remind the clinician of various cognitive strategies available for therapeutic intervention.

Selected List of Self-Help Treatment Manuals That Can Be Assigned When Educating a Client into the Cognitive Model and Treatment of Anxiety

1. Abramowitz, J. S. (2009). *Getting over OCD: A 10-step workbook for taking back your life.* New York: Guilford Press.

2. Antony, M. M., & McCabe, R. E. (2004). *10 simple solutions to panic: How to overcome panic attacks, calm physical symptoms and reclaim your life.* Oakland, CA: New Harbinger.

3. Antony, M. M., & Norton, P. J. (2008). *The anti-anxiety workbook: Proven strategies to overcome worry, phobias, panic and obsessions.* New York: Guilford Press.

4. Antony, M. M., & Swinson, R. P. (2000b). *The shyness and social anxiety workbook: Proven techniques for overcoming your fears.* Oakland, CA: New Harbinger.

5. Barlow, D. H., & Craske, M. G. (2007). *Mastery of your anxiety and panic: Workbook* (4th ed.). Oxford, UK: Oxford University Press.

6. Butler, G., & Hope, T. (2007). *Managing your mind: The mental fitness guide.* Oxford, UK: Oxford University Press.

7. Clark, D. A., & Beck, A. T. (2010). *Defeat fear and anxiety: A cognitive therapy workbook.* Manuscript in preparation. Department of Psychology, University of New Brunswick, Canada.

8. Craske, M. G., & Barlow, D. H. (2006). *Mastery of your anxiety and worry: Workbook* (2nd ed.). Oxford, UK: Oxford University Press.

9. Hope, D. A., Heimberg, R. G., Juster, H. R., & Turk, C. L. (2000). *Managing social anxiety: A cognitive-behavioral therapy approach. Client workbook.* Oxford, UK: Oxford University Press.

10. Hope, D. A., Heimberg, R. G., & Turk, C. L. (2006). *Managing social anxiety: A cognitive-behavioral therapy approach.* Oxford, UK: Oxford University Press.

11. Kabat-Zinn, J. (1990). *Full catastrophe living: Using the wisdom of your body and mind to face stress, pain, and illness.* New York: Bantam Dell.

12. Leahy, R. L. (2005). *The worry cure: Seven steps to stop worry from stopping you.* New York: Harmony Books.

13. Leahy, R. L. (2009). *Anxiety free: Unravel your fears before they unravel you.* Carlsbad, CA: Hay House.

14. Purdon, C., & Clark, D. A. (2005). *Overcoming obsessive thoughts: How to gain control of your OCD.* Oakland, CA: New Harbinger.

15. Rygh, J. L., & Sanderson, W. C. (2004). *Treating generalized anxiety disorder: Evidenced-based strategies, tools, and techniques.* New York: Guilford Press.

Testing Anxious Appraisals: Looking for Evidence

Name: _____ Date: _____

1. Briefly state the anxious thought or appraisal: _____

2. State how likely this outcome feels to you when you are most anxious from 0% (won't happen) to 100% (certain): _____ %

3. State how serious the outcome feels to you when you're anxious from 0 (not serious) to 100 (a catastrophe): _____ %

Evidence for the Anxious Thought or Appraisal	Evidence against the Anxious Thought or Appraisal
1.	1.
2.	2.
3.	3.
4.	4.
5.	5.
6.	6.

* Use additional pages to list evidence for and against.

4. State how likely this outcome appears after looking at the evidence from 0% (won't happen) to 100% (certain): _____ %

5. State how serious the outcome appears after looking at the evidence from 0 (not serious) to 100 (a catastrophe): _____ %

Cost–Benefit Form

Name: _____   Date: _____

1. Briefly state the anxious thought, belief, or appraisal: _____

_____

Immediate and Long-Term Advantages	Immediate and Long-Term Disadvantages
1.	1.
2.	2.
3.	3.
4.	4.
5.	5.
6.	6.

Circle the costs and benefits that are most important to you.

2. Briefly state an alternative perspective: _____

_____

Immediate and Long-Term Advantages	Immediate and Long-Term Disadvantages
1.	1.
2.	2.
3.	3.
4.	4.
5.	5.
6.	6.

Circle the costs and benefits that are most important to you.

Alternative Interpretations Form

Name: _____ Date: _____

1. Briefly state the most dreaded outcome (worst-case scenario) associated with your anxiety: _____

2. Briefly state the most desirable outcome (best possible scenario) associated with your anxiety: _____

3. Briefly state the most realistic (probable) outcome associated with your anxiety: _____

Evidence for the Dreaded Outcome (catastrophic view)	Evidence for the Most Desired Outcome (most desired goal)	Evidence for the Most Probable Outcome (alternative view)
1.	1.	1.
2.	2.	2.
3.	3.	3.
4.	4.	4.
5.	5.	5.

Empirical Hypothesis-Testing Form

Name: _____   Date: _____

1. State the threat interpretation associated with your anxiety: _____

2. State the alternative interpretation proposed in therapy: _____

3. State the hypothesis (predicted outcome) for this exercise: _____

Description of the Exercise	Record How Exercise Was Conducted	Describe Outcome of the Exercise

Chapter 6 Quick Reference Summary: Cognitive Interventions

I. Education Phase (sessions 1–2)
Define anxiety and fear; fear adaptive; cognitive basis of anxiety (handout Fig. 6.1) and use client examples from assessment; negative consequences of anxiety; role of avoidance and safety seeking (use client examples); establish treatment goals and CT rationale (turn off, deactivate the "anxiety program").

II. Identifying the First Apprehensive Thoughts (sessions 2–3)
1. Review client's "Situational Analysis Form" (Appendix 5.2); probe for immediate, automatic, first anxious thought. If needed use illustration of "walk alone and hear a noise."
2. Emphasize the exaggerated probability and severity of threat appraisals in first anxious thinking.
3. Assign "Apprehensive Thoughts Self-Monitoring Form" (Appendix 5.4) as homework.
4. Emphasize importance of homework (see explanation in Chapter 6, pages 199–200) and therapeutic benefits of understanding one's anxiety.

III. Standard Cognitive Interventions (sessions 3 to end)
1. *Evidence Gathering*—first use "Testing Anxious Appraisals: Looking for Evidence" form (Appendix 6.2) in session; use client anxiety episode from past week or from "Situational Analysis Form." Assign "Testing Anxious Appraisals" form as homework.
2. *Cost–Benefit Analysis*—first use "Cost–Benefit Form" (Appendix 6.3) in session; list advantages/ disadvantages of "threat perspective" first and then repeat for "alternative perspective."
3. *Decatastophizing*—explore with client his worst outcome; go through preparation, catastrophe description, and problem-solving stage; have client imagine the worst possible outcome or write down its description.
4. *Identify Thinking Errors*—provide client handout of "Common Errors and Biases in Anxiety" (Appendix 5.6) and go over recent anxious thinking for possible errors; assign "Identifying Anxious Thinking Errors" as homework.
5. *Generating Alternative Explanation*—first work on generating alternative thinking to recent anxious episode; use "Alternative Interpretations Form" (Appendix 6.4); work on evidence for worst outcome, then most desired outcome, and finally most realistic outcome. Assign as homework if another anxiety concern is evident.
6. *Empirical Hypothesis Testing (homework assignment)*—provide rationale; specific statement of threat appraisal and its competing alternative; plan the experiment (write down instructions); client uses "Empirical Hypothesis-Testing Form" (Appendix 6.5) to record actual experiment (write down threat interpretation, alternative, and expected outcome when setting up experiment); explore outcome of experiment in following sessions (consolidation phase); write out a summary of conclusions about the experiment for client.

IV. Alternative Cognitive Interventions (latter part of therapy)
1. *Attentional Training Technique (ATT)*—counters self-focused attention, rumination, and worry; trained attention to three neutral sounds in office, then three sounds outside office, then three sounds in distance, use ATT rating scale after each; therapist calls out different sounds to practice alternating attention; homework assignment is 10–15 minutes of ATT practice twice daily.
2. *Metacognitive Intervention*—assess whether client engaged in faulty appraisals and beliefs about her thoughts; use standard cognitive interventions to challenge metacognitive appraisals and beliefs; encourage cessation of any counterproductive thought control strategies; allow anxious thinking to "fade naturally."

(cont.)

3. ***Imaginal Reprocessing and Expressive Writing***—have client generate script or imagery of traumatic or troubling imagery or memory; develop an alternative, more adaptive version and repeatedly expose; client instructed to write out a detailed description of thoughts and feelings associated with past troubling memory or imagery in form of expressive writing.

4. ***Mindfulness and Acceptance***—utilize self-monitoring and mindfulness exercises to train clients in a nonjudgmental, observational, and objectifying acceptance of anxious thoughts, feelings, and bodily sensations in order to reduce experiential avoidance of anxiety.

Chapter 7

Behavioral Interventions
A Cognitive Perspective

Courage is resistance to fear, mastery of fear—
not absence of fear.
—MARK TWAIN (19th-century American author
   and humorist, 1835–1910)

Maria had struggled with severe and incapacitating generalized social phobia since the age of 13. After 18 years of poor response to various medication regimens, hospitalization, and false starts with different psychotherapists, Maria's anxiety disorder had worsened to the point where she was practically housebound, unable to work or socialize in a meaningful way. Although there was evidence of a past comorbid bipolar I disorder, it was the social anxiety that was the primary diagnosis at the time of assessment. She did not meet diagnostic criteria for current mania or depression, so the intervention focused on her social anxiety symptoms and associated panic attacks.

Maria had an intense fear of negative evaluation from others, especially familiar people. She was concerned that others would stare at her and conclude that she was "nothing" because of her poor physical appearance or because she had achieved so little with her life. She became preoccupied with her physical appearance and attire, afraid that others would think she was wearing a "horrible outfit" and so conclude that she was unable to take care of herself. She developed an intense fear of meeting people from her past who she feared would remember her inappropriate behavior during past manic episodes and this would contribute to their harsh judgment of her. When in public settings, Maria would frequently experience panic attacks that included chest pain, numbness, smothering sensations, dizziness, and heart palpitations.

In an effort to reduce her heightened state of anxiety, Maria developed a number of behavioral coping strategies. She avoided all social gatherings and most public places, leaving her practically housebound. She spent hours getting ready in the morning in order to look "just perfect" and would compulsively check her appearance in the mirror and seek reassurance from family members on whether she looked neat and tidy. She was convinced that if she looked perfect, people would think she was competent and this would make her feel more confident and less anxious. When she started to feel panicky around others, Maria would engage in an exaggerated form of controlled breathing that was so extreme that others could not help but notice an unusual breathing pattern that bordered on hyperventilation. She was also so internally focused on her anxiety that she had difficulty maintaining a conversation. She engaged in extensive postevent processing in which she would spend considerable time ruminating about her performance in a social situation. In the end she performed poorly in social encounters because of her heightened anxiety, panic, and preoccupation. This daily battle against anxiety and perceived social incompetence left Maria feeling hopeless and pessimistic, drained of all self-confidence and sense of self-worth.

This case provides a good illustration of the importance of behavior change in alleviating anxiety disorders. Avoidance, compulsive checking, reassurance seeking, hyperventilation, and social skills deficits were just some of the maladaptive behavioral responses that actually contributed to the persistence of Maria's social anxiety. It was clear from the case formulation that an effective cognitive intervention must focus on behavioral change. Graded exposure, behavioral experimentation, and social skills training through use of videotaped feedback and role plays would be critical therapeutic ingredients in her treatment plan.

In this chapter we discuss the role of behavioral interventions in cognitive therapy for anxiety disorders. We begin by considering the importance of behavioral strategies in cognitive therapy of anxiety and how these interventions are restructured to facilitate change in anxious thoughts and beliefs. Attention is then turned to exposure as the single most effective intervention for therapeutic change across the anxiety disorders. General guidelines and procedures for implementing exposure-based treatment are considered along with its three main areas of focus: situations, imagery, and physical sensations. We then consider the importance of response prevention in eliminating maladaptive safety seeking and other forms of ineffective coping responses. Relaxation and breathing retraining are discussed as possible supplementary elements of cognitive therapy for anxiety.

IMPORTANCE OF BEHAVIORAL INTERVENTION

Given the prominence of escape and avoidance responses in most forms of pathological anxiety, it is not surprising that behavioral change is a critical aspect of cognitive therapy for anxiety. Beck et al. (1985, 2005) devoted an entire chapter to behavioral strategies and behavioral change is emphasized in CBT protocols for specific anxiety disorders like panic (D. M. Clark, 1997; Craske & Barlow, 2001), social phobia (D. M. Clark, 2001; Rapee & Heimberg, 1997), OCD (D. A. Clark, 2004; Rachman, 2006; Salkovskis, 1999; Salkovskis & Wahl, 2003), and PTSD (Ehlers & Clark, 2000; Taylor, 2006). In addition, empirical research indicates that behavioral interventions like exposure and response prevention have their own direct significant effects on reducing anxiety (Abramowitz, Franklin, & Foa, 2002; Fava, Zielezny, Savron, & Grandi, 1995; Feske & Chambless, 1995; Riggs, Cahill, & Foa, 2006). Thus behavioral intervention strategies are a central therapeutic ingredient of cognitive therapy for anxiety.

Cognitive Perspective on Behavioral Interventions

In cognitive therapy behavioral strategies are employed as interventions for modifying faulty threat and safety appraisals and beliefs. Thus the cognitive therapist conceptualizes behavioral-oriented assignments quite differently from a strictly behavioral perspective. Instead of viewing behavioral interventions in terms of strengthening inhibition or habituation of an anxiety response, cognitive therapy views the interventions in terms of its effect on changing threat-related cognition, which in turn will lead to a reduction in anxious symptoms. This cognitive reconceptualization of behavioral treatment has several practical implications for how behavioral interventions are implemented in the following steps. (See the section on empirical hypothesis testing in the previous chapter for a discussion of issues relevant to the use of behavioral interventions in cognitive therapy.)

Rationale

As with any therapeutic intervention, the client should be provided a rationale for the behavioral assignment that is based on the cognitive model of anxiety presented during the psychoeducational phase of treatment (see Figure 6.1). There are two essential ideas about behavioral interventions that should be communicated to clients. First, the cognitive therapist explains that one of the most effective ways to change anxious thinking is through direct experience with anxiety-provoking situations. In our case example it was explained to Maria that the experience she gained from exposure to actual social situations was the most potent way to learn whether other people were evaluating her as harshly as she imagined.

Second, a cognitive rationale for behavioral interventions should include a discussion of potentially maladaptive behavioral coping strategies. It is explained that modification of these coping strategies is an essential component of cognitive therapy. Another reason for behavioral interventions, then, is the modification of dysfunctional coping responses and the acquisition of more effective responses that will lead to a reduction in anxiety.

Identify Target Thought/Belief

The cognitive therapist always introduces a behavioral intervention as a means for achieving cognitive change. Thus a specific anxious thought, appraisal, or belief is identified as the primary target for the behavioral intervention. In order for the behavioral exercise to be effective, the client must be clear on the anxious thought or belief that is under evaluation by the intervention. For Maria three core beliefs were particularly critical in her cognitive therapy: "If I happen to meet familiar people, they will consider that I have little worth or value, that I'm a real failure in life," "Familiar people will view me as emotionally unstable because they will remember my 'crazy' behavior when

I was manic," and "If my physical appearance is perfect, people will think I am more competent and in control."

Behavioral Prescription

The client is always provided specific information on how to perform a behavioral exercise, something analogous to a behavioral prescription. A schedule indicating when to do the exercise, where, and for how long should be worked out. It should be clearly spelled out whether there are restrictions on the use of safety cues (e.g., a person with agoraphobia can take a trusted friend to the shopping mall but must spend 30 minutes in the mall alone). Moreover, the therapist should discuss with the client what coping responses are considered healthy when performing the behavioral task and what responses would undermine the success of the intervention (see section on planning behavioral experiments in previous chapter).

Self-Monitoring

Clients should record the outcome of any behavioral exercise performed as a homework assignment. Specific self-monitoring forms should be used such as the assessment or thought record forms reproduced in the appendices of Chapters 5 and 6 or the behavioral forms that can be found later in this chapter. Although some clients insist on keeping less formal, more open-ended records of their homework, it is important that sufficient information is recorded to allow an evaluation of the behavioral assignment (see previous chapter on recording in behavioral experiments).

Evaluation

The postintervention follow-up is perhaps the most critical component of the behavioral exercise in cognitive therapy. The therapist should review in detail the information recorded on the self-monitoring form. It is critical to highlight how the client's experience with the behavioral intervention disconfirmed the anxious appraisal and supported an alternative interpretation. This could even be written down on a "coping card" that clients use to counter their anxious thoughts in subsequent anxious episodes.

In our case example Maria was asked to accompany a friend to a café and sit with her for at least 20 minutes while they had a drink and chatted about their daily lives. Maria was asked to self-monitor her anxiety level throughout the behavioral assignment, taking particular notice of her automatic thoughts and any social cues that she picked up from those around her. She made two important observations. First, her anxiety escalated even further as she became more and more preoccupied with her internal anxious state and worried that others noticed that she looked uncomfortable. And second, there was no objective evidence that anyone even noticed her in the café. No one was looking at her or showed the least interest in her presence. Thus the behavioral experiment disconfirmed her maladaptive belief that her anxiety was due to others looking at her, of being the "center of their attention," and supported the alternative explanation that her anxiety was due to heightened self-focused attention on her internal state. Based on the results of this assignment, therapy then focused on various cognitive strategies to counter the deleterious effects of heightened self-focused attention when in social situations.

Clinician Guideline 7.1

Behavioral interventions are a critical therapeutic ingredient of cognitive therapy of anxiety. These interventions are used to directly test the dysfunctional thoughts and beliefs that maintain anxiety. Behavioral interventions are introduced early in treatment and used throughout therapy in a highly structured and organized fashion as within-session demonstrations and between-session homework assignments.

EXPOSURE INTERVENTIONS

Exposure involves systematic, repeated, and prolonged presentation of objects, situations, or stimuli (either internal or external) that are avoided because of their anxiety-provoking properties. The effectiveness of *in vivo* exposure has been clearly demonstrated for panic disorder, with situational exposure essential when agoraphobic avoidance is present (van Balkom, Nauta, & Bakker, 1995; Gould, Otto, & Pollack, 1995). In addition, exposure is an effective intervention strategy for OCD (see Foa, Franklin, & Kozak, 1998; Foa & Kozak, 1996), social phobia (Heimberg & Juster, 1995), and PTSD (Foa & Rothbaum, 1998; Riggs et al., 2006). Exposure, then, is one of the most powerful therapeutic tools available to the therapist for the reduction of fear and anxiety.

Exposure procedures are effective because they modify fear memory structures. Foa and Kozak (1986) contend that exposure must present fear-relevant information that fully activates the fear memory structure. Exposure information that is sufficiently incompatible with meaning and response elements of the fear structure will lead to a decrease in fear and anxiety, whereas information compatible with the fear structure will have the opposite effect. Two important therapeutic implications can be drawn from this analysis.

1. *Effective exposure must activate fear schemas* (i.e., memory structures). In other words, individuals must be moderately anxious during the exposure exercise in order to attain therapeutic threshold.
2. *Effective exposure must present disconfirming information*. The success of an exposure experience will depend on whether the individual is fully attentive to and processes incompatible information that disconfirms exaggerated threat and vulnerability elements of the fear schema.

In addition to a solid theoretical and empirical basis for exposure, these procedures serve multiple functions within cognitive therapy for anxiety. Table 7.1 presents a summary of the reasons for using exposure in cognitive therapy of anxiety.

Three types of exposure interventions can be utilized in fear reduction: *in vivo* or situational, imaginal, and internal exposure. Situational exposure involves contact with physical objects or actual situations that are avoided in the external environment,

TABLE 7.1. Purpose of Exposure in Cognitive Therapy of Anxiety

Reasons for including exposure procedures in cognitive therapy

- To provide assessment information on the anxiety response in avoided situations
- To provide corrective information that disconfirms perceived threat and vulnerability
- To test catastrophic beliefs through behavioral experimentation
- To confirm alternative, more adaptive appraisals and beliefs
- To reinforce adaptive coping strategies and challenge the utility of maladaptive responses
- To weaken reliance on safety-seeking cues and behavior
- To provide new learning experiences about fear and anxiety
- To reduce or eliminate escape and avoidance behavior

whereas internal self-focused procedures involve exposure to feared physical sensations (Antony & Swinson, 2000a). Imaginal exposure involves presentation of symbolic fear stimuli. Later we will discuss the implementation of each of these exposure procedures, but first we consider a number of issues that must be addressed when undertaking an exposure-based intervention.

General Guidelines for Exposure Procedures

Probably no other psychotherapeutic intervention has been misjudged more often than exposure-based treatment. The intervention appears deceptively simple and yet most therapists can attest to the difficulty of its implementation. Ensuring that clients receive sufficient "dosage" to be therapeutically effective is a challenge in its own right. Many individuals give up after one or two exposure attempts so their experiences only heighten rather than reduce anxiety. The following issues must be taken into account when planning an exposure intervention. (For an expanded discussion of guidelines for implementing exposure procedures, see Antony & Swinson [2000a]; Craske & Barlow [2001]; Foa & Rothbaum [1998]; Kozak & Foa [1997]; Steketee [1993]; and Taylor [2000, 2006].)

Rationale and Planning

The cognitive therapist explains exposure procedures as effective interventions that provide direct experience with information that disconfirms anxious appraisals and beliefs. It is emphasized that learning from experience has a much more powerful effect on changing emotion-based thinking than logical persuasion. However, some clients might express skepticism about the therapeutic benefits of exposure-based treatment by pointing out that they already encounter fear situations and yet remain anxious. This potential objection can be addressed by discussing the differences between naturally occurring exposure and therapeutic exposure. Table 7.2 lists some of the differences between natural and therapeutic exposure noted by Antony and Swinson (2000a).

It is important that between-session exposure exercises (i.e., homework assignments) be highly structured and well planned. Antony and Swinson (2000a) note that individuals with panic disorder may be inclined to carry out exposure on less anxious

TABLE 7.2. Differences between Naturally Occurring Exposure and Therapeutic Exposure

Naturally occurring exposure	Therapeutic exposure
Unpredicted and unsystematic	Predicted, planned, and systematic
Brief duration → perceived defeat	Prolonged duration → perceived victory
Infrequent and sporadic	Frequent and repeated
Threat information exaggerated and safety information ignored	Threat information evaluated and safety information is processed
Intolerance of anxiety and heightened anxiety control efforts	Increased tolerance of anxiety and reduced control efforts
Reliance on escape and avoidance	Elimination of escape and avoidance

Note. Based on Antony and Swinson (2000a).

days than on days when anxiety is especially elevated. If the exercises are planned in advance, this will reduce the chance that clients will save homework for their "good days."

Within Session versus Between Sessions

Exposure exercises can be conducted with therapist assistance as part of the session agenda or, more often than not, they are assigned as between-session homework. It is recommended that the first few exposure exercises be completed with the therapist present as part of the therapy session. This gives the cognitive therapist opportunity to observe the client's response to exposure and correct any problems that might arise. Select a low to moderately difficult situation so a client's initial experiences with exposure are successful. The therapist first demonstrates how to carry out the exposure task (i.e., modeling) and then coaches clients in the correct performance of the task, providing lots of praise and encouragement for confronting their fear and avoidance. In addition the cognitive therapist probes for any automatic anxious thoughts during the exposure demonstration and uses cognitive restructuring strategies to generate alternative interpretations. In this way a within-session exposure exercise can become an empirical hypothesis-testing experiment of exaggerated threat appraisals and beliefs.

There are practical reasons for beginning exposure-based treatment with some therapist-assisted within-session exposure. If the therapist moves too quickly into self-directed exposure homework assignments, the client might become overwhelmed with anxiety, resort to escape and avoidance responses, and then give up on the procedure. There are many pressures on therapists to proceed quickly because often clients have limited health insurance coverage. Nevertheless, this does not change the risks of introducing self-directed exposure too quickly. Although clients will differ on the amount of therapist-assisted within-session exposure required in the early phase of treatment, it would be the rare individual who could proceed directly into self-directed exposure without requiring at least some practice with the therapist.

Graduated versus Intense Exposure

Most clinicians conduct exposure in a graduated fashion guided by an exposure hierarchy. The hierarchy lists 10–20 situations relevant to the individual's anxious concerns that are associated with fear and avoidance ranging from mild to severe intensity. An expected anxiety level rated on a 0–100 scale is estimated for each situation in the hierarchy. Therapists begin exposure with one of the moderately distressing situations and proceed as quickly as possible to increasingly more difficult situations (Antony & Swinson, 2000a; Kozak & Foa, 1997). Table 7.3 presents an illustrative exposure hierarchy that could have been used with Maria in treating her social anxiety.

In this case example the cognitive therapist would begin with a moderately distressing situation such as "walking downtown alone on a busy street" or "meet with friend at a café" and repeatedly assigns these exposure tasks until there was a significant reduction in anxiety. Treatment would then progress to the next most distressing situation (e.g., "go shopping with a friend"). Appendix 7.1 presents an Exposure Hierarchy form for use in developing graduated exposure programs for anxious individuals. Clients rank their experiences from least to most difficult in terms of associated anxiety and avoidance. In addition, individuals are asked to note the core anxious thought associated with each situation, although this might not be accessible until the individual initially confronts the situation. Appendix 7.2 is then used to record both within- and between-session exposure practice sessions. The information from the Exposure Practice Record can be summarized on the Empirical Hypothesis-Testing Form (see Appendix 6.5) and used as a behavioral experiment for evaluating exaggerated threat-related appraisals and beliefs and their alternative perspective.

TABLE 7.3. Maria's Illustrative Exposure Hierarchy of Social Situations

Items in fear hierarchy	Level of anxiety (0= no anxiety to 100 = maximum anxiety/panic)
Sitting at home talking to family	10
Going for a drive	15
Going for a walk around unfamiliar neighborhood (minimal risk of meeting a familiar person)	25
Going for a walk around my neighborhood (greater risk of meeting a familiar person)	35
Walk downtown by myself on busy street	40
Go to movies with a friend	55
Meet with friend in a café	55
Go shopping with a friend	60
Go shopping alone	75
Go grocery shopping alone	80
Go to a party with familiar people	90
Participate in a class or group	95
Make a speech	100

There have been reports of success in using very intensive, massed exposure in which individuals begin with the most difficult items in the hierarchy. In fact this ungraded, intensive exposure has been found to be highly successful in treating panic disorder with agoraphobic avoidance (see discussion by Craske & Barlow, 2001; White & Barlow, 2002). However, graduated exposure is usually more acceptable to individuals with anxiety disorders who already are concerned about elevated anxiety as a result of exposure. The prospect of confronting their "worst fears" from the outset is too risky for most individuals who then might be inclined to refuse further exposure-based treatment (Antony & Swinson, 2000a). No doubt graduated exposure is the preferred *modus operandi*, although the therapist must guard against progressing too slowly up the exposure hierarchy.

Frequency and Duration

Behavioral manuals on situational exposure recommend daily sessions on a 5-day per week basis over 3–4 week time intervals with each exposure lasting up to 90 minutes (e.g., Kozak & Foa, 1997; Steketee, 1993, 1999). At its most intense, exposure procedures have been prescribed 3–4 hours a day, 5 days a week (Craske & Barlow, 2001). Although this latter procedure represents an extreme upper limit, it is probably true that the exposure-based treatments offered in specialized behavioral centers probably involve more exposure work than what is often seen in more generic naturalistic clinical settings. Failure to achieve within-session and between-session decrements in fear response with exposure therapy is a significant predictor of poor treatment response (e.g., Foa, 1979; Foa, Steketee, Grayson, & Doppelt, 1983; Rachman, 1983). Although a number of factors may be responsible for poor treatment outcome, it is possible that individuals may have received an insufficient number of exposure sessions especially when considering the treatment regimens often provided in mental health centers.

There is some evidence that a concentrated presentation of exposure is more effective than spacing exposure sessions so they occur more sporadically (Antony & Swinson, 2000a; Foa & Kozak, 1985), although there is considerable inconsistency in the research on this question (see Craske & Barlow, 2001). Antony and Swinson (2000a) recommend three to six longer practice sessions per week interspersed with brief practices throughout the day. No doubt the most prudent clinical advice would be to encourage at least daily exposure practice when this is a primary intervention strategy in the treatment plan. Every effort should be made to avoid the negative effects of insufficient exposure practice on treatment response.

It would appear that prolonged exposure sessions are better than short presentations (Foa & Kozak, 1985), with decreases in anxiety evident after 30 to 60 minutes of exposure. Foa and Kozak (1986) argue that longer exposure intervals may be necessary for more pervasive, intense, and complex fears such as agoraphobia. Individual differences in response to exposure can be expected, so the clinician relies on reductions in subjective anxiety to indicate when to end an exposure session. Antony and Swinson (2000a) suggest a decrease in anxiety to a mild or moderate level (30 to 50/100) as indicated by self-report and observer ratings as the criteria for successful completion of an exposure session. Taylor (2006) considers a 50% reduction in anxiety indicative of successful exposure. Although differing in their specific findings, the behavioral literature is clear that frequent, intense, and prolonged exposure is needed to bring about significant and enduring fear reduction.

Attention versus Distraction

Foa and Kozak (1986) argued that use of distraction strategies that involve cognitive avoidance such as pretending to be somewhere else, distorting a fear image, concentrating on nonfearful elements of a situation, and generating fear-irrelevant thoughts or images will diminish encoding of fear-relevant information, impede fear activation, and so lead to failure in emotional processing. Thus it is recommended that clients fully attend to the fear elements of a situation during exposure and to minimize distraction as much as possible (Craske & Barlow, 2001).

The empirical research on the effects of attention versus distraction in exposure-based treatment has not been consistent (for reviews, see Antony & Swinson, 2000a; Craske & Barlow, 2001). The best conclusion is that distraction may not have a particularly negative effect in the short term but it does appear to undermine treatment effectiveness in the long term. Based on Antony and Swinson (2000a), we make the following recommendations for enhancing the effectiveness of exposure:

1. Instruct clients to fully attend to the fear elements of the situation or image. This is accomplished by having clients verbally describe elements of the situation, their reaction to these features, and their interpretations of what they see or feel. Taylor (2006) notes that the intensity of the exposure experience can be adjusted by altering the amount of detail the client describes in the fear situation.

2. Minimize overt and covert sources of distraction as much as possible. Frequently ask clients what they are thinking about at this moment. Remind clients to refocus on the task at hand if attention becomes distracted.

3. Encourage clients not to fight their anxiety by trying to suppress their feelings. Antony and Swinson (2000a) note that efforts to suppress anxious feelings or even the attempt to reduce discomfort could paradoxically maintain or increase discomfort. Thus "accepting the fear" is probably the most beneficial attitude to maintain during exposure.

Controlled Escape versus Endurance

Standard exposure-based protocols assume that clients should continue (i.e., endure) with an exposure exercise until there is a significant reduction in anxiety (e.g., Foa & Kozak, 1985). An alternative view is that exposure should continue until individuals feel their anxiety level is "too high" or intolerable, at which point they can escape from the situation as long as there is an immediate return to the fear situation a few minutes later (Craske & Barlow, 2001).

If one adheres to a behavioral view of anxiety reduction, then endurance is the preferred method in order to ensure within-session habituation of anxiety (Foa & Kozak, 1986). On the other hand, if anxiety reduction is explained in terms of increased self-efficacy or the incorporation of safety signals, then controlled escape would be permissible (Craske & Barlow, 2001). Once again the empirical research is not entirely consistent on this issue (see review by Craske & Barlow, 2001). From a cognitive perspective, controlled escape may be problematic because it could reinforce beliefs that the situation is fraught with danger, high anxiety is intolerable, and the best response is escape. For these reasons we believe that encouraging clients to endure exposure sessions until there is a significant reduction in anxiety will provide the best disconfirmatory evidence against exaggerated appraisals of threat and personal vulnerability.

Collaboration and Client-Oriented Control

Perceived predictability and control are important for individuals engaged in exposure-based treatment (Antony & Swinson, 2000a). Consistent with the cognitive therapy orientation, there should be a strong collaborative atmosphere, with clients directly involved in setting their exposure homework assignment. Individuals should be assured that they will never be asked to do something they don't "want" to do and that the pace of the exposure treatment is under their own control. Naturally the therapist will be encouraging clients to challenge themselves, but there should be no hint of a coercive or heavy-handed approach. Some cognitive restructuring may be necessary before a reluctant client agrees to undertake some aspect of the exposure hierarchy. It may also be useful to ask the client for an expected timetable for progressing through the hierarchy. That way the therapist can correct any faulty expectations about speed of progress in light of the client's actual pace of exposure treatment.

Antony and Swinson (2000a) noted that some exposure situations will be inherently unpredictable such as social situations (e.g., the socially anxious client asked to initiate a brief conversation with work colleagues). In such cases the therapist might have to work on preparing the client for possible negative outcomes. At other times one might want to build some unpredictability into later exposure exercises so the client is better prepared to handle all the vicissitudes inherent in naturalistic daily life experiences.

Safety Signals and Partner-Assisted Exposure

Most behavioral therapists recommend that reliance on safety signals be eliminated during exposure (e.g., Taylor, 2000: White & Barlow, 2002). Some of these behaviors can be quite subtle such as the production of automatic responses like tensing or holding one's breath. Dealing with safety cues during exposure means that the therapist must first identify these responses, wean clients off the safety signals by building this into the exposure exercises, and encouraging the client to refrain from safety seeking (Taylor, 2000). Eliminating safety signals is important in therapy, because their continued presence is a form of avoidance that undermines disconfirmation of the threat and vulnerability beliefs. In the illustrative case example, Maria believed that maintaining a neat and tidy appearance would guarantee protection against the negative evaluation of others. This served a safety-seeking function that was targeted in therapy through cognitive restructuring conducted concurrently with social situation exposure assignments.

In some anxiety disorders, like agoraphobia, a particular family member or friend may be a powerful safety cue for the anxious client. When reviewing exposure homework, the therapist must always inquire whether the task was completed alone or with partner assistance. If there is excessive reliance on a partner, this should be built into the exposure hierarchy so that clients are gradually weaned off their dependence on others as they progress up the hierarchy. Individuals who can not venture into an anxious situation without support of a friend, family member, or spouse are unlikely to maintain long-term gains in anxiety reduction (Antony & Swinson, 2000a).

Anxiety Management during Exposure

Given the importance of frequent and prolonged exposure to fear stimuli, one might assume that any form of anxiety management has no place in exposure-based treatment. Is it not better that the client remains in a heightened state of anxiety so that the full effects of the disconfirming evidence can be processed and a natural reduction in anxiety is achieved? In most instances it would be better to refrain from deliberate anxiety management. However, there are times when some anxiety management may be necessary in order to encourage prolonged and repeated exposure to high anxiety-provoking situations. For example, clients who experience extreme levels of anxiety in a wide range of situations or others who have exceptionally low tolerance for anxiety could be taught some anxiety management strategies to reduce anxiety to the moderate range, which is more optimal for successful exposure.

Steketee (1993) describes four types of anxiety management strategies that can be used in exposure-based treatment to reduce subjective anxiety. The first is cognitive restructuring in which individuals challenge their exaggerated threat appraisals by noting evidence in the exposure situation that the danger is not as great as they expect and that anxiety eventually declines naturally. Beck et al (1985, 2005) list a number of "coping statements" that can be used by clients to encourage endurance in the anxious situation. The aim of these cognitive strategies is to alter the appraisals and beliefs responsible for the elevated anxiety in the situation. With Maria, cognitive interventions focused on her erroneous beliefs about the source of her anxiety (e.g., "that other people are looking at me").

A second anxiety management approach is to provide the client relaxation training such as progressive muscle relaxation, controlled breathing, or meditation. These coping responses could then be used during exposure to reduce anxiety. However, Steketee (1993) warns that relaxation has been shown not to be particularly effective in moderate to high anxiety. Also relaxation could easily be transformed into an avoidance or safety-seeking response. For these reasons, relaxation training is rarely incorporated into exposure-based treatment. Occasionally, however, it could be taught as a means of bolstering perceived control for anxious individuals who initially refuse exposure intervention because of low self-efficacy expectations. In other cases, like with Maria, reliance on controlled breathing can prove detrimental because her breathing rate was so exaggerated during peak anxiety that it actually bordered on hyperventilation and probably drew attention from others.

A third approach is to use paradoxical intention in which a person is instructed to exaggerate her anxious response in a fear situation. Asking people to exaggerate their fear often highlights the absurdity and improbability of the fear, which has the intended paradoxical effect of causing a reevaluation of the actual threat and vulnerability associated with the situation (Steketee, 1993). For example, a person with panic disorder and agoraphobic avoidance might be reluctant to take a walk five blocks from home. Assuming proper medical clearance was obtained, the person could be instructed to jog when he feels intensely panicky from an accelerated heart rate. The jogging, of course, would elevate the heart rate even further but it would cause its reattribution to increased physical activity. This would probably result in a reduction of subjective anxiety to a more tolerable level.

A final anxiety management strategy involves calling the therapist, a family member, or a friend for reassurance and support (Steketee, 1993). Given our previous discussion on safety seeking, this form of intervention could quickly undermine the effectiveness of exposure and so should be used sparingly. Any evidence that this form of support seeking has become an entrenched coping style would require that it be immediately faded from treatment. On the other hand, it may be that the provision of some support may be needed for a brief interval, especially in the early phase of treatment, to encourage participation in the exposure sessions. Beck et al. (1985, 2005) recommended the use of significant others to serve as auxiliary therapists in carrying out behavioral exercises. White and Barlow (2002) concluded from their review of the empirical literature that attending to the client's social support system and utilizing significant others in homework assignments might actually enhance the effectiveness of exposure treatment, especially for individuals with agoraphobia. In the early stage of treatment, family members accompanied Maria to long avoided social situations but their presence was quickly faded as soon as possible. At the very least, then, the role of partners, family, and close friends should be considered when setting between-session exposure assignments.

Clinician Guideline 7.2

Effective exposure interventions must activate fear schemas and provide disconfirming threat information that will result in modification of the client's fear structure. This is best accomplished by providing frequent, moderately intense, and prolonged within-session and between-session exposure that is implemented in a planned, systematic, and graduated manner. Clients should be given a cognitive rationale for the exercises with a therapeutic orientation that emphasizes exposure as a direct, experiential evaluation of anxious appraisals and beliefs. To enhance exposure assignments safety seeking, distraction, and escape/avoidance should be eliminated. Clients should engage in daily exposure between sessions.

Situational (In Vivo) Exposure

The most common form of exposure-based treatment involves repeated, systematic presentation of real-life experiences (Craske & Barlow, 2001). We see situational or *in vivo* exposure used most often with specific phobias, panic disorder with agoraphobic avoidance, OCD, and social phobia. In such cases the exposure hierarchy consists of a range of real-life situations that elicit varying degrees of avoidance. Taylor (2006) notes that exposure should not be used if the client has poor impulse control, uncontrolled substance use disorder, suicidal ideation or urges, or engages in stress-induced self-injurious behavior. Furthermore, clients should have a physical examination by a physician to determine if there are any medical contraindications for engaging in certain types of exposure interventions.

As discussed previously, exposure is introduced as a powerful "learning through experience" intervention that can reduce anxiety. However, the therapist will have to take special consideration of clients who had a past negative experience with exposure.

Antony and Swinson (2000a) suggest that the therapist focus on highlighting the differences between "bad" exposure and "good" exposure (see Table 7.2). In the end the therapist must provide a convincing rationale for exposure that will encourage the client's full participation in the exposure procedures.

When implementing exposure, begin with therapist-assisted demonstrations in the treatment session followed by well-planned, structured, and graduated between-session self-directed exposure assignments that evoke moderate anxiety. Exposure should be done daily with many of the sessions at least 30–60 minutes long and continued until there is a 50% reduction in subjective anxiety. Each session begins with a 0–100 rating of initial anxiety level and recording any anticipatory anxious thoughts about the exposure task. The individual then enters the fear situation and provides an anxiety rating every 10–15 minutes. In addition clients should take note of any specific anxiety symptoms experienced during the exposure session and their interpretation of the symptoms. As well, any apprehensive thoughts or images should be noted and clients should be encouraged to use cognitive restructuring strategies to correct their thinking. A final anxiety rating is completed at the end of the exposure session and observations noted about the outcome of the exposure session. One of the core beliefs targeted in Maria's exposure assignments was "People are looking at me and will notice that I am anxious, that I can't breath, and conclude there is something wrong with me."

The postexposure evaluation session is perhaps the most important part of the intervention from a cognitive perspective (see previous chapter on consolidation and summary stages of behavioral experiments). The cognitive therapist reviews in detail the Exposure Practice Form and other materials that document the client's thoughts, feelings and behavior during the exposure exercise. In cognitive therapy, exposure is viewed as a behavioral experiment or empirical hypothesis-testing exercise. Thus the client's observations of the exposure exercise can be recorded on the Empirical Hypothesis-Testing Form (see Appendix 6.5) and this can be used to emphasize those features of the exposure experience that disconfirmed core anxious appraisals and beliefs. It is expected that repeated evaluation of multiple exposure experiences will ultimately provide the disconfirming evidence needed to modify the client's anxious thoughts and beliefs and lead to long-term reduction in anxiety. Examples of graded *in vivo* exposure can be found in various behavioral treatment manuals (e.g., Antony & McCabe, 2004; Kozak & Foa, 1997; Foa & Rothbaum, 1998; Steketee, 1993), as well as in Chapter 6 on empirical hypothesis testing.

Clinician Guideline 7.3

In vivo exposure is perhaps the most powerful behavioral intervention for fear reduction. Whenever possible, employ this therapeutic tool in the treatment of anxiety disorders.

Imaginal Exposure

The goal of any exposure intervention is to provoke anxiety or distress and allow it to decrease spontaneously without recourse to avoidance, neutralization, or other forms of safety seeking. There is considerable empirical evidence that this objective can be achieved with imaginal exposure, although most behavior therapists recommend the use of *in vivo* exposure whenever possible because it appears to yield more potent and generalizable treatment effects (e.g., Antony & Swinson, 2000a; Foa & Kozak, 1985; Steketee, 1993). Foa and McNally (1996) stated that imaginal scripts can not be as effective as real-life exposure, because they provide improvished informational input and so are less evocative of the fear memory structure. However, there are times when imaginal exposure is the preferred modality because *in vivo* exposure is impractical (or impossible), or the addition of imaginal exercises enhances treatment maintenance of externally based exposure (Kozak & Foa, 1997). The following is a list of occasions when imaginal exposure might be the more appropriate therapeutic modality.

- When the object of fear is a thought, image, or idea, imaginal exposure may be the only possible therapeutic approach (e.g., in OCD thinking of the end of the world, of eternal damnation, of committing the "unpardonable sin").
- Imaginal exposure is used when it is impractical or unethical to utilize *in vivo* exposure (e.g., fear of shouting obscenities in church, thoughts of accidentally causing harm or injury to another, fear of natural disasters).
- In PTSD imaginal exposure is often utilized when fear is associated with memory of a trauma that happened in a distant geographic location or at an earlier time of life (Keane & Barlow, 2002).
- Borkovec (1994) has argued that worry is a conceptually based cognitive strategy used to avoid aversive imagery and the physiological arousal associated with threatening topics. Imaginal exposure has become an important component of CBT protocols for GAD (Brown, O'Leary, & Barlow, 2001; Rygh & Sanderson, 2004).
- Imaginal exposure is effective as a preparatory skills exercise such as in treating public speaking anxiety where imagery and role-play rehearsal are utilized for skills acquisition prior to *in vivo* exposure.
- Finally, imaginal exposure may be employed initially when a client refuses to engage in real-life exposure in order to facilitate the eventual acceptance of *in vivo* exposure exercises (Antony & Swinson, 2000a).

Implementation

The general guidelines previously discussed under situational exposure are applicable to imaginal exposure, although the following caveat should be taken into account. First, flooding or abrupt exposure procedures, which involve the immediate presentation of the most feared scenario, are used more often in imaginal than in *in vivo* exposure. This is particularly true for the imagery exposure used in PTSD or GAD where a hierarchical approach to trauma or "worst-case scenario" may not be necessary. Since flooding is more efficient and equally (or more) effective to hierarchical exposure (Foa & Kozak, 1985; White & Barlow, 2002), clinicians should consider whether an intensive form of imaginal exposure can be applied.

Second, imaginal exposure sessions are usually no more than 30 minutes and so are much shorter in duration than situational exposure. Sustained imagery exercises require a great deal of attentional resources so most individuals would not be able to maintain their full concentration on the imagery task for prolonged periods. However, it is likely that the number of imaginal exposure sessions is no more or less than for *in vivo* exposure.

Third, cognitive avoidance is more difficult to control in imaginal than real-life exposure sessions (Foa & Kozak, 1986). Individuals can distract themselves from the fear image by replacing it with another thought or image, or they can imagine less threatening versions of the fear scenario. This will weaken the effectiveness of exposure by undermining the image's capacity to activate fear schemas (see Foa & McNally, 1996).

To overcome this inherent limitation with symbolic representation, behavior therapists have introduced certain modifications in order to enhance the effectiveness of imaginal exposure. One procedure is to require the client to write down a full description of the *fear imagery script* (e.g., Kozak & Foa, 1997; Rygh & Sanderson, 2004). (See discussion on imaginal reprocessing and expressive writing in Chapter 6.) For the scripted narrative to be effective it must include details that have emotional significance to the client as well as the client's anxiety response (e.g., increased tension, heart palpitations) to the fear scenario (Kozak & Foa, 1997). Developing an effective fear narrative can be difficult, so this is usually done in the session with the therapist using guided discovery to help the client come up with an effective imagery script. Once a script has been developed, the first imaginal exposure sessions should be conducted in the therapy session. The exposure exercise begins by having the client read the narrative aloud and then closing her eyes to generate a full and complete image of the fear scenario. If the image starts to fade, the client should open her eyes and reread sections of the narrative to reestablish the image. This process continues for the duration of the exposure session. After repeated presentations of the fear imagery, it may be necessary to modify the narrative in order to maintain its evocative properties. The following is an example of a narrative script for a 55-year-old man with GAD who was terrified of financial ruin even though he had attained a high level of financial security.

"You wake up on a Thursday morning feeling particularly anxious. You've had very little sleep because you've been tossing and turning all night long, worried about your finances. You finally crawl out of bed feeling tired, exhausted. You have a low-grade headache, your muscles ache, and you can hardly walk as you shuffle to the kitchen. The house feels quite cool as you are the first up on this particular morning. It is dark and dreary outside with a light rain spattering on the window pane. You sit at the kitchen table, your mind continuing to race about your investments and whether you made the right decision while doing some online trading. You have a sickening feeling that you left yourself financially vulnerable by overinvesting in that tech stock. You notice that you are feeling tense, your chest aches, and your heart is racing. You try to get control but the more you try the worse it gets. You are now convinced that you've made a terrible mistake. How could you be so stupid as to invest so much money in a high-risk stock? You can feel yourself becoming more and more agitated, you get up and start pacing, wringing your hands as you walk. All you can think about is that stupid investment when suddenly you notice that the mail has come for that day. You try to distract yourself by going to the mailbox. There is quite a bite of correspondence but your eye immediately drops to an envelope from your bank. You notice that it is from your discount brokerage firm. You know this is the monthly statement of your investments. With trembling hands, and a feeling of nausea in your stomach you tear open the envelop. Your eyes immediately fix on the monthly balance. You can't believe what you see; your investments have been practically wiped out! A couple of important investments have gone sour and your hard-earned investments have been decimated. You feel your legs weaken, your hands are shaking, and you think you are going to be sick. You drop into the chair, your heart feels like it is going to explode, and you feel sharp chest pains. You can't believe what you see and so you keep looking at the numbers. And yet, there it is; you've lost thousands and thousands of dollars. You realize you are finished, your investment portfolio is ruined. What will you do now?"

Another procedure that has been introduced to enhance imaginal exposure is *audio habituation training*. A recording of the fear scenario is made on a CD so that the fear script is presented repeatedly without interruption. The client is instructed to listen to the CD and to get into the scenario depicted as fully as possible. The CD is allowed to play repeatedly for 20–30 minute exposure sessions. It is important that clients make the CD recording themselves so that they are listening to their own voice. A number of single-case reports have described the effectiveness of audiotaped exposure for obsessional fears in which the audiotape not only enhances the imaginal exposure experience but reduces the opportunity for clients to engage in covert neutralizing responses that would undermine the exposure experience (e.g., Headland & McDonald, 1987; Salkovskis, 1983; Thyer, 1985).

Clinician Guideline 7.4

Imaginal exposure is particularly useful in the treatment of OCD, GAD, and PTSD where the source of anxiety is a thought, image, or memory. Abrupt forms of exposure or flooding are more often used along with narrative scripts or audiorecordings of the imaginal fear to ensure sufficient fear activation and reduction in cognitive avoidance.

Exposure to Bodily Sensations

Certain physical sensations such as chest pain, shortness of breath, dizziness, nausea, and the like can elicit, or at least further exacerbate, anxiety because they are erroneously misinterpreted in a threatening manner. This catastrophic misinterpretation of bodily sensations is especially characteristic of panic disorder (Beck, 1988; Beck & Greenberg, 1988; D. M. Clark, 1986a). As with any fear stimulus, it is important that clients experience repeated exposure to their anxiety-provoking bodily sensations. This is accomplished by conducting various "panic induction exercises" that involve deliberate activation of bodily sensations such as overbreathing or hyperventilating, breathing through a straw, running on the spot, and so on. In cognitive therapy the purpose of these exposure exercises is to activate fear schemas, in this case fear of bodily sensations, and provide anxious individuals with experiences that correct their erroneous symptom equation (e.g., that chest pain = elevated risk of heart attack; Beck & Greenberg, 1987).

Exposure to bodily sensations in cognitive therapy bears some resemblance to Barlow's interoceptive exposure that involves repeated reproduction and exposure to uncomfortable arousal-related bodily sensations (White & Barlow, 2002; Taylor, 2000). The purpose of interoceptive exposure is fear reduction of specific bodily cues through repeated exposure (Craske & Barlow, 2001). However, in cognitive therapy these exercises are used differently to activate the fear schemas associated with bodily sensations and provide corrective evidence against the catastrophic misinterpretations of physical symptoms. Although interoceptive exposure is most often used in cognitive therapy for panic disorder, it is relevant for any anxious individual who fears a particular body sensation (Antony & Swinson, 2000a). A more detailed account of this type of exposure can be found in the next chapter on panic disorder.

Clinician Guideline 7.5

Use exposure to bodily sensations to activate the client's fear schema by intentionally producing the body sensations associated with anxiety in order to provide corrective evidence against the catastrophic misinterpretation of the sensation. The procedure is used most frequently in the treatment of panic disorder.

RESPONSE PREVENTION

Response prevention involves the deliberate suppression of any coping strategy, such as a compulsion, neutralization, or other control response performed to alleviate anxiety or discomfort (D.A. Clark, 2004). As a behavioral intervention, response prevention is most often used in conjunction with exposure interventions, especially in the treatment of OCD. However, when viewed more broadly as the prevention of maladaptive coping responses that contribute to the persistence of anxiety, response prevention can be an important treatment component for any of the anxiety disorders. For instance, with Maria it was important to reduce her reliance on "controlled" breathing when she became anxious because it actually intensified her anxious state.

Response prevention is most relevant for addressing the deliberate safety-seeking strategies that anxious individuals employ during the elaborative phase of anxiety (see Chapter 2, Figure 2.1). In Chapter 5 we listed 34 behavioral and emotional coping responses that might be used to neutralize anxiety (see Appendix 5.7). Moreover, highly anxious individuals often engage in effortful cognitive strategies aimed at alleviating discomfort such as deliberate thought suppression, rationalization, and the like (see Appendix 5.9). Response prevention, then, is a robust intervention strategy designed to eliminate problematic behavioral, that is, emotional and cognitive responses that lead to premature termination of exposure to a fear stimulus.

In essence any therapeutic intervention that seeks to suppress the expression of safety-seeking responses in the context of anxiety arousal is a form of response prevention. The goal is to help clients become more aware of their maladaptive coping responses, suppress these responses, and engage in more adaptive responses to ensure continued exposure to the fear-eliciting situation. Initially the therapist can model response prevention in the therapy session and then proceed to coaching the client in similar coping strategies. The eventual goal is for the client to engage in self-directed response prevention in the naturally occurring anxious situation.

Implementing Response Prevention

There are a number of steps involved in implementing response prevention. (See also Rygh & Sanderson, 2004, for a description of response prevention for GAD.)

Identify Maladaptive Coping and Neutralization

In order to implement response prevention, the therapist must first identify the cognitive, behavioral, and emotional responses used to terminate exposure to fear stimuli and reduce anxiety. The assessment forms in Appendixes 5.7 and 5.9 are quite useful for this purpose. In addition direct observation of the client during exposure to fear situations may identify other more subtle automatic safety-seeking responses that should be addressed in the exposure and response prevention sessions. For example, Maria would frequently interrupt therapy sessions by asking the therapist if he thought she looked alright and she would also frequently leave her seat in order to check on her appearance in the mirror. Response prevention of these safety-seeking responses and their underlying beliefs was an important part of the therapy. In most cases it is helpful to assign homework that requires self-monitoring of safety-seeking and other coping responses in order to heighten the client's awareness of these strategies. Repeated self-monitoring of one's anxiety responses and control efforts can help bring fairly automatic processes under more elaborative, conscious control.

Provide Rationale for Response Prevention

It must be explained to clients why the prevention of maladaptive coping responses is a critical component of cognitive therapy. Often the rationale for response prevention is presented when educating the client about exposure-based interventions. Rygh and Sanderson (2004) suggest that a cost–benefit approach can be used in which the short-term anxiety reduction associated with maladaptive coping and neutralization responses is offset by the long-term persistence of anxiety. It should be explained that long-term anxiety reduction will only occur when the underlying faulty appraisals and beliefs about exaggerated threat and vulnerability are truly modified. The most effective strategy for changing these attitudes is learning to tolerate anxiety and then letting it decline naturally.

Preventing maladaptive responses that prematurely terminate anxiety is an important part of this treatment approach. The following is a clinical excerpt that illustrates educating a client with panic disorder on the importance of response prevention.

THERAPIST: Derek, I notice from the behavioral checklist [Appendix 5.7] that whenever you feel anxious about chest pains you immediately stop all activity, rest, and try to control your breathing in an effort to relax yourself.

CLIENT: Yeah, I've done this for so long it is kinda automatic now. I keep thinking it is really important to relax and get control of myself.

THERAPIST: I also notice that on other occasions, when the anxiety gets really bad, you'll look on the Internet for medical information, make an appointment with your family doctor, or even go to the hospital emergency department. These all look like ways of seeking reassurance that you are alright and not having a heart attack.

CLIENT: I've been doing these things for years but the anxiety seems to always come back.

THERAPIST: Derek, that's an important observation that you just made. So you find that trying to relax or seeking medical advice calms your anxiety for a while but then it comes back just as strong as ever.

CLIENT: That's exactly what happens.

THERAPIST: It's kind of like the old adage in reverse "short-term gain but long-term pain." Responses like trying to relax or seeking reassurance may work in the short term but over time they actually contribute to the persistence of anxiety. They prevent you from learning to tolerate anxiety and that nothing terrible will happen to you because of the physical symptoms of anxiety. By artificially cutting short the anxiety, it doesn't have a chance to disappear naturally and you never have a chance to learn that your fearful thoughts about chest pain and heart attacks are based on exaggerated misunderstandings about risks to your health.

CLIENT: Are you saying that going to the doctor or trying to relax are bad, that these things actually make me more anxious?

THERAPIST: Yes, that is exactly what I am saying. These coping strategies prevent you from actually learning ways to deal with faulty beliefs about risks to your health. And so the anxiety you have over chest pain and heart attacks continues unabated. You recall that earlier we talked about the exposure exercises as an important way to learn how to let anxiety decline naturally. It is also very important to eliminate some of these coping strategies like rest, trying to relax, or seeking medical reassurance that artificially interrupt the anxiety response. So while you are doing the exposure exercises, I would also like to work with you on ways to reduce these problematic coping behaviors. We use procedures called response prevention which focus on suppressing certain maladaptive responses. Would you like to look at some strategies we could use to reduce or even eliminate these problem behaviors and build up better responses to the anxiety?

CLIENT: Sure, this sounds like a good idea.

Prepare Client for Heightened Anxiety

Individuals must be forewarned to expect an immediate increase in anxiety with prevention of safety-seeking responses and prolonged exposure to fear stimuli. Although individuals will differ in the duration of peak anxiety, some reduction in anxiety should be evident after 30–60 minutes of exposure. However, continued prevention of maladaptive coping and neutralization may be necessary for several hours after an exposure session. For example, individuals with obsessive fears of contamination can engage in washing and cleaning rituals that take hours to complete. In such cases the response prevention phase of an exposure homework assignment can extend over a 2–3 hour time period. The approximate duration of a response prevention session should be discussed with clients. Most often clients will be encouraged to continue with their response prevention until their anxiety reaches the mild range.

There are times when an individual's anxiety is so intense over a prolonged period of time that she refuses to engage in exposure and response prevention. In such cases certain anxiety management strategies such as distraction, controlled breathing, and progressive muscle relaxation can be temporarily introduced. It is important that these strategies be employed briefly because they can interfere with full exposure to the fear stimuli. In the end the effectiveness of exposure and response prevention will be weakened if clients continue to rely on anxiety management. This would suggest that the individual's exaggerated threat appraisal of the physical symptoms of anxiety remains intact.

Instruct Client about "Blocking" Strategies

A number of strategies can be used to suppress maladaptive coping behavior and other forms of safety-seeking responses. First, the client can write down a list of *self-instructional coping statements* that can be used as reminders of the benefits of preventing maladaptive responses and the costs of continued reliance on problematic safety-seeking behavior. Second, individuals could develop a repertoire of *competing activities* that interfere with performance of the maladaptive coping behaviors. For example, individuals who hold their breath when anxious could practice diaphragmatic breathing or those who tend to overbreathe when anxious could focus on holding their breath between exhalations. To compete with compulsive checking, an individual could immediately leave the situation so that repeating a check becomes more difficult. For instance, Maria was restricted to using mirrors only at certain times of the day and to refrain from carrying a mirror in her purse. Considerable exploration will be necessary to develop a repertoire of competing activities that would effectively block safety-seeking behavior. It is likely that these competing responses will be quite idiosyncratic to the individual and the specific safety-seeking behavior under consideration.

A third response prevention strategy that is probably the most effective in blocking problematic coping responses is *paradoxical intention*. This involves having the client engage in behaviors that are completely opposite to the safety-seeking response. For example, a person who tries to rest whenever he feels anxious for fear that his pulse rate is too high could engage in a high-energy physical activity when he feels anxious. Someone who uses cognitive avoidance or distraction to deal with her anxiety could be instructed to fully attend to the fear stimulus. And of course the person who relies on escape and avoidance would be encouraged to remain in the fear situation. The client who suppresses anxious feelings would be instructed to openly express his emotions, whether they be fear or anger. It is likely that the deliberate performance of a behavior that is opposite to the coping response will provide the most effective response prevention.

And finally, the *support and encouragement of family and friends* can be a powerful incentive to refrain from problematic responses to anxiety. With proper instruction from the therapist family members can serve as "coaches" to encourage exposure and response prevention. Given Maria's excessive reassurance seeking, family members would need to be instructed on how to handle her requests for reassurance about her physical appearance. Of course, involvement of significant others has to be monitored carefully so that the person does not become a safety cue. Furthermore, the therapist should provide verbal encouragement and be available by phone between sessions to assist clients who might have difficulty blocking their maladaptive coping responses.

Develop Alternative Coping Responses

The adaptive alternative that is promoted in cognitive therapy is continued exposure to the fear stimulus. Any coping responses that encourage the client to wait for anxiety to dissipate naturally is considered an adaptive approach. For example, a client with a long-standing panic disorder was very terrified of panic attacks. The core belief was she might lose control and eventually go insane. Any signs of anxiety, especially trembling, shaking, or crying, were misinterpreted as loss of control. She responded by tensing her muscles, distracting herself, and trying to suppress her anxious feelings. To counter these futile attempts at anxiety control, a form of paradoxical response prevention was formulated. Whenever she noticed the first signs of anxiety, she was to go to her bedroom, stand before a full-length mirror, and purposefully shake and cry as hard as possible. She was to watch herself do this in the mirror until her anxiety level dropped significantly. This plan for coping with anxious episodes served several functions. It encouraged direct exposure to the physical symptoms that frightened her. It also blocked her maladaptive coping responses and it usually ended with a good laugh, which initiated an emotional state contrary to anxiety. In sum, effective response prevention should not only specify the safety-seeking responses that should be blocked or suppressed, but also alternative ways of responding that promote adaptive exposure.

Challenge Problematic Cognitions

The cognitive therapist is always attentive to any faulty thoughts or beliefs that might lead to continued reliance on safety-seeking responses and undermine response prevention. This can be done by questioning clients on their automatic thoughts about perceived need to avoid or control anxiety as well as by examining self-monitoring records for maladaptive safety-seeking cognitions that occurred during exposure assignments. Once such thinking is identified, cognitive restructuring can be employed to modify the anxious appraisals and beliefs (see Chapter 6).

Certain themes are common in the automatic thoughts and beliefs that maintain safety seeking and interfere with response prevention. These include an intolerance of anxiety and uncertainty, a need to maintain control, the importance of minimizing risk, and the maintenance of safety and security. Individuals with anxiety will often express beliefs like "I can't stand the anxiety," "I need to be certain that I haven't left the stove burners on and could cause a fire," "If I don't maintain strict control over my emotions, people will notice there is something wrong with me," "I can't stand to take risks; it's better to be safe than sorry," "The more I feel peace and comfort the better my physical and mental health," or "If I look perfect, I can avoid the negative evaluation of familiar people [Maria]." In many cases response prevention of maladaptive coping and safety seeking will not be accepted as long as the anxious person endorses this way of thinking. Thus the cognitive therapist should probe for problematic cognitions whenever clients fail to follow through on response prevention.

Record and Evaluate

As with any intervention, it is essential that clients maintain some record of their response prevention efforts between sessions. The Response Prevention Record in Appendix 7.3

can be used for this purpose. This form can be completed when clients engage in exposure homework assignments or when they prevent maladaptive coping during spontaneous, naturally occurring anxiety episodes. Although the form collects data on anxiety levels and urge to engage in the "prevented response," the cognitive therapist should always probe for clients' cognitions about response prevention and safety-seeking behavior when reviewing the form.

Clinician Guideline 7.6

Preventing maladaptive coping behavior and other forms of safety-seeking responses is an important component of cognitive therapy that promotes exposure to information that disconfirms the client's faulty threat and vulnerability beliefs.

DIRECTED BEHAVIORAL CHANGE

As previously discussed, individuals with anxiety disorders often exhibit problematic behaviors that require modification or they may present with behavioral deficits that actually contribute to their anxious state. An individual with social phobia may have performance deficits in interpersonal and communication skills, although Antony and Swinson (2000b) remind us that most people with social anxiety have better interpersonal skills than they think. However, social behavioral performance deficits may also be evident in other anxiety disorders. It can occur in the person with panic disorder and agoraphobic avoidance who has shunned social settings for many years, or the individual with chronic OCD who might avoid others because of obsessions of doubt or contamination. Moreover, individuals with PTSD often have significant social withdrawal and other interpersonal difficulties (Turner, Beidel, & Frueh, 2005). In such cases a skills-training component might be included in the treatment plan.

Directed behavioral change refers to intervention strategies that teach individuals how to change specific behaviors in order to improve their personal effectiveness at home, at work, and in interpersonal relations. In the anxiety disorders behavioral change strategies typically focus on improving prosocial skills, assertiveness, or verbal and nonverbal communication (see Antony & Swinson, 2000a, 2000b, for further discussion). Table 7.4 presents the steps normally involved in behavioral change interventions.

TABLE 7.4. Therapeutic Elements in Direct Behavioral Change Interventions

- Didactic instruction or psychoeducation
- Modeling specific behaviors
- Behavioral rehearsal
- Corrective feedback and reinforcement
- *In vivo* homework assignments
- Self-monitoring and evaluation

When initiating a behavioral change intervention, the therapist begins with *didactic instruction* aimed at preparing the client for behavioral rehearsal. Goldfried and Davison (1976) comment that this didactic introduction is necessary for ensuring that the client recognizes that behavioral change is needed, to accept behavioral rehearsal as an important step in learning new behaviors, and to overcome any anxiety about role playing. In addition, the therapist provides specific information that helps clients learn the difference between their maladaptive behaviors and more effective prosocial behaviors.

In cognitive therapy a rationale should be given for shifting therapy from a focus on the cognitive basis of anxiety to this more behavioral orientation. Clients should be informed that these interventions are not intended as a direct anxiety-reduction strategy, but rather their aim is to improve one's functioning and confidence in social situations. Improved social functioning might have an indirect anxiolytic effect by increasing the frequency of positive responses from others, which in turn would increase a person's motivation to expose himself to anxiety-provoking encounters with others.

Modeling plays an important role in teaching anxious clients how to engage in more effective interpersonal behavior. The therapist demonstrates the skill that is to be learned and then discusses with the client how to perform the behavior in question. Even though didactic explanations of new behaviors are important, nothing can substitute for actually showing a client how to respond. For example, a person with social anxiety had a tendency to talk too quickly when conversing at work. Even though it ensured quicker escape from an anxious social interaction, it interfered in the quality of her communication and actually intensified her subjective anxiety. This acceleration of her speech actually occurred in the therapy session. The therapist was able to interrupt the conversation, point out that her speech was accelerating, and then demonstrate a more appropriate rate of speech. This modeling led naturally into the next phase of the behavioral change intervention.

Behavioral rehearsal is really the core therapeutic ingredient of direct behavioral change interventions. Within-session role plays are conducted in which the client practices executing the new behavior in a variety of possible situations. The therapist might begin by modeling in the role play the target behavior such as initiating a conversation with a stranger, making a request, maintaining eye contact, refusing an unreasonable request, or the like. The client is then asked to practice the behavior within the role play. Throughout the role play the therapist provides coaching in the form of *corrective feedback* as well as *reinforcement and encouragement* for attempts to perform the target behavior. Since many individuals are uncomfortable with acting and may find these behavioral practice sessions tedious, it is important to keep the atmosphere light or informal and use humor to put individuals at ease. In the treatment of social phobia videotaped in-session role plays with therapist and client or with additional "actors" can be used to enhance behavioral rehearsal (e.g., Antony & Swinson, 2000a; D. M. Clark, 2001). In such cases the therapist provides feedback and correction while reviewing the tape with the client.

Beck at al. (1985, 2005) also notes that important dysfunctional thoughts and beliefs may become apparent in the course of behavioral rehearsal. Once identified these automatic thoughts and beliefs would be addressed with cognitive restructuring strategies. For example, during behavioral rehearsal that targeted eye contact with a person suffering from chronic social phobia, the therapist noticed that the client had great difficulty maintaining eye contact. The role play was stopped and the therapist asked the client "When we were role-playing just now, what was going through your mind?" The client stated that he was thinking "I am staring at the person; he is going to get angry if I just keep staring like this." So, automatically the client would break off his gaze and look away, which meant that he did not perform the behavioral rehearsal correctly. Identifying and correcting faulty cognitions that arise in the course of behavioral rehearsal is an important use of this strategy in cognitive therapy for anxiety.

The effectiveness of any behavioral change intervention will depend on whether behavioral rehearsal is followed by systematic and repeated practice of these new skills as *in vivo homework assignments*. As with any intervention the generalizability and maintenance of any new learning achieved within session depends on completion of homework assignments. Individuals should also *self-monitor* their behavioral homework assignments by keeping a record of the situations in which they practiced the new behavior, their anxiety level, the outcome, and their evaluation of their performance. In the follow-up session the therapist would review the homework self-monitoring form. Examples of positive behavioral change would be praised and any problematic cognitions or behavioral responses would be targeted for further intervention.

Clinician Guideline 7.7

Direct behavioral change interventions are often employed in cognitive therapy to address performance deficits in social functioning that may exacerbate withdrawal and isolation from others and interfere with the client's participation in crucial between-session exposure assignments.

RELAXATION TRAINING

Relaxation training has had a long and venerable history in behavior therapy for anxiety. At one time it was the cornerstone of behavioral treatment for anxiety and considered critical for inhibiting conditioned anxiety responses (i.e., Wolpe & Lazarus, 1966). Recently cognitive-behavior therapists have questioned the wisdom and effectiveness of relaxation therapy for anxiety. White and Barlow (2002), for example, argued that any behavior that minimizes panic symptoms or provides escape/distraction from these symptoms would be maladaptive. Teaching individuals to relax via progressive muscle relaxation or breathing retraining could undermine exposure and be tantamount to "teaching avoidance as a coping strategy" (White & Barlow, 2002, p. 317). In many respects relaxation training is also incompatible with the objectives of CT for anxiety. Empirical hypothesis testing of faulty appraisals and beliefs depends on exposure to anxiety situations in order to gather disconfirming information. If relaxation was invoked whenever a person felt anxious, then that person would forfeit an opportunity to learn that the anxious concerns were unfounded. In this way relaxation as an anxiety management response would undermine the effectiveness of cognitive therapy.

So, is there a place for relaxation training in cognitive therapy of anxiety? We would only recommend relaxation techniques as an adjunctive intervention if an individual's anxiety level was so extreme that the client refused to engage in any exposure or refused to tolerate even the slightest amount of anxiety. In such cases relaxation training could be taught to lower anxiety level so the individual would engage in exposure and other behavioral experiments designed to modify the faulty appraisals and beliefs of threat, vulnerability, and the need for safety. For the cognitive therapist, it is the deactivation of the fear schemas that is considered essential for long-lasting reduction in anxiety and not the acquisition of a relaxation coping strategy.

Despite these concerns with its conceptual basis, relaxation training continues to be advocated as an effective intervention for inhibiting the physical tension of anxiety (e.g., Bourne, 2000; Craske & Barlow, 2006). However, the empirical research indicates that relaxation training has a far more limited role in treatment of anxiety than once envisioned. Progressive muscle relaxation, for example, continues to be an important therapeutic ingredient in CBT protocols for GAD (e.g., Brown, O'Leary, & Barlow, 2001; see Conrad & Roth, 2007, for review of empirical status) and PTSD (Foa & Rothbaum, 1998), but it appears to have less value for social anxiety (Heimberg & Juster, 1995) and OCD (Foa et al., 1998; Steketee, 1993), and has produced mixed results, at best, for panic disorder (see D. M. Clark, 1997; Craske & Barlow, 2001, for reviews).

Progressive Muscle Relaxation

In 1938 Edmund Jacobson published his work on relaxation that was based on a rather unique theory of anxiety. Jacobson argued that the core experience of anxiety is muscle tension, which involves contraction or shortening of the muscle fibers. In order to reduce this tension and subjective anxiety, progressive muscular relaxation (PMR) was introduced as a method that eliminates tension by lengthening muscle fibers (Jacobson, 1968; see also Bernstein & Borkovec, 1973). By systematically tensing and releasing various muscle groups, Jacobson found that muscle contractions could be practically eliminated and a state of deep relaxation induced. The only problem is his method of relaxation was extremely time consuming, involving 50–200 sessions of training (see Wolpe, 1958; Wolpe & Lazarus, 1966).

Jacobson's relaxation procedure was adopted and refined by the pioneers of behavior therapy as an incompatible response that could inhibit fear and anxiety. Wolpe (1958) concluded from Jacobson's writings that his relaxation method had anxiety-countering effects, because individuals were taught to use differential relaxation in their day-to-day lives in which muscle groups not directly in use were relaxed. This will lead to reciprocal inhibition of any anxiety-evoking stimuli encountered and with repeated occurrences a conditioned inhibition of the anxiety response gradually develops. However, Wolpe (1958) introduced two major modifications to improve the efficiency and effectiveness of differential relaxation. First, he was able to drastically reduce the number of relaxation training sessions to six 20-minute sessions and two 15-minute daily practice sessions at home (Wolpe & Lazarus, 1966). And second, in subsequent sessions relaxation was paired with systematic graduated imaginal evocation of a fear stimulus in a treatment procedure called *systematic desensitization*. The result was the introduction of a highly effective behavioral treatment for fears and phobias.

The induction of deep relaxation became an essential tool in the behavior therapist's armamentarium for inhibiting anxiety. Wolpe discovered that the autonomic effects of relaxation can only counter a weak anxiety response, but once a weak stimulus is no longer anxiety-provoking a slightly stronger anxiety-provoking stimulus can be repeatedly paired with relaxation until it too ceases to arouse anxiety (Wolpe & Lazarus, 1966). Gradually, with repeated presentations, deep relaxation will inhibit successively stronger anxiety responses until even the most intense anxiety-provoking situation no longer elicits anxiety.

The systematic tensing and releasing of specific muscle groups that was pioneered by Edmund Jacobson is still the most common approach to relaxation training used in CBT. Clients are instructed to tense a specific muscle group "as hard as possible without causing pain," to hold the tension for 5–7 seconds, to notice the tension in the muscle group, then to relax and release the tension, and to notice the feeling of relaxation that occurs when the tension is released (Bernstein & Borkovec, 1973). The purpose of this "tense–release" cycle is to facilitate tension detection and sharpen the client's ability to discriminate between sensations of tension and relaxation. Although many different PMR variations exist, we present a 10-muscle group protocol in Table 7.5 that can be initially taught to clients. It is derived from lengthier protocols described in Bernstein and Borkovec (1973), and Cautela and Groden (1978).

Rationale and Instructions

Before initiating a relaxation training session, it is important to provide a rationale for the procedure. The following is one possible explanation and set of instructions for PMR that can be used with clients. (For other examples of rationales and instructions for PMR, see Bernstein & Borkovec, 1973; Bourne, 2000; Cautela & Groden, 1978; Craske & Barlow, 2006; Foa & Rothbaum, 1998; Goldfried & Davison, 1976.)

> "Today I am going to teach you how to use relaxation to mange your anxiety. This procedure, called deep muscle relaxation, was first introduced 75 years ago by a Harvard University physiologist, Dr. Edmund Jacobson. He found that individuals could learn to induce a state of deep relaxation by tensing and then releasing specific groups of muscles. The important part of this procedure is learning the difference between feeling tense and feeling relaxed, so you will be coached on how to pay especially close attention to the feelings and physical sensations associated with your muscles being tense and then relaxed. Do you recall from the earlier assessment session that one of the anxiety symptoms that you noticed was muscle tension? Could you remind me of what that is like for you. [Have client describe the discomfort associated with feeling physically tense or uptight when anxious.] When you feel tense, certain muscles in your body tighten; that is, the muscle fibers actually contract, producing that tense feeling. Progressive muscle relaxation is a technique that interrupts the anxiety process by relaxing the muscles. It literally reverses one of the main symptoms of anxiety, physical tension, by releasing unwanted muscle contraction or tension. Once you've mastered the skill of inducing deep relaxation, you can use it in a variety of situations to interrupt a rise in your anxiety level.

TABLE 7.5. A 10-Muscle-Group Protocol for Progressive Muscle Relaxation

Muscle group	Tense–release procedure
1. Dominant arm	"Extend your right arm (i.e., dominant) straight out, make a tight fist, and tighten whole arm from hand to shoulder. Notice tension in biceps, forearm, elbow, wrist, and fingers. Then relax, bending arm at elbow and resting it on your lap."
2. Nondominant arm	"Extend your left arm (i.e., nondominant) straight out, make a tight fist, and tighten whole arm from hand to shoulder. Notice tension in biceps, forearm, elbow, wrist, and fingers. Then relax, bending arm at elbow and resting it on your lap."
3. Forehead	"Wrinkle forehead by lifting the eyebrows as high as you can, push your eyebrows up, putting tension in the forehead and scalp areas. Then slowly relax, letting your eyebrows drop and notice the release of tension in the forehead."
4. Eyes and nose	"Close your eyes very tightly, squint them hard so you can feel tension around your eyes. At the same time, wrinkle your nose, again pushing your nose hard against your face. Notice the tension around the eyes, nose, and upper cheeks. Slowly relax, release the tension around your eyes and nose by not squinting your eyes or wrinkling your nose. Keep your eyes closed and focus on the relaxed feelings around your eyes and nose."
5. Jaw and neck	"Tense the mouth, jaw, and neck regions by making an exaggerated grin, clench the teeth, and tighten your neck by drawing your mouth and chin inward. Notice the tightness of your muscles around the mouth, jaw, and front part of the neck. As you release the tension, focus on the feeling of relaxation in these regions of the face and neck."
6. Shoulders and back	"Move forward in the chair and bring the elbows up and back so that you can feel your shoulder blades being pushed together. At the same time the chest is being pulled out. Notice the tension in the shoulders and upper back. Gradually release the tension by sitting back in the chair, placing your arms in your lap and allowing the shoulders to fall back into their normal position. Focus on the release of tension in the shoulders and down the middle of the back."
7. Chest	"Tighten the chest by taking a deep breath and then hold it. Feel the tension in the chest as you constrict and pull it in. As you relax focus on how loose the chest muscles now feel."
8. Stomach	"Tighten the stomach by pulling it in and making it as hard as a board. Notice the tension in your stomach and how hard it feels. As you release the tightness in your stomach, notice how it feels to switch from tension to relaxation."
9. Dominant leg	"Lift your right (i.e., dominant) leg off the floor so that your leg is fully extended outward, bend your toes inward toward you, and tighten your whole leg as much as possible. Notice the tension in your foot, calf, knees, and thighs. Gradually relax, lowering your leg back to the floor and bending your knee slightly so that your foot is squarely on the floor. Notice the feeling of relaxation that now permeates through the entire length of the leg."
10. Nondominant leg	"Lift your left (i.e., nondominant) leg off the floor so that your leg is fully extended outward, bend your toes inward toward you, and tighten your whole leg as much as possible. Notice the tension in your foot, calf, knees, and thighs. Gradually relax, lowering your leg back to the floor and bending your knee slightly so that your foot is squarely on the floor. Notice the feeling of relaxation that now permeates through the entire length of the leg."

Note. Based on Bernstein and Borkovec (1973) and Cautela and Groden (1978).

"The best way to learn deep muscle relaxation is through demonstration, coaching, and practice. I am going to ask you to produce tension in particular muscle groups, hold the tension for 5–7 seconds, and then release this tension. I will instruct you on how to tense and release various muscles. Throughout the procedure I will be prompting you to focus on the feelings of tension and relaxation. This is a very important part of the technique because you need to learn how it feels to be relaxed. We will begin by tensing and relaxing 10 different muscle groups and the whole procedure will take about 20 minutes. I will be asking you to tense and then relax particular muscles. For example, let's quickly run through the procedure with each of the muscles so you will know what to expect. Take your right arm, extend it in front of you, make a tight fist, and hold it. Do you notice any tension or tightness in your arm? [Ask client to indicate whether tension was felt in hands, forearm, elbow, and bicep of the arm.] Now tense the arm again and this time release the tension by letting your arm fall back into your lap, with the arm slightly bent at the elbow. How does it feel now? [Client is asked to describe the feeling of relaxation in the arm.] Now I am going to demonstrate for you how to tense and relax the other 9 muscle groups. Each time I would like you to watch how I do it and then try for yourself. I do need to warn you we'll be making some funny faces in order to tense the facial muscles. Are you okay with that? [Therapist then demonstrates how to tense and relax muscles based on Table 7.5.]

"[After demonstrating the 10-muscle tense–release procedure, the therapist continues with the introduction.] It is important that you realize that deep muscle relaxation is a skill that takes repeated practice to learn. Just like learning to ride a bicycle or drive a car, the technique may at first feel unnatural to you. You may not feel very relaxed. However, the more you practice it, the easier it will become and you will get better and better at inducing a deeper level of relaxation. Also once you've mastered the 10 muscle technique, I will teach you how to do the abbreviated version of muscle relaxation so that you can literally induce relaxation in a few minutes anywhere, anytime. But to get to that point, you will need to practice relaxation twice a day, every day for 15 minutes. I will be giving you a CD with relaxation instructions that should help you do the homework practice. Also I will ask that you complete a Weekly Progressive Muscle Relaxation Record [see Appendix 7.4] so we can monitor your progress. Do you have any questions? Okay, let's begin with our first relaxation training session."

It is important to emphasize that the effectiveness of relaxation training depends on a conducive setting. Bourne (2000) offers a number of practical suggestions for enhancing the relaxation experience. Choose a quiet location, a dimly lit room, and a comfortable chair or sofa. Practice on an empty stomach and loosen any tight-fitting garments. Remove shoes, watches, and glasses, and keep eyes closed. Tell the client to assume a passive, detached attitude in which "you let everything, all thoughts, feelings, and behavior, just happen. Don't try to control what you are thinking or evaluate how you are performing. Just 'let yourself go' and don't worry about whether you are doing the procedure correctly." If the person has difficulty relaxing a particular muscle group, he or she should just skip to the next group of muscles. Not all muscle groups have to achieve the same level of deep relaxation. Emphasize that it is important to practice twice a day for 15 minutes preferably at a regular time.

The following example illustrates how to coach a client on the tense–release cycle. We have chosen the stomach muscle group to illustrate the instructional set that should be employed with each muscle group.

"Now I would like you to tense your stomach muscles. Tighten your stomach by pulling it in and making is as hard as a board. NOW, tighten your stomach muscles [therapist uses firm, moderately loud voice]. HOLD IT! Feel the tension, the tightness of your stomach muscles, HOLD IT, HOLD IT! Focus your attention on the hardness of your stomach [5–7 seconds after the NOW] And noowww, RELAXXXX! [Therapist drags out the "now relax" in a lower, soothing voice.] Let all the tension go from your stomach, let it flow out of your muscles, and notice the difference between feeling tense and relaxed. You feel your stomach muscles go further and further into relaxation. [For 30–40 seconds therapist makes suggestive statements about relaxation.] You focus all your attention on the pleasant feeling of relaxation. You notice how the stomach muscles now feel slack, loosened, and smoothed out compared to their hard, stiff, and tight state when you were tensing them. Continue to focus your attention on the feeling of relaxation as we move to your right leg."

In the first training session of PMR, it may be advisable to repeat each muscle group twice before proceeding to the next set of muscles. Also allow a few seconds of silence between muscle groups so that the whole process does not become too hurried. During each phase of release the client should subvocally repeat the word "relax" or "calm." Furthermore, the therapist can add a pleasant imagery suggestion at the end of the relaxation session in order to enhance the experience of deep relaxation.

Abbreviated PMR

If PMR is to have any utility as a coping response for anxiety in the naturalistic setting, clients must quickly learn more efficient, abbreviated relaxation protocols that can be employed anytime and in any place. If the client has mastered 10-muscle deep relaxation after 2 weeks of daily practice, the therapist can proceed with a *4-muscle group protocol* described in Bernstein and Borkovec (1973). This consists of the following procedure:

1. *Tense and release the arms*—both arms are held out in front of the person with a 45° bend at the elbow. Make a tight fist in each hand and hold the tension.
2. *Face and neck*—all of the face and neck muscles are tensed simultaneously by making a frown, squinting the eyes, wrinkling the nose, clenching the teeth, making an exaggerated grin, and pulling the chin downward to the chest.
3. *Chest and abdomen*—take a deep breath and then hold it while at the same time sitting forward, pull the shoulders back so that the shoulder blades are being pushed together, and tighten the stomach.
4. *Both legs*—lift both legs off the floor, point the toes up, and rotate the feet inward.

If deep muscular relaxation can be achieved after 2 weeks of daily practice, the client is ready to proceed to the final stage of PMR, *release-only relaxation*. Here the tense part of the exercise is omitted and the client simply focuses on releasing tension in various muscle groups starting at the top of the head and progressing downward to the toes (Taylor, 2000). Having daily practiced deep muscle relaxation for at least a month, individuals are now so well accustomed to the relaxed state that they are able to feel relaxed simply through recall (Bernstein & Borkovec, 1973). When asked to release the tension from particular muscle groups, this can be done by recalling their previous relaxed state. In release-only relaxation, the client is first instructed to breathe calmly and then to relax the various muscles of the face, neck, shoulders, arms, stomach, back, and legs (see Öst, 1987a, for detailed instructions). Once again individuals should practice release-only relaxation twice per day for at least 1 week. The protocol can be recorded to assist with homework practice and then faded out as the client masters this skill (Taylor, 2000). Clients who have mastered release-only relaxation now have a coping skill that can be used in almost any situation involving naturally occurring anxiety. It is a highly portable, efficient technique that enables the individual to achieve a relaxed state in 5–7 minutes (Öst, 1987a).

Clinician Guideline 7.8

Progressive muscle relaxation is an adjunct intervention that can be used by the cognitive therapist as preliminary skills training to reduce extreme levels of anxiety so the client will engage in self-directed exposure or to provide coping strategies for individuals with severe intolerance of anxiety. However, any relaxation training must be carefully monitored to ensure it is not used to avoid anxiety or to undermine the benefits of exposure-based behavioral experimentation.

Applied Relaxation

Applied relaxation (AR) is an 8- to 10-week treatment program developed by Lars-Göran Öst (1987a) at the Psychiatric Research Center, University of Uppsala, Sweden. It is an intensive, systematic, graded form of relaxation training that builds from PMR through cue-controlled relaxation to the application of rapid relaxation skills to anxiety elicited in natural situations. Because the final stage of AR involves within- and between-session practice in applying relaxation to anxiety-arousing situations, AR actually involves repeated brief situational and interoceptive exposure and so can not be considered a purely relaxation-based intervention for anxiety (Taylor, 2000). Nevertheless, what makes AR of interest is its conceptualization in terms of a coping perspective on anxiety and empirical evidence of its effectiveness for GAD in particular (e.g., see meta-analysis by Gould, Safren, Washington, & Otto, 2004). Öst (1987a) states that the purpose of AR is to teach individuals how to recognize the early signs of anxiety and learn to cope with anxiety rather than feel overwhelmed by their anxiousness. Table 7.6 presents a breakdown of the AR procedure as described by Öst (1987a).

Öst (1987a) reviewed 18 controlled outcome studies from his own lab that utilized AR and concluded that 90–95% of individuals were able to acquire the relaxation skill, with AR significantly more effective than no treatment or nonspecific treatment comparisons. The strongest empirical evidence for the effectiveness of AR comes from

TABLE 7.6. Applied Relaxation Treatment Protocol

Sessions	Intervention	Instructions
Session 1	Psychoeducation	Explain nature of anxiety, rationale for AR, graduated homework in identifying and recording symptoms of anxiety.
Sessions 1–4	14-muscle PMR	Complete body relaxation based on the 14-muscle PMR protocol of Wolpe & Lazarus (1966). Twice daily homework practice assigned.
Sessions 5–6	Release-only relaxation	Teach relaxation of muscle groups directly without tension instructions. Reduce relaxation induction time to 5–7 minutes. Takes 1 or 2 sessions with daily homework practice.
Sessions 6–7	Cue-controlled relaxation	Purpose is to create conditioned association between word "relax" and the relaxation state. Focus is on controlled breathing, relaxation induced via release-only method, and repeated pairing of subvocalization of word "relax" with every exhale. Homework practice assigned for 1–2 weeks.
Sessions 8–9	Differential relaxation	Purpose is to teach individuals to relax in other situations such as seating at a desk or walking and to remove tension from muscles not in use for an activity.
Sessions 10	Rapid relaxation	Teach client to relax in 20–30 seconds in multiple nonstressful daily situations by controlled breathing, think "relax," and scan body for tension and release by relaxation.
Sessions 11–13	Application training	Brief exposure (10–15 minutes) to wide range of *in vivo* anxiety-arousing situations, physical sensations (i.e., hyperventilation, physical exercise), or imagery in order to practice applying relaxation as coping response to anxiety.
Sessions 14–15	Maintenance program	Client encouraged to scan body at least daily and use rapid relaxation to get rid of any tension. Differential and rapid relaxation to be practiced twice a week on a regular basis.

clinical trials of GAD. In a variety of outcome studies AR produced significant post-treatment effects for GAD and maintenance of gains over follow-up that equalled cognitive therapy (Arntz, 2003; Borkovec & Costello, 1993; Borkovec, Newman, Lytle, & Pincus, 2002; Öst & Breitholz, 2000). However, Butler, Fennell, Robson, and Gelder (1991) found that standard PMR was less effective than cognitive therapy for GAD and barely more effective than a wait-list control. Moreover D. M. Clark and colleagues found that cognitive therapy was somewhat superior to AR in the treatment of panic disorder (D. M. Clark et al., 1994) and clearly superior to AR plus exposure in the treatment of social anxiety (D. M. Clark, Ehlers, Hackmann, McManus, Fennell et al., 2006). Öst and Westling (1995), on the other hand, found that CBT and AR were equally effective in treatment of panic disorder. In summary, it would appear that AR is an alternative treatment for GAD that can produce results equivalent to cognitive therapy, but its effectiveness for the other anxiety disorders remains less certain.

> **Clinician Guideline 7.9**
>
> Applied relaxation (AR) is an intensive, systematic, and graded relaxation training protocol that can be effective in the treatment of GAD, although it may be less effective for other anxiety disorders. AR is a viable alternative to cognitive therapy for GAD when the latter may not be acceptable to a client.

Breathing Retraining

Training in controlled breathing is considered a form of relaxation that is often included in relaxation procedures for stress and anxiety (e.g., Bourne, 2000; Cautela & Groden, 1978). Individuals often engage in rapid shallow breathing when in anxious or stressful situations. Controlled breathing procedures train individuals to become more aware of their dysfunctional breathing and to replace this with a slower, more paced diaphragmatic breathing of approximately 8–12 breaths per minute. This slower, deeper rate of breathing promotes a greater sense of relaxation, thereby reducing the anxious state. It is a quick and fairly simple intervention strategy that can give anxious individuals a limited sense of control over their emotional state. Because breathing retraining has been used most extensively in CBT of panic disorder, further discussion of this procedure is presented in the next chapter.

> **Clinician Guideline 7.10**
>
> Controlled breathing is a relatively quick and simple relaxation strategy that can be used to counter the rapid, shallow overbreathing that often contributes to heightened anxiety. In recent years clinical research has questioned the therapeutic role of controlled breathing, particularly in the treatment of panic disorder.

SUMMARY AND CONCLUSION

Behavioral interventions play a critical role in cognitive therapy of anxiety disorders. In fact it is difficult to imagine an effective cognitive treatment for anxiety that does not include a significant behavioral component. There is a large empirical literature demonstrating the effectiveness of exposure interventions in the treatment of all types of fear and anxiety. When utilized as a therapeutic ingredient of cognitive therapy, exposure-based exercises provide the most powerful forms of corrective information for the faulty threat and vulnerability appraisals and beliefs that sustain heightened anxiety. Exposure in the form of empirical hypothesis-testing experiments should be a focal point in all cognitive therapy interventions offered to treat the anxiety disorders.

Greater attention should be given to response prevention and correction of safety-seeking cognitions and behaviors in cognitive interventions for anxiety (e.g., D. M. Clark et al., 1999; Salkovskis, Clark, & Gelder, 1996). Without intervention that directly reduces reliance on safety-seeking cues and coping responses, it is likely that any reduction in anxiety will be incomplete and place the individual at high risk for relapse.

The role of relaxation training in treatment of anxiety disorders continues to generate considerable debate. The long-established tradition of teaching progressive muscle relaxation to relieve anxiety may still have some efficacy for the treatment of GAD and possibly panic disorder, especially when the more systematic and intense applied relaxation protocol is employed. However, relaxation training for OCD and social phobia is unwarranted, although it may still have some value in PTSD for those with heightened generalized anxiety. Breathing retraining is often used in treatment of panic disorder but as discussed in the next chapter its therapeutic effectiveness has been called into question. A Quick Reference Summary is provided in Appendix 7.5 as a brief overview of the behavioral interventions that are useful in treating the anxiety disorders.

Exposure Hierarchy

Name: _____ Date: _____

Instructions: On a blank sheet of paper write down 15–20 situations, objects, physical sensations, or intrusive thoughts/images that are relevant to your anxious concerns. Select experiences that fall along the full range from those that trigger only slight anxiety and avoidance to experiences that elicit moderate and then severe anxiety and avoidance. Next rank-order these experiences from least to most anxious or avoidant and transfer the list into the second column on this form. In the first column record the level of anxiety you expect with each entry. In the third column write down the core anxious thought associated with each situation if this is known to you.

	A. Expected level of anxiety/ avoidance (0–100)	**B. Briefly describe the anxious/ avoided situation, object, sensation, or intrusive thought/image**	**C. Note the most prominent anxious or apprehensive thought associated with this entry**
LEAST	1.		
	2.		
	3.		
	4.		
	5.		
	6.		
	7.		
	8.		
	9.		
	10.		
	11.		
	12.		
	13.		
	14.		
	15.		
	16.		
MOST	17.		

Exposure Practice Record

Name: _____ Date: _____

Instructions: Keep a record of your daily exposure practice sessions using this form. Be sure to record the initial, middle, and final anxiety rating as well as the type of exposure task completed and its duration.

Date and Time	Exposure Task	Duration (minutes)	Initial Anxiety (0–100)	Midpoint Anxiety (0–100)	End-point Anxiety (0–100)

Response Prevention Record

Name: _____   Date: _____

Instructions: Keep a record of your daily response prevention practice sessions using this form. Be sure to record the initial and endpoint "urge to engage in response" and anxiety level.

Date and Time	Describe Response That Was Prevented	Initial Urge to Engage in Response (0–100)	Initial Anxiety (0–100)	Endpoint Urge to Engage in Response (0–100)	Endpoint Anxiety Level (0–100)

List "blocking strategies" used for response prevention: _____

_____

_____

Weekly Progressive Muscle Relaxation Record

Name: _____   Date: _____

Instructions: Two 15-minute relaxation sessions should be scheduled daily. Use the chart below to record your progress in achieving a relaxed state with each of the muscle groups. Make a check mark (✓) if you successfully relaxed a muscle group during a practice session and mark an (**X**) if you had difficulty relaxing the muscle group. At the bottom of the column, rate the overall level of relaxation achieved in the practice session from 0 ("unable to relax at all") to 50 ("moderately relaxed but conscious of some tension") to 100 ("so completely relaxed that I fell asleep").

Day of Week:	Day One		Day Two		Day Three		Day Four		Day Five		Day Six		Day Seven	
Practice session:	1	2	1	2	1	2	1	2	1	2	1	2	1	2
1. Dominant arm														
2. Nondominant arm														
3. Forehead														
4. Eyes and nose														
5. Jaw and neck														
6. Shoulders and back														
7. Chest														
8. Stomach														
9. Dominant leg														
10. Nondominant leg														
11. Rate overall level of relaxation (0–100)														

Chapter 7 Quick Reference Summary: Behavioral Interventions

I. **Adopt a Cognitive Perspective**
   1. *Rationale*—based on Figure 6.1 (client handout of cognitive therapy model), explain use of behavioral assignment to examine validity of anxious thoughts and their alternatives.
   2. *Identify Target Thought*—write down the anxious thought challenged by the behavioral exercise.
   3. *Behavioral Prescription*—write out specific instructions on how to do exercise, what thoughts are evaluated, and the outcome criteria.
   4. *Self-Monitoring*—client records how the exercise was conducted, its outcome, anxiety level, automatic thoughts, evidence for and against target thoughts.
   5. *Evaluation*—extensive evaluation of outcome of exercise; review self-monitoring form; conclusions reached about target thought (belief) and its alternative; write out a summary of exercise in form of a "coping card."

II. **Graded Exposure**
   1. For *situational exposure,* review the Situational Analysis Form (Appendix 5.2) and hierarchically arrange anxiety-provoking situations from mildly to intensely anxious.
   2. Begin with moderately anxious situation; initially demonstrate exposure within session.
   3. Obtain 0–100 anxiety ratings before exposure, every 10 minutes during exposure, and finally at conclusion of the exercise.
   4. Assign exposure as homework, at least 30–60 minutes daily. Use Exposure Practice Record (Appendix 7.2) to record outcome.
   5. *Imaginal exposure* begins with development of a fear script, within-session demonstration, and then 30 minutes of daily homework. Audio habituation training should be considered when cognitive avoidance is present.
   6. *Exposure to bodily sensations* involves extensive within-session demonstration prior to homework assignment. Table 8.8 (panic disorder chapter) provides a description of various interoceptive exercises.

III. **Response Prevention**
   1. *Identify maladaptive cognitive and behavioral coping strategies* or other forms of neutralization (see Behavioral Responses to Anxiety Checklist, Appendix 5.7, and Cognitive Responses to Anxiety Checklist, Appendix 5.9).
   2. Provide **treatment rationale** for response prevention.
   3. Instruct client on *"blocking strategies"* (e.g., self-instructional coping statements, competing responses, paradoxical intention, encouragement).
   4. Develop *alternative coping strategies* for anxiety.
   5. Challenge *problematic cognitions*.
   6. *Record and evaluate* success of intervention using the Response Prevention Record (Appendix 7.3).

IV. **Other Behavioral Interventions**
   1. *Direct behavioral change* involves teaching specific behaviors that improve personal effectiveness through methods of didactic instruction, modeling, behavioral rehearsal, reinforcement, and self-monitoring.
   2. *Relaxation training* can be progressive muscle or applied relaxation training; most useful for GAD. A rationale for PMR can be found in Chapter 7, pages 260–262. Instructions for 10-muscle PMR are in Table 7.5 and an outline for AR is described in Table 7.6. Assign PMR as homework and record daily practice on the Weekly Progressive Muscle Relaxation Record (Appendix 7.4).
   3. *Breathing retraining*—Table 8.9 on page 324 (panic disorder chapter) contains diaphragmatic breathing retraining protocol.

COGNITIVE THEORY AND TREATMENT OF SPECIFIC ANXIETY DISORDERS

In the last two decades psychotherapy innovation and research has focused increasingly on the development and evaluation of treatment protocols that target specific DSM-IV-TR (APA, 2000) disorders. The growth of disorder-specific manualized treatment has been particularly evident in the anxiety disorders. The generic cognitive model of anxiety presented in Part I and the core cognitive assessment and intervention strategies described in Part II can be readily adapted to target the shared and distinct symptom features of the more common types of anxiety disorders. This final part of the book provides disorder-specific cognitive models, hypotheses, case conceptualizations, and treatment protocols for five different types of anxiety disorder. Chapter 8 discusses the cognitive model and treatment of panic disorder with its emphasis on threat misinterpretations of internal states and loss of reappraisal capacity, whereas Chapter 9 presents the cognitive theory and treatment of social phobia that focuses on fear of negative evaluation of others and presence of maladaptive coping responses. Chapter 10 provides a cognitive model and treatment of generalized anxiety and worry, Chapter 11 discusses the cognitive appraisal perspective on theory and treatment of obsessive–compulsive disorders, and Chapter 12 presents a cognitive model and treatment that focuses on the faulty appraisals and beliefs associated with the trauma-related intrusive thoughts and memories of posttraumatic stress disorder.

Chapter 8

Cognitive Therapy of Panic Disorder

Of course, we were afraid and fear isn't always a wise counselor, let's go back, for our greater safety we ought to barricade the door of the wards....
—JOSÉ SARAMAGO (Portuguese novelist and 1998 Nobel Laureate in Literature, 1922–)

Helen is a 27-year-old single woman who worked in the insurance industry and presented with an 11-year history of panic disorder and moderate agoraphobic avoidance. At the time of assessment she was experiencing approximately eight full-blown panic attacks daily with elevated levels of generalized anxiety, considerable apprehension about having panic attacks, and avoidance of routine activities such as travel outside her community, not maintaining close proximity to medical facilities, highway driving, air travel, and the like. The first onset of panic occurred when she was 16 years old but the panic attacks were few and far between until she took her first business trip to New York City at age 22. She described 4 days of terrifying acute anxiety involving chest pain, heart palpitations, tingling in the extremities, abdominal distress, and agitation. These bodily sensations were accompanied by an intense fear that she might die from a heart attack. However, she did not seek medical intervention at the time but instead coped by resting, taking Gravol, and trying to remain calm. Upon returning home the panic attacks continued. In the intervening 5 years she has been treated with citalopram, lorazepam, and relaxation training with minimal effectiveness.

Pretreatment assessment revealed that heart palpitations, chest pain, sweating, shortness of breath, feelings of choking, nausea, and hot flushes were the main bodily sensations during her panic attacks. Although fears of a heart attack or of going crazy were still present, her main misinterpretation of threat had shifted to a focus on breathlessness, with a fear that she would stop breathing and suffocate. Extensive reliance on safety seeking emerged such that Helen became preoccupied with maintaining close geographic proximity to medical facilities, frequently making trips to her family physician and hospital emergency department whenever she felt intense panic or concern about her respiration or cardiac functioning. As a result she became increasingly reluctant to venture more than a few miles from a hospital for fear that she would be trapped without access to medical facilities. Avoidance, reassurance seeking and self-monitoring of physical symptoms (e.g., repeated pulse checking) became the main coping strategies for her daily battle with panic attacks.

A structured diagnostic interview revealed that Helen met DSM-IV criteria for panic disorder with agoraphobic avoidance of moderate severity. She did not have any other current comorbid condition but did report two previous episodes of major depression with suicidal ideation. Her pretreatment symptom scores were BDI-II = 8, BAI = 22, PSWQ = 64, Agoraphobic Cognitions Questionnaire (ACQ) = 33, and Body Sensations Questionnaire (BSQ) = 48. Her main threat-related thoughts concerned "What if I can't get my breath and I suffocate?", "Could this chest pain mean that I am having a heart attack?", "What if I can't get to the hospital in time?", "What if this builds into another panic attack and it eventually drives me crazy?", and "Is this ever going to end?" In short, Helen revealed a pattern of anxious thinking and misinterpretation that reflected an intolerance of anxiety and reliance on maladaptive avoidance and safety-seeking strategies in a desperate attempt to control her anxiety and prevent the much dreaded panic attacks.

Helen's clinical state exemplifies a fairly typical presentation of panic disorder. Twelve individual sessions of CBT followed by four booster sessions over an 8-month period proved highly effective in reducing panic frequency, generalized anxiety, and agoraphobic avoidance. Treatment focused on (1) psychoeducation in the cognitive therapy model, (2) intentional activation of bodily sensations and underlying fear schemas, (3) cognitive restructuring and reattribution of misinterpretations of bodily sensations, (4) graded situational exposure homework, and (5) increased tolerance and acceptance of anxiety, risk, and uncertainty with a corresponding reduction in intentional control efforts. In this chapter we begin with a description of the phenomenology and diagnosis of panic and agoraphobia, followed by a discussion of the cognitive model of panic, and its empirical status. The remainder of the chapter discusses issues of assessment, case formulation, the cognitive therapy treatment protocol, and its efficacy.

DIAGNOSTIC CONSIDERATIONS AND CLINICAL FEATURES

The Nature of Panic

Panic attacks are discrete occurrences of intense fear or discomfort of sudden onset that are accompanied by a surge of physiological hyperarousal. Barlow (2002) considers panic the clearest clinical presentation of fear. In addition to strong autonomic arousal, panic is characterized by a faulty verbal or imaginal ideation of physical or mental catastrophe (e.g., dying, going insane), intense uncontrollable anxiety, and a strong urge to escape (Barlow, 2002; Beck et al., 1985, 2005; Ottaviani & Beck, 1987). So aversive is the panic experience that many patients have a strong apprehension about having another attack and develop extensive avoidance of situations thought to trigger panic. As a result panic and agoraphobia are closely associated, with most individuals with panic disorder presenting with some degree of agoraphobic avoidance and 95% of people with agoraphobia reporting a past or current panic disorder (Antony & Swinson, 2000a; APA, 2000). In the latest epidemiological study panic disorder had a 12-month prevalence of 2.7%, whereas agoraphobia without panic disorder was much less common at 0.8% (Kessler et al., 2005).

DSM-IV-TR defines *panic attacks* as "a discrete period of intense fear or discomfort in which four (or more) of the following symptoms developed abruptly and reached a peak within 10 minutes" (APA, 2000, p. 432). The typical panic attack lasts between 5 and 20 minutes, although a heightened state of anxiety can linger long after the panic episode subsides (Rachman, 2004). According to DSM-IV-TR, the defining symptoms of panic are:

- Elevated heart rate or palpitations
- Sweating
- Trembling or shaking
- Smothering sensation or shortness of breath
- Feeling of choking
- Chest tightness, pain, or discomfort
- Abdominal distress or nausea
- Dizziness, lightheadedness, faintness, or feeling unsteady
- Feelings of unreality (derealization) or detachment from oneself (depersonalization)
- Numbness or tingling sensations
- Chills or hot flushes
- Fear of losing control or going crazy
- Fear of dying

Table 8.1 lists a number of prominent features that characterize panic attacks.

Situational Triggers

Even though DSM-IV specifies that two unexpected panic attacks must occur to meet diagnostic criteria for panic disorder, the majority of panic episodes are anticipated because they are provoked by exposure to an identifiable stressor (Rachman, 2004). Theaters, supermarkets, restaurants, department stores, buses, trains, airplanes, sub-

---

TABLE 8.1. Critical Features of Panic Attacks

- Situational triggers
- Abrupt onset of physiological arousal
- Heightened self-focus, hypervigilance of bodily sensations
- Perceived physical, mental, or behavioral catastrophe
- Apprehension, fear of future panic attacks
- Extensive safety seeking (escape, avoidance, etc.)
- Perceived lack of controllability
- Qualitatively distinct from anxiety

---

ways, driving in the car, walking on the street, staying alone at home, or being far away from home are all examples of external situations that individuals with panic disorder report may trigger a panic attack. As a result these situations are often avoided in order to minimize the possibility of triggering a panic episode. More recently, researchers have argued that internal cues such as thoughts, images, feelings, or bodily sensations can trigger panic and avoidance (Barlow, 2002; McNally, 1994; White et al., 2006).

Acute Physiological Arousal

Although an abrupt onset of physiological symptoms is one of the hallmarks of panic attacks, it is clearly not a defining feature of the disorder. Individuals with panic disorder are not more autonomically hyperactive to standard laboratory stressors than nonpanickers (Taylor, 2000). Furthermore, even though 24-hour ambulatory heart rate monitoring of panic patients indicates that most panic attacks involve a distinct elevation in heart rate, a significant minority of self-reported attacks (i.e., 40%) are not associated with actual increase in heart rate or other physiological responses and most episodes of physiological hyperarousal (i.e., tachycardia) occur without self-reported panic episodes (e.g., Barsky, Cleary, Sarnie, & Rushkin, 1994; Lint, Taylor, Fried-Behar, & Kenardy, 1995; Taylor et al., 1986). Moreover, individuals with panic disorder do not have more cardiac arrhythmias in a 24-hour period than nonpanic patients investigated for heart palpitations (Barsky et al., 1994). As discussed below, it is not the presence of physiological symptoms that is critical in the pathogenesis of panic but rather how these symptoms are interpreted.

Hypervigilance of Bodily Sensations

Empirical studies are inconsistent on whether panic disorder is characterized by heightened interoceptive acuity especially in terms of cardiac perception (e.g., Pollock, Carter, Amir, & Marks, 2006), although individuals may be more sensitive to the particular body sensations linked to their central fear (e.g., increased pulse rate for those afraid of heart attacks; Taylor, 2000). As McNally (1999) noted, fearing bodily sensations does not mean that a person will necessarily be better at detecting interoceptive cues. On the other hand, individuals with panic have heightened anxiety sensitivity (see Chapter 4) and greater vigilance for the physical sensations associated with anxiety (e.g., Kroeze & van den Hout, 2000a; Schmidt, Lerew, & Trakowski, 1997). We can conclude from this that panic is characterized by a heightened vigilance and responsiveness to specific physical symptoms linked to a core fear but it is unclear whether individuals with panic disorder are better at detecting changes in their physical state.

Catastrophic Interpretations

A key feature of panic episodes is the tendency to interpret the occurrence of certain bodily sensations in terms of an impending biological (e.g., death), mental (i.e., insanity), or behavioral (e.g., loss of control) disaster (Beck, 1988; Beck & Greenberg, 1988; D. M. Clark, 1986a). For example, individuals with panic disorder may interpret (a) chest pain or a sudden increase in heart rate as sign of a possible heart attack, (b) shaking or trembling as a loss of control, or (c) feelings of unreality or depersonalization as a sign of mental instability or "going crazy." Catastrophic misinterpretations are discussed more fully in our review of the cognitive research.

Apprehension of Panic

Individuals with panic disorder report extreme distress, even terror, during panic attacks and so quickly develop considerable apprehension about having future attacks. This fear of panic is a distinguishing feature of the disorder and is included in DSM-IV-TR as a diagnostic criterion (APA, 2000). Presence of fear and avoidance of panic attacks differentiates panic disorder from other anxiety disorders in which panic attacks occur but the "fear of panic" is missing.

Extensive Safety Seeking and Avoidance

Safety-seeking behavior and avoidance of panic-related situations are common responses to panic attacks and may be seen as coping strategies to prevent the impending disaster (e.g., overwhelming panic, a heart attack, loss of control). Phobic avoidance is common in panic disorder and is elicited by the anticipation of panic attacks in particular (Craske & Barlow, 1988). The phobic situations associated with agoraphobia are quite variable across individuals because the avoidance is elicited by the anticipation of panic attacks and not by the situations themselves (White & Barlow, 2002). White et al. (2006) reported that 98% of panic disorder cases have mild to severe situational avoidance, 90% experiential avoidance (i.e., use safety signals or thought strategies to withdraw or minimize contact with a phobic stimulus), and 80% interoceptive avoidance (i.e., refusal of substances or activities that could produce the physical sensations associated with panic). Furthermore, they found that severity of agoraphobic avoidance was predicted by elevated fear of physical symptoms of anxiety (i.e., anxiety sensitivity) and low perceived control over threat. Together these findings indicate a close but complicated relationship between panic attacks and the development of avoidance responses.

Perceived Lack of Control

Beck et al. (1985, 2005) noted that a striking characteristic of panic attacks is the feeling of being overwhelmed by uncontrollable anxiety. This apparent loss of control over one's emotions and the anticipated threat causes a fixation on the panicogenic sensations and a loss of capacity to use reason to realistically appraise one's physical and emotional state (Beck, 1988; see also Barlow, 2002).

Panic Distinct from Anxiety

McNally (1994) argues that panic should not be seen as an extreme form of anxiety involving the anticipation of future threat but rather as an immediate "fight-or-flight" response to perceived imminent danger. In the cognitive model of anxiety presented in Chapter 2, panic attacks would fall within the "immediate fear response" (Phase I), whereas apprehension about panic, avoidance, and safety-seeking would constitute secondary processes (Phase II) that maintain a state of heightened anxiety about having panic attacks.

Clinician Guideline 8.1

Panic attacks involve a sudden onset of intense fear of certain activated physical sensations that are misinterpreted as indicating an imminent, even catastrophic, threat to one's physical or mental health. The misinterpretations of threat increases apprehension of and vigilance regarding these physical symptoms, and leads to avoidance and safety-seeking responses to reduce the possibility of future panic attacks.

Varieties of Panic

It is generally recognized that there are different types of panic attacks or episodes. Table 8.2 presents five types of panic experience that may have distinct functional characteristics with implications for treatment.

Spontaneous and Situationally Cued Panic

DSM-IV-TR recognizes three types of panic. With *spontaneous or unexpected (uncued) panic attacks* "the individual does not associate onset with an internal or external situational trigger (i.e., the attack is perceived as occurring spontaneous 'out of the blue'), [whereas] *situationally bound (cued) panic attacks* are defined as those that almost invariably occur immediately on exposure to, or in anticipation of, the situational cue or trigger" (APA, 2000, pp. 430–431). Examples of situationally cued panic include the woman who always has a panic attack whenever she goes alone to a large department store, the man who always has a panic episode whenever he drives outside the city limits, or the young person who panics at night when left alone in the house. *Situationally predisposed panic attacks* are similar to situationally bound episodes but are not always associated with the situational cues or do not necessarily occur immediately upon exposure to the situational trigger (APA, 2000). An example would be sometimes experi-

TABLE 8.2. **Various Types of Panic Attacks**

Type of panic attack	Description
Spontaneous panic	Unexpected ("out of the blue") panic attacks that are not associated with external or internal situational triggers (DSM-IV-TR; APA, 2000).
Situationally cued panic	Panic attacks that occur *almost* invariably with exposure or anticipated exposure to a particular situation or cue (DSM-IV-TR; APA, 2000).
Nocturnal panic	A sudden awaking from sleep in which the individual experiences a state of terror and intense physiological arousal without an obvious trigger (e.g., a dream, nightmares).
Limited-symptom panic	A discrete period of intense fear or discomfort that occurs in the absence of a real danger but involves less than four panic attack symptoms.
Nonclinical panic	Occasional panic attacks reported in the general population that often occur in stressful or evaluative situations, involve fewer panic symptoms, and are associated with less apprehension or worry about panic (McNally, 1994).

encing a panic attack while waiting in a bank line or attending the movies. As Taylor (2000) noted, many factors can determine whether a situation increases the probability of a panic attack including temperature, access to exits, crowding, familiarity, and the like.

The distinction between uncued versus cued panic has important diagnostic implications in distinguishing panic disorder from other types of anxiety disorders. Although panic attacks are present in the majority of anxiety disorders (over 80%), they are usually associated with specific situations (e.g., anticipation of or exposure to a social encounter in social phobia; see review by Barlow, 2002). For this reason DSM-IV-TR (APA, 2000) requires the presence of at least two uncued or spontaneous panic attacks in order to make a diagnosis of panic disorder. However, it can be difficult to determine if a panic episode is entirely unexpected because we are dependent on the client's retrospective report and observational skills (McNally, 1994). The unexpectedness of panic probably falls along a continuum, thereby making it difficult to assign panic attacks to a discrete category of either expected or unexpected. Moreover, truly unexpected, uncued panic attacks may be relatively infrequent, even in panic disorder (Brown & Deagle, 1992; Street, Craske, & Barlow, 1989).

Clinician Guideline 8.2

Assessment for panic disorder should include a thorough evaluation of the frequency, severity, subjective probability, and contextual factors associated with spontaneous and situationally cued panic attacks.

Nocturnal Panic Attacks

Nocturnal panic attacks (NPs) are a frequent occurrence, with 25–70% of individuals with panic disorder reporting at least one sleep panic attack, and 18–33% reporting frequent, recurrent NPs (Barlow, 2002; Craske & Rowe, 1997; Mellman & Uhde, 1989). NPs, though phenomenologically similar to daytime panic attacks (Craske & Rowe, 1997), are characterized by an abrupt waking from sleep in a state of panic, especially during the transition from Stage 2 to Stage 3 sleep (Barlow, 2002; Hauri, Friedman, & Ravaris, 1989; Taylor et al., 1986). NPs are distinct from other sleep-related conditions such as night terrors, sleep apnea, sleep seizures, or sleep paralysis (Craske, Lang, Aikins, & Mystkowski, 2005). There is some evidence that individuals with NPs have more severe panic attacks than those with panic disorder without NPs, and many patients with frequent NPs become fearful of sleep (Barlow, 2002; Craske & Rowe, 1997).

Craske and Rowe (1997; see also Aikins & Craske, 2007) proposed that the same cognitive factors responsible for panic attacks in wakefulness are implicated in NPs. Thus fear of change in physical state during sleep or relaxation, heightened vigilance for and perception of changes in bodily state, and catastrophic appraisal of physiological changes immediately upon waking are considered important in the pathogenesis of NPs. In NP distress about sleep and relaxation may reflect a fear of losing vigilance for bodily changes during sleep (Aikins & Craske, 2007). In support of this cognitive-behavioral explanation, studies have found an increase in physiological changes in the minutes before panicky awaking (Hauri et al., 1989; Roy-Byrne, Mellman, & Uhde, 1988) and experimental manipulation of individuals' expectations and interpretations of the physiological arousal symptoms associated with sleep can influence their level of anxiety and presence of panic attacks upon abrupt awaking (Craske et al., 2002; see also Craske & Freed, 1995, for similar results). In addition Craske et al. (2005) reported significant posttreatment gains at 9-month follow-up in a sample of panic disorder patients with recurrent NPs who were offered 11 sessions of CBT. NPs, then, are common in panic disorders and can be accommodated within the cognitive perspective.

Limited-Symptom Panic

DSM-IV-TR recognizes that limited-symptom attacks are common in panic disorder and are identical to full-blown attacks except they involve fewer than 4 of 13 symptoms (APA, 2000). The usual profile is for individuals to experience full-blown panic attacks interspersed with frequent minor attacks, with both showing similar functional and phenomenological characteristics (Barlow, 2002; McNally, 1994).

Nonclinical Panic

Contrary to expectations, panic attacks are actually quite common in the general population. Questionnaire studies indicate that over one-third of nonclinical young adults experience at least one panic attack within the past year (Norton, Dorward, & Cox, 1986; Norton, Harrison, Hauch, & Rhodes, 1985), but only 1–3% report three or more panic attacks in the last 3 weeks (i.e., Salge et al., 1988). Unexpected panic attacks are less common, ranging from 7 to 28%, and far fewer (approximately 2%) meet diagnostic criteria for panic disorder (Norton et al., 1986; Telch, Lucas, & Nelson, 1989). Structured interviews produce much lower rates (i.e., 13%) of nonclinical panic (Brown & Deagle, 1992; Eaton, Kessler, Wittchen, & Magee, 1994; Hayward et al., 1997; Norton, Cox, & Malan, 1992). However, the infrequent panic attacks of infrequent nonclinical panickers are less severe, less pathological, and more situationally predisposed than the unexpected, "crippling" attacks found in diagnosable panic disorder (Cox, Endler, Swinson, & Norton, 1992; Norton et al., 1992; Telch et al., 1989), leading to the possibility that a history of infrequent panic attacks might be a possible risk factor for panic disorder (e.g., Antony & Swinson, 2000a; Brown & Deagle, 1992; Ehlers, 1995).

Clinician Guideline 8.3

The dimensional quality to panic attacks should be recognized when assessing this clinical phenomenon. Clients should be evaluated for past and current experiences with less severe, "partial" panic episodes as well as the occurrence of nocturnal panic attacks. An exclusive focus on "full-blown" panic attacks may not capture the total impact of panic experiences on individual clients.

Agoraphobic Avoidance

Agoraphobia is the avoidance or endurance with distress of "places or situations from which escape might be difficult (or embarrassing) or in which help may not be available in the event of having a panic attack or panic-like symptoms" (DSM-IV-TR; APA, 2000, p. 432). The anxiety usually leads to pervasive avoidance of a variety of situations such as being at home alone, crowds, department stores, supermarkets, driving, enclosed places (e.g., elevators), open spaces (e.g., crossing bridges, parking lots), theaters, restaurants, public transportation, air travel, and the like. In some cases agoraphobia is mild and confined to a few specific places, whereas for others it is more severe in which a "safe zone" may be defined around the home with travel outside this zone highly anxiety-provoking (Antony & Swinson, 2000a). In extreme cases, the person may be completely housebound.

Panic attacks most often precede the onset of agoraphobia (Katerndahl & Realini, 1997; Thyer & Himle, 1985) and individuals with panic disorder are more likely to develop agoraphobic avoidance to situations associated with the first panic attack (Faravelli, Pallanti, Biondi, Paterniti, & Scarpato, 1992). Furthermore, the development of agoraphobic avoidance is less dependent on the frequency and severity of panic attacks and more likely due to high anticipatory anxiety about the occurrence of panic, elevated anxiety sensitivity, diminished sense of control over threat, and a tendency to use avoidance as a coping strategy (Craske & Barlow, 1988; Craske, Rapee, & Barlow, 1988; Craske, Sanderson, & Barlow, 1987; White et al., 2006). The close association between panic attacks and agoraphobia is also confirmed by the low prevalence of agoraphobia without panic disorder (AWOPD). In the NCS-R AWOPD had a 12-month prevalence rate of only 0.8% compared to 2.7% for panic disorder (Kessler et al., 2005) and rates among treatment-seeking samples may be even lower because individuals with AWOPD may be less likely to seek professional treatment (e.g., Eaton, Dryman, & Weissman, 1991; Wittchen, Reed, & Kessler, 1998). Although relatively rare, AWOPD may be more severe and associated with less favorable treatment outcome than panic disorder, but the studies are divided on whether it is characterized by greater impaired functioning (Buller, Maier, & Benkert, 1986; Buller et al., 1991; Ehlers, 1995; Goisman et al., 1994; Wittchen et al., 1998).

Clinician Guideline 8.4

Expect some form of agoraphobic avoidance in most cases of panic disorder. It can vary from mild, even fluctuating, forms of situational avoidance to severe cases of being housebound. The clinician should adopt a broad, dimensional assessment perspective, with a focus on recording the variety of situations, body sensations, feelings, and experiences that the client avoids.

Diagnostic Features

Table 8.3 presents the DSM-IV-TR (APA, 2000) diagnostic criteria for panic disorder.
There are three possible diagnoses relevant to panic disorder; panic disorder without agoraphobia (300.01), panic disorder with agoraphobia (300.21), and agoraphobia

TABLE 8.3. DSM-IV Diagnostic Criteria for Panic Disorder

Criterion A. Both (1) and (2):

(1) recurrent unexpected Panic Attacks (i.e., at least two)
(2) at least one of the attacks has been followed by 1 month (or more) of one (or more) of the
    following:
    (a) persistent concern about having additional attacks
    (b) worry about the implications of the attack or its consequences (e.g., losing control, having a
        heart attack, "going crazy")
    (c) a significant change in behavior related to panic attacks

Criterion B.

Presence of agoraphobia is necessary for a diagnosis of Panic Disorder with Agoraphobia (300.21)
or absence of agoraphobia for a diagnosis of Panic Disorder without Agoraphobia (300.01)

Criterion C.

The Panic Attacks are not due to the direct physiological effects of a substance (e.g., drug of abuse,
a medication) or a general medical condition (e.g., hyperthyroidism)

Criterion D.

The Panic Attacks are not better accounted for by another mental disorder, such as Social Phobia
(e.g., occurring on exposure to feared social situations), Specific Phobia (e.g., on exposure to a
specific phobic situation), Obsessive–Compulsive Disorder (e.g., on exposure to dirt in someone
with an obsession about contamination), Posttraumatic Stress Disorder (e.g., in response to stimuli
associated with a severe stressor), or Separation Anxiety Disorder (e.g., in response to being away
from home or close relatives).

Note. From American Psychiatric Association (2000). Copyright 2000 by the American Psychiatric Association.
Reprinted by permission.

without a history of panic disorder (AWOPD; 300.22). The first two diagnoses are distinguished on the basis of presence or absence of situational avoidance. If a more inclusive definition of agoraphobic avoidance is used to include experiential and interoceptive (internal) cues (White et al., 2006), then practically no one would receive a diagnosis of panic disorder without agoraphobia.

Psychiatric Comorbidity

Panic disorder is associated with a high rate of diagnostic comorbidity. Based on a large clinical sample (N = 1,127), Brown, Campbell, et al. (2001) found that 60% of individuals with a principal diagnosis of panic disorder with agoraphobia (n = 360) had at least one other Axis I disorder. The most common comorbid conditions were major depression (23%), GAD (22%), social phobia (15%), and specific phobia (15%). PTSD (4%) and OCD (7%) were relatively less common comorbid disorders. In the NCS 55.6% of individuals with lifetime panic disorder met criteria for lifetime major depression, whereas only 11.2% of those with lifetime major depression were comorbid for lifetime panic disorder (Roy-Byrne et al., 2000). Panic disorder is more severe in those with comorbid major depression (Breier, Charney, & Heninger, 1984). In terms of temporal relationships, another anxiety disorder is more likely to precede panic with or without agoraphobia (Brown, DiNardo, Lehman, & Campbell, 2001; Newman et al., 1996).

Substance abuse is also common in panic disorder (e.g., Sbrana et al., 2005). Results of the National Epidemiologic Survey on Alcohol and Related Conditions ($N = 43,093$ respondents) indicate that panic disorder with agoraphobia and GAD were more likely associated with a substance use disorder than other mood and anxiety disorders (Grant et al., 2004). Rates of Axis II personality disorders range from 25 to 75%, with particular concentration in the Cluster C disorders (Diaferia et al., 1993; Renneberg, Chambless, & Gracely, 1992). Presence of borderline, dependent, schizoid, or schizotypal personality disorder by age 22 significantly predicted elevated risk for panic disorder by age 33 (Johnson, Cohen, Kasen, & Brook, 2006). This finding is consistent with the observed trend for nonpanic conditions to precede the development of panic disorder when individuals have multiple diagnoses (Katerndahl & Realini, 1997).

Clinician Guideline 8.5

Presence of comorbid conditions, especially major depression, GAD, substance abuse, and personality disorder, should be determined when conducting a diagnostic evaluation for panic disorder.

Panic and Suicide Attempts

Although findings from the ECA suggested that individuals with panic disorder were 2.5 times more likely to attempt suicide than individuals with other psychiatric conditions (Weissman, Klerman, Markowitz, & Ouellette, 1989), later studies contradicted this finding, showing that suicide attempts are practically nonexistent in panic disorder (e.g., Beck, Steer, Sanderson, & Skeie, 1991; Swoboda, Amering, Windhaber, & Katschnig, 2003). More recently Vickers and McNally (2004) reanalyzed the NCS data set and concluded that any suicide attempts in panic disorder were due to psychiatric comorbidity and that panic itself did not directly increase risk for suicide attempts.

Increased Medical Morbidity and Mortality

A number of medical conditions are elevated in panic disorder such as cardiac disease, hypertension, asthma, ulcers, and migraines (Rogers et al., 1994; Stewart, Linet, & Celentano, 1989). Panic sufferers are more likely to first seek medical evaluation of their symptoms than attend a mental health setting (e.g., Katerndahl & Realini, 1995). A significant number of individuals with cardiac complaints (9–43%) have panic disorder (Barsky et al., 1994; Katon et al., 1988; Morris, Baker, Devins, & Shapiro, 1997). Moreover, higher rates of cardiovascular disease, even fatal ischemic heart attacks, have been found in men with panic disorder (Coryell, Noyes, & House, 1986; Haines, Imeson, & Meade, 1987; Weissman, Markowitz, Ouellette, Greenwald, & Kahn, 1990). In addition postmenopausal women who experience full-blown panic attacks have a threefold increased risk of coronary heart disease or stroke (Smoller et al., 2007). In a recent cohort study based on analysis of the British General Practice Research Database, men and women with panic disorder had a significantly higher incidence of coronary heart disease and those younger than 50 years of age had a higher incidence of myocardial infarction (Walters, Rait, Petersen, Williams, & Nazareth, 2008). Mitral valve prolapse (MVP), a malformation of the leaflets of the heart's mitral valve that causes symptoms like chest pain, tachycardia, faintness, fatigue, and anxiety (see Taylor, 2000), is twice as common in individuals with panic disorder as in nonpanic controls (Katerndahl, 1993). However, most individuals are asymptomatic and not at high risk for serious health consequences (Bouknight & O'Rourke, 2000), so there is no clinical significance in distinguishing panic patients with or without the condition (Barlow, 20002).

Panic disorder is associated with higher mortality rates possibly due to elevated risk of cardiovascular and cerebrovascular diseases, especially in men with panic disorder (Coryell et al., 1986; Weissman et al., 1990). Moreover, panic disorder and respiratory diseases such as asthma (Carr, Lehrer, Rausch, & Hochron, 1994) and chronic obstructive pulmonary disease (Karajgi, Rifkin, Doddi, & Kolli, 1990) show a high rate of incidence, although these diseases usually precede the onset of panic episodes. Panic disorder is only diagnosed when there is clear evidence that the patient holds exaggerated negative beliefs about the dangerousness of unpleasant but harmless sensations like breathlessness (Carr et al., 1994; Taylor, 2000).

There are a number of medical conditions that can produce physical symptoms similar to panic disorder. These include certain endocrine disorders (e.g., hypoglycemia, hyperthyroidism, hyperparathyroidism), cardiovascular disorders (e.g., mitral valve prolapse, cardiac arrhythmias, congestive heart failure, hypertension, myocardial infarction), respiratory disease, neurological disorders (e.g., epilepsy, vestibular disorders), and substance use (e.g., drug/alcohol intoxication, or withdrawal) (see Barlow, 2002; Taylor, 2000, for further discussion). Again, presence of these disorders does not automatically exclude the possibility of diagnosing panic disorder. If panic attacks precede the disorder, occur outside the context of substance use, or the physical symptoms are misinterpreted in a catastrophic fashion, than a diagnosis of comorbid panic disorder should be considered in those with a medical condition (DSM-IV-TR; APA, 2000; Taylor, 2000). Other characteristics such as onset of panic attacks after age 45, presence of unusual symptoms such as loss of bladder or bowel control, vertigo, loss of consciousness, slurred speech, and the like, and brief attacks that stop abruptly suggest a general medical condition or substance use may be causing the panic (DSM-IV-TR; APA, 2000; see Taylor, 2000). It is possible that physiological irregularities and ill health experiences could contribute to a heightened sensitivity to body sensations in panic disorder (e.g., Hochn-Saric et al., 2004). For example, Craske, Poulton, Tsao, and Plotkin (2001) found that experience with respiratory ill health or disturbance during childhood and adolescence predicted the subsequent development of panic disorder with agoraphobia at 18 or 21 years. Thus medical conditions can play either a contributing cause and/or effect role in many cases of panic disorder.

Clinician Guideline 8.6

Most individuals with panic disorder have sought medical consultation prior to referral to mental health services. However, a thorough medical examination should be obtained in cases where a self-referral was made in order to rule out a co-occurring medical condition that might mimic or exacerbate panic symptoms.

Descriptive Characteristics

Epidemiological studies indicate that panic disorder with or without agoraphobia have 1-year prevalence rates ranging from 1.1 to 2.7% and lifetime prevalence rates of 2.0–4.7% (Eaton et al., 1991; Kessler et al., 1994; Kessler, Berglund, et al., 2005; Kessler, Chiu, et al., 2005; Offord et al., 1996). This makes panic disorder second only to OCD as the least common of the anxiety disorders discussed in this volume. As expected, prevalence of panic disorder is much higher in primary care settings than in the general population (Katon et al., 1986; Olfson et al., 2000). Moreover, there do not appear to be significant ethnic differences in the prevalence of panic disorder (e.g., Horwath, Johnson, & Hornig, 1993; Kessler et al., 1994), although cultural factors do influence which panic symptoms are more commonly reported and how they are labeled (see discussion by Barlow, 2002; Taylor, 2000).

Panic attacks as well as panic disorder with or without agoraphobia are approximately twice as common in women as in men (Eaton et al., 1994; Gater et al., 1998; Kessler et al., 1994). Moreover, agoraphobia may be particularly gendered, with women representing approximately 75% of the agoraphobic population (Bourdon et al., 1988; Yonkers et al., 1998). Panic disorder appears to take a more severe course in women as indicated by more severe agoraphobic avoidance, more catastrophic thoughts, more threatening interpretations of bodily sensations, and higher recurrence of panic symptoms (Turgeon, Marchand, & Dupuis, 1998; Yonkers et al., 1998). Women in general may show a heightened tendency to report more physical symptoms, fear, and panic in response to acute distress (Kelly, Forsyth, & Karekla, 2006). Furthermore, it is possible that increased panic disorder and agoraphobic avoidance in women is linked to a higher rate of childhood physical and sexual abuse which could lead to increased hypervigilance and overpredictions of threat (Stein, Walker, et al., 1996). Craske (2003), however, notes that the main difference between men and women is in their reliance on avoidance rather than in the number of reported panic attacks, which could be due to socialization into the traditional feminine gender role.

Panic disorder usually begins in young adulthood with the ECA reporting a mean onset age of 24 years (Burke, Burke, Regier, & Rae, 1990) and 75% of panic disorder cases having first onset by age 40 in the NCS-R survey (Kessler, Berglund, et al., 2005). Despite a relatively early onset, there is usually considerable delay between onset and first treatment contact. In the NCS-R a median duration of 10 years occurred between onset of panic disorder and first treatment contact (Wang, Berglund, et al., 2005). Despite lengthy delays in seeking treatment, the vast majority of individuals with panic disorder eventually do make treatment contact (Wang, Berglund, et al., 2005).

Like other anxiety disorders, onset of panic is often associated with stressful life events such as separation, loss or illness of significant other, being a victim of an assault, financial problems, work difficulties, personal health problems, unemployment, and the like (e.g., Faravelli & Pallanti, 1989; Franklin & Andrews, 1989; Pollard, Pollard, & Corn, 1989). In other studies a high incidence of past childhood sexual and physical abuse has been found in panic disorder and agoraphobia, especially among women (Pribor & Dinwiddie, 1992; Saunders, Villeponteaux, Lipovsky, Kilpatrick, & Veronen, 1992; Stein et al., 1996), although it is still uncertain whether rates of adverse early childhood events are any higher in panic disorder compared to major depression or even schizophrenia (Friedman et al., 2002). In an analysis of the NCS data set women with panic disorder without comorbid PTSD were six times more at risk of having childhood physical or sexual abuse, and individuals with comorbid panic and PTSD were significantly more likely to have survived rape (43%) than those with panic alone (7.5%) (Leskin & Sheikh, 2002). These findings indicate that lifetime trauma may act as a risk factor for panic disorder, especially in women. Moreover, social environmental factors may also affect clinical course, with factors such as childhood separation, lower socioeconomic status, and marital breakup significant predictors of poor outcome 7 years after initial treatment (Noyes et al., 1993).

Relationship problems may be more common in panic disorder than in other conditions, both as a contributing cause and a consequence of the disorder (Marcaurelle, Bélanger, & Marchand, 2003). However, the empirical evidence is inconsistent in whether panic disorder with agoraphobia is associated with more marital problems and quality of marital relationship at pretreatment is not a significant predictor of treatment prognosis (Marcaurelle et al. 2003).

If left untreated, panic disorder typically takes a chronic course with only 12% of patients achieving complete remission after 5 years (Faravelli, Paterniti, & Scarpato, 1995). In a 1-year prospective study Ehlers (1995) found that 92% of panic patients continued to experience panic attacks and 41% of the initially remitted patients relapsed. However, in an 11-year follow-up of 24 patients with panic disorder treated in an 8-week clinical trial of imipramine, alprazolam, or placebo, 68% had no panic attacks over the follow-up period and 90% showed no or only mild disabilities (Swoboda et al., 2003). This suggests that with treatment, the long-term prognosis for panic disorder may be more optimistic.

Panic disorder is also associated with significant functional impairment and decrements in quality of life, especially when comorbid with depression (Massion, Warshaw, & Keller, 1993; Roy-Byrne et al., 2000; Sherbourne et al., 1996). Furthermore, greater functional impairment can significantly increase the likelihood of panic recurrence in previously recovered individuals (Rodriguez, Bruce, Pagano, & Keller, 2005). In a meta-analytic review of 23 quality of life studies, panic disorder was similar to the other anxiety disorders in showing significant decrements in physical health, mental health, work, social functioning, and family functioning (Olatunji et al., 2007), although poor subjective quality of life is worse in major depression than in panic disorder (Hansson, 2002).

Panic disorder with agoraphobia can be a costly disorder both in terms of human suffering and increased burden on health care services (e.g., Eaton et al., 1991). In the NCS-R panic disorder and PTSD had the highest annual rates of mental health utilization compared to the other anxiety disorders, and panic disorder had a much higher rate of accessing general medical care (Wang, Lane, et al., 2005; see also Deacon, Lickel, & Abramowitz, 2008). The health care costs associated with panic disorder, then, are substantial. The number of annual medical visits by individuals with panic disorder is seven times that of the general population, resulting in an annual medical cost that is twice the American population average (Siegel, Jones, & Wilson, 1990).

Clinician Guideline 8.7

Negative life events, past and current stressors, negative coping style, and psychosocial impairment will have a significant impact on the course of panic disorder. The clinician must take these factors into consideration during assessment and treatment of panic.

COGNITIVE THEORY OF PANIC DISORDER

Description of the Model

Panic attacks are an immediate fear response and so the psychogenic processes primarily responsible for the onset and persistence of panic occur within Phase I of the cognitive model depicted in Chapter 2 (see Figure 2.1). The key cognitive processes of panic, then, occur at an automatic level of activation. The Phase II processes, representing deliberate, elaborative efforts to cope with heightened anxiety and the anticipation of panic, are secondary contributors to the persistence of the disorder. In this way the cognitive basis of panic is entirely different from that of GAD where Phase II processes play a more critical role in the disorder. The cognitive model of panic was first articulated in the mid- to late 1980s by Beck and colleagues (Beck, 1988; Beck et al., 1985; Beck & Greenberg, 1988; D. M. Clark & Beck, 1988) and further elaborated by D. M. Clark (1986a, 1988, 1996; D. M. Clark et al., 1988). Derived from these earlier accounts, Figure 8.1 illustrates the current cognitive explanation for panic based on the generic cognitive model (i.e., Figure 2.1). It should be noted that the cognitive model was formulated to explain the pathogenesis of recurrent panic attacks or panic disorder. It has less relevance for understanding the occasional panic attacks found in the general population or the occurrence of nonfearful panic-like somatic symptoms prominent in medical settings (D. M. Clark, 1997; see also Eifert, Zvolensky, & Lejuez, 2000).

Activation and Attention

Changes in internal states such as the occurrence or intensification of certain physical sensations (e.g., chest tightness, breathlessness, increased heart rate, nauseous feelings) or mental processes (e.g., mind goes blank, sense of derealization) are the primary triggers for panic attacks. In most cases of recurrent panic external stimuli or situations will become triggers, but only because they have the capacity to elicit bodily sensations that are perceived as threatening (D. M. Clark, 1986a). In our case example Helen's primary trigger for panic was a sense of breathlessness. However, she perceived changes in her breathing whenever she was in novel situations and so unfamiliar settings such as travel outside her community, visiting new people, and so on began to trigger heightened anxiety and anticipated panic. Naturally she started avoiding these situations because they elicited the threatening somatic sensation, breathlessness. In severe agoraphobia a wide variety of external situations can trigger panic but only because they elicit some feared internal state. The physical and mental processes that are misperceived as an imminent threat are most often due to anxiety, and less often due to other emotional states, stress, physical exertion, ingestion of substances with caffeine or other chemicals, or even the natural ebb and flow of physiological function (D. M. Clark, 1986a, 1988, 1996).

As noted in Figure 8.1, individuals prone to panic are oriented toward selectively attending to internal somatic or mental processes. They are hypervigilant for the experience of these sensations and focus their attention on any change in functioning that might seem abnormal (Beck, 1988). The orienting mode in panic disorder is primed toward rapid detection of interoceptive cues that could represent an immediate and imminent danger to survival. This early detection process is automatic and nonconscious, resulting in a hypersensitivity to bodily sensations.

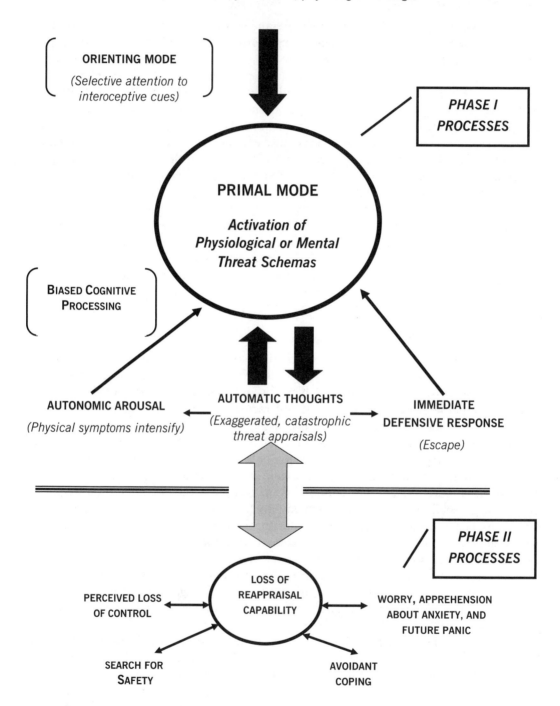

FIGURE 8.1. Cognitive model of panic disorder.

Schematic Activation

In the cognitive model recurrent panic attacks occur because of the activation of enduring schemas (beliefs) about the dangerousness of particular physiological changes. These physiological and mental threat schemas are consistent with the primal threat mode that dominates in anxiety. Some examples of panicogenic schemas are "My heart palpitations and chest pain might be signs that I am having a potentially fatal heart attack," "My episodes of breathlessness could lead to suffocation and death," "Dizzy spells might be caused by a brain tumor," "This feeling of nausea could cause me to be violently sick and vomit controllably," "Feeling tense and a little nervous could lead to loss of control and overwhelming panic," or "I could lose control of my emotions and go crazy." The physiological and mental threat schemas predispose certain individuals to experience recurrent panic attacks and involve themes of personal vulnerability, helplessness, the dangerousness of particular internal states, and the rapid escalation of anxiety (Beck & Greenberg, 1988).

There is a close association between specific bodily or mental sensations and the panicogenic beliefs that underlie the catastrophic misinterpretation of interoceptive cues. Table 8.4 presents connections between some common internal sensations and the corresponding physiological or mental threat schemas often seen in panic disorder.

Panic-relevant schemas are quite idiosyncratic and can be highly variable so that some individuals will hold exaggerated threat beliefs for only certain internal sensations, others will misinterpret a wide range of somatic and mental phenomena as threatening,

TABLE 8.4. Links between Panic-Relevant Internal Sensations and Their Corresponding Physiological or Mental Threat Schema

Internal sensation	Physiological/mental threat schema
Chest tightness, pain, heart palpitations	Belief of vulnerability to heart attacks.
Breathlessness, smothering sensation, irregular breathing	Belief of possible suffocation and death.
Dizziness, lightheadedness, faintness	Belief of losing control and doing something embarrassing or of going crazy, or presence of a brain tumor.
Nausea, abdominal cramps	Belief of vomiting uncontrollably.
Numbness, tingling in extremities	Belief in the possibility of having a stroke or losing one's sanity.
Restless, tense, agitation	Belief that these symptoms are an indication of losing control which could lead to a severe panic attack and eventual loss of function.
Feel shaky, trembling	Belief these symptoms indicate a loss of control and are often a precursor to severe panic.
Forgetful, inattentive, loss of concentration	Belief of losing control over one's mental functioning and ending up losing cognitive function.
Feelings of unreality, depersonalization	Belief that these symptoms may indicate a seizure or of going crazy.

Note. Based on Taylor (2000).

and still others may show a shift in which only certain physiological threat schemas are dominant at any particular time (D. M. Clark, 1986a). Acquisition of particular physiological threat schemas (e.g., "Heart palpitations are dangerous") will depend on prior learning history and the circumstances associated with the first panic attack (D. M. Clark, 1997). For example, it is common for individuals who experience chest pain to first go to emergency departments where they receive a full cardiac assessment. Such experiences can reinforce beliefs that "chest pain represents a highly imminent danger of heart attack and possible death." It is obvious how such experiences can lead to hypervalent schemas about the dangerousness of chest pain and the pathogenesis of panic disorder.

In order to activate physiological and mental threat schemas, the corresponding internal sensations must reach a certain threshold of intensity (Beck, 1988). For example, Helen did not experience heightened anxiety until her sense of breathlessness was sufficiently intense that she began to wonder if she was getting enough air. Furthermore, once schematic activation occurs, the main consequence is the catastrophic misinterpretation of the internal sensation. Once Helen's beliefs about the danger of breathlessness, suffocation, and lack of oxygen were activated by attention to her respiratory sensations, she made a rapid, automatic catastrophic misinterpretation. "There is something wrong with my breathing and I am not getting enough oxygen; I could suffocate to death." Thus the cognitive basis of the catastrophic misinterpretation of bodily sensations is the activation of prepotent and enduring threat-oriented schemas about the imminent danger associated with certain somatic or mental sensations.

Catastrophic Misinterpretation of Internal Sensations

The central cognitive process in the persistence of panic is the catastrophic misinterpretation of somatic or mental sensations (see Beck, 1988; Beck et al., 1985; D. M. Clark, 1986a). Often the catastrophic outcome associated with physical sensations is death caused by heart attack, suffocation, seizure, or the like. However, the imagined catastrophe can also involve a loss of control that leads to insanity (i.e., "I'll go crazy"), or acting in an embarrassing or humiliating manner in front of others. In addition, fear of panic attacks can be so intense that the catastrophe might be the possibility of experiencing another severe full-blown panic episode. Whatever the actual nature of the dreaded catastrophe, the sensations are misinterpreted as representing an imminent physical or mental disaster (D. M. Clark, 1988). In order to precipitate panic, the catastrophic threat must be perceived as imminent; if the misinterpretation is merely exaggerated threat, then anxiety rather than panic will be roused (Rachman, 2004). The occurrence of the catastrophic misinterpretation is the cognitive basis for the remaining processes that contribute to panic disorder (see Figure 8.1). In cued or situational panic attacks sensations associated with heightened anxiety are misinterpreted, whereas in spontaneous (uncued) panic attacks the sensations arise from a variety of nonanxious sources (e.g., exercise, stress, emotional reactions). D. M. Clark (1988) argued that the catastrophic misinterpretation of bodily sensations is necessary for the production of a panic attack and represents an enduring cognitive trait (vulnerability) that is evident even when individuals with panic disorder are not anxious.

As a Phase I process that is elicited by activation of panicogenic schemas, the catastrophic misinterpretation is an involuntary, automatic, and rapid response to the detection of certain internal sensations. D. M. Clark (1988) argued that catastrophic misinterpretations can be rapid and outside conscious awareness so the panic attack appears spontaneous. Once activated the panicogenic schemas and catastrophic misinterpretations tend to dominant the information-processing apparatus during panic. It is highly biased, giving processing priority to danger cues and minimizing or ignoring schema-incongruent safety information.

Symptom Intensification and Defense

The catastrophic misinterpretation of bodily sensations will cause an intensification of the feared internal sensations by heightening vigilance and an internal focus on interoceptive cues (Beck, 1988; D. M. Clark, 1997). A vicious cycle occurs in which the escalating intensity of the physiological or mental sensation further reinforces the misinterpretation that indeed a physical or mental disaster is imminent. Helen, for example, would notice that her breathing was a little irregular and felt like she was not getting enough air. Her initial appraisal "I am not breathing normally, I don't think I am getting enough air" (*exaggerated threat interpretation*) led to an increased focus on her breathing. She would breathe deeply and try to establish a more controlled breathing rate. But the heightened focus on her breathing intensified her sense of breathlessness (*symptom intensification*) that in turn deepened her conviction that her respiratory problem was getting worse and even more likely to lead to suffocation (*catastrophic misinterpretation*).

In addition to an automatic intensification of symptoms, the catastrophic misinterpretation will result in immediate attempts to escape. Again, efforts to escape are viewed as an automatic and involuntary response to panicogenic schema activation and the catastrophic misinterpretation of the bodily sensation. A person fearful of chest tightness may quickly cease a particular activity when the somatic sensation is detected. A patient who had a profound sense of derealization in his hotel room after driving in heavy traffic in New York City immediately laid down and then had several alcoholic drinks in order to relax. His responses were an attempt to escape from the sense of derealization which he interpreted as a symptom of going crazy. When in a state of heightened anxiety and panic, the escape response triggered by the catastrophic misinterpretation can occur quite automatically without deliberate, effortful planning. As noted in Figure 8.1, the intensification of physical sensations and escape responses will contribute to the continued activation of the panic-relevant schemas.

Loss of Reappraisal Capability

According to Beck (1988), the dissociation of the higher level reflective processes (Phase II) from the automatic cognitive processing (Phase I) is a necessary condition for a panic attack. Thus we consider the loss of reappraisal capability the central process at the secondary, elaborative phase that is responsible for the persistence of anxiety and panic. Activation of the physiological threat schemas and subsequent catastrophic misinterpretation of bodily sensations dominates information processing and inhibits the panic-stricken patient's ability to generate alternative, more realistic, and benign interpretations of the fearful sensations. If reappraisal of the perceived threat is possible, the catastrophic misinterpretation would be challenged and the escalation into panic would be thwarted.

This loss of reappraisal capability is clearly illustrated in a young man with panic disorder who was fearful of sudden increases in his heart rate. On some occasions, such as sitting at his computer, he would perceive an increase in heart rate that elicited the apprehensive thought "Why is my heart racing?" His underlying physiological threat schemas were "I am vulnerable to heart attacks," "If I let my heart rate get too high, I could have a heart attack," and "After all, I do have a cardiac condition" (he had a diagnosed congenital cardiac condition that was benign). Once activated, he generated a catastrophic misinterpretation ("My heart is racing, I might be having a heart attack"). At this point he was unable to generate an alternative explanation for this increased heart rate, and so he became panicky. On other occasions, such as when working out at the gym (as recommended by his physician), he would notice his heart rate increase, wonder if it could be a sign of a cardiac problem, but immediately reappraised the sensations as due to the demands of his physical activity. One of the main objectives of cognitive therapy for panic is to improve the patient's ability to reappraise fearful internal sensations with more realistic, plausible, and benign alternative interpretations.

Other Secondary Elaborative Processes

As illustrated in Figure 8.1 there are a number of other secondary cognitive and behavioral processes that occur as a result of the dissociation of elaborative reasoning from the automatic catastrophic threat appraisals. Beck et al. (1985) noted that a striking characteristic of panic attacks is the experience of anxiety as an overwhelming and uncontrollable state. The individual with recurrent panic attacks thinks of anxiety as a rapidly escalating and uncontrollable experience that she learns to dread.

A second cognitive process at the elaborative phase is apprehension and worry about mounting anxiety and the recurrence of panic attacks. The worry in panic disorder is focused almost exclusively on panic attacks and the intolerance of heightened states of anxiety. After a number of CT sessions, Helen's panic attacks remitted. However, her apprehension and worry over a possible relapse remained high. For example, she was considering a change of jobs and a move to a new city but was very reluctant to make any changes for fear it would heighten her anxiety and trigger a new round of panic attacks.

With elaborative information processing dominated by perceptions of uncontrollable and escalating anxiety, constant apprehension and worry about panic, and loss of higher order reflective reasoning to counter the domination of catastrophic thinking, it is little wonder that the person with panic disorder deliberately turns to avoidance and other safety-seeking strategies to exert better control over his negative emotional state. However, there is now considerable evidence that agoraphobic avoidance actually contributes to the persistence and increased severity of panic disorder (see previous discussion). Moreover, reliance on safety-seeking behaviors such as carrying anxiolytic medication in case of emergency, being accompanied by a family member or friend, or suppressing strong emotions and unwanted thoughts, can actually contribute to the persistence of panic by maintaining the person's belief that certain internal sensations are dangerous (D. M. Clark, 1997, 1999).

As can be seen from Figure 8.1, there is a strong reciprocal relationship between the panic-relevant cognitive processes that occur early at the automatic, catastrophic interpretation level and those that occur later at the secondary, elaborative phase. However, the inability of secondary elaborative thinking to correct the automatic catastrophic threat appraisals of bodily sensations accounts for the persistence of panic and the development of panic disorder. Cognitive therapy of panic, then, focuses on redressing the dissociation between the two levels of processing so that a more benign interpretation of previously feared interoceptive sensations is accepted.

EMPIRICAL STATUS OF THE COGNITIVE MODEL

The proposition that panic attacks are caused by the catastrophic misinterpretation of bodily sensations has generally received strong empirical support from a large number of correlational and experimental studies conducted over the past two decades, although inconsistencies and limitations have also been noted (for reviews, see Austin & Richards, 2001; Casey, Oei, & Newcombe, 2004; D. M. Clark, 1996; Khawaja & Oei, 1998; McNally, 1994). In this section we expand our review of the empirical status of the cognitive model to include additional cognitive processes that are important in the pathogenesis of panic. Table 8.5 presents six hypotheses that capture the main tenets of the cognitive model of panic (see Figure 8.1).

TABLE 8.5. Core Hypotheses of the Cognitive Model of Panic

Hypotheses	Statement
1. Interoceptive hypersensitivity	Individuals with panic disorder will exhibit selective attention to and greater vigilance for internal somatic and mental sensations than individuals without panic disorder.
2. Schematic vulnerability	Panic-prone individuals will endorse more beliefs about the dangerousness of specific physiological or mental sensations than nonpanic comparison groups.
3. Catastrophic misinterpretations	Panic attacks are characterized by a misinterpretation of bodily or mental sensations as signifying an imminent physical, mental, or social catastrophe. Production of the catastrophic misinterpretation will increase panic symptoms in panic disorder individuals, whereas correction of the misinterpretation will prevent panic attacks.
4. Interoceptive amplification	The production of a catastrophic misinterpretation of internal cues will heighten the intensity of the feared sensations in panic but not in nonpanic states.
5. Dissociation	Individuals with panic disorder will exhibit diminished ability to employ higher order reflective thinking to generate more realistic and benign interpretations of their fearful internal sensations compared to nonpanic individuals.
6. Safety seeking	Avoidance and maladaptive safety-seeking behavior will intensify anxiety and panic symptoms in those with panic disorder relative to nonpanic controls.

Hypothesis 1. Interoceptive Hypersensitity

Individuals with panic disorder will exhibit selective attention to and greater vigilance for internal somatic and mental sensations than individuals without panic disorder.

If panic disorder is characterized by heightened vigilance and response to bodily sensations, at the very least one would expect individuals with panic disorder to report greater response to physical sensations on questionnaire and interview measures. In several studies individuals with panic disorder and agoraphobia scored significantly higher on the Body Sensations Questionnaire (BSQ), which assesses fear of 17 physical and mental sensations common in anxiety and panic, compared to individuals with other anxiety disorders or nonclinical control groups (e.g., Chambless & Gracely, 1989; Kroeze & van den Hout, 2000a; Schmidt et al., 1997). Similarly McNally et al. (1995) found that individuals with panic reported more severe physical sensations than nonclinical controls, with fear of dying, fear of heart attack, fear of losing control, and tingling being the best discriminators. However, individuals with panic disorder may have heightened discomfort intolerance, as indicated by a reduced ability to withstand unpleasant physical sensations and pain more generally (Schmidt & Cook, 1999; Schmidt, Richey, & Fitzpatrick, 2006). Overall there is fairly consistent evidence that individuals who experience recurrent panic attacks report greater sensitivity to physical sensations and are more likely to interpret these symptoms negatively (see also Taylor, Koch, & McNally, 1992).

Stronger support for the interoceptive hypersensitivity hypothesis comes from experimental studies that induce physical sensations through various biological challenges such as hyperventilation, inhalation of CO_2-enriched or O_2-enriched air, lactate infusion, and the like. A consistent finding across these experimental studies is that panic disorder patients evidence a significantly greater subjective response to the sensations produced by the inductions as indicated by higher ratings on the intensity, severity, and anxiousness associated with the bodily sensations produced by the induction manipulations (e.g., Antony, Coons, McCabe, Ashbaugh, & Swinson, 2006; J. G. Beck, Ohtake, & Shipherd, 1999; Holt & Andrews, 1989; Rapee, 1986; Schmidt, Forsyth, Santiago, & Trakowski, 2002; Zvolensky et al., 2004).

If panic disorder is characterized by increased vigilance for physical sensations, we might expect panic disorder patients to demonstrate greater acuity or perception of their physiological responding. A number of studies have investigated heart rate perception in panic disorder. In an early study by Pauli et al. (1991) panic disorder individuals who wore an ECG recorder over 24 hours did not report significantly more cardiac perceptions than healthy controls but significantly more self-reported anxiety was associated with the perceptions. Moreover, heart rate acceleration occurred after cardiac perceptions that were associated with intense anxiety whereas cardiac perceptions associated with no anxiety led to heart rate deceleration.

Some studies have used a "mental tracking" procedure in which individuals silently count felt heartbeats without taking their pulse. Early findings suggested that individuals with panic disorder had better heartbeat perception than other patient groups or nonclinical controls (e.g., Ehlers & Breuer, 1992; Ehlers, Breuer, Dohn, & Fiegenbaum, 1995), but a later reanalysis of pooled data across different studies found that accurate heartbeat perception was more often evident in panic disorder compared to depressed and normal controls but not when compared to patients with other anxiety disorders (van der Does, Antony, Ehlers, & Barsky, 2000). Moreover, only a minority of the panic disorder patients was classified as accurate perceivers (17%). Thus accurate heartbeat perception appears to be a characteristic of having frequent episodes of clinical anxiety as opposed to panic attacks per se.

An automatic, preconscious attentional processing bias for physical cue words should be apparent if panic is characterized by hypervigilance for bodily sensations. Lundh and colleagues (1999) found that panic disorder patients had significantly higher Stroop interference effects to panic-related words than nonclinical controls at both a subliminal and a supraliminal level but this biasing effect was also evident for interpersonal threat words. In addition the panic disorder group identified more panic-related words presented at perceptual threshold (see also Pauli et al., 1997). Using a novel variant of the dot probe detection task in which response latency was assessed to a letter preceded by a snapshot sample of ECG heart rate data or a moving line, Kroeze and van den Hout (2000a) found evidence that the panic group was more fully attentive to the ECG trials than the control group (see Kroeze & van den Hout, 2000b, for contrary finding).

In a study involving 20 individuals with claustrophobia, those told to concentrate on their bodily sensations while in an enclosed chamber reported significantly higher fear and panic scores, and experienced a higher rate of panic attacks than individuals in the control (distraction) group (Rachman, Levitt, & Lopatke, 1988). Strenuous physical exercise is a naturalistic situation that normally increases attention to physical state. Furthermore, vigorous exercise increases blood lactate levels, which individuals with panic might find less tolerable given their heightened reactivity to sodium lactate infusion (Liebowitz et al., 1985). So, one might expect panic patients to be less tolerant of strenuous physical exercise. Interestingly, it appears that individuals with panic disorder are able to engage in vigorous physical exercise without experiencing thoughts or feelings indicative of panic even though the exercise produces blood lactate levels that are equal to or greater than those attained in lactate infusion studies (Martinsen, Raglin, Hoffart, & Friis, 1998).

Although individuals with panic disorder may have greater physiological reactivity such as a elevated respiratory rate, heart rate, and blood pressure, and lower skin temperature during biological provocations that induce bodily sensations (J. G. Beck et al., 1999; Craske, Lang, Tsao, Mystkowski, & Rowe, 2001; Holt & Andrews, 1989; Rapee, 1986; Schmidt et al., 2002), the physiological differences are relatively modest and inconsistent across studies, with some even reporting negative results (Zvolensky et al., 2004). On the other hand, differences in perceived intensity and distress of the physical sensations produced by these biological challenges have been robust and quite consistent across studies (e.g., J. G. Beck et al., 1999; Holt & Andrews, 1989; Rapee, 1986). In a recent study Story and Craske (2008) found that individuals at risk for panic (high anxiety sensitivity and a history of panic attacks) reported significantly more panic symptoms following false elevated heart-rate feedback than low-risk individuals, even though there were no group differences in actual heart rate. Together these findings provide strong evidence for the cognitive perspective on panic disorder, suggesting that the main difference is in the perception and interpretation of physical changes rather than in actual physiological responses.

In summary, there has been fairly consistent empirical support from self-report and biological challenge experiments that panic disorder is characterized by a heightened sensitivity or perceptual bias to physical sensations, even though they may not have enhanced physiological reactivity (Ehlers, 1995). The findings of greater perceptual acuity for interoceptive cues (e.g., enhanced cardiac awareness), however, remains uncertain. Moreover, it is clear that contextual factors affect response to physical sensations and their interpretation. When bodily sensations occur in unexpected or anxious situations, individuals with panic disorder are likely to be more vigilant and responsive to changes in their physical or mental state.

Hypothesis 2. Schematic Vulnerability

Panic-prone individuals will endorse more beliefs about the dangerousness of specific physiological or mental sensations than nonpanic comparison groups.

In their critical review of the cognitive perspective on panic disorder, Roth, Wilhelm, and Pettit (2005) noted that if individuals with panic disorder did not exhibit enduring "catastrophic beliefs" when panic attacks are absent, then this would be problematic for the theory. According to the schema vulnerability hypothesis, individuals with panic disorder are expected to exhibit stronger endorsement of thoughts, assumptions, and beliefs that reflect activation of physiological threat schemas than nonpanic disorder individuals even in the absence of a panic attack. Unfortunately, very little research has specifically focused on beliefs in panic disorder. Khawaja and Oei (1992) developed the 50-item Catastrophic Cognitions Questionnaire to assess misinterpretations of the dangerousness of specific physical, emotional, and mental states but the measure failed to differentiate panic from other anxiety disorders (Khawaja, Oei, & Baglioni, 1994). Greenberg (1989) constructed the 42-item Panic Belief Questionnaire (PBQ) to assess level of agreement to maladaptive panic-related beliefs. The PBQ had a moderate correlation with the ASI ($r = .55$) and panic disorder patients scored higher on the total score than a social phobia group, although the difference was not statistically significant (Ball, Otto, Pollack, Uccello, & Rosenbaum, 1995). More recently Wenzel et al. (2006) reported that the PBQ Physical Catastrophes subscale had strong correlations with other panic symptom questionnaires and that scores on the measure declined significantly with treatment. Inspection of the PBQ item content indicates that only seven items (17%) tap into beliefs about physical sensations. Thus at present we do not have a self-report measure that specifically assesses the enduring physiological and mental threat schemas proposed by the cognitive model.

Currently the strongest self-report evidence for the schema vulnerability hypothesis comes from research on anxiety sensitivity (see discussion in Chapter 4). Even though the ASI is not a belief measure per se, it does assess an enduring tendency to interpret physical sensations in a threatening manner, which is relevant to the nature of preexisting physiological threat schemas. Evidence that individuals with panic disorder score significantly higher than other anxiety groups, especially on the ASI Physical Concerns subscale, and that high ASI scores predict response to biological challenge experiments as well as development of panic attacks is entirely consistent with the schema vulnerability hypothesis for panic disorder. However, the same type of research that has been conducted on the ASI needs to be extended to a specific panic belief measure like the

PBQ in order to determine if physiological and mental threat schemas play a critical role in the development of panic disorder.

If beliefs about the threatening nature of internal states are preexisting cognitive structures, then individuals prone to panic disorder should evidence biased processing of panic-relevant information even during nonanxious or nonpanic states. In fact there is a large body of information-processing research that is consistent with activation of physiological or mental threat schemas in panic disorder. Experiments employing the emotional Stroop task have shown that compared to nonclinical control groups, individuals with panic disorder exhibit a specific color-naming interference for physical threat or catastrophe words (Hayward et al., 1994; McNally et al., 1994; Teachman, Smith-Janik, & Saporito, 2007) even at subliminal presentation rates (Lim & Kim, 2005; Lundh et al., 1999). However, some studies have found that the interference effect in panic is evident for all threat words in general (Ehlers, Margraf, Davies, & Roth, 1988; Lundh et al., 1999; McNally, Kaspi, Riemann, & Zeitlin, 1990) or even all emotionally valenced words (Lim & Kim, 2005; McNally et al., 1992). A few studies have reported no specific color-naming interference for physical threat words in panic disorder (Kampman, Keijsers, Verbraak, Näring, & Hoogduin, 2002; McNally et al., 1992). Nevertheless, the general findings from the emotional Stroop experiments are consistent with the presence of prepotent physiological and mental threat schemas in panic disorder.

Evidence has also been found for an interpretation bias for internal stimuli in panic disorder. Harvey et al. (1993) found that panic disorder patients chose threat explanations for ambiguous interoceptive scenarios more than social phobics, although there was no statistical significance between the groups in how often they made threat interpretations. In a covariation bias experiment Wiedemann, Pauli, and Dengler (2001) found that individuals with panic disorder but not healthy controls overestimated the association between emergency room pictures (i.e., panic-relevant stimuli) and a negative consequence (i.e., harmless shock to forearm). However, this finding was not replicated in a later study (Amrhein, Pauli, Dengler, & Wiedemann, 2005), although electrophysiological evidence for a covariation bias in panic disorder was found. Coles and Heimberg (2002) in their review concluded that panic disorder is characterized by an explicit but not an implicit memory bias for threatening information, especially when deep processing is encouraged at the encoding stage. Moreover, the explicit memory bias may be especially pronounced with physical threat information (Becker et al., 1994; Cloitre et al., 1994; Pauli, Dengler, & Wiedermann, 2005), although others have failed to find a specific memory bias (Baños et al., 2001; Lim & Kim, 2005). Finally, Teachman et al. (2007) found that individuals with panic disorder produced faster response times to self-evaluative panic-relevant associations on an Implicit Association Test, which reflects involuntary processing of stimuli congruent with underlying threat schemas.

Overall there is strong empirical support for the schema vulnerability hypothesis from the information-processing literature. Findings of an automatic threat-processing bias in nonpanic states are consistent with our contention of a prepotent, enduring schematic threat organization in panic disorder. However, it is still unclear whether the schematic content in panic disorder is highly specific to physiological and mental sensations or more reflective of general threat themes, and whether activation of these schemas is responsible for the catastrophic interpretation of bodily sensations. We also await the development of a more specific panic belief questionnaire that can test the predictive validity of the schema vulnerability hypothesis in prospective research designs.

Hypothesis 3. Catastrophic Misinterpretation

Panic attacks are characterized by a misinterpretation of bodily or mental sensations as signifying an imminent physical, mental, or social catastrophe. Production of the catastrophic misinterpretation will increase panic symptoms in individuals with panic disorder, whereas correction of the misinterpretation will prevent panic attacks (see D. M. Clark, 1996).

Over the years various reviews of the relevant literature have concluded that there is strong support that individuals with panic disorder are significantly more likely to misinterpret bodily sensations in terms of a serious impending threat or danger than nonpanic comparison groups (for reviews, see Austin & Richards, 2001; Casey et al., 2004; Khawaja & Oei, 1998). Moreover, there is considerable empirical evidence that panic disorder is characterized by elevated scores on the ASI Fear of Somatic Sensations subscale, a finding entirely predicted by the catastrophic misinterpretation hypothesis (e.g., Deacon & Abramowitz, 2006a; Rector et al., 2007; Taylor, Zvolensky, et al., 2007; see also discussion of anxiety sensitivity in Chapter 4). And yet, dissenting views have been expressed stating that a number of key aspects of the catastrophic misinterpretation hypothesis remain in doubt (McNally, 1994; Roth et al., 2005). Three types of research provide a critical test of the catastrophic misinterpretation hypothesis: self-report measures of catastrophic cognitions, clinical studies of the relation between misinterpretations of bodily sensations and subsequent panic symptomatology, and evidence of cognitive mediation in biological challenge experiments.

Various clinical studies indicate that most individuals with panic disorder report thoughts or images of physical or mental catastrophe in response to internal stimuli during panic episodes (e.g., Argyle, 1988; Beck et al., 1974; Ottaviani & Beck, 1987). The Agoraphobic Cognitions Questionnaire (ACQ) assesses the frequency of maladaptive thoughts about catastrophic consequences (e.g., fainting, choking, heart attack, loss of self-control) when feeling anxious (Chambless, Caputo, Bright, & Gallagher, 1984). Individuals with panic disorder score significantly higher than depressed and other anxiety disorder groups on the ACQ Physical Concerns but not the Social/Behavioral Consequences factor (Chambless & Gracely, 1989).

D. M. Clark et al. (1997) developed the Body Sensations Interpretation Questionnaire (BBSIQ) to assess endorsement rates and belief in threatening, positive, or neutral explanations for ambiguous panic body sensations and external events (control items). Analysis revealed that panic disorder patients ranked negative interpretations of panic body sensations as significantly more probable and believed the negative explanation more than GAD, social phobia, or nonclinical comparison groups. Furthermore, the BBSIQ correlated .49 with the ACQ Physical Concerns subscale (for similar findings, see Austin, Richards, & Klein, 2006; Teachman et al., 2007). However, Austin et al. (2006) found that panic patients rarely made a subsequent harm-related interpretation (e.g., "I'm having a heart attack") to their initial anxiety-related interpretation (e.g., "I'm having a panic attack"). Studies that examined interpretations to ambiguous scenarios also found evidence of a threat interpretation bias for physical sensations in panic disorder compared to nonclinical controls (Kamieniecki et al., 1997; McNally & Foa, 1987; see also Uren et al., 2004), although it appears the panic disorder individuals generated more anxiety interpretations for both internal and external threats. Generally the self-report studies have supported the catastrophic misinterpretation hypothesis of bodily sensations, although most found that the interpretation bias is not specific to internal sensations alone and that anxiety interpretations (i.e., an expectation of becoming more anxious) are much more common than truly harm-related catastrophes (i.e., appraisals of dying from suffocation or a heart attack).

A few studies have investigated the presence of catastrophic misinterpretations in panic disorder samples that have been exposed to fear situations. Occurrence of a panic attack leads to greater expectation of subsequent fear or a heightening of anticipatory anxiety, which increases the likelihood that individuals will consider their anxious symptoms highly threatening (i.e., Rachman & Levitt, 1985). Moreover, when panic occurs during exposure to a fear situation, panic disorder individuals experience more bodily sensations and catastrophic cognitions than during the nonpanic exposure trials, although 27% (n = 8/30) of the panic episodes were not associated with any fearful cognitions (Rachman, Lopatka, & Levitt, 1988). In a further analysis of these data, Rachman, Levitt, and Lopatka (1987) found that individuals with panic disorder were four times more likely to have a panic attack when the bodily sensation was accompanied by catastrophic cognitions. Street et al. (1989) also found a high rate of catastrophic thinking when individuals recorded their next three panic attacks, especially when the attacks were expected. In addition there were many moderate correlations between the expected disturbing cognitions and their corresponding physical sensations (see Rachman et al., 1987, for similar finding).

Kenardy and Taylor (1999) had 10 women with panic disorder use a computer diary to self-monitor onset of panic attacks over a 7-day period. Analysis revealed that individuals overpredicted panic attacks; in 70% of cases the expectation of an attack never materialized. Moreover, catastrophic cognitions and somatic symptoms were common before expected but not unexpected panic attacks, indicating that catastrophic thoughts were associated with prediction or expectation of a panic attack rather than its actual occurrence. Finally, a small pilot study of panic disorder found that 3.25 hours of belief disconfirmation exposure resulted in significantly greater improvement in frequency and belief of agoraphobic cognitions as well as symptom measures than the group who received habituation exposure training only (Salkovskis, Hackmann, Wells, Gelder, & Clark, 2006). This suggests that reductions in catastrophic interpretations lead to an improvement in anxious and panic symptoms. Overall, these studies support the catastrophic misinterpretation hypothesis with two caveats. First, Rachman et al. (1987) did find a small number of "noncognitive panic attacks" that are difficult to explain from the catastrophic misinterpretation perspective. And second, some of the expected combinations of bodily sensations and catastrophic cognitions were not found such as heart palpitations, fear of heart attack, and various combinations of symptoms could lead to the same catastrophic cognition.

The strongest evidence for the catastrophic misinterpretation hypothesis comes from experiments involving panic induction via biological challenge (e.g., lactate fusion, CO_2 enriched air, hyperventilation, or exercise). There is considerable evidence that some form of cognitive mediation is a critical factor that influences the frequency of panic induction and heightened anxiety produced by these biological challenge experiments (D. M. Clark, 1993). In order to separate the effects of the induction and individuals' cognitions, participants typically are randomly assigned to receive instructions to expect that the induction would lead to unpleasant reactions or that the induction would be a pleasant or benign experience. Findings from these studies indicate that type of information provided, expectations, perceived control, and presence of safety cues influence individuals' anxiety and arousal to the induction (Khawaja & Oei, 1998). For example, in a study of healthy individuals who received sodium lactate and a placebo on two different days, only those who received the lactate infusion and anxious instructions experienced a significant increase in anxiety (van der Molen, van den Hout, Vroemen, Lousberg, & Griez, 1986).

Over the years numerous studies have demonstrated that individuals with panic disorder show greater reactivity to inhaled carbon dioxide (CO_2) than other anxiety disorder groups and healthy controls by experiencing more intense bodily sensations, and greater likelihood of panic symptoms and elevated anxiety as indicated by subjective measures, even though there are few differences in physiological functioning (e.g., Perna, Barbini, Cocchi, Bertani, & Gasperini, 1995; Perna et al., 2004; Rapee et al., 1992; Verburg, Griez, Meijer, & Pols, 1995). Furthermore, individuals with panic disorder report that the symptoms produced by CO_2 inhalation are similar to real-life panic attacks (Fyer et al., 1987; van den Hout & Griez, 1984; see review by Rapee, 1995a). It appears that affective response to CO_2 inhalation may even have etiological significance. In a 2-year follow-up study, Schmidt, Maner, and Zvolensky (2007) found that CO_2 reactivity predicted the later development of panic attacks. However, there are individual differences even among panic disorder individuals in their response to CO_2 inhalation, with 55–80% reporting a panic attack (Perna et al., 1995, 2004; Rapee et al., 1992). Rapee (1995a) noted that individuals who respond to a biological challenge are more likely to experience symptoms that are similar to their real-life panic symptoms and to report thoughts of impending catastrophe. He concluded that individuals will exhibit a greater affective response to biological challenges if they associate an immediate impending physical or mental catastrophe (threat) with the induced sensations and perceive diminished control over the aversive experience (e.g., Rapee et al., 1992; Sanderson, Rapee, & Barlow, 1989). Consistent with this conclusion Rapee et al. (1992) found that the only significant predictor of fear associated with hyperventilation and CO_2 inhalation was ASI Total Score (see also Rassovsky et al., 2000). Overall these findings are entirely consistent with the catastrophic misinterpretation hypothesis.

Additional support for the hypothesis is evident in recent studies that investigated information processing of physical stimuli and induction of physical symptoms. Using a modified semantic priming experiment, Schneider and Schulte (2007) found that individuals with panic disorder exhibited a significantly higher automatic (but not strategic) priming effect for idiographically selected anxiety symptom primes followed by catastrophic interpretations than nonclinical controls. The authors interpret this automatic priming effect as a consequence of strong idiographic associations produced by the relation of catastrophic thoughts to bodily symptoms during panic attacks. More specifically, there is evidence that imposing a respiratory load influences processing bias for negative physical words in those with fear of suffocation (Kroeze et al., 2005; see also Nay, Thorpe, Robertson-Nay, Hecker, & Sigmon, 2004).

In summary there is strong empirical support for the catastrophic misinterpretation hypothesis (see Austin & Richards, 2001; Khawaja & Oei, 1998; Casey et al., 2004; Rapee, 1995a). Misinterpreting physical or mental sensations as signifying an imminent threat has been consistently found in self-report, clinical, and experimental studies and its presence influences the intensity of panic symptoms. However, there are a number of issues that remain unresolved. First, there is evidence that catastrophic misinterpretations of bodily sensations may not be necessary to experience a panic attack, a finding that directly challenges a major tenet of the catastrophic cognition model of D. M. Clark (1988). (For further discussion of this criticism, see Hofmann, 2004a; McNally, 1994; Rachman, 2004; Roth et al., 2005.) Second, there is considerable evidence that catastrophic misinterpretations are not sufficient in themselves to produce panic. Rapee (1995a) has argued that perceived uncontrollability is an important cognitive variable in panic symptoms and Casey et al. (2004) have proposed an integrated model in which the ongoing occurrence of panic is influenced by catastrophic misinterpretations of bodily sensations and panic self-efficacy (i.e., positive cognitions that emphasize control or coping). We would argue that a more comprehensive cognitive model of panic is needed (see Figure 8.1) in which the extent of dissociation between an automatic catastrophic misinterpretation and a more realistic, benign interpretation of bodily sensations will determine the occurrence of panic attacks (Beck, 1988). In other words, the persistence of panic symptoms may not only depend on the occurrence of catastrophic misinterpretations but also on the inability to self-correct with a more realistic explanation of the physical changes at the elaborative stage.

Two other criticisms of the catastrophic misinterpretation model must be mentioned. Defining what is meant by "catastrophe" has proven difficult. If a narrow definition is adopted in which catastrophe means an "imminent physical or psychological harm" (e.g., heart attack, fainting, suffocation), than these types of interpretations are relatively infrequent in panic disorder. Instead the most common threat interpretations associated with physical symptoms is "fear of losing control" or "fear of an impending panic attack," or even some social threat such as being embarrassed in front of others (Austin & Richards, 2001). Austin and Richards suggest that a much broader range of outcomes should be included as "catastrophes." Finally, more research is needed on the causal links between body sensations, catastrophic cognitions, and panic symptoms. Rachman (2004) has argued that it is difficult to determine if catastrophic cognitions are the cause, the consequence, or merely a correlate of panic, although the biological challenge experiments have been most informative in this regard.

Hypothesis 4. Interoceptive Amplification

The production of a catastrophic misinterpretation of internal cues will heighten the intensity of the feared sensations in panic but not in nonpanic states.

According to the cognitive model, a positive feedback loop occurs with the automatic catastrophic misinterpretation of bodily sensations directly contributing to a further intensification of the physical or mental changes that were the initial source of threat schema activation. An escalation in the feared sensations will fuel continued activation of the physiological threat schemas, ensuring that the individual with panic disorder becomes fixated on the catastrophic misinterpretation (Beck, 1988).

Few studies have directly investigated this hypothesis. Evidence of a moderate positive correlation between catastrophic cognitions and their corresponding bodily sensation (i.e., breathless–fear of suffocation) is consistent with the interoceptive amplification hypothesis (e.g., Rachman et al., 1987; Street et al., 1989). D. M. Clark et al. (1988) commented on a study conducted in their laboratory in which panic patients but not recovered patients or healthy controls experienced a panic attack after reading word pair associates consisting of bodily sensations and catastrophes (e.g., palpitations-dying; nausea-numbness). In their cardiac monitoring study of panic disorder, Pauli et al. (1991) found that anxiety elicited by cardiac perceptions led to an increase in patients' heart rate during the period immediately after the cardiac perception. In another study involving a panic disorder sample, scores on the ASI Physical subscales predicted subjective fear during a hyperventilation challenge (Brown et al., 2003). Although these studies provide only indirect support, there is sufficient evidence to encourage further research that bodily sensations are experienced more intensely after catastrophic misinterpretations.

Hypothesis 5. Dissociation

Individuals with panic disorder will exhibit diminished ability to employ higher order reflective thinking to generate more realistic and benign interpretations of their fearful internal sensations compared with individuals without panic disorder.

A critical difference between a catastrophic misinterpretation model of panic and the cognitive model of panic proposed by Beck (1988) is the central role that dissociation of higher order reflective thinking plays in the pathogenesis of the anxiety attack. Beck stated: "The next state which is crucial to the experience of panic, as contrasted to simple severe anxiety, is the loss of the capacity to appraise the symptoms realistically, which is associated with the fixation on the symptoms" (1988, p. 94). Thus panic attacks occur because the individual with panic disorder is unable to retrieve a more realistic explanation for the sensations that counters the catastrophic misinterpretation. Unfortunately this aspect of the cognitive model has generated little research attention as most of the focus has been on the role of catastrophic misinterpretations of bodily sensations.

In a questionnaire study comparing individuals with panic disorder and nonclinical groups, Kamieniecki et al. (1997) found that individuals with panic disorder provided significantly more anxious interpretations of ambiguous internal scenarios which were not followed by benign alternative explanations for the elevated physical sensations described in the scenario. The authors conclude that the panic disorder patients were unable to reinterpret their physical state in an innocuous manner. Wenzel et al. (2005) reported that individuals successfully treated for panic disorder scored higher on items that reflected an ability to reason about and evaluate their anxious thoughts and symptoms more realistically than individuals who still experienced difficulties with panic. There is also evidence that providing a more benign explanation for experimentally induced physical sensations or safety information can reduce anxiety and increase a feeling of safety (Rachman & Levitt, 1985; Rachman, Levitt, & Lopatka, 1988; Schmidt, Richey, Wollaway-Bickel, & Maner, 2006). If a feeling of safety is a critical factor in the offset or termination of a panic episode (Lohr, Olatunji, & Sawchuk, 2007; Rapee, 1995a), then generating a corrective interpretation of physical arousal might be an important factor in engendering safe feelings. The inability to self-correct catastrophic misinterpretations would be a major obstacle to acquiring safe feelings. At the very least these preliminary findings suggest that further investigation of the dissociation of automatic physical threat appraisals and more realistic reinterpretations would be a fruitful area of research.

Hypothesis 6. Safety Seeking

Avoidance and maladaptive safety-seeking behavior will intensify anxiety and panic symptoms in those with panic disorder relative to nonpanic controls.

Since *safety seeking* is any cognitive or behavioral strategy that is intended to prevent or minimize a feared outcome, it includes escape as well as all forms of avoidance (Salkovskis, 1988, 1996b). Any cognitive or behavioral strategy (e.g., controlled breathing, relaxation, sitting, being accompanied by a friend, distraction) that subverts access to information that would disconfirm the catastrophic belief is considered maladaptive and will contribute to the persistence of panic symptoms (D. M. Clark, 1999; Salkovskis, 1988). Lohr et al. (2007) argue that safety signals may reduce the immediate experience of fear but ultimately contribute to the maintenance of pathological fear.

As noted previously, there is an extensive research literature showing that safety-seeking behavior and avoidance contribute to the persistence of anxiety (see Chapter 3, Hypotheses 2 and 10). Schmidt et al. (2006), for example, found that the provision of safety cues undermined the effectiveness of safety information in reducing anxiety to a CO_2 inhalation challenge, whereas other studies found a strong link between safety behaviors and catastrophic misinterpretations (e.g., Salkovskis et al., 1996). Lundh et al. (1998) found that a recognition bias for safe faces correlated with avoidance of fear situations, which suggests a strong link between pursuit of safety and avoidance. In a naturalistic self-monitoring study, Radomsky, Rachman, and Hammond (2002) found that individuals with panic disorder used a variety of safety-seeking strategies to hasten the end of a panic attack, the most common being an effort to calm down. Individuals believed that these strategies helped terminate panic as indicated by a reduction in bodily sensations and fearful cognitions. Even though individuals believed that the safety-seeking behaviors made them feel somewhat safe and reduced the likelihood of another immediate panic attack, Radomsky and colleagues employed a repeated hyperventilation challenge test to show there was, in fact, no panic-safe refractory period. Thus individuals may believe that safety seeking helps terminate a panic attack and reduce the likelihood of an immediate recurrence even though the prophylactic effect of safety seeking is highly unlikely.

Furthermore, there is evidence that a reduction in safety seeking can have positive therapeutic effects on anxiety and panic symptoms (see Salkovskis et al., 1999; Salkovskis et al., 2006). And yet Rachman found that the provision of safety-signal training increased predictions of safety, reduced expectations of fear, and inhibited panic when individuals were exposed to their fear situations (Rachman & Levitt, 1985; Rachman, Levitt, & Lopatka, 1988b). Similarly Milosevic and Radomsky (2008) found that snake-fearful individuals had significant reductions in subjective anxiety and fearful cognitions as well as increased approach behavior with a single 45-minute exposure session whether or not they were allowed to rely on safety behavior during the exposure session.

In summary, research on safety seeking indicates that a distinction must be made between safety-seeking behavior and feelings of safety. Producing a sense of safety appears to be important in terminating, and possibly inhibiting, panic (Lohr et al., 2007; Rapee, 1995a). However, there are clearly healthy and unhealthy ways to achieve this state of safety (Schmidt et al., 2006). Helping individuals with panic disorder adopt stronger beliefs in safety explanations for bodily sensations may be the most effective approach in panic disorder, whereas reliance on actual safety-seeking behavior (e.g., distraction, avoidance) may block access to disconfirming evidence and contribute to the persistence of panic symptoms, though this latter conclusion still requires considerable investigation in light of more recent findings that safety behavior may not be as deleterious as once thought.

COGNITIVE ASSESSMENT AND CASE FORMULATION

Diagnosis and Symptom Measures

Assessment for panic disorder should begin with a structured diagnostic interview like the SCID-IV (First et al., 1997) or ADIS-IV (Brown et al., 1994) given that panic attacks per se are highly prevalent in all the anxiety disorders. The ADIS-IV is recommended for the diagnosis of panic disorder because it has high interrater reliability for the disorder ($\kappa = .79$; Brown, Di Nardo, & Barlow, 2001) and provides a wealth of information on panic symptoms. It distinguishes between situationally cued and unexpected panic attacks and severity ratings are obtained on all the DSM-IV symptoms for both full-blown unexpected panic attacks and limited symptom attacks. In addition information is collected on extent of worry over future panic attacks, situational triggers, avoidance, interoceptive sensitivities, safety signals, and negative impact associated with recurrent panic attacks. The module on agoraphobia provides ratings on the degree of apprehension and avoidance associated with 20 situations commonly avoided in agoraphobia.

Various self-report panic symptom measures should also be administered as part of the cognitive assessment. In Chapter 5 we reviewed evidence that the BAI (Beck & Steer, 1990) assesses the physiological symptoms of anxiety (e.g., Beck, Epstein, et al., 1988; Hewitt & Norton, 1993), thus making it a particularly sensitive measure for panic disorder. Leyfer, Ruberg, and Woodruff-Borden (2006) calculated that a BAI Total Score cutoff of 8 would identify 89% of individuals with panic disorder and exclude 97% without panic disorder. The ASI is another measure that is highly relevant for panic (see Chapter 4) given that individuals with panic disorder score significantly higher than individuals with all other anxiety disorders. Below we briefly discuss four panic symptom measures that are especially useful when assessing panic disorder.

Agoraphobic Cognitions Questionnaire

The Agoraphobic Cognitions Questionnaire (ACQ) is a 15-item self-report questionnaire that assesses thoughts of perceived negative or threatening consequences (i.e., fear of fear) associated with the physical symptoms of anxiety (Chambless et al., 1984). Individuals with agoraphobia score significantly higher than those with other anxiety disorders, especially on the ACQ—Physical Concerns subscale (Chambless & Gracely, 1889), and the instrument is sensitive to treatment effects (Chambless et al., 1984). Individuals with panic attacks report higher ACQ scores than those without panic attacks (Craske, Rachman, & Tallman, 1986). The mean ACQ Total score for panic disorder is approximately 28, with posttreatment scores dropping to 19 (e.g., D. M. Clark et al., 1994).

Body Sensations Questionnaire

The Body Sensations Questionnaire (BSQ) is a 17-item questionnaire also developed by Chambless et al. (1984) to assess intensity of fear associated with physical symptoms of arousal (Antony, 2001a). The BSQ and ACQ are normally administered together and both have been used extensively in the research literature. Individuals with agoraphobia or panic disorder score significantly higher on the BSQ (Chambless & Gracely, 1989) with panic disorder samples (M = 46.3; SD = 8.7) scoring significantly higher than healthy (M = 28.4, SD = 6.5) controls (e.g., Kroeze & van den Hout, 2000b). The BSQ also is sensitive to treatment effects, with posttreatment scores dropping within the normal range (i.e., D. M. Clark et al., 1994). The clinician will find the ACQ useful for assessing exaggerated threat appraisals of physical symptoms and the BSQ useful for assessing fear of panic-relevant bodily sensations. A copy of both measures can be found in Antony (2001a, Appendix B).

Mobility Inventory for Agoraphobia

The Mobility Inventory for Agoraphobia (MI) is a self-report questionnaire that assesses the severity of agoraphobic avoidance, frequency of panic attacks, and size of safety zone (Chambless, Caputo, Jasin, Gracely, & Williams, 1985). The first section of the questionnaire lists 26 situations often avoided in agoraphobia and individuals rate the extent of avoidance of each situation on a 5-point scale (1 = "never avoid"; 5 = "always avoid") when accompanied and when alone. They then circle the five situations that cause the greatest amount of concern or impairment. The most recent version of the MI also instructs individuals to indicate the frequency of panic attacks in the past 7 days as well as in the past 3 weeks, and to rate the severity of their panic attacks on a 1 ("very mild") to 5 ("extremely severe") scale (see Antony, 2001b). The modified MI added a fourth section in which individuals report on the location and size of their safety zone. Most research on the MI has focused on the first section of the questionnaire in which two summed scores are calculated, an Avoidance Accompanied and an Avoidance Alone score.

Individuals with agoraphobia score significantly higher on the MI Avoidance Alone and Avoidance Accompanied subscales than do those with other anxiety disorders and nonclinical controls (Chambless et al., 1985; Craske et al., 1986) and the factorial structure of the MI showed high stability over a 5-year period (Rodriguez, Pagano, & Keller, 2007). For the clinician the MI yields valuable information on the nature and extent of agoraphobic avoidance often associated with panic disorder. The original MI was reproduced in an appendix of Chambless et al. (1985) and the modified MI can be found in Antony (2001b, Appendix B).

Albany Panic and Phobia Questionnaire

The Albany Panic and Phobia Questionnaire (APPQ) is a 27-item questionnaire that assesses level of fear (0–8 scale) associated with physical and social activities that produce somatic sensations (Rapee, Craske, & Barlow, 1994–1995). Three subscales are derived; Social Phobia (10 items), Agoraphobia (nine items), and Interoceptive (eight items). Although the factorial structure of the APPQ has been supported, contrary to expectation APPQ Agoraphobia was more strongly related to fear of panic than APPQ Interoceptive (Brown, White & Barlow, 2005). Until more is known about the APPQ's psychometric properties, it is recommended for research purposes only.

Clinician Guideline 8.8

A standard pretreatment assessment of panic disorder should include the ADIS-IV for diagnostic information as well as the BAI, ASI, ACQ, and BSQ to determine frequency and intensity of panic symptoms. The MI should be administered when agoraphobia is present.

Case Conceptualization

Although diagnostic and symptom measures are helpful in developing a case conceptualization, idiographic assessment of key cognitive and behavioral features of panic is essential in making a case formulation. Table 8.6 provides a summary of the key elements in a cognitive assessment and case formulation for panic disorder.

TABLE 8.6. Key Elements of a Cognitive Assessment and Case Formulation of Panic Disorder

Cognitive construct assessed	Assessment instruments
Context and frequency of panic	ADIS-IV, Weekly Panic and Acute Anxiety Log (Appendix 8.1), Situational Analysis Form (Appendix 5.2)
Heightened sensitivity and vigilance of bodily/mental sensations	BSQ, Physical Sensations Self-Monitoring Form (Appendix 5.3), Expanded Physical Sensations Checklist (Appendix 5.5)
Catastrophic misinterpretation(s)	ACQ, Physical Sensations Self-Monitoring Form (Appendix 5.3), Apprehensive Thoughts Self-Monitoring Form (Appendix 5.4)
Beliefs, apprehension, and intolerance of anxiety and discomfort	ASI, Identifying Anxious Thinking Errors (Appendix 5.6), Worry Self-Monitoring Form A (Appendix 5.8)
Escape, avoidance, and other safety-seeking cognitive and behavioral strategies	MI, Behavioral Response to Anxiety Checklist (Appendix 5.7), Cognitive Responses to Anxiety (Appendix 5.9), Exposure Hierarchy (Appendix 7.1)
Accessibility of reappraisal schemas	Symptom Reappraisal Form (Appendix 8.2), Weekly Panic and Acute Anxiety Log (Appendix 8.1)
Outcome of panic attacks; sense of safety and perceived coping ability	Weekly Panic and Acute Anxiety Log (Appendix 8.1), Symptom Reappraisal Form (Appendix 8.2), Anxious Reappraisal Form (Appendix 5.10)

Note. ADIS-IV, Anxiety Disorders Interview Schedule for DSM-IV; BSQ, Body Sensations Questionnaire; ACQ, Agoraphobic Cognitions Questionnaire; ASI, Anxiety Sensitivity Index; MI, Mobility Inventory.

Weekly Panic Log

One of the most important instruments in any assessment of panic is a daily self-reported measure of panic attacks called the *panic log* (Shear & Maser, 1994). The panic log should be introduced at first contact with the client and utilized as a weekly homework assignment throughout the course of therapy. Appendix 8.1 provides a weekly panic log that is tailored to the cognitive therapy discussed in this chapter. If completed correctly it will give the clinician most of the basic information that is needed to develop a cognitive case formulation of panic. The panic log provides crucial contextual information about panic attacks, their symptom expression, anxious interpretation, extent of reappraisal capacity, and coping resources. To maximize the clinical utility of the panic log, the therapist should provide instructions on how to use the panic log. The following points should be covered in the explanation.

1. Complete the log as soon as possible after experiencing a panic or anxiety attack to ensure greater accuracy of self-observations.
2. Record a broad range of panic experiences including full-blown panic attacks, partial attacks, and acute anxiety attacks. In the Severity/Intensity column, label each anxiety episode as a full-blown panic attack (i.e., abrupt onset involving four or more physical symptoms), a limited panic attack (i.e., abrupt onset involving one-to-three physical symptoms), or an acute anxiety episode (i.e., sudden onset of apprehension or nervousness).
3. Duration of panic (column 1) is defined as the length of time the panic lasts at its peak intensity (i.e., Brown et al., 1994).
4. In the second column briefly note the circumstances or context in which the anxiety or panic occurred. Make particular note of any specific external or internal stimulus that may have triggered the panic (e.g., "you are driving alone in the car and notice that you are breathing more deeply than usual"). Also indicate whether the attack is expected or unexpected.
5. Briefly describe the physical and mental symptoms that characterized the panic attack. Make special note of the symptoms that were particularly intense or most distressing.
6. In the column labeled "Anxious Interpretation," answer "What concerned you most while having the panic attack?", "What were you afraid might happen?", "When you were most anxious, what was the worst consequence or outcome that crossed you mind? (e.g., heart attack, loss of control, embarrassment or humiliation)."
7. The sixth column, labeled "Evidence for the Alternative," inquires whether the client was able to find any evidence or explanation that the panic attack was less serious than first thought. "Was there anything about the anxiety or panic that made you think it was not a serious threat?" "Or did you recall anything that made you question the seriousness of the anxiety or panic experience?"
8. In the last column indicate how the panic or anxiety episode terminated. "Did you do anything that ended the panic attack?" "How effective were you at bringing an end to the anxiety or panic episode?" "To what extent was a sense or feeling of safety restored at the termination of the episode?"

Important contextual and phenomenological information on panic can also be obtained from the panic disorder module of the ADIS-IV. The Situational Analysis Form (Appendix 5.2) is an alternative measure that can be used to gather data on the situational triggers, primary symptoms, and anxious interpretation of panic. Whether this form is used or the weekly panic log, arriving at a valid case formulation depends on obtaining this "online assessment" of multiple instances of panic that occur in naturalistic settings. Individuals who refuse to fill in the panic log or who provide insufficient information will hamper treatment.

Helen, who was introduced at the beginning of this chapter, recorded one to two daily panic and anxiety episodes on her weekly panic log at pretreatment. Only one to two of these weekly episodes were considered full-blown panic attacks. The remainder were limited-symptom attacks or acute anxiety over physical symptoms associated with a heightened degree of worry that a panic attack might occur. A variety of situations were identified that triggered anxiety and panic including public settings, staying overnight away from home, driving alone in the car outside her community, being in locations that were distant from medical facilities, and the like. Evidence of mild to moderate agoraphobic avoidance indicated that *in vivo* exposure should be a prominent feature of the treatment plan.

Interoceptive Hypersensitivity

Two issues are particularly important when assessing hypersensitivity to bodily sensations. What is the first physical or mental sensation experienced in the sequence of sensations that leads to panic? And which physical or mental sensation is the focus of the catastrophic misinterpretation?

Although the BSQ can be helpful in assessing responsiveness to bodily sensations, the idiographic rating forms such as the Physical Sensation Self-Monitoring Form (Appendix 5.3) or the Expanded Physical Sensations Checklist (Appendix 5.5) will have the greatest clinical utility along with the weekly panic log. The cognitive therapist should review completed forms with clients, extracting from the discussion the temporal order of the internal sensations and the primary sensation that is considered most threatening. For example, a review of Helen's panic logs revealed that the first sensation she often noticed during a panic episode was a sense that maybe her breathing was a little irregular followed by other sensations such as tension, weakness, restlessness, and lightheadedness. This culminated very rapidly in the physical symptom that was the focus of her catastrophic misinterpretation and the apex of the panic experience: shortness of breath. Based on this information we included symptom amplification exercises in our treatment plan in order to increase Helen's exposure to the breathlessness sensation and decatastrophize her interpretation of the sensations.

Catastrophic Misinterpretation

A critical part of the cognitive assessment is to identify the primary catastrophic misinterpretation of internal sensations. The clinician focuses on discovering the impending immediate physical or mental catastrophe that underlies the panic episode (e.g., fear of heart attack, suffocation, going crazy). Often a fear of anxiety or dread of future panic attacks replaces the somatic catastrophe for those with a history of recurrent panic attacks. For others, fear of panic, loss of control, and intolerance of anxiety are associated features of the catastrophic misinterpretation. Although Helen's catastrophic misinterpretation remained fear of suffocation, in later sessions she expressed greater anxiety and apprehension about the return of panic attacks rather than of dying from suffocation. In the early stage of treatment it is important to obtain a full description of the various negative consequences that clients think about when they are anxious or panicky. Helen's treatment plan required that we target both her catastrophic misinterpretation of chest pain and breathlessness (i.e., fear of heart attack or suffocation) and her apprehension about panic and intolerance of anxiety.

As noted in Table 8.6, the ACQ can provide some initial indication of the patient's misinterpretation of anxious symptoms. However, self-monitoring forms that instruct individuals to record their symptom appraisals during peak anxiety will be most helpful. These include the weekly panic log, the Physical Sensations Self-Monitoring Form (Appendix 5.3), and the Apprehensive Thoughts Self-Monitoring Form (Appendix 5.4). It may be necessary to use a panic induction exercise during the session to identify the client's faulty appraisal process. This may be especially true for individuals who have limited insight into their anxious cognitions.

Apprehension and Intolerance of Anxiety

It is important to identify the panic individual's faulty cognitions and beliefs about anxiety, panic, and physical discomfort more generally. The ASI will provide an indication of an individual's tolerance of anxiety, especially its physical symptoms. Faulty beliefs about anxiety can also be deduced from the types of cognitive errors that individuals commit when anxious (use Identifying Anxious Thinking Errors, Appendix 5.6) and the focus of their worries (use Worry Self-Monitoring Form, Appendix 5.8). Individuals with panic disorder often worry about being anxious and panicky, so their worry content may reveal their beliefs about anxiety and its consequences. Helen had a very good response to cognitive therapy for panic but continued to endorse a number of beliefs that ensured recurrent states of heightened anxiety such as "If I have some unexpected physical discomfort, there must be something wrong," "I have to deal with this discomfort, or it could escalate into anxiety and panic," "I can't stand feeling anxious, I have to get rid of the feeling," and "If I don't stop the anxiety, it will escalate into panic." Thus the latter sessions shifted focus from the catastrophic misinterpretation to normalization exercises designed to increase her tolerance of anxiety.

Avoidance and Safety-Seeking

A cognitive assessment of panic must also include a list of all the situations and stimuli, both external and internal, that are avoided for fear of elevated anxiety or panic. For each situation the patient should rate degree of anxiety associated with the situation (0–100) and extent of avoidance (0= never avoided to 100= always avoided). In addition the cognitive therapist identifies all the subtle cognitive and behavioral safety cues that may be used to reduce anxiety. The Behavioral Responses to Anxiety Checklist (Appendix 5.7) and the Cognitive Responses to Anxiety Checklist (Appendix 5.9) forms can be helpful in this regards, whereas the Mobility Inventory and Exposure Hierarchy (Appendix 7.1) may be used to explore avoidance behavior. If the concept of avoidance is broadened to include interoceptive and experiential states (i.e., White et al., 2006), then the clinician should take a wide-ranging perspective when describing the avoidance component of the case formulation. As noted previously, Helen continued to use avoidance to manage her anxiety so *in vivo* exposure was a critical component of her treatment plan.

Reappraisal Capacity

In the current cognitive model of panic disorder, loss of reappraisal capability is an important factor in the persistence of panic attacks. Therefore it is important to assess an individual's ability to generate alternative, nonthreatening explanations for her physical sensations. The Symptom Reappraisal Form (Appendix 8.2) can be used to assess critical components of reappraisal capability that might be present prior to treatment. Three particular questions need to be addressed.

1. Is the client able to offer a number of alternative non-threat explanations for the physical sensations?
2. How much does he believe these explanations when anxious or panicky and when not anxious?
3. Is the client able to recall these explanations when anxious and if so, what effect does this have on the anxious state?

The weekly panic log can be a useful starting point for a discussion on possible alternative explanations for unpleasant or anxious physical sensations. Even if an individual is unable to generate an alternative explanation to the catastrophic misinterpretation, this will be valuable clinical information for treatment planning.

In our case illustration, Helen's initial apprehensive thoughts after noticing an unexpected physical sensation were "What's wrong with me?", "Why am I feeling this way?" She immediately generated a catastrophic misinterpretation such as "Could this be a heart attack?" (i.e., if she felt chest pain), "What if I can't catch my breath and then start to suffocate?" (i.e., if she experienced a breathless sensation), or "Will I have a terrible panic attack?" At pretreatment she was able to generate two less-threatening alternative explanations for the sensations (e.g., the sensation could be a symptom of anxiety or stress that will eventually subside). Occasionally she could attribute the symptoms to physical activity or a state of ill health (e.g., having a cold, flu symptoms). However, she had difficulty believing these alternative explanations or even being able to access them when she felt intense anxiety or panic. Also she became intolerant of anxiety, so interpreting the sensations as symptoms of anxiety provided no relief for her. It was clear from the assessment that strengthening her reappraisal capability would be an important focus of treatment.

Perceived Panic Outcome

A final component of the case conceptualization is to determine the "natural" outcome of panic attacks. It is expected that individuals will engage in escape, avoidance, and safety-seeking behaviors in an effort to control the anxiety and panic. The clinician should assess the perceived effectiveness of these strategies. To what extent is an individual able to achieve a sense of safety after the occurrence of an anxiety or panic episode? How long does this sense of safety last before the patient is again concerned about the recurrence of panic? What is the individual's degree of self-efficacy in her ability to cope with panic? Information on panic outcome can be obtained from the weekly panic log, the Symptom Reappraisal Form (Appendix 8.2), and the Anxious Reappraisal Form (Appendix 5.10).

Helen was able to achieve a reasonably high level of safety after her episodes of acute anxiety and panic but these tended to be relatively short-lived (e.g., 12–24 hours). She engaged in extensive reassurance seeking from family members and searching for her symptoms on the Internet, as well as avoiding perceived triggers. She believed that avoidance was quite effective in curbing the anxiety and ensuring that it did not escalate into panic. The reassurance seeking was considered moderately effective in reducing current states of anxiety over unexplained physical sensations. Helen also relied heavily on self-reassurance in which she repeated to herself "Everything will be okay, nothing is wrong with me." Again she thought this helped "calm her down" to a certain extent. Treatment, then, had to target Helen's beliefs about the effectiveness of her avoidance and safety-seeking strategies to ensure the elimination of maladaptive coping that contributed to the persistence of panic.

Clinician Guideline 8.9

A cognitive case formulation of panic should include a contextual analysis of the panic attacks as well as an assessment of (1) physiological hypervigilance, (2) catastrophic misinterpretation of bodily sensations, (3) presence of maladaptive beliefs about anxiety tolerance, (4) role of avoidance and safety-seeking strategies, (5) accessibility of reappraisal schemas, and (6) perceived outcome of anxiety and panic episodes. The case formulation will be the basis of treatment planning and implementation of an individualized cognitive intervention.

DESCRIPTION OF COGNITIVE THERAPY FOR PANIC DISORDER

There are five main treatment goals in cognitive therapy for panic disorder. The first two goals pertain to the automatic schematic threat processing that occurs during the immediate fear response (Phase I), whereas the remaining goals refer to responses that occur during elaborative processing (Phase II) (see Figure 2.1). The primary treatment goals are:

1. Reduce sensitivity or responsiveness to panic-relevant physical or mental sensations
2. Weaken the catastrophic misinterpretation and underlying hypervalent threat schemas of bodily or mental states
3. Enhance cognitive reappraisal capabilities that result in adoption of a more benign and realistic alternative explanation for distressing symptoms
4. Eliminate avoidance and other maladaptive safety-seeking behaviors
5. Increase tolerance for anxiety or discomfort and reestablish a sense of safety

Table 8.7 presents the main treatment components of cognitive therapy employed to achieve these goals.

TABLE 8.7. Main Treatment Components of Cognitive Therapy for Panic

- Education into the cognitive therapy model of panic
- Schematic activation and symptom induction
- Cognitive restructuring of catastrophic misinterpretation
- Empirical hypothesis testing of alternative explanation
- Graded *in vivo* exposure
- Symptom tolerance and safety reinterpretation
- Relapse prevention
- Breathing retraining (optional)

Educating Clients into the Cognitive Therapy Model of Panic

The first treatment session focuses on educating the client into the cognitive explanation for recurrent panic attacks. If the cognitive assessment strategy has been followed, then the therapist already has much of the critical information available for educating the client such as the situational triggers for panic, distressing physical sensations, catastrophic misinterpretations, and maladaptive avoidance/safety-seeking responses. Normally clients have started keeping a weekly panic log (see Appendix 8.1) and so a typical panic episode can be selected from the log. Using Socratic questioning, the cognitive therapist explores the client's experience during this panic episode and his interpretation of the symptoms. The therapist and client collaboratively complete the Vicious Cycle of Panic form found in Appendix 8.3. It is important that the therapist records specific thoughts and feelings associated with the panic episode and that the cognitive explanation is presented as "one possible explanation of the origins of panic that needs to be tested."

At this initial stage of treatment it is unlikely the client is ready to abandon her catastrophic misinterpretation and embrace the cognitive explanation. Instead the goal of the educational session is to merely introduce an alternative explanation for panic that provides a treatment rationale. The session normally ends with a homework assignment in which clients continue with their panic logs but this time they examine whether their anxiety and panic experiences are consistent or not with the cognitive explanation. When reviewing homework in the subsequent session, it is important that the therapist deal with anxiety experiences that appear contrary to the model and reinforce the client's observations that are consistent with the cognitive explanation.

In our case illustration a Vicious Cycle of Panic form (see Appendix 8.3) was completed at the outset of cognitive therapy. Helen identified a number of triggers from her panic log such as being at a work meeting and sitting beside the guest speaker, not being in close proximity to a hospital, flying, and driving alone some distance from home. Her initial physical sensations were feeling lightheaded, sensing that her breathing was a little irregular, and experiencing an unusual feeling of pressure in her chest. This was followed by some initial anxious cognitions such as "What's wrong with me?", "Why am I feeling this way?", "Something is not right," "I don't like this," "I am beginning to feel anxious," "I feel trapped," and so on. These anxious thoughts often led to an escalation in a few physical sensations such as feelings of suffocation or heart palpitations. Once these intense physical sensations occurred, Helen identified a number of catastrophic cognitions like "I'm not getting enough air, I'm going to die of suffocation," "What if I'm having a heart attack?", or "If I don't stop I'm going to have a full-blown panic attack." The catastrophic misinterpretation led to various control efforts such as escape, reassurance seeking from others, controlled breathing, or distraction, which together often ended in intense anxiety or panic attacks. After completing the Vicious Cycle of Panic form, the therapist emphasized that catastrophic misinterpretations and maladaptive control efforts were the main catalysts for panic rather than the real possibility of some imminent threat (e.g., possible heart attack). Helen was given a copy of the completed Vicious Cycle of Panic form and asked to record her anxiety and panic experiences over the next week with particular focus on whether the cognitive model was a good explanation for her anxious experiences.

Clinician Guideline 8.10

Use the Vicious Cycle of Panic form (Appendix 8.3) to begin educating clients to the cognitive model and highlight the central role of catastrophic misinterpretations in the persistence of panic.

Schema Activation and Symptom Induction

A critical feature of cognitive therapy for panic is the use of within-session exercises to induce the client's feared physical sensations (Beck, 1988; Beck & Greenberg, 1988; D. M. Clark, 1997; D. M. Clark & Salkovskis, 1986). When cognitive therapy of panic was first developed, patients were always given a 2-minute breathing hyperventilation exercise followed by instruction in controlled breathing in order to introduce overbreathing as a possible alternative explanation for the occurrence of intense physical sensations (D. M. Clark & Salkovskis, 1986). However, it is now known that hyperventilation probably plays a less prominent role in panic, so controlled breathing is no longer recommended in most cases of panic disorder (see discussion below). Furthermore, cognitive therapists are more likely to use a variety of induction exercises repeatedly throughout treatment based on the positive effects of interoceptive exposure on panic reduction (see White & Barlow, 2002).

Symptom induction exercises are important in cognitive therapy of panic disorder because they allow direct activation of threat schemas and opportunity to challenge catastrophic misinterpretations of bodily sensations. Usually the intentional production of symptoms like dizziness, heart palpitations, breathlessness, and so on in the presence of the therapist is less intense and better tolerated by the patient than in real life. In this way the client learns that certain physical sensations are not always frightening, that the physical sensations do not lead to the catastrophic outcome, and that an exacerbation of unwanted sensations can be due to other, more benign causes. Often the within-session symptom induction is the first direct experiential evidence that challenges the catastrophic misinterpretation. After engaging in symptom induction, the cognitive therapist always reviews the experience with clients in terms of whether the experience confirms or disconfirms the catastrophic misinterpretation of bodily sensations. Symptom induction exercises are introduced by the second or third session and they are repeated often throughout treatment. Eventually symptom induction is assigned as homework with clients instructed to practice intentionally producing their feared physical sensations first in neutral and then in anxiety-provoking situations.

Before introducing symptom induction it is important to determine if the client has any medical contraindications for engaging in the exercise. Of course clients must be physically able to do the exercise and willing to endure a moderate level of discomfort. Any medical problems that could be worsened by an induction exercise must be taken into account by possibly consulting with the client's family physician. Taylor (2006) lists various health conditions that would warrant extreme caution when using certain induction exercises (e.g., lower back pain, pregnancy, postural hypotension, chronic obstructive lung disease, severe asthma, or cardiac disease).

Table 8.8 presents a list of the most common symptom induction exercises, the physical sensations evoked by the exercise, and an example of a typical threat misinterpretation associated with the symptom. See also Taylor (2000, 2006) and Antony, Rowa, Liss, Swallow, and Swinson (2005) for a similar list of symptom induction and exposure exercises.

As can be seen from this table, most of these exercises are very brief and must be repeated frequently both as within-session demonstrations and as homework assignments. Antony et al. (2005) found that breathlessness/smothering sensations, dizziness or feeling faint, and pounding/racing heart were the most common physical sensations elicited by the exercises. Although two-thirds of the panic disorder group in their study reported at least moderate fear to one or more of the symptom induction exercises, most exercises produced only a low intensity of symptoms with spinning, hyperventilation, breathing through a straw, and use of a tongue depressor the most potent exercises. Other exercises such as quickly raising the head, staring at a light, tensing muscles, running on the spot, or sitting close to a heater were relatively ineffective.

Hyperventilation and breath holding were the two main symptom induction exercises used with Helen. These proved highly effective because of her fear of suffocation. Breath holding, in which Helen was encouraged to hold her breath until she felt absolutely compelled to breathe, was a particularly effective intervention that was first demonstrated in session and then assigned whenever she felt anxious about her breathing. By holding her breath, Helen was challenging her catastrophic view "I can't breathe" and by exaggerating the sense of breathlessness the sensation became less frightening. The intense urge to breathe after a period of holding her breath was powerful evidence that "not breathing" was extremely difficult to do even when it was intentional. Her panicogenic belief that "I might just stop breathing and die" was weakened by realizing that she possessed an intense automatic physiological urge to breathe.

Clinician Guideline 8.11

Within-session symptom induction is a critical therapeutic ingredient for activating panic-relevant fear schemas and directly challenging the catastrophic misinterpretation of physical sensations. A solid rationale for symptom induction must be provided. The exercises are utilized repeatedly throughout treatment and eventually assigned as homework. Some exercises are more effective than others in provoking physical sensations that are somewhat similar to naturally occurring panic attacks.

TABLE 8.8. Symptom Induction Exercises Commonly Used in the Treatment of Panic Disorder

Exercise	Evoked physical sensation	Example of misinterpretation of threat
1. Hyperventilate for 1 minute	Breathlessness, smothering sensation	"I can't stand this; I think I am going to faint if I continue."
2. Hold breath for 30 seconds	Breathlessness, smothering sensation	"What if I can't breathe normally? I could suffocate."
3. Breathe through narrow straw for 2 minutes	Breathlessness, smothering sensation	"I need to get more air or I'll suffocate."
4. Spin around at medium pace while standing for 1 minute	Dizzy or faint	"If I let myself feel nauseous, I might vomit."
5. Place head between knees for 30 seconds and then raise head quickly	Dizzy or faint	"When I feel lightheaded, could this be a sign of a stroke?"
6. Shake head rapidly from side to side for 30 seconds	Dizzy or faint	"When feeling dizzy I am losing contact with reality which could lead to insanity."
7. Tense all body muscles for 1 minute	Trembling, shaking	"People will notice that I am trembling and think there is something wrong with me."
8. Run on spot for 1 minute	Pounding, racing heart	"I could have a heart attack."
9. Sit facing a heater for 2 minutes	Breathless, smothering sensation, sweating	"People will be disgusted by my sweating."
10. Place tongue depressor at back of tongue for 30 seconds	Choking sensation	"This choking feels so bad it could cause me to vomit."
11. Stare continuously at fluorescent light for 1 minute and then try to read	Dizzy or faint; feeling of unreality	"My environment is feeling weird. This could mean that I am starting to go insane."
12. Stare continuously at self in mirror for 2 minutes	Feeling unreal, dreamy; dizzy or faint	"If I feel spacey I could lose contact with reality."
13. Stare continuously at spot on wall for 3 minutes	Feeling unreal, dreamy; dizzy or faint	"Feelings of unreality means that I could be having a stroke."

Cognitive Restructuring of Catastrophic Misinterpretation

Cognitive restructuring fulfills two functions in cognitive therapy of panic: it introduces conflicting evidence for the catastrophic misinterpretation and it offers an alternative explanation for internal sensations. In panic disorder evidence gathering, identifying cognitive errors (i.e., exaggerating the probability and severity of imminent danger), and generating alternative explanations will be most helpful. See Chapter 6 for a detailed discussion of these cognitive intervention strategies.

It is often useful to begin cognitive restructuring with a very clear description of the most feared catastrophic outcome and then generate a list of possible alternative explanations for the physical sensations. The Symptom Reappraisal Form (Appendix

8.2) can be used to focus the client on alternative explanations for fearful sensations. Most clients have considerable difficulty generating alternative explanations for their most feared sensations so this will take a considerable amount of guided discovery. A variety of alternative explanations for the symptoms can be raised such as (1) response to heightened anxiety; (2) reaction to stress; (3) product of physical exertion; (4) fatigue; (5) side effects of coffee, alcohol, or medication; (6) heightened vigilance of bodily sensations; (7) strong emotions like anger, surprise, or excitement; (8) random occurrence of benign internal biological processes; or (9) other context-specific possibilities.

Another aspect of the alternative explanation that is emphasized is the role that catastrophic thoughts and beliefs play in exacerbating symptoms (D. M. Clark, 1996). For example, "Is an underlying cardiac condition your problem so that chest pains could signal a heart attack (catastrophic interpretation) or is your problem that you *believe* there is something wrong with your heart and so you are preoccupied with your heart rate" (alternative cognitive explanation)? At this point the therapist simply raises these alternative explanations as possibilities or hypotheses and invites the client to investigate the validity of each explanation by gathering confirming and disconfirming evidence. This can be done by using information recorded on the Weekly Panic Log (Appendix 8.1) or one of the cognitive forms provided in Chapter 6 (e.g., Appendices 6.2 or 6.4). The goal of cognitive restructuring is for individuals with panic to realize that their anxiety and panic symptoms are due to their erroneous beliefs that certain physical sensations are dangerous. Although patients may find it difficult to accept this alternative because of their heightened anxiety, they are repeatedly encouraged to focus on the evidence, not on how they feel.

A major part of Helen's cognitive therapy for panic was the gathering of evidence for alternative explanations for her symptoms of breathlessness, which had become the primary dreaded physical sensation. Gradually, with accumulating evidence based on repeated experiences, she began to accept that her sense of breathlessness was most likely due to excessive monitoring of her breathing and the possibility that she was actually suffocating was entirely remote at best. Over time she found evidence that other physical sensations were probably due to stress, anxiety, fatigue, or alcohol consumption was much more compelling than the automatic catastrophic interpretation. At this point therapy shifted away from challenging the catastrophic interpretation toward increasing her tolerance of anxiety and its physical manifestations.

Clinician Guideline 8.12

In panic disorder cognitive restructuring focuses on gathering evidence (1) that the client automatically generates a highly unlikely and exaggerated misinterpretation of unwanted physical or mental sensations, and (2) that alternative, benign explanations are more plausible. The role of catastrophic thoughts and beliefs in perpetuating anxiety and panic symptoms is emphasized throughout treatment.

Empirical Hypothesis-Testing Experiments

Behavioral experiments play a particularly important role in the treatment of panic. They often take the form of deliberate exposure to anxiety-provoking situations in order to induce fearful symptoms and their outcome. The outcome of the experiment is observed and provides a test of the catastrophic versus the alternative explanation for bodily sensations. D. M. Clark and Salkovskis (1986) describe various behavioral experiments that can be used in the treatment of panic disorder.

A number of behavioral experiments were used to test Helen's catastrophic interpretations and beliefs. In one homework assignment she was asked to hold her breath whenever she felt breathless sensations in order to amplify the sensations. After a few seconds of breath holding, she was told to breathe normally and note differences between breath holding and breathing. "Was there any evidence that she was exaggerating the sense of breathlessness prior to breath holding?" "Was she able to breathe normally after holding her breath?" From these experiences Helen found evidence that indeed she was exaggerating breathlessness and her breathing was much more normal than she thought. In another behavioral experiment Helen was encouraged to induce physical sensations while in fear situations by increasing her physical activity level. These experiments provided evidence that physical sensations themselves do not automatically lead to anxiety or panic (e.g., "Even when anxious, increasing my heart rate by running up stairs does not increase my anxiety level"). Instead she discovered that how she interprets the symptoms determines whether anxiety escalates into panic (e.g., "When I know my heart is pounding fast because of exercise I don't feel anxious").

Clinician Guideline 8.13

Behavioral experiments provide a critical test of the role that catastrophic thoughts and beliefs play in the persistence of anxiety and panic symptoms. The experiments are designed to show that the mere occurrence of physical sensations is not the primary cause of anxiety but rather it is their catastrophic misinterpretation that leads to panic attacks.

Graded In Vivo Exposure

Given that most individuals with panic disorder exhibit at least mild forms of agoraphobic avoidance, graded *in vivo* exposure is a major component of cognitive therapy for panic disorder. When agoraphobic avoidance is severe, *in vivo* exposure must be introduced early in treatment and become the main focus of therapy. However, the cognitive therapist uses exposure to challenge the catastrophic cognitions and beliefs of the agoraphobic individual. Since Chapter 7 provided an extensive discussion of graded *in vivo* exposure and its implementation, the reader is encouraged to consult that section when employing exposure exercises in cognitive therapy of panic.

In our case illustration Helen presented with fairly extensive avoidance of external situations because of her fear of panic attacks and of being too distant from a hospital in case she suffered a heart attack or episode of suffocation. A fear hierarchy was constructed involving 23 situations ranging from taking a bus trip to a nearby city (rated 10 on a scale of 0–100) to taking a transcontinental flight (rated 100). Helen engaged in repeated exposure to a variety of situations on her fear hierarchy, gathering evidence against her most feared outcomes, and confirming the role of catastrophic thinking in the genesis of panic. Furthermore, the exposure suggested more benign, alternative explanations for her physical sensations, thereby enhancing her ability to reappraise unwanted feelings and sensations.

Clinician Guideline 8.14

Graded *in vivo* exposure is important in the treatment of agoraphobic avoidance and in disconfirming the catastrophic thoughts and beliefs pathogenic to panic attacks and their fear.

Symptom Tolerance and Safety Reinterpretation

As stated earlier, cognitive therapy seeks to increase the panic individual's tolerance of unexpected physical sensations and discomfort as well as subjective anxiety and to instill a greater sense of safety and coping ability. This can be accomplished by intentionally focusing on the client's ability to tolerate the physical symptoms of anxiety during within-session and between-session behavioral exposure exercises. For example, a client who is anxious about chest tightness and heart palpitations could be asked to monitor his physical sensations while doing a cardio workout in the gym. Not only would repeated experiences of physiological activation provide evidence that physical symptoms can be tolerated, but the panic-prone individual will be learning that mere occurrence of physical symptoms is not dangerous. However, for these experiences to be therapeutic the cognitive therapist must repeatedly emphasize the idea that "clearly you are able to tolerate these physical sensations just like everyone else."

Therapy must also focus on increased tolerance for physical discomfort and anxiety. Clients could be asked to keep a diary of their experiences of physical discomfort that are not associated with anxiety such as episodes of headaches, sore muscles, fatigue, and the like. Individuals can be asked to rate the degree of discomfort associated with these symptoms and their level of anxiety. The point of this exercise is for the panic-prone individual to learn that she is capable of tolerating discomfort without feeling anxious. By reinforcing this observation, the therapist can strengthen the client's beliefs in her ability to cope with the physical discomfort associated with anxiety. Moreover, tolerance of anxiety can be improved through graded *in vivo* exposure exercises in which the therapist gradually increases the level of anxiety so individuals learn they can cope with even high anxiety states.

The cognitive therapist can increase the client's sense of safety by helping him reinterpret anxiety-provoking situations encountered during homework assignments. At every opportunity, the therapist redirects the client's attention by asking questions such as "What aspects of this situation suggested safety?", "Was there anything about this situation that made you think it was less dangerous and more safe than you initially thought?", or "As you look back on the situation, what safety cues were present that you just didn't notice at the time?" An important goal of cognitive therapy is to "train" the individual with panic disorder to intentionally reconsider the safety features of an anxiety-provoking situation in order to counter his automatic catastrophic interpretation. The Symptom Reappraisal Form (Appendix 8.2) can be used for this purpose. In addition it is helpful to have clients rate the "realistic" level of danger associated with the situation (e.g., 0–100 rating scale) as well as the "realistic" level of safety after recording danger and safety features on the panic log (Appendix 8.1). It is important to ensure that clients' ratings are based on a "realistic" assessment rather than on "how they feel" because emotion-based ratings will always be distorted because of a heightened anxiety state.

Given Helen's relative youth and good physical health, she was encouraged to increase her physical activity level and record her physiological arousal. This proved quite effective in helping Helen realize she could tolerate chest tightness and breathless sensations, and that these sensations could be evoked without danger. Also the breath-holding exercises when anxious again provided evidence of tolerance and safety. Later in the therapy sessions cognitive restructuring always focused on processing the safety features of anxious experiences. Helen was repeatedly asked questions such as "Looking back, what aspects of the situation indicate that it was safer than you originally thought"? Toward the end of treatment, Helen would spontaneously generate safety reinterpretations of anxiety-provoking situations and reported a greater sense of safety in her daily life.

Clinician Guideline 8.15

A perceived sense of safety and tolerance of the physical symptoms of anxiety are important goals for cognitive therapy of panic. They are achieved by cognitive restructuring and behavioral exercises that emphasize the client's natural tolerance of discomfort and the reinterpretation of safety features associated with anxiety-provoking situations.

Relapse Prevention

As is done in the treatment of other anxiety disorders, relapse prevention should be built into the final sessions of cognitive therapy for panic. The therapist must ensure that the client realizes that occasional panic attacks will occur, that unexpected physical sensations may occur from time to time, and that anxiety is a normal part of life. Relapse can be minimized if the client has realistic expectations of treatment outcome and adopts a healthy perspective on anxiety and panic. In addition, significant reduction in the client's "fear of fear" can improve the chance of reduced relapse and recurrence of panic. The client who continues to fear panic attacks (e.g., "I just hope I never have to experience those terrible panic attacks again") is probably most vulnerable to relapse when the physical symptoms of anxiety reoccur.

In addition to correcting unrealistic expectations about treatment and the "return of fear," a number of other measures can be taken to prevent relapse. Therapy sessions can be gradually faded and booster sessions scheduled. An intervention protocol can be written down that clearly specifies what to do if unexpected physical symptoms return or the individual experiences a resurgence in anxiety. However, the most important relapse prevention strategy for panic may involve having panic disorder patients intentionally produce their feared physical sensations when in anxiety-provoking situations. Those individuals who progress to the point where they can exaggerate their physical symptoms while feeling highly anxious may be better inoculated against future unexpected resurgences of anxiety and panic.

Clinician Guideline 8.16

Relapse prevention is enhanced when cognitive therapy clients are prepared for the unexpected return of fear and panic. In addition relapse and recurrence of panic disorder may be less likely in individuals who can engage in exaggerated physiological activation when experiencing high levels of anxiety.

Breathing Retraining (Optional)

Breathing retraining is a relaxation strategy that was incorporated into early versions of cognitive therapy for panic disorder (e.g., Beck, 1988; Beck & Greenberg, 1988; D. M. Clark, 1986a). Based on the notion that hyperventilation, which involves deep and rapid breathing, is an important factor in the production of panic attacks, it was proposed that training in slow, shallow breathing should counter panic symptoms (D. M. Clark, Salkovskis, & Chalkley, 1985; Salkovskis, Jones, & Clark, 1986). Key elements of D. M. Clark and Salkovskis's (1986) early cognitive treatment protocol for panic included:

1. A 2-minute voluntary hyperventilation exercise of breathing at a rate of 30 breaths per minute.
2. Observation of the physical sensations caused by hyperventilation and their similarity to panic symptoms.
3. Education on the physiology of hyperventilation and how it can produce the physical sensations of a panic attack.
4. Reattribution of the physical symptoms of panic to stress-induced hyperventilation (or overbreathing) rather than to a misperceived catastrophic health threat (e.g., "I am having a heart attack").
5. Training in slow breathing in order to provide a coping response that is incompatible with hyperventilation. Controlled breathing also becomes a behavioral experiment by demonstrating that physical symptoms must be due to overbreathing rather than the catastrophic threat because the symptoms are so quickly reduced when slow, shallow breathing is established.

The hyperventilation exercise and breathing retraining became key elements of the cognitive therapy treatment protocol for panic offered at the Center for Cognitive Therapy in Philadelphia from the mid-1980s to the late 1990s (Beck & Greenberg, 1988). Together they provided a critical empirical hypothesis-testing experiment indicating that the catastrophic misinterpretation of symptoms was incorrect, and that the physical symptoms were actually a harmless consequence of overbreathing or even hyperventilation (Beck & Greenberg, 1987).

Breathing Retraining Exercise

Abdominal or diaphragmatic breathing has been the most common form of breathing retraining used in the treatment of anxiety disorders. It assumes a key role for hyperventilation in the etiology of panic by causing an acute decrease in arterial partial pressure carbon dioxide ($_pCO_2$), called hypocapnia, that in turn results in a wide range of unpleasant bodily sensations (e.g., dizziness, heart palpitations, tingling in extremities, breathlessness), which the individual misinterprets as representing a serious medical threat (Meuret, Ritz, Wilhelm, & Roth, 2005; D. M. Clark et al., 1985). Various studies have found other breathing abnormalities in anxiety disorders such as shallow and rapid overbreathing, disorganized breathing patterns, and frequent sighing (see Meuret et al., 2005; Meuret, Wilhelm, Ritz, & Roth, 2003; Salkovskis et al., 1986). Individuals are trained in slow, deep abdominal breathing to eliminate hypocapnia and its uncomfortable physical sensations thereby reducing the anxious state. Table 8.9 presents a typical diaphragmatic breathing retraining protocol.

Current Status of Breathing Retraining

There is currently considerable debate over the role of breathing retraining in CBT for panic disorder. There are three reasons why cognitive-behavioral therapists are now questioning the use of breathing retraining. The first is a very practical, clinical concern. Like using other forms of relaxation, a person with panic disorder might use controlled breathing as a safety response or coping strategy to escape from an anxious state (Antony & McCabe, 2004; Salkovskis et al., 1996; White & Barlow, 2002). This, of course, would undermine the effectiveness of cognitive therapy by reinforcing a fear of the anxiety and the client's faulty evaluation of the dangerousness of the physical sensations. If there is any evidence that the client is using controlled breathing because of a fear of anxiety and its symptoms, then the coping response should be discontinued immediately.

Second, the rationale for offering breathing retraining in panic disorder has been called into question with evidence that hyperventilation and hypocapnia are often not present even in panic attacks that occur in the natural setting (see review by Meuret et al., 2005; Taylor, 2000). And third, the therapeutic effectiveness of breathing retraining has been questioned (e.g., Salkovskis, Clark, & Hackman, 1991; D. M. Clark et al., 1999). Schmidt and colleagues conducted a dismantling study that compared the effectiveness of 12 sessions of group-administered CBT plus breathing retraining, CBT without breathing retraining, and a wait list condition at posttreatment and 12-month follow-up (Schmidt, Woolaway-Bickel, et al., 2000). At posttreatment both active treatments were significantly improved over the wait list condition but there was no statistically significant difference between the CBT and CBT + breathing retraining conditions. At 12-month follow-up 57% of the CBT group met recovery criteria compared with 37% for the CBT + breathing retraining group. The authors concluded that the addition of diaphragmatic breathing does not add any therapeutic benefits to CBT for panic beyond the standard treatment components of education, cognitive restructuring, and exposure. They recommended that respiratory-control techniques be used only as a behavioral experiment to provide corrective information for the catastrophic misinterpretation of bodily sensations and that therapists refrain from using them as an anxiety management technique. Based on these findings we conclude that breathing retraining should be considered optional in cognitive therapy for panic.

Clinician Guideline 8.17

Breathing retraining should be limited to individuals who clearly hyperventilate during a panic attack. In most cases breathing retraining will not be necessary. If it is included in the treatment protocol, careful monitoring is needed to ensure it does not become a safety-seeking response.

TABLE 8.9. Diaphragmatic Breathing Retraining Protocol for Cognitive Therapy of Panic

PHASE I. BASELINE PREPARATION

Rationale: Review physical sensations and cognitions of most recent panic attack. Obtain belief ratings at varying levels of anxiety to show how same sensations can be interpreted differently at different times.

Instructions: Ask client to describe the physical sensations and the catastrophic misinterpretation associated with the panic attack; client rates belief in the misinterpretation now and when most anxious.

PHASE II. HYPERVENTILATION INDUCTION

Rationale: To demonstrate the production of physical sensations similar to a panic attack through overbreathing.

Instructions: Individuals are asked to overbreathe at rate of 30 breaths per minute for 2 minutes or until it becomes too difficult to continue. They are instructed in use of paper bag to rebreathe expired CO_2. They are also instructed to focus on the physical sensations produced by hyperventilation.

PHASE III. REATTRIBUTION

Rationale: To introduce possibility that physical sensations during panic are wrongly attributed to a health threat and instead could be due to overbreathing.

Instructions: Clients are asked to review the physical sensations during hyperventilation and the sensations described during panic. Rate their degree of similarity and discuss how the overbreathing symptoms might be worse in a naturalistic setting.

PHASE IV. EDUCATION AND TREATMENT RATIONALE

Rationale: Explain the physiology of hyperventilation and how it causes uncomfortable physical sensations

Instructions: Discuss how hyperventilation can cause an abrupt drop in arterial $_pCO_2$ that causes uncomfortable physical sensations. When these symptoms are misinterpreted as indicating a life-threatening danger like a heart attack, going crazy, or suffocation, panic sets in. Learning to counter overbreathing with a slower, moderate breathing rate will reduce the intensity of the physical sensations and provide new evidence that the sensations are due to overbreathing and not the catastrophic health threat.

PHASE V. DIAPHRAGMATIC BREATHING

Rationale: Learn a relaxation coping skill to counter hyperventilation and other breathing irregularities that cause the production of physical sensations that are misinterpreted in a threatening manner.

Instructions:

1. Place one hand on chest with thumb just below neck and the other hand on stomach with little finger just above naval.
2. Have client take short, shallow breaths through nose. Notice how hand on chest slightly rises but hand on stomach hardly moves.
3. Now have client take slower, normal breaths through the nose and notice how the abdomen moves slightly outward with each inhale and then deflates with each exhale.
4. Practice for 2–3 minutes with the client focusing on the movement of the abdomen with each inhale and exhale.
5. Proceed to work on slowing the breathing rate down to 8 or 12 breaths per minute. Introduce a paced breathing rate in which therapist demonstrates a 4 second inhale–4 second exhale cycle. This can be done by counting 1–2–3–4 with each inhale, and then 1–2–3–4 with each exhale. A short pause occurs at the end of each inhale and exhale. As the client exhales the word "relax" should be repeated. After the therapist and client practice this slow, moderate breathing, the client should continue with the diaphragmatic breathing with a particular focus on the slow steady rhythm of breathing and the rise and fall of the stomach with each inhale and exhale.
6. Homework assignments begin with two to three daily 10-minute diaphragmatic breathing practice sessions with or without a pacing audiotape. This is followed by daily sessions of 1–2 minutes of hyperventilation followed by slow breathing.
7. The final phase of homework involves application of diaphragmatic breathing in a variety of anxious everyday situations.

EFFICACY OF COGNITIVE THERAPY FOR PANIC DISORDER

Cognitive behavior therapy for panic disorder falls within the American Psychological Association's well-established category of empirically supported treatments (Chambless et al., 1998; Chambless & Ollendick, 2001). The American Psychiatric Association Practice Guidelines for the treatment of panic disorder concluded that CBT was a proven effective treatment for panic, with a 78% completer response rate that was at least equal or superior to the effectiveness of antipanic medication (American Psychiatric Association, 1998).

Numerous reviews of the clinical outcome research have concluded there is strong support for the efficacy of CBT for panic disorder. After reviewing more than 25 independently conducted clinical trials, Barlow and colleagues concluded that 40–90% of patients treated with CBT are panic-free at end of treatment (Landon & Barlow, 2004; White & Barlow, 2002). Other reviewers have also concluded that the effectiveness of CBT for panic is strongly supported by the outcome literature (Butler, Chapman, Forman, & Beck, 2006; DeRubeis & Crits-Christoph, 1998; Otto, Pollack, & Maki, 2000) and that treatment gains endure beyond termination more than with medication (Hollon, Stuart, & Strunk, 2006). In the following section we provide a brief review of selected key clinical outcome studies for CBT as well as dismantling studies that investigate the mechanism of change in the treatment package.

CBT Outcome Studies

Several meta-analyses have determined that CBT for panic is associated with superior effect sizes. For example in a meta-analysis based on 13 studies Chambless and Peterman (2004) obtained an average effect size of .93 for panic and phobic symptoms, with 71% of CBT patients panic-free at posttreatment compared to 29% for the control conditions (i.e., wait list or attention placebo). Furthermore, significant treatment gains were evident in other symptom domains such as the cognitive symptoms of panic, generalized anxiety, and, to a lesser extent, depression (see also Gould et al., 1995, for similar conclusions).

One of the earliest reports on cognitive therapy for panic disorder was a naturalistic outcome study of 17 patients treated with a mean of 18 individual sessions of cognitive therapy that focused on misinterpretations of the physical symptoms of anxiety, exposure, and cognitive restructuring of panic-relevant fears (Sokol, Beck, Greenberg, Wright, & Berchick, 1989). At posttreatment panic frequency declined to zero and was maintained at 1-year follow-up, and significant reductions were achieved on the BAI and BDI. In addition improvement was made in patients' ability to reappraise their fears in a more realistic manner. In a later randomized clinical trial in which 33 patients with panic disorder were assigned to 12 weeks of individual cognitive therapy or 8 weeks of brief supportive psychotherapy, Beck, Sokol, Clark, Berchick, and Wright (1992) found that at 8 weeks the cognitive therapy group had significantly fewer self-reported and clinician-rated panic attacks than the comparison group. In addition the cognitive therapy group had less generalized anxiety and fear but not less depression, and 71% were panic-free compared to 25% in the psychotherapy condition. At 1-year follow-up 87% of the cognitive therapy group remained panic-free.

In a major outcome study 64 panic patients were randomly assigned to an average of 10 weekly individual sessions of cognitive therapy, applied relaxation, imipramine only, or a 3-month wait list control followed by random assignment to one of the active treatments (D. M. Clark et al., 1994). At posttreatment (i.e., 3 months), cognitive therapy was significantly more effective than applied relaxation and imipramine in reduction of panic symptoms (i.e., panic composite score), agoraphobic avoidance, misinterpretation of bodily sensations, and hypervigiliance for body symptoms. In addition 80% of the cognitive therapy patients reached high-end functioning at 3 months compared to 25% for applied relaxation and 40% for imipramine. Moreover, at 15-month follow-up cognitive therapy remained superior to applied relaxation and imipramine on six measures of panic/anxiety, with 85% of cognitive therapy patients still panic-free compared with 47% of applied relaxation and 60% of imipramine patients.

In a large multisite randomized placebo-controlled clinical trial involving 77 patients with panic disorder (Barlow, Gorman, Shear, & Woods, 2000) intent-to-treat analyses revealed that CBT and imipramine were superior to placebo, but there were no significant differences between imipramine and CBT at posttreatment, although there was a trend favoring CBT at 6-month follow-up. Overall, then, major treatment outcome studies have clearly established that CBT for panic disorder is at least as effective as medication, although there is little advantage in combining CBT with pharmacotherapy. Comparisons of CBT with applied relaxation (i.e., Öst & Westling, 1995) indicate that CBT is probably more effective for panic disorder (Siev & Chambless, 2007).

Outcome studies indicate that CBT can be effective for more difficult cases of panic disorder. CBT can produce enduring treatment effects even with comorbid diagnoses, with significant improvement evident in both panic and comorbid symptoms (e.g., Craske et al., 2007; Tsao, Mystkowski, Zucker, & Craske, 2005). In fact Craske and colleagues found more generalized symptom improvement in panic-focused CBT than in a condition in which therapists were allowed to stray onto issues related to the comorbid condition. CBT has also been shown to be effective in drug-refractory individuals with panic disorder (Heldt et al., 2006) and in reducing both day and nighttime panic symptoms in patients with nocturnal panic attacks (Craske et al., 2005). Finally, brief versions of CBT (e.g., intensive 2-day intervention), as well as computerized adaptations, can be highly effective for panic disorder (D. M. Clark et al., 1999; Deacon & Abramowitz, 2006b; Kenardy et al., 2003). Although these findings are preliminary, they do suggest that more efficient and cost-effective cognitive interventions may be available for panic disorder.

CBT Process Studies

Exposure is an important component of cognitive therapy for panic disorder, especially when agoraphobic avoidance is prominent. Given our emphasis on cognitive intervention, how critical is cognitive restructuring to the effectiveness of CBT for panic disorder? In their meta-analysis, Gould et al. (1995) found that cognitive restructuring plus interoceptive exposure (i.e., symptom induction or schema activation) yielded the largest effect sizes, but cognitive restructuring alone produced highly variable results. In an early study Margraf and Schneider (1991) found cognitive restructuring without exposure as effective as pure exposure or combined exposure plus cognitive restructuring.

In a series of multiple baseline single cases Salkovskis et al. (1991) found that two sessions of cognitive restructuring focused on evidence gathering for and against the patient's catastrophic interpretation of physical symptoms produced significant reduction in panic frequency in six out of seven patients, whereas nonfocal treatment had little effect on panic symptoms. In a more recent multivariate time series single-case analysis both cognitive restructuring with empirical hypothesis testing versus exposure alone produced equivalent changes in dysfunctional beliefs and self-efficacy that preceded improvements in panic apprehension (Bouchard et al., 2007). The authors concluded that the findings add to growing empirical evidence that cognitive changes precede improvement in panic symptoms whether treatment is primarily cognitive or behavioral. Other studies have found that exposure alone is as effective as exposure plus cognitive restructuring (Bouchard et al., 1996; Öst, Thulin, & Ramnerö, 2004), although Van den Hout, Arntz, and Hoekstra (1994) found that cognitive therapy alone reduced panic attacks but not agoraphobia. In a recent study of group CBT for panic, 20% of patients experienced a sudden gain (i.e., rapid symptom reduction) after two sessions and this predicted better symptom outcome at posttreatment (Clerkin, Teachman, & Smith-Janik, 2008). Overall, these studies indicate that CBT can produce rapid and effective symptom reduction in panic disorder and that cognitive restructuring is an important component of the treatment package.

The therapeutic effects of cognitive restructuring suggest that targeting the catastrophic misinterpretations of bodily sensations is a central mechanism of change in cognitive therapy of panic disorder. In their clinical trial D. M. Clark at al. (1994) found a significant correlation between BSIQ scores at 6 months and panic symptoms and relapse rates at 15 months. This relation between a continued tendency to misinterpret bodily sensations and worst outcome at follow-up was supported in the authors' outcome study of brief cognitive therapy (D. M. Clark et al., 1999). However, comparison of standard cognitive therapy that focused on interpersonal beliefs relevant to generalized anxiety versus focused cognitive therapy that targeted catastrophic misinterpretations of bodily sensations showed that both were equally effective in reducing panic symptoms, although reduction in panic-related cognitions and beliefs was correlated with changes in panic frequency at termination (Brown, Beck, Newman, Beck, & Tran, 1997). In their descriptive and meta-analytic review of 35 CBT studies on panic disorder, Oei, Llamas, and Devilly (1999) concluded that the therapy is effective for panic disorder and does produce change in cognitive processes, although it is unclear whether change in catastrophic misinterpretations is the central change mechanism in CBT for panic disorder. Overall it would appear that change in catastrophic misinterpretations of the physical symptoms of anxiety is an important part of the treatment process in panic but whether a specific focus on these symptoms is necessary remains unclear.

Clinician Guideline 8.18

Cognitive therapy involving cognitive restructuring, symptom induction, and empirical hypothesis-testing exposure exercises is a well-established empirically based treatment for panic disorder with or without agoraphobic avoidance. Cognitive strategies and exposure-oriented homework are both central ingredients in the treatment's efficacy for panic attacks.

SUMMARY AND CONCLUSION

The problem of recurrent panic attacks provides the clearest example of the cognitive conceptualization of fear. Occurrence of at least two unexpected panic attacks, apprehension or worry about further attacks, and avoidance of situations thought to trigger panic are hallmarks of panic disorder.

A revised cognitive model of panic disorder was presented in Figure 8.1. The essential components of this model are (1) increased attention or hypervigilance for certain physical or mental sensations, (2) activation of physiological or mental threat schemas, (3) the catastrophic misinterpretation of physical symptoms as indicating an imminent dire threat to self, (4) further intensification of the physical symptoms of anxiety, (5) loss of ability to reappraise symptoms in a more realistic, benign manner, and (6) reliance on avoidance and safety seeking to reduce heightened anxiety and terminate the panic episode. Empirical evidence, reviewed for the model's six key hypotheses, found strong support for increased responsiveness to internal states, the activation of prepotent physiological or mental threat schemas, the catastrophic misinterpretation of bodily sensations, and the functional role of avoidance and safety seeking in the persistence of panic attacks.

Table 8.7 summarized the main components of cognitive therapy for panic disorder. Reduction in hypervigilance for feared bodily sensations, reversal of the catastrophic misinterpretation of internal states, increased ability to produce more realistic and balanced reappraisals of the feared symptoms of anxiety, reduction in avoidance and safety seeking, and an increased sense of safety are the primary goals of cognitive therapy. These are achieved using within-session symptom induction to activate threat schemas, cognitive restructuring to weaken catastrophic misinterpretations and improve reappraisal capacity, and systematic situational and interoceptive exposure assignments in a hypothesis-testing context. Over the last two decades a number of well-designed randomized clinical trials have established cognitive therapy as a highly efficacious treatment for panic disorder with or without agoraphobic avoidance.

There are a number of issues that remain for cognitive theory and therapy of panic disorder. Panic disorder is characterized by increased responsiveness to changes in internal state, although the specific processes that contribute to this interoceptive hypersensitivity are not well understood. It is still not clear whether a catastrophic misinterpretation of bodily sensations is necessary for the production of all panic attacks, whether it is a cause or a consequence of repeated panic attacks, and whether the concept should be broadened to include imminent social and emotional threats such as fear of further panic attacks. Moreover, there is insufficient research on whether loss of reappraisal capacity is a major determinant of recurrent panic attacks and the role played by panic self-efficacy or perceived effectiveness in terminating panic episodes. In terms of treatment effectiveness, comparative outcome studies of cognitive therapy versus the newer SSRIs are needed as well as longer follow-up periods to determine the enduring benefits of treatment. Nevertheless, cognitive therapy/CBT is now considered a well-established and efficacious treatment for panic disorder with or without agoraphobia and should be the first-line treatment choice in most cases of the disorder.

APPENDIX 8.1

Weekly Panic and Acute Anxiety Log

Name: _____   Date: _____

Instructions: Please use this form to record any panic attacks, limited panic attacks or acute anxiety episodes that you experienced in the past week. Try to complete the form as close to the anxiety episode as possible in order to increase the accuracy of your remarks.

Date, Time, and Duration of Episode	Situational Triggers (Label E or UE)*	Severity/Intensity of Anxiety (0–100); (Label FPA, LPA, AAE)*	Description of the Anxious Physical or Mental Sensations	Anxious Interpretation of the Sensations	Evidence for an Alternative Interpretation of Sensations	Outcome (Coping Responses and Sense of Safety)+
1.						
2.						
3.						
4.						
5.						

* E = expected to have panic in this situation; UE = panic occurred unexpectedly, completely out of the blue; FPA = full-blown panic attack; LPA = limited symptom attack; AAE = acute anxiety episode (sudden onset of anxiety but not panic)

+ rate sense of safety after panic ceases from 0 = don't feel at all safe from panic to 100 = feel absolutely safe from further panic

Symptom Reappraisal Form

Name: _____ Date: _____

Instructions: Please use this form to write down any alternative explanations you can think for why you are experiencing a variety of physical sensations that make you feel anxious or panicky.

State the Physical Sensation Experienced (e.g., racing heart, breathlessness, nausea)	List a Number of Alternative Explanations for the Sensations Other Than the Worst Outcome (i.e., the feared catastrophe)	Rate Belief in Each Explanation When Not Anxious (0–100)*	Rate Belief in Each Explanation When in Anxious State (0–100)*	Effectiveness of Explanation in Countering Anxiety (0–100)+
1.				
2.				
3.				
4.				
5.				

* For belief ratings, 0 = absolutely no belief in the explanation, 100 = absolutely certain that this is the cause of the physical sensations.

+ For effectiveness ratings, 0 = explanation has absolutely no positive effect on anxiety, 100 = explanation is completely effective in eliminating anxious feelings.

Vicious Cycle of Panic

Name: _____   Date: _____

Situational Triggers
1. _____
2. _____
3. _____

⬇

Initial Physical, Mental, Emotional Symptoms
1. _____
2. _____
3. _____

⬇

First Anxious (Apprehensive) Thoughts/Images
1. _____
2. _____
3. _____

⬇

Main Escalating Symptoms
1. _____
2. _____

⬇

Thoughts/Images of Imminent Danger (catastrophe)
_____
_____
_____

Attempts to Cope/Control
_____
_____
_____

→ **PANIC**

Chapter 9

Cognitive Therapy of Social Phobia

Nothing so much prevents our being natural
as the desire to seem so.
—FRANÇOIS, DUC DE LA ROCHEFOUCAULD
(French writer and aristocrat, 1613–1680)

Gerald is a 36-year-old man who has worked as an accountant for a large multinational trucking firm for the past 12 years and who has a long history of severe social anxiety. SCID assessment revealed that he met DSM-IV diagnostic criteria for generalized social phobia. He reported intense anxiety in most social situations with an overwhelming fear that other people will notice him. His main concern was that they would notice that he was hot and flushed and would think "What's wrong with him?", "He doesn't look normal," and "He must have low self-esteem or some serious mental problem." Gerald believed that people "could look right through him" and so he was always hypervigilant when around others. He was also concerned that others would think he was boring and wasting their time. Gerald noted that he is almost always anxious when around other people and recognized that his anxiety is excessive. Over the years he got to the point where he avoids social contact as much as possible, spending most of his time outside of work alone and isolated. He has never had an intimate relationship and no close friends. He prefers to avoid people because of the anxiety and a fear that social interaction will result in obligations to others even though he realizes the avoidance has been detrimental to his career. A year ago he joined a health club for a few months but found it too anxiety-provoking to attend. Gerald rated participating in meetings, taking a course, meeting an unfamiliar person, answering the telephone, taking public transportation, or even visiting an acquaintance as very anxiety-provoking. Gerald indicated that he has been socially anxious since childhood and that it has severely limited his life. In fact the anxiety and self-imposed loneliness have been so great that he commented "I'm tired of waiting for life to start; sometimes I just want to get it over with."

Gerald's clinical presentation is fairly typical of someone with a chronic and severe generalized social phobia. In fact he met criteria for an Axis II avoidant personality disorder as indicated by (1) his attempt to avoid signifi-

332

cant interpersonal contact at work (he would start work at 7:00 A.M. and quit at 2:00 P.M. in order to minimize contact with others), (2) unwillingness to get involved with people, (3) fear of intimate relationships, (4) inhibition in new interpersonal relationships because of inadequacy feelings, (5) perceived inferiority to others, and (6) reluctance to engage in any new, even relatively mundane, social activities for fear of embarrassment. Gerald received 19 sessions of cognitive therapy that focused specifically on his social evaluative anxiety, inhibitory behavior, and extreme avoidance. Therapy targeted Gerald's maladaptive beliefs about negative social evaluation by others, his reliance on escape and avoidance to manage anxiety, and graded *in vivo* exposure to moderately anxious social situations.

This chapter presents the cognitive theory and treatment of generalized social phobia as first described in Beck et al. (1985, 2005). We begin with a discussion of the diagnostic and phenomenological characteristics of social phobia. This is followed by a description of a more elaborated cognitive theory of social phobia as well as a review of its empirical support. We then propose a cognitive approach to assessment and treatment of social phobia. The chapter concludes with a review of the empirical status of cognitive therapy and CBT for generalized social phobia.

DIAGNOSTIC CONSIDERATIONS

Diagnostic Overview

The core feature of social phobia is a "marked and persistent fear of social or performance situations in which embarrassment may occur" (DSM-IV-TR; APA, 2000, p. 450). Although anxious feelings are common to most people when they enter novel, unfamiliar, or social-evaluative situations like a job interview, the person with social phobia invariably experiences intense fear or dread, even when anticipating the possibility of exposure to various common social situations. The anxiety stems from a fear of scrutiny and negative evaluation from others that will lead to feelings of embarrassment, humiliation, and shame (Beck et al., 1985, 2005). The perceived cause of the embarrassment usually centers on some aspect of self-presentation such as exhibiting a symptom(s) of anxiety, speaking awkwardly, making a mistake, or acting in some other humiliating manner (Heckelman & Schneier, 1995). As a result the person with social phobia tends to be highly self-conscious and self-critical in the feared social situation, often exhibiting involuntary inhibitory behaviors such as appearing stiff and rigid or being verbally inarticulate, which results in detrimental social performance and the unwanted attention of others.

Social phobia is closely related to simple phobia because the fear occurs only in situations in which the person must do something in the context of being observed and possibly evaluated by others (Hofmann & Barlow, 2002). The person with social phobia who experiences intense anxiety while eating, speaking, or writing in front of unfamiliar people has no difficulty engaging in these behaviors when alone or with family and close friends. Although Marks and Gelder (1966) first described the syndrome of social phobia (see also Marks, 1970), it was not until DSM-III (American Psychiatric Association, 1980) that it was incorporated as a separate diagnostic entity. The core diagnostic criteria have remained constant throughout subsequent DSM revisions with the exception that a generalized subtype of social phobia was introduced in DSM-III-R (American Psychiatric Association, 1987) and the exclusionary rule for avoidant personality disorder was removed. Although an alternate label, *social anxiety disorder,* has been recommended (Liebowitz, Heimberg, Fresco, Travers, & Stein, 2000), we retain use of the term "social phobia" because it captures the strong urge to avoid anxiety-provoking situations that is the hallmark of the disorder. Table 9.1 presents the DSM-IV-TR diagnostic criteria for social phobia.

Fear of Negative Evaluation

Fear of negative evaluation by others is a core feature of social phobia that is not only recognized in cognitive models of the disorder (Beck et al., 1985, 2005; D. M. Clark, 2001; Rapee & Heimberg, 1997; Wells & Clark, 1997), but it is the basis of the marked and persistent fear in social evaluative situations described in DSM-IV-TR Criterion A. Individuals with social phobia may hold excessively high standards of social performance, wanting to make a particular impression on others but doubting their ability to actually make a positive impression (Beck et al., 1985, 2005; Hofmann & Barlow, 2002). They also believe they draw the attention of others in social situations and live in fear that in this social evaluative context they will embarrass or humiliate themselves

---

TABLE 9.1. DSM-IV-TR Diagnostic Criteria for Social Phobia

A. A marked and persistent fear of one or more social or performance situations in which the person is exposed to unfamiliar people or to possible scrutiny by others. The individual fears that he or she will act in a way (or show anxiety symptoms) that will be humiliating or embarrassing.

B. Exposure to the feared social situation almost invariably provokes anxiety, which may take the form of a situationally bound or situationally predisposed Panic Attack.

C. The person recognizes that the fear is excessive or unreasonable.

D. The feared social or performance situations are avoided or else are endured with intense anxiety or distress.

E. The avoidance, anxious anticipation, or distress in the feared social or performance situation(s) interferes significantly with the person's normal routine, occupational (academic) functioning, or social activities or relationships, or there is marked distress about having the phobia.

F. In individuals under 18 years of age, the duration is at least 6 months.

G. The fear or avoidance is not due to the direct physiological effects of a substance (e.g., drug of abuse, medication), or a general medical condition, and is not better accounted for by another mental disorder (e.g., Panic Disorder With or Without Agoraphobia, Separation Anxiety Disorder, Body Dysmorphic Disorder, a Pervasive Developmental Disorder, or Schizoid Personality Disorder).

H. If a medical condition or another mental disorder is present, the fear in Criterion A is unrelated to it (e. g., the fear is not of Stuttering, trembling in Parkinson's disease, or exhibiting abnormal eating behavior in Anorexia Nervosa or Bulimia Nervosa).

Specify if:

Generalized: if the fears include most social situations (also consider the additional diagnosis of Avoidant Personality Disorder)

Note. From American Psychiatric Association (2000). Copyright 2000 by the American Psychiatric Association. Reprinted by permission.

by acting or appearing foolish, less intelligent, or visibly anxious (Beidel & Turner, 2007). There is considerable empirical evidence that fear of negative evaluation is a core feature of social phobia (e.g., Ball et al., 1995; Hackmann et al., 1998; Hirsch & Clark, 2004; Mansell & Clark, 1999; Voncken, et al., 2003). However, individuals with social phobia may fear any social evaluation, either positive or negative, that involves feelings of conspicuousness or self-consciousness (Weeks, Heimberg, Rodebaugh, & Norton, 2008). Moreover, the negative evaluation feared by those with social phobia is not simply some mildly negative impression on others but a much more extreme experience of dreaded humiliation or shame (Beck et al., 1985, 2005). Shame is a painful affect in which personal attributes, characteristics, or behavior are perceived as causing a loss of social standing or attractiveness to others, or even worse, their outright criticism or rejection (Gilbert, 2000).

Social Situations

The majority of individuals with social phobia experience marked anxiety in a variety of social situations (Rapee, Sanderson, & Barlow, 1988; Turner, Beidel, Dancu, & Keys, 1986). Rachman (2004) noted that the most common situations feared in social phobia are public speaking, attendance at parties or meetings, and speaking to authority figures. Beidel and Turner (2007) reported that formal speaking (the most distressing situation), parties, initiating and maintaining conversations, and informal speaking and meetings were rated as distressing and avoided by more than 75% of patients with social phobia. Dating was rated as distressing and something avoided by half of the sample, whereas eating and drinking in public, using public washrooms, and writing in public was feared by 25% or less of social phobic individuals. The anxiety-provoking situations in social phobia have been categorized as those dealing with social interaction versus those concerned with performance (Rapee, 1995b). Table 9.2 presents a list of interpersonal and performance situations from Antony and Swinson (2000b) that are rated for level of fear and avoidance when assessing social phobia.

TABLE 9.2. Common Interpersonal and Performance Situations Feared in Social Phobia

Interpersonal situations	Performance situations
• Initiating a date or appointment with someone • Being introduced to unfamiliar person • Attending a party or social gathering • Having friend for dinner • Starting a conversation • Talking on phone to a familiar person • Talking on phone to an unfamiliar person • Expressing your personal opinion to others • Having job interview • Being assertive with others • Returning a purchased item • Making eye contact • Expressing dissatisfaction with restaurant food • Talking to authority figures	• Making a toast or speech • Speaking in meetings • Playing sports in front of an audience • Participating in a wedding party or public ceremony • Singing/performing to an audience • Eating/drinking in a public setting • Using public washrooms • Writing in front of others • Making a mistake in public (e.g., mispronouncing a word) • Walking/running in busy public place • Introducing yourself to others • Shopping in a busy store • Walking in front of a large group of people (e.g., walking up aisle of church, theater)

Note. Based on Antony and Swinson (2000b).

Anxious Arousal and Panic

The second diagnostic criterion in DSM-IV-TR is that exposure to the feared social situation will invariably provoke anxiety, which may involve a situationally bound or situationally predisposed panic attack (American Psychiatric Association, 2000). Individuals with social phobia often experience panic attacks when in feared social situations or even when anticipating a social event (Kendler, Neale, Kessler, Heath, & Eaves, 1992c). Although the physical symptoms of these situationally triggered attacks are identical to those in panic disorder (Beidel & Turner, 2007), physical symptoms of anxiety that can be observed by others, such as twitching muscles or blushing, may be more prominent in the anxiety experienced in social phobia (Amies, Gelder, & Shaw, 1983). Furthermore, individuals with social phobia experience greater physiological arousal during exposure to a distressing social situation than nonphobic individuals (e.g., Turner et al., 1986). It is little wonder that fear of having a panic attack in a social situation is a major concern of many people with social phobia (Hofmann, Ehlers, & Roth, 1995). In fact fear of losing control over any emotional responses, especially anxiety symptoms, is a critical aspect of the perceived social threat (Hofmann, 2005). Even though fear of anxiety is common across the anxiety disorders, it is particularly germane to social phobia because any display of anxiety in social settings is perceived to increase the likelihood of negative evaluation by others.

Awareness, Avoidance, and Inhibition

To meet DSM-IV-TR diagnostic criteria for social phobia, the person must have some awareness of the excessive or unreasonable nature of her social fears (i.e., Criterion C). This criterion helps distinguish social phobia from other diagnoses such as paranoid personality disorder in which the person actually believes others are trying to embarrass or humiliate him (Beidel & Turner, 2007).

Given the experience of intense anxiety when anticipating or entering feared social situations, the urge to avoid social situations can be intense in social phobia. Compared to other anxiety disorders, individuals with social phobia are more likely to engage in avoidance of social situations even though they may be convinced it is detrimental for them (i.e., Rapee, Sanderson, & Barlow, 1988). Assessment of the frequency and extent of avoidance associated with various social evaluative situations (see Table 9.2) is an important part of the diagnostic assessment of social phobia (Hope, Laguna, Heimberg, & Barlow, 1996–1997).

Individuals with social phobia are highly inhibited when encountering social interactions. They often appear rigid and stiff, their face taut with forced expression. When trying to speak they can appear inarticulate because of stumbling over their words, being "tongue-tied," or having difficulty thinking of the right word. All of these involuntary behaviors are detrimental to their performance and increase the probability of a negative evaluation by others—the very essence of their social anxiety.

Individuals with social phobia also rely on subtle avoidance or safety behaviors in an attempt to conceal their anxiety which they assume will cause others to evaluate them negatively (Beck et al., 1985; Wells & Clark, 1997). Individuals with social phobia may try to conceal their anxiety by avoiding eye contact or trying to keep physically cool so that one's face does not look red or flushed, wearing certain clothes or makeup to hide blushing, give an excuse for one's red face by blaming it on a hot room or not feeling well, or the like (D. M. Clark, 2001). These concealment strategies (i.e., safety behaviors) are problematic because they can directly exacerbate anxious symptoms (e.g., person wears a heavy sweater to conceal sweating but this raises body temperature and tendency to sweat). In addition the behaviors prevent disconfirmation of the feared outcome (e.g., attributes nonoccurrence of negative evaluation to performance of the safety behavior), maintain a heightened self-focused attention, and draw greater negative attention from others (Wells & Clark, 1997). There is some evidence that socially anxious individuals realize the negative social effects of trying to conceal anxiety (Voncken, Alden, & Bögels, 2006) but still tend to engage in safety behaviors (Alden & Bieling,1998).

Marked Distress and Interference

Anxiety or nervousness in social situations is common in the general population. In a randomized community telephone survey of 526 adults, 61% reported feeling nervous or uncomfortable in at least one of seven social situations with public speaking being the most frequently endorsed situation (Stein, Walker, & Forde, 1994). Thus the marked distress or interference criterion in DSM-IV-TR is needed to distinguish the more severe, clinical forms of social phobia disorders from the milder subclinical variants of social anxiety found throughout the nonclinical population (Heckelman & Schneier, 1995).

Clinician Guideline 9.1

Social phobia is characterized by a marked and persistent anxiety, even panic, most often across numerous interpersonal and/or performance situations in which the person fears scrutiny and negative evaluation by others that will lead to embarrassment, humiliation, or shame. A key concern is that one's interpersonal behavior, appearance, or expression of anxiety will be negatively judged by others. Anticipatory anxiety can be intense, leading to extensive avoidance of feared social situations, as well as production of involuntary inhibitory responses and attempts to conceal anxiety when social interaction is unavoidable.

Shyness and Social Phobia

There is considerable confusion about the relationship between shyness and social phobia, with some emphasizing their common characteristics of high social anxiety and fear of negative evaluation by others (Stravynski, 2007), whereas others note there are important quantitative differences so that the two should not be considered synonymous (Bruch & Cheek, 1995). Like social phobia, shyness has been described as anxiety, discomfort, and inhibition in social situations and fear of negative evaluation by others, especially authority figures (Heiser, Turner, & Beidel, 2003). Some have concluded that social phobia is very similar to chronic shyness (Henderson & Zimbardo, 2001; Marshall & Lipsett, 1994). Moreover, delineating clear boundaries between shyness and social phobia has been difficult because (1) there is no consensus on the definition of shyness; (2) they have many shared behavioral, cognitive, and physiological features; (3) they arise from different research traditions with shyness studied by social, personality, and counseling psychologists whereas social phobia is a research topic in clinical psychology; and (4) their differences may be more quantitative than qualitative in nature (Bruch & Cheek, 1995; Heckelman & Schneier, 1995; Rapee, 1995b).

Shyness is a normal personality trait that involves some degree of nervousness, inhibition, and self-consciousness in social interaction. Butler (2007) described shyness as a sense of shrinking back from social encounters and retreating into one's self due to physical discomfort (e.g., tension, sweating, trembling), feeling anxious, inhibition, or inability to express yourself, and excessive self-focused attention. Zimbardo defined shyness as "a heightened state of individuation characterized by excessive egocentric preoccupation and overconcern with social evaluation … with the consequence that the shy person inhibits, withdraws, avoids, and escapes" (cited in Henderson & Zimbardo, 2001, p. 48). Despite the similarities with social phobia, there are important differences. Compared to social phobia, shyness is much more pervasive in the general population, it may be less chronic or enduring, it is associated with less avoidance and functional impairment, and shy individuals may be more able to engage in social interaction when necessary (Beidel & Turner, 2007; Bruch & Cheek, 1995).

Table 9.3 presents some important differences between shyness and social phobia (Turner, Beidel, & Townsley, 1990).

Social phobia is undoubtedly a more severe condition than shyness, with severe and pervasive avoidance of social situations being one of the most important distinctions. Although the differences are more quantitative than qualitative in nature (Rapee, 1995b), Beidel and Turner (2007) concluded in their review that social phobia should not be considered an extreme form of shyness. Studies that have directly compared prevalence of shyness and social phobia confirm the distinctiveness of the two syndromes. Chavira, Stein, and Malcane (2002) found that only 36% of individuals who had high levels of shyness met criteria for generalized social phobia compared to 4% of individuals with average or normative shyness. In another study only 17.7% of shy university students met diagnostic criteria for social phobia (Heiser et al., 2003) and analysis of the NCS data set revealed a lifetime prevalence for social phobia of 28% for women and 21% for men who reported excessive childhood shyness (Cox, MacPherson, & Enns, 2005). Conversely only 51% of women and 41% of men with lifetime complex (generalized) social phobia had excessive childhood shyness. Together these findings

TABLE 9.3. **Distinguishing Features of Shyness and Social Phobia**

Shyness	Social phobia
• Normal personality trait	• Psychiatric disorder
• Primarily social inhibition and reticence	• Presence of marked anxiety, even panic, in social evaluative situations
• Can socially engage when necessary	• More likely to exhibit poor social performance
• Less likely to avoid social situations	• Avoidance of social situations more frequent and pervasive
• Highly prevalent in population	• Lower prevalence rate
• More transitory course for many individuals	• Longer duration, more chronic, and unremitting
• Earlier onset perhaps in preschool years	• Later onset in early to midadolescence
• Less impairment in daily living	• Greater social and occupational impairment

indicate that shyness and social phobia, though significantly related, can not be considered synonymous.

Social Phobia Subtypes: Generalized versus Specific

DSM-IV-TR (APA, 2000) allows for the distinction between a generalized and a specific or circumscribed subtype of social phobia. Unfortunately the criteria for making this distinction are not at all clear. Generalized social phobia (GSP) can be specified when individuals fear most social situations including both public performance and social interaction situations. However, the number of feared situations needed to qualify for GSP is not stated. The "specific subtype" of social phobia is even less clearly defined. DSM-IV-TR states that this subtype may be quite heterogeneous including people who fear just a single performance situation (i.e., public speaking) as well as those who fear most performance situations but not social interaction situations. In their prospective community study, Wittchen, Stein, and Kessler (1999) reported a lifetime prevalence of 5.1% for specific social phobia and 2.2% for GSP among 14- to 24-year-old, with the specific subtype mostly characterized by fears of test performance and speaking in front of people.

There is considerable debate in the literature on the validity of the generalized versus specific distinction in social phobia. Not only are the DSM-IV-TR descriptions of generalized and specific social phobia ambiguous, but researchers employ different definitions of the specific subtype from reserving the term for fear of public speaking only to a broader definition that includes fear of multiple situations within one social domain such as social performance situations only (see Hofmann & Barlow, 2002). Furthermore, a more fundamental problem for subtyping is that social phobia appears to lie on a continuum of severity with no clear-cut boundaries to delineate subtypes. Taxometric analyses indicate that social anxiety favors a dimensional model of severity (Kollman, Brown, Liverant, & Hofmann, 2006) and community-based studies have failed to find a clear demarcation of subtypes based on the number of feared social situations (e.g., Stein, Torgrud, & Walker, 2000; Vriends, Becker, Meyer, Michael, & Margraf, 2007a). These findings suggest that the generalized distinction may be confounded with symptom severity so that the specifier may be arbitrarily selecting out the most severe on the social anxiety continuum.

Others, however, have argued that specifying a generalized subtype is a clinically useful distinction. The majority of individuals with social phobia who seek treatment will meet criteria for the generalized subtype (see Beidel & Turner, 2007; e.g., Kollman et al., 2006), whereas specific social phobia may be more prevalent in community samples (Wittchen et al., 1999). In addition GSP is associated with greater symptom severity, depression, avoidance, and fear of negative evaluation, as well as greater functional impairment, earlier onset, greater chronicity, and increased rate of comorbid Axis I and II diagnoses (e.g., Herbert, Hope, & Bellack, 1992; Holt, Heimberg, & Hope, 1992; Kessler, Stein, & Berglund, 1998; Mannuzza et al., 1995; Turner, Beidel, & Townsley, 1992; Wittchen et al., 1999). Overall, the findings indicate that the generalized versus specific subtype of social phobia is really capturing a severity distinction based on the number of feared social situations, with GSP the more severe form of social phobia that is most often seen in treatment settings. For this reason the cognitive perspective described in this chapter is most relevant to GSP.

Clinician Guideline 9.2

Rather than forming distinct subtypes, social phobia varies along a continuum of severity with milder forms involving fear of a limited range of social situations and more severe, generalized social phobia characterized by fear of a wider number of both social interaction and performance situations.

Social Phobia and Avoidant Personality Disorder

A high degree of diagnostic overlap exists between GSP and avoidant personality disorder (APD) which has led researchers to question whether they really are two separate conditions as currently described in DSM-IV (Sanderson, Wetzler, Beck, & Betz, 1994; Tyrer, Gunderson, Lyons, & Tohen, 1997; van Velzen, Emmelkamp, & Scholing, 2000; Widiger, 1992). As can be seen from the diagnostic criteria for APD in Table 9.4, both GSP and APD share much in common because essentially both are characterized by a pervasive pattern of discomfort, inhibition, and fear of negative evaluation across a variety of social or interpersonal contexts (Heimberg, 1996).

In his review Heimberg (1996) concluded that approximately 60% of individuals with GSP will meet criteria for APD compared with 20% of nongeneralized social phobias. Moreover, almost all individuals with APD will meet diagnostic criteria for social phobia (Brown, Heimberg, & Juster, 1995; Herbert et al., 1992; Turner et al., 1992). Given this close relationship between GSP and APD, an assessment for APD should be made whenever individuals meet diagnostic criteria for social phobia.

Comparison of the clinical presentation between GSP with and without APD have generally revealed that those with GSP and APD have greater symptom severity, diagnostic comobidity, functional impairment, social skills deficiencies, and possibly less motivation and response to CBT (e.g., Holt et al., 1992; van Velzen et al., 2000; see also Beidel & Turner, 2007; Heimberg, 1996). More recently Chambless, Fydrich, and

---

TABLE 9.4. DSM-IV-TR Diagnostic Criteria for Avoidant Personality Disorder

A pervasive pattern of social inhibition, feelings of inadequacy, and hypersensitivity to negative evaluation, beginning by early adulthood and present in a variety of contexts, as indicated by four (or more) of the following:

(1) avoids occupational activities that involve significant interpersonal contact, because of fears of criticism, disapproval, or rejection

(2) is unwilling to get involved with people unless certain of being liked

(3) shows restraint within intimate relationships because of the fear of being shamed or ridiculed

(4) is preoccupied with being criticized or rejected in social situations

(5) is inhibited in new interpersonal situations because of feelings of inadequacy

(6) views self as socially inept, personally unappealing, or inferior to others

(7) is unusually reluctant to take personal risks or to engage in any new activities because they may prove embarrassing

Note. From American Psychiatric Association (2000). Copyright 2000 by the American Psychiatric Association. Reprinted by permission.

Rodebaugh (2006) found that GSP with APD was characterized by a more severe form of social phobia and poorer social skills compared to GSP without APD, with low self-esteem in the APD group the only qualitative difference. The authors concluded that DSM-IV APD should be considered a severe form of GSP rather than a separate diagnosis.

Beidel and Turner (2007) raise a number of treatment implications that may argue for the clinical utility of retaining the APD diagnosis. They note that individuals with APD may have less tolerance for exposure-based treatment and so a more gradual approach may be necessary. They also indicate that individuals with APD may have more social skills deficits and lower social/occupational functioning, thereby making social skills training an essential treatment ingredient when APD is present. Despite these clinical observations, the empirical research to date suggests that social anxiety should be conceptualized as a continuum of severity with specific or circumscribed social phobia at the milder end, GSP without APD in the moderate range, and GSP with APD the most severe form of the disorder (McNeil, 2001).

Clinician Guideline 9.3

Avoidant personality disorder (APD) is a severe form of GSP associated with greater psychopathology and functional impairment. Given the treatment complications that may be associated with this diagnosis, include an assessment of APD in the diagnostic protocol for social phobia.

EPIDEMIOLOGY AND CLINICAL FEATURES

Prevalence

Social phobia is the most common of the anxiety disorders and third most common over all mental disorders. The NCS employed DSM-III-R criteria for social phobia and found that 12-month prevalence was 7.9% and lifetime prevalence was 13.3% (Kessler et al., 1994). Moreover, approximately two-thirds of these individuals had GSP, with the remainder having purely speaking fears that were less persistent and impairing (Kessler et al., 1998). The more recent NCS-R based on DSM-IV diagnostic criteria reported a 12-month prevalence of 6.8% and lifetime prevalence of 12.1% for social phobia (Kessler, Berglund, et al., 2005; Kessler, Chiu, et al., 2005). The high prevalence for social phobia has been found in other epidemiological and large community studies (e.g., Newman et al., 1996). There is also some evidence that the incidence of social phobia may be increasing over time (Rapee & Spence, 2004).

As noted previously, milder forms of social anxiety are more prevalent in the general population than social phobia. Social inhibition, fear of negative evaluation, anxiousness, and feelings of inadequacy when in social situations are reported to occur occasionally to moderately often by the majority of nonclinical individuals. Moreover, fear and avoidance of social situations is common in panic disorder, GAD, and agoraphobia (Rapee et al., 1988). What distinguishes social phobia is the number of social situations feared and the degree of functional impairment (Rapee et al., 1988; Stein et al., 2000).

Gender and Cross-Cultural Differences

Unlike the other anxiety disorders, the gender ratio for social phobia is not as highly skewed toward women. There is an approximate 3:2 ratio of women to men with social phobia. In the NCS the lifetime prevalence for women was 15% and for men 11.1% (Kessler et al., 1994). However, Rapee (1995b) notes that an equal number of men and women seek treatment for social phobia, although nonclinical questionnaire studies suggest women may feel greater social anxiety and shyness than men (e.g., Wittchen et al., 1999). Cross-cultural differences may also be apparent in the gender ratio for social phobia. In a study conducted on a Turkish sample of 87 individuals with DSM-III-R social phobia, 78.2% were men (Gökalp et al., 2001).

Cross-national differences have also been reported in the prevalence of DSM-III or DSM-IV social phobia. In the Cross-National Epidemiological Surveys there was a fourfold increase of social phobia in English-speaking Western countries compared to East Asian countries like Taiwan and South Korea (see Chapman, Mannuzza, & Fyer, 1995). The authors question whether this reflects real differences in the rates of social phobia across cultures. They note that the interview questions may have lacked cultural relevance outside Western countries. Also there are conditions analogous to social phobia that are specific to certain Asian countries that were not included in the survey such as "taijin kyofu-sho" (TKS) in Japan, which is a persistent and irrational fear of causing offense, embarrassment, or harm to others because of some personal inadequacy or shortcoming (Chapman et al., 1995).

Even within Western countries where rates of social phobia may be quite similar, the clinical presentation of the disorder can be affected by cultural factors. For example, a study that compared social phobia in American, Swedish, and Australian samples found that the Swedish sample was significantly more fearful of eating/drinking in public, writing in public, meetings, and speaking to authority figures (Heimberg, Makris, Juster, Öst, & Rapee, 1997). Thus social phobia may be found in most countries around the world but the social concerns, symptom presentation, and even threshold for disorder may vary across cultures (Hofmann & Barlow, 2002; Rapee & Spence, 2004). As well, the mediating variables for social anxiety may differ between cultures. For example, shame has a stronger mediating role in social anxiety for Chinese than American samples (Zhong et al., 2008).

Age of Onset and Course

Social phobia typically begins in early to mid-adolescence which gives it a later onset than specific phobias but an earlier onset than panic disorder (Öst, 1987b; Rapee, 1995a). In the NCS-R, 13 years old was the median age of onset for social phobia which was substantially younger than the onset age for panic disorder, GAD, PTSD, and OCD (Kessler, Berglund, et al., 2005). In fact many individuals with social phobia report a lifelong struggle, with 50–80% reporting an onset of the disorder in childhood (Otto et al., 2001; Stemberger, Turner, Beidel, & Calhoun, 1995). Early onset is associated with a more chronic and severe course of the disorder (Beidel & Turner, 2007).

It is commonly believed that untreated social phobia takes a chronic and unremitting course (Beidel & Turner, 2007; Hofmann & Barlow, 2002; Rapee, 1995b). This appears to be supported by a number of longitudinal studies in which the majority of individuals with social phobia report a chronic course that can last for years, if not decades (Chartier, Hazen, & Stein, 1998; Keller, 2003; see Vriends et al., 2007b, for contrary findings). As with other disorders, it is likely that a greater preponderance of those with the more chronic form of social phobia will be represented among treatment seekers.

A number of variables predict chronicity in social phobia. Presence of a comorbid personality disorder, especially APD, is associated with a lower probability of remission (Massion et al., 2002), and the generalized subtype of social phobia is characterized by greater chronicity. Consistent with other anxiety disorders, greater symptom severity and psychopathology as well as increased functional impairment is associated with a more enduring and stable course of social phobia (e.g., Chartier et al., 1998; Vriends et al., 2007b).

Detrimental Effects of Social Phobia

Social phobia is associated with lower educational attainment, lost work productivity, lack of career advancement, higher rates of financial dependency, and severe impairment in social functioning (e.g., Keller, 2003; Schneier, Johnson, Hornig, Liebowitz, & Weissman 1992; Simon et al., 2002; Turner, Beidel, Dancu, & Keys, 1986; Zhang, Ross, & Davidson, 2004). In the NCS individuals with social phobia reported significantly more role impairment than those with agoraphobia but fewer days absent from work (Magee, Eaton, Wittchen, McGonagle, & Kessler, 1996). As with the other anxiety disorders social phobia with comorbid anxiety (e.g., panic, GAD) or depression has greater functional impairment (Magee et al., 1996).

Individuals with social phobia also judge their quality of life to be significantly poorer than nonclinical individuals (Safren, Heimberg, Brown, & Holle, 1996–1997). A meta-analysis of quality of life in the anxiety disorders revealed that social phobia had similar negative effects on social, work, and family/home as panic disorder and OCD (Olatunji et al., 2007). In sum, social phobia is a serious mental disorder that can have enduring negative effects on life satisfaction and daily living.

Treatment Delay and Service Utilization

Despite many negative effects of the disorder, individuals with social phobia have some of the lowest rates of treatment utilization of the anxiety disorders. The vast majority of individuals with social phobia never seek treatment for their condition. In the NCS individuals with social phobia had lower rates of seeking professional help than those with simple phobia or agoraphobia (Magee et al., 1996). Moreover, only 24.7% of individuals who met DSM-IV criteria for social phobia in the NCS-R made at least one visit to a mental health specialist in a 12-month period (Wang, Lane, et al., 2005). In the same study, the median duration of delay in first treatment contact was 16 years for social phobia, a length of delay that was substantially longer than those for panic disorder, GAD, PTSD, or major depression (Wang, Berglund, et al., 2005). They also make fewer general medical visits than individuals with panic disorder (Deacon et al., 2008). In sum individuals with social phobia are less likely to seek treatment and the minority who do eventually make an initial contact only after many years with the disorder. Furthermore, social phobia tends to go undetected by physicians and other health professionals, thereby compounding the problem of low service utilization (Wagner, Silvoe, Marnane, & Rouen, 2006). In fact analysis of the NCS-R data set also confirms that the disorder is undertreated, with some evidence that those who have the greatest need for treatment are least likely to receive it (Ruscio, Brown, et al., 2007).

Clinician Guideline 9.4

Social phobia is the most prevalent of the anxiety disorders, affecting slightly more women than men, with cultural differences in rate and clinical presentation. The disorder commonly arises in late childhood or adolescence and takes a chronic and unremitting course that results in significant decrement in social and occupational functioning. Despite these negative effects, individuals typically delay seeking treatment.

Comorbidity

Social phobia can be difficult to distinguish from other anxiety disorders because social anxiety is a common symptom in all the anxiety disorders and comobidity rates are high in those with a principal diagnosis of social phobia (Turner & Beidel, 1989). Rapee et al. (1988) found that 80% of individuals with panic disorder, GAD, or simple phobia reported at least slight fear in one or more social situations and over 50% reported moderate fear and avoidance. At the same time, rates of more serious secondary social phobia that meet diagnostic criteria are high among those with another primary anxiety disorder or major depression. In the large clinical study by Brown et al. (2001), secondary social phobia was present in large numbers of patients with panic disorder (23%), GAD (42%), OCD (35%), specific phobia (27%), PTSD (41%), and major depression (43%).

The comorbidity rate for those with a principal diagnosis of social phobia appears similar to the overall rates found in the other anxiety disorders. Lifetime rates of comorbid disorder range from 69 to 88% (Brown et al., 2001; Kessler, Berglund, et al., 2005; Schneier et al., 1992; Wittchen et al., 1999), with approximately three-quarters of individuals with social phobia currently meeting criteria for another major disorder. In most cases social phobia precedes onset of the other disorder (e.g., Brown et al., 2001; Schneier et al., 1992) and is associated with greater functional impairment than uncomplicated cases of social phobia (Wittchen et al., 1999).

The highest rates of comorbid conditions in social phobia are major depression, substance abuse, GAD, and, to a lesser extent, panic disorder. In the NCS, 56.9% of individuals with social phobia had a comorbid anxiety disorder, the most common being simple phobia (37.6%), agoraphobia (23.2%), and GAD (13.3%) (Magee et al., 1996). Major depression occurred in 37.2% and substance abuse in 39.6% of social phobia cases. In the NCS-R social phobia correlated most highly with GAD, PTSD, major depression, attention-deficit/hyperactivity disorder, and drug dependence (Kessler, Chiu, et al., 2005).

One might expect high rates of alcohol consumption in social phobia as a form of self-medication (Rapee, 1995b), but findings from the epidemiological studies suggest the rates of comorbid substance disorder are no greater in social phobia than in the other anxiety disorders or major depression (Grant et al., 2004). However, in a recent review Morris, Stewart, and Ham (2005) concluded that individuals with generalized social phobia have high rates of comorbid alcohol use disorders that may be linked to fears of negative evaluation and expectancies that alcohol will reduce social anxiety.

Given the significant decline in function associated with social phobia, a large number of individuals with social phobia also develop major depression as well as elevated rates of suicidal ideation and attempts (Schneier et al., 1992). In fact both simple (24.3%) and social phobia (27.1%) had the highest lifetime rates of secondary major depression within the anxiety disorders in the NCS, with the occurrence of major depression approximately 11.9 years after the onset of social phobia (Kessler et al., 1996). Finally, Axis II disorders are commonly associated with social phobia, the most frequent being APD, although elevated rates of dependent and obsessive–compulsive personality disorders have also been reported (see Beidel & Turner, 2007; Heimberg & Becker, 2002; Turner, Beidel, Borden, Stanley, & Jacobs, 1991).

According to DSM-IV-TR, a diagnosis of social phobia is not made when the social anxiety and avoidance concern the potential embarrassment arising from a general medical condition such as tremors due to Parkinson's disease, facial scarring, obesity, stuttering, or the like (APA, 2000). However, this prohibition may be too stringent. Stein, Baird, and Walker (1996), for example, found that 44% of patients seeking treatment for stuttering met diagnostic criteria for social phobia when the diagnosis was made only when the social anxiety was in excess to the severity of their dysfluency. Thus a careful assessment of the context and severity of the social anxiety is needed to determine if it is a reasonable or exaggerated response to the general medical condition.

Clinician Guideline 9.5

Given the high rate of comorbid major depression, generalized anxiety, specific phobias, agoraphobia, and substance abuse in social phobia, the clinician must include a thorough diagnostic assessment for these conditions when treating social phobia. In addition frequency, intensity, and duration of panic attacks and suicidal ideation should be assessed prior to treatment.

Negative Life Events and Social Adversity

Like other anxiety disorders, social phobia is associated with an increased rate of childhood adversities, though the relationship is not as strong as seen in the mood disorders (Kessler, Davis, & Kendler, 1997). In their etiological model of social phobia, Rapee and Spence (2004) proposed that negative life events and more specific learning experiences can contribute to increased risk of pathological social anxiety for individuals with a genetically mediated high social anxiety "set point." In the present context we are more interested in whether certain adverse interpersonal events in childhood or adolescence might play an etiological role in social phobia or whether individuals with social phobia experience more adverse, even traumatic, interpersonal events that could reinforce their social anxiety.

Heritability estimates suggest that 30% of the disease liability in social phobia is due to genetic factors, leaving considerable room for the influence of environmental factors (Kendler et al., 1992b). In fact a significant association has been found between traumatic events in childhood such as physical or sexual abuse as well as childhood adversities such as lack of a close relationship with an adult, marital conflict in family of origin, frequent moving, running away from home, failing grades, and the like and increased risk for anxiety disorders in adulthood including social phobia (Chartier, Walker, & Stein, 2001; Kessler et al., 1997; Stemberger et al., 1995). Rates of social phobia among survivors of child physical or sexual assault range from 20 to 46%, with PTSD, GAD, and specific phobias being more prevalent (Pribor & Dinwiddie, 1992; Saunders et al., 1992). Higher levels of childhood emotional abuse (Gibb, Chelminski, & Zimmerman, 2007) and adverse childhood life events such parental marital breakup; family conflict; negative parenting styles such as overprotection, verbal aggression, and rejection; and parental psychopathology have been linked to an increased risk for social phobia (e.g., Lieb et al., 2000; Magee, 1999).

If fears of social situations are acquired, we might expect social phobia to be associated with a higher rate of adverse social experiences. In their review paper Alden and Taylor (2004) concluded that individuals with social phobia have fewer and more negative social relationships throughout their life and their interpersonal style elicits more negative responses from others that create a self-perpetuating interpersonal cycle of events. Whether adverse social events play a defining role in the etiology of social phobia is less certain. Certainly other people tend to judge socially anxious individuals more negatively and less desirably than nonsocially anxious individuals (Alden & Taylor, 2004). Harvey, Ehlers, and Clark (2005) administered a Learning History Questionnaire to 55 individuals with social phobia, 30 individuals with PTSD, and 30 nonpatient controls. The social phobia group reported that their parents were significantly less likely to encourage them to engage socially, were more emotionally cold, and were less likely to warn them about the dangers of social events than the nonclinical group. Furthermore, problems with peer group and not fitting in with their peers were among the most common experiences that participants reported with the development of social phobia. Interestingly, only 13% of the social phobia sample said that a conditioning event was a primary reason for the onset of their social phobia and only four out of 12 variables investigated were significant to social phobia versus PTSD. Kimbrel (2008) concluded it is unclear whether peer neglect and exclusion are a cause or a consequence of social anxiety.

In summary, negative social experiences, particularly during the formative years of childhood and adolescence, probably contribute to the development of social phobia. It is also likely that shy and socially anxious individuals experience more negative social events than less anxious individuals, in part because their interpersonal style elicits less positive response from others (Alden & Taylor, 2004). However, it is doubtful that socially phobic individuals experience more qualitatively traumatic interpersonal events or become socially phobic in response to a single traumatic social event. Instead of environmental or social factors, we contend that cognitive responses to social experiences will be the distinguishing feature of social phobia. In other words, the most critical factor in the etiology of social phobia may be the negative interpretation that shy or socially anxious individuals generate about their social interactions with others.

Social Skills Deficits

There has been much debate in the literature on whether social phobia is characterized by deficits in social skills or whether the main difference is that individuals with social phobia perceive their performance in social situations more negatively (Hofmann & Barlow, 2002). Various etiological models of social phobia have included impaired social performance as an important maintenance factor (Beck et al., 1985, 2005; D. M. Clark & Wells, 1995; Kimbrel, 2008; Rapee & Heimberg, 1997; Rapee & Spence, 2004). In the cognitive models, impaired social performance is considered a consequence of anxiety in the social situation. For example, D. M. Clark and Wells (1995) mention a number of negative social behaviors that result from feeling anxious around others such as gaze avoidance, an unsteady voice, shaky hands, behaving less friendly toward others, avoiding self-disclosure, and the like. Beck et al. (1985, 2005) mention various automatic inhibitory behaviors that will negatively affect social performance. Rapee and Spence (2004) distinguish between interrupted social performance that is due to heightened anxiety versus poor social skills, which is a fundamental lack of social ability (e.g., poor conversational skills, unassertiveness, passivity, submissiveness). The role of social skill deficits has an important treatment implication. If positive social skills are absent, then social skills training will be an important component in treatment.

There is little doubt that the experience of heightened anxiety in social evaluative situations significantly disrupts social performance. What is less certain is whether individuals with social phobia either lack social knowledge or an internalized ability to perform socially which itself contributes to the development of social phobia (Rapee & Spence, 2004). Certainly individuals with social phobia perceive themselves to be less effective socially than nonanxious individuals (e.g., Alden & Philips, 1990; Stangier, Esser, Leber, Risch, & Heidenreich, 2006). Also when performance in social situations is rated by external observers, individuals with social phobia tend to exhibit less warmth and interest, are more visibly anxious, are less dominant, generate fewer positive verbal behaviors, and generally exhibit poorer overall performance than nonanxious comparison groups (e.g., Alden & Bieling, 1998; Alden & Wallace, 1995; Mansell, Clark, & Ehlers, 2003; Rapee & Lim, 1992; Stopa & Clark, 1993; Walters & Hope, 1998). However, individuals with social phobia consistently appraise their social performance more negatively than external observers (e.g., Abbott & Rapee, 2004; Alden & Wallace, 1995; Mellings & Alden, 2000; Rapee & Lim, 1992; Stopa & Clark, 1993). Also, it is well established that socially anxious individuals do not always exhibit maladaptive social behavior. Alden and Taylor (2004) note that occurrence of maladaptive behaviors depends on the social context, with socially anxious individuals more likely to exhibit poor social performance when anticipating an evaluative or ambiguous situation.

We can conclude that actual deficits in social skills probably play, at most, a minor role in the etiology of social phobia (Rapee & Spence, 2004). At the same time it is clear that socially anxious individuals do perform more poorly in certain social settings, primarily as a consequence of their heightened anxiety and automatic inhibitory behavior. However, the situational specificity of this performance deficit as well as the well-documented negative self-evaluative bias indicates that cognitive factors play a greater role in the development and maintenance of social phobia than behavioral deficits.

Clinician Guideline 9.6

Individuals with social phobia may have more negative social experiences because of less positive reactions from others due to deficiencies in their social behaviors when anxiety is elevated in social evaluative or unfamiliar social settings. However, their negative subjective evaluation of their social performance is greatly exaggerated and is the main contributor to the persistence of their social anxiety.

COGNITIVE THEORY OF SOCIAL PHOBIA

Description of the Model

A theoretical account of social phobia must consider three features that are unique to this disorder. First, feelings of embarrassment and shame are often the dominant negative emotions that result from a social encounter rather than anxiety alone (Beck et al., 1985, 2005; Hofmann & Barlow, 2002). Second, the intense anxiety associated with social situations often elicits automatic inhibitory behaviors and attempts to conceal anxiety that has the unfortunate effect of disrupting social performance and causing the catastrophe the socially phobic person fears most: the negative evaluation of others (Beck et al., 1985, 2005). Unlike panic disorder in which the catastrophe repeatedly fails to occur (e.g., a heart attack), the perceived catastrophe in social phobia often happens because of the disruptive effects of anxiety. And third, anxiety itself becomes a secondary threat as individuals with social phobia believe they must conceal anxiety in order to avoid negative evaluation by others. The theoretical account discussed below proposes a number of cognitive processes and structures that can explain these features of social phobia and its persistence. The model draws heavily on the cognitive theory of evaluative anxieties described in Beck et al. (1985, 2005) as well as the significant contributions of D. M. Clark and Wells (1995), and Rapee and Heimberg (1997). The following account recognizes three phases to social anxiety; the anticipatory phase, actual exposure to the social situation, and postevent processing. Figure 9.1 illustrates this refined and elaborated cognitive model of social phobia.

The Anticipatory Phase

In most instances there is some forewarning of an impending social encounter that for individuals with social phobia can elicit almost as much anxiety as exposure to the actual social interaction. This anticipatory phase could be triggered by a variety of informational or contextual cues such as being told of a future social task, reviewing the entries in one's work diary, or being in a location that reminds a person of a future social event (e.g., walking past the boardroom where the meeting will be held). The length of the anticipatory phase could vary from a few minutes to many days or even weeks. We would expect anxiety to intensify as the feared social event becomes more imminent, which is consistent with Riskind's (1997) concept of looming maladaptive style. Moreover, the more intense the anticipatory anxiety, the more likely it is that avoidance will be the preferred outcome. Pervasive avoidance of social interaction is the hallmark of social phobia because it is considered the most effective way to eliminate anticipatory anxiety. Consequently, individuals feel a strong urge to avoid when anticipating a future social event even though they recognize its detrimental effects (e.g., failing to return a call from your investment broker).

In our case illustration Gerald frequently experienced intense anticipatory anxiety whenever he even suspected the possibility of a social encounter. He would immediately begin strategizing how he could avoid the social situation and maintain his isolation from others. However, avoidance is not always possible and so the anxiety experienced during this phase will mean that the socially phobic individual enters the social situation in a state of heightened anxiety.

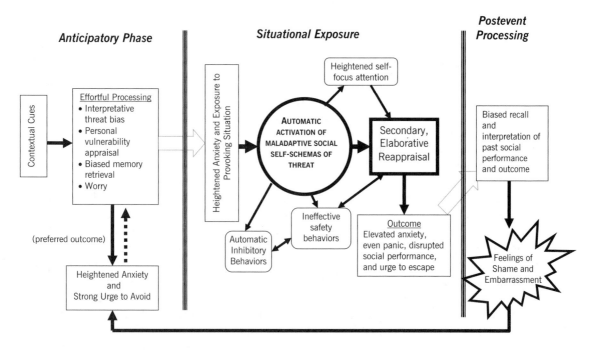

FIGURE 9.1. Cognitive model of social phobia.

The cognitive basis of anticipatory social anxiety will primarily involve effortful, elaborative processes as the individual intentionally thinks about the approaching social event. Preexisting maladaptive social self-schemas will be activated that involve beliefs of perceived social inadequacy, the distressing nature of anxiety, the imagined negative judgments of others, and the inability to meet expected social performance standards. The negative social self-schemas will tend to dominate the socially anxious person's thinking of the impending social event. His thinking will selectively focus on the possible threatening aspects of the situation. Gerald, for example, would think about people looking at him and trying to initiate conversations with him which he interpreted as highly threatening. The possibility of acceptance by others and positive social performance were completely discounted. At the anticipatory phase socially anxious individuals also evaluate themselves as vulnerable and incapable of meeting the perceived social performance expectations of the impending task. Memory of past social situations, especially those similar to the future event, will be biased for retrieval of experiences that involved intense social anxiety and embarrassment, leading to an exaggerated expectation of threat and personal vulnerability in the anticipated social event. This will initiate a worry process as the individual becomes preoccupied with the threat and danger of the approaching social event. The expected probability and severity of a negative outcome will become magnified the longer the individual is stuck in this anxious ruminative process. Gerald experienced intense worry when a meeting was scheduled at work. All he could think about was the terrible anxiety he felt in past meetings and the relief experienced when he was able to find an excuse for not attending.

Situational Exposure

Of course individuals with social phobia often find themselves in social situations that are unavoidable and this is when anxiety will be the most intense. Both automatic and effortful cognitive processes will be activated during exposure to the feared social situation. The central cognitive process is the automatic activation of maladaptive social self-schemas of threat and vulnerability that result in an attentional bias for threat, heightened focus on internal cues of anxiety, automatic inhibitory behaviors, secondary negative evaluation of one's emotional state and performance, and ineffective use of safety behaviors. Table 9.5 provides a list of key maladaptive schemas that characterize social phobia.

The schemas that characterize social phobia are highly specific to social situations and will not be apparent in nonsocial situations. It is anticipated or actual exposure to a fearful social situation that will activate the maladaptive social self-schema cluster. This cluster includes dysfunctional core self-beliefs (e.g., "I'm boring," "I'm different from others," "I'm not a likeable person"), faulty conditional assumptions (e.g., "If people get to know me, they won't like me"; "If I blush, people will notice I am anxious and think there is something wrong with me"), and rigid rules of social performance (e.g., "I must not show any sign of anxiety or weakness", "I must take control by being outgoing and witty") (D. M. Clark, 2001; D. M. Clark & Wells, 1995).

A number of consequences follow from automatic activation of the maladaptive social self-schemas. The first is an automatic attentional shift for processing internal

TABLE 9.5. Maladaptive Social Self-Schemas in Social Phobia

Schema content	Examples
Core beliefs of helpless, weak, or inferior social self	"I'm boring", "I'm not a friendly person", "People don't tend to like me", "I'm socially awkward", "I don't fit in."
Beliefs about others	"People are critical of others", "In social situations people are always forming evaluations of each other", "Individuals are constantly scrutinizing other people, looking for their flaws and weaknesses."
Beliefs about disapproval	"It is awful when others disapprove of you", "It would be horrible if others thought I was weak or incompetent", "To embarrass yourself in front of others would be unbearable, a personal catastrophe."
Beliefs about social performance standards	"It is important not to show any signs of weakness or loss of control to others", "I must appear confident and interpersonally competent in all my social interactions", "I must always sound intelligent and interesting to others."
Beliefs about anxiety and its effects	"Anxiety is a sign of emotional weakness and loss of control", "It is important not to show any signs of anxiety around others", "If people see that I'm blushing, perspiring, have shaking hands, etc., they will wonder what is wrong with me", "If I am anxious, I won't be about to function in this social situation", "I can't stand to feel anxious around others."

and external cues of social threat. External feedback in the form of verbal and non-verbal cues from others that can be interpreted as signs of possible negative evaluation will be given attentional processing priority (Rapee & Heimberg, 1997), whereas external social cues indicative of safety (i.e., approval) or "benign acceptance" will be ignored or minimized. In addition internal information such as symptoms of anxiety or an "online" negative evaluation of one's social performance will be given attentional priority because they are consistent with the maladaptive social self-schemas and negative mental representation of how socially phobic individuals think they are perceived by others in the social situation. In fact the *"mental representation of the self as seen by the audience"* which "is based on how the individual believes the audience views him or her at any given moment" (Rapee & Heimberg, 1997, p. 744) is a core cognitive construct in Rapee and Heimberg's model of social phobia.

A second consequence of schema activation is a heightened self-focused attention during social interaction (see D. M. Clark, 2001; D. M. Clark & Wells, 1995). Activation of the social threat schemas results in hypervigilance and observation of one's internal state, especially any physical, emotional, or behavioral cues that might be interpreted as signs of anxiety and loss of control. Socially anxious individuals assume other people also notice these anxiety symptoms which then become the basis of their negative evaluation. In this way interoceptive information reinforces the socially anxious person's mental representation of how she assumes she is seen by others. D. M. Clark and Wells (1995) highlight two additional consequences associated with heightened self-focused attention. Because most of the attentional resources are devoted to self-monitoring, very little attention is available for processing external information from individuals in the social setting. As a result individuals fail to process social information that might disconfirm their maladaptive threat schemas. Furthermore, the intense self-monitoring results in a type of emotional reasoning or "ex-consequentia reasoning" (Arntz et al., 1995) so that socially anxious individuals assume that others must also observe what they feel. This *processing of the self as a negative social object* is a key concept in D. M. Clark and Wells's (1995) model in which socially phobic individuals are considered "trapped in a closed system in which most of their evidence for their fears is self-generated and disconfirmatory evidence (such as other people's responses) becomes inaccessible or is ignored" (D. M. Clark, 2001, p. 408). As an example, Gerald's hands and legs would shake when he felt intensely anxious in social situations. Because he was so aware of these physical sensations, he assumed others would notice his shaking, conclude that he must be nervous, and wonder if he might have some mental illness that was causing him to behave so strangely.

Occurrence of involuntary inhibitory behaviors is another important consequence of negative social self-schema activation in social situations. Socially phobic individuals are actually inhibited in social encounters as indicated by their stiff and rigid posture, taut face expression, and often inarticulate speech such as stuttering, stammering, having difficulty finding the right word, or appearing tongue-tied. Socially phobic individuals realize they tend to behave in this manner when socially anxious and that these inhibitory behaviors are not only noticed by others but are probably interpreted by them in a negative manner. Feeling unable to counter the negative effects of inhibition on social performance, this tendency for inhibition in social phobia leads to a perceived loss of control, heightened perception of personal vulnerability and social ineptitude, and hence increased anxiety. The direct relationship between social threat and the occurrence of inhibition is readily apparent in the fact that socially phobic individuals can be casual and articulate in nonthreatening situations.

A fourth consequence of social schema threat activation is reliance on safety-seeking or concealment behaviors in order to minimize or even prevent negative evaluation. Although safety seeking may have a less negative impact on anxiety than involuntary inhibition, their contribution to the persistence of anxiety should not be overlooked. D. M. Clark (2001) noted that safety-seeking strategies include both overt behaviors (e.g., avoid eye contact, tense arm or leg muscles to control shaking,) and mental processes (e.g., memorize what to say in a social setting, give brief or curt responses in conversation). However, these coping strategies can paradoxically increase the very symptoms that the person fears or that draw the attention of others, thereby causing an actual increase in the risk of negative evaluation by others (D. M. Clark, 2001).

Maladaptive schema activation and its associated consequences will also disrupt conscious elaborative thought processes during the social encounter. The socially anxious person will experience an increased frequency and salience of social threat thoughts and images. A conscious and deliberate evaluation and reevaluation of internal and external social cues will reinforce the threatening inference. The socially phobic person's perceived discrepancy between what she thinks is the expected standard of performance held by others and her actual behavior will contribute to the conclusion that she is being judged negatively by those around her. The stronger a socially anxious person believes that others in a particular social situation have formed a negative impression of her, the greater her anxiety level and the more pervasive its adverse effects on her social performance.

Postevent Processing

Like other cognitive-behavioral theories of social phobia, the current model posits that postevent processing, a cognitive process involving the detailed recall and reevaluation of one's performance following a social situation, plays a pivotal role in the maintenance of social anxiety (Brozovich & Heimberg, 2008). Social phobics can not entirely escape their anxiety when exposure to a social situation ceases because they often engage in a "post-mortem" review and evaluation of their social performance and its outcome (D. M. Clark & Wells, 1995). Of course their recall and reevaluation of the social event and their performance is biased for schema-congruent information of social threat and ineptitude. In the end they are likely to conclude that their performance and reception by others was much more negative than was actually the case. Often a ruminative process occurs at the postevent phase so that the more one thinks about the social interaction, the worse the outcome because of the selective focus and elaboration of possible disapproval and failure (Brozovich & Heimberg, 2008). Gerald had a tendency to look back on activities with friends and conclude that he felt such intense anxiety and discomfort that it was hardly worth the effort. It was much better to stay at home alone and be depressed but feel comfortable. As with Gerald, postevent processing for most individuals with social phobia yields schema-congruent evaluations of social threat and vulnerability that leads to feelings of embarrassment and shame about past social encounters and, in turn, heightens anticipatory anxiety and the urge to avoid future social interaction.

EMPIRICAL STATUS OF THE COGNITIVE MODEL

Over the last decade the volume of correlational and experimental research that has demonstrated an information-processing bias for social threat information in social phobia has grown exponentially (for reviews, see Alden & Taylor, 2004; Bögels & Mansell; 2004; D. M. Clark, 2001; D. M. Clark & McManus, 2002; Heimberg & Becker, 2002; Heinrichs & Hofmann, 2001; Hirsch & Clark, 2004; Wilson & Rapee, 2004). Critics argue that the role of biased cognitive processes in social anxiety remains unclear, especially as it pertains to etiological significance (Beidel & Turner, 2007; see also Stravynski, Bond, & Amado, 2004). In their review Heinrichs and Hofmann (2001) concluded there was partial support for the cognitive model, especially for biased attention and interpretation of self-referent social information. From our own review we believe there is strong empirical support for cognitive dysfunction in social phobia, although we agree that prospective studies and more sophisticated laboratory-based experimental research is needed to determine the causal status of cognitive factors (see also D. M. Clark & McManus, 2002). In the discussion that follows we focus on six hypotheses that are central to the reformulated cognitive model of social phobia. Although considered a key factor in social phobia, there is not enough research on involuntary inhibition to include this concept in our review of the literature.

Hypothesis 1

Social phobia is characterized by an explicit elaborative interpretation and recall bias for self-referent social threat information that is evident in the anticipatory, exposure, and postprocessing phases of social anxiety.

If a deliberate and intentional information-processing bias for social threat is evident in all three phases of social phobia, then we predict that socially phobic individuals will exhibit a tendency to exaggerate the probability and severity of negative consequences in socially relevant situations. Various studies have administered mildly positive and negative self-referent hypothetical social events and found that socially anxious individuals overestimate the probability and/or the consequences of negative social events compared to individuals with other anxiety disorders and nonclinical controls (e.g., Foa et al., 1996; Lucock & Salkovskis, 1988; McManus, Clark, & Hackmann, 2000). Wilson and Rapee (2005) used a more refined questionnaire of hypothetical social events to show that the threat judgment bias is specifically related to social phobia and consists of beliefs that others would perceive you negatively, that the event was an indication of negative self-characteristics, and that the event would have long-term adverse consequences (see also Wenzel, Finstrom, et al., 2005). This negative judgmental bias is specific to all social events whether positive or negative (Brendle & Wenzel, 2004; Voncken et al., 2003) and is significantly reduced by CBT (Foa et al., 1996; Lucock & Salkovskis, 1988; McManus et al., 2000).

Individuals with social anxiety have a significantly greater tendency to choose negative interpretations to self-referent social but not nonsocial ambiguous hypothetical events compared to people with other anxiety disorders or nonclinical groups (Amir et al., 1998b; Constans et al., 1999; Stopa & Clark, 2000). However, more recent studies suggest that when individuals with social phobia make "online inferences" (i.e., inferences made when social information is first encountered), the main problem is a failure to exhibit a positive inferential bias for hypothetical ambiguous social scenarios that was characteristic of the nonanxious group (Amir et al., 2005; Hirsch & Mathews, 1997, 2000). Moreover, individuals with high social anxiety can be trained to make positive or benign interpretations of ambiguous social scenarios and this trained interpretation bias reduces levels of predicted anxiety to an anticipated social encounter but not levels of current state anxiety (Murphy, Hirsch, Mathews, Smith, & Clark, 2007). These findings suggest that the interpretation bias evident when social phobics first encounter a social situation is characterized by an inability to access positive or benign inferences whereas later, more reflective interpretations that are based on preexisting maladaptive beliefs show the enhanced negative threat bias (D. M. Clark, 2001; see also Hirsch & Clark, 2004; Hirsch et al., 2006).

A final prediction of the first hypothesis is that individuals with social phobia will exhibit a recall bias for negative or threatening information associated with past social situations and their performance. However, Coles and Heimberg (2002) concluded in their review that there was little support for an explicit memory bias for threat information in social phobia with only 2 of 11 studies showing the predicted effect. In most studies socially phobic individuals did not exhibit a clear recall bias for negative social threat words compared to nonanxious controls (e.g., Lundh & Öst, 1997; Rapee et al., 1994; Rinck & Becker, 2005). Moreover, a threat recall bias is not apparent when socially phobic individuals recall more complex social passages (Brendle & Wenzel, 2004; Wenzel & Holt, 2002) or positive and negative social evaluative video vignettes (Wenzel, Finstrom, et al., 2005). In addition memory bias for threat has not been apparent in response to autobiographical memory cueing to social threat words (Rapee et al., 1994; Wenzel et al., 2002; Wenzel, Werner, Cochran, & Holt, 2004).

In summary, there is strong and consistent empirical support for Hypothesis 1 from studies of interpretation bias to mildly negative or ambiguous social information. However, it is still unclear whether a threat interpretation bias only occurs when socially phobic individuals reflect back on their social experiences, with absence of a self-enhancing positive interpretation bias characterizing the more immediate inferences that occur when individuals encounter a social situation. Also there is little support for an explicit memory bias in social phobia, but this could be due to failure to use externally valid stimuli or to prime the relevant emotional state at the time of retrieval (Coles & Heimberg, 2002; Mansell & Clark, 1999).

Clinician Guideline 9.7

Cognitive therapy targets the socially phobic individuals' tendency to make exaggerated threat inferences when they reflect on their social experiences and their inability to access positive inferences during exposure to social situations.

Hypothesis 2

The schematic organization in social phobia consists of core beliefs of an inadequate social self, the threatening nature of social interaction, and a negative mental representation of how one is perceived by others in the social situation.

In social phobia the maladaptive schema activated by anticipated or actual exposure to a social evaluative situation involve negative beliefs about the inadequacy of one's
social ability, the threatening or critical nature of social interactions, and a negative self-
image in which socially anxious individuals assume they make a negative impression
on others (D. M. Clark, 2001). In essence, the schematic organization in social phobia
revolves around issues related to the social self. Evidence of an explicit interpretation
bias for social threat on retrospective measures (see Hypothesis 1) supports the predictions of activated negative social self-schemas in Hypothesis 2. However, there are three
other lines of research that have directly addressed this issue.

First, a number of early questionnaire studies have reported a significant increase in
negative social evaluative cognitions that is specific to social phobia compared to other
anxiety disorders or nonclinical controls (e.g., Becker et al., 2001; Beidel et al., 1985;
Turner & Beidel, 1985; Turner et al., 1986). Based on think-aloud and questionnaire
measures of thoughts generated by socially anxious individuals after they participated
in a 7–8 minute conversation, Stopa and Clark (1993) found that the socially anxious
group had significantly more negative self-evaluative cognitions and believed their negative thoughts more than individuals with other anxiety disorders (see also Magee &
Zinbarg, 2007). A more recent questionnaire study suggests that any experience that
involves conspicuousness or heightened self-consciousness, whether positive or negative,
might be related to social anxiety (Weeks et al., 2008).

A second body of research has shown that social phobia may be characterized by
implicit (i.e., automatic or unintended encoding and retention processes) memory and
associative bias that reflects activation of negative social self-schemas. Using a variety of
experimental paradigms, socially anxious individuals have shown an implicit memory
bias for social threat sentences or videos (Amir et al., 2003; Amir, Foa, & Coles, 2000)
but not previously presented social threat words (Lundh & Öst, 1997; Rapee et al.,
1994; Rinck & Becker, 2005). Too few studies have employed the Implicit Association
Test (IAT) to provide clear results but there is some suggestion that high social anxiety is
associated with less positive implicit self-esteem (Tanner et al., 2006), although de Jong
(2002) did not find this difference. At this point, we can only conclude that support for
Hypothesis 2 from research on implicit processes is weak and inconsistent at best.

Much of the research relevant to Hypothesis 2 has investigated the presence of a
negative self-image in social phobia which involves "processing of the self as a social
object" (D. M. Clark & Wells, 1995, p. 72). In the current model this negative social
self-image reflects activation of maladaptive social self-schemas. A number of findings
are consistent with this formulation. Based on a semistructured interview, individuals
with social phobia reported significantly more spontaneous negative images of how they
might appear to others when recalling a recent episode of social anxiety than low socially
anxious individuals (Hackmann et al., 1998). Mansell and Clark (1999) found that only
high socially anxious individuals had a significant correlation between perceived body
sensations while giving a speech and self-ratings of how anxious they thought they
appeared to others. When socially anxious volunteers were randomly assigned to hold
a negative or control image in their mind while interacting briefly with a confederate,
the negative self-image condition elicited significantly more anxiety, greater use of safety
behaviors, poorer social performance, and beliefs that they appeared more anxious and
performed less well with the confederate (Hirsch, Meynen, & Clark, 2004; see also
Hirsch, Clark, Williams, & Morrison, 2005).

Other studies have found that individuals with social phobia are more likely than nonanxious controls to take an observer perspective (i.e., seeing oneself from an external point of view) when recalling more threatening social situations or immediately after completing a social interaction role play (Coles, Turk, Heimberg, & Fresco, 2001; Coles, Turk, & Heimberg, 2002). They are also more likely to engage in upward social comparisons (Antony et al., 2005) and to experience the "spotlight effect" (i.e., tendency to overestimate the extent that others see and attend to one's external appearance) in high social-evaluative situations (Brown & Stopa, 2007). All of these processes are relevant to generation of a negative self-image in social phobia which reflects activation of negative social self-schemas (i.e., "how I think I appear to others").

Overall there is emerging evidence that a negative self-image involving the perspective of the other (i.e., "how I think others see me") is a basic cognitive process in social phobia. More recent studies suggest that manipulation of this social self-schema may have causal effects on social threat inferences, subjective anxiety, and safety behaviors that are central processes in the maintenance of social phobia. However, research on the more automatic or implicit aspects of schema activation in social phobia have produced inconsistent findings. At this point support for Hypothesis 2 is modest with many unanswered questions remaining about the structure and interrelations of the negative social self schemas in social phobia.

Clinician Guideline 9.8

A central feature of cognitive therapy of social phobia is the precise specification and restructuring of negative social self-schemas. This requires correction of the socially anxious person's inaccurate assumptions about how she thinks she appears to others.

Hypothesis 3

During situational exposure, individuals with social phobia will exhibit an automatic attentional bias for internal and external social threat information.

A central prediction of the cognitive model is that individuals with social phobia are hypervigilant to social threat information that is congruent with their negative social self-schemas (Beck et al., 1985, 2005). Thus attentional resources will be preferentially directed toward schema-congruent social threat information, especially during exposure to social situations.

Some of the earliest research on automatic attentional bias for threat in social phobia employed the emotional Stroop task. As predicted, most studies found significantly greater interference for social threat words (Becker et al., 2001; Grant & Beck, 2006; Hope et al., 1990; Mattia et al., 1993), although negative results have also been reported (e.g., Gotlib, Kasch, et al., 2004). Findings from dot probe detection experiments indicate that social phobia is characterized by faster response latencies to probes followed by social threat cues (Asmundson & Stein, 1994; Vassilopoulos, 2005). Moreover, these results have been confirmed in a modified version of the experiment in which the probe is preceded by an angry or threatening, happy, or neutral facial expression (Mogg, Philippot, & Bradley, 2004; Mogg & Bradley, 2002), although Gotlib, Kasch, et al. (2004)

failed to find a significant effect for angry faces. Based on the face-in-the-crowd identification task, Gilboa-Schechtman et al. (1999) also found that individuals with GSP had an attentional bias for angry faces. Other studies using a modified visual dot probe task in which pairs of faces are shown found that high social anxiety is associated with attention away from emotional faces (Chen et al., 2002; Mansell et al., 1999). Furthermore, Vassilopoulos (2005) found a vigilance-avoidance pattern with high social anxiety associated with an initial attentional preference for social threat words at 200 milliseconds exposure, followed by attentional bias away from the same stimulus word type at 500 milliseconds (see Amir et al., 1998a, for similar results). Recently Schmidt et al. (2009) reported that training individuals with GSP to attend to neutral rather than disgusted faces on a modified dot probe task results in significant reduction in social anxiety. This suggests that attentional threat may have a causal role in social phobia.

In summary, there is strong support that socially anxious individuals exhibit an automatic attentional bias for social threat. Recent studies indicate that attentional bias for threat may be particularly evident when socially phobic individuals process angry faces, a stimulus highly salient for individuals with fear of negative evaluation (Stein, Goldin, Sareen, Eyler Zorrilla, & Brown, 2002). However, a more complex vigilance-avoidance pattern may best characterize the attentional bias for threat in social phobia (Heimberg & Becker, 2002). Moreover, it is still unclear whether individuals with social phobia are hypervigilant for external social threat cues or instead direct their attention away from external social stimuli in favor of heightened self-focused attention.

Clinician Guideline 9.9

In cognitive therapy of social phobia deliberate and effortful processing of positive social cues is encouraged to correct the negative effects of the client's automatic attentional bias for social threat.

Hypothesis 4

For social phobia exposure to social situations is associated with a heightened self-focused attention on internal cues of anxiety and its adverse effects on performance and the perceived negative impression of others.

According to the cognitive model (see Figure 9.1), a heightened focus on one's thoughts, images, physiological responses, behaviors, and feelings will occur during situational exposure because of activation of the maladaptive social self-schemas. There is now consistent empirical support for this hypothesis. Individuals with social phobia attend less to the external environment and more to their negative, self-focused cognitions when confronting a social-evaluative experience (e.g., Daly et al., 1989; Mansell & Clark, 1999). Other studies have reported an information-processing bias for internal physiological cues rather than external social threat stimuli (Mansell et al., 2003; Pineles & Mineka, 2005). When giving an impromptu speech, high socially anxious individuals reported significantly greater perceived physiological activity than low anxious individuals, even though the groups did not differ significantly in level of self-reported anxiety or actual physiological response (Mauss et al., 2004). In a series of experimental studies, Bögels and Lamers (2002) found that focusing attention on the self increases social anxiety whereas focusing attention on the task reduces social anxiety. Similarly socially phobic individuals told that their pulse rate had increased while anticipating a social interaction experienced greater anxiety and more negative beliefs during a threatening social encounter (Wells & Papageorgiou, 2001; see Bögels et al., 2002, for contrary findings). More recently George and Stopa (2008) used a mirror and a videocamera to manipulate self-awareness during a standard conversation and found that high socially anxious students could not shift their attention away from internal aspects of themselves during the conversation in the same manner as evident in the low socially anxious group. Overall, then, there is considerable evidence that socially anxious individuals engage in excessive self-monitoring and misinterpret this interoceptive information in a manner that increases their social anxiousness (see Hofmann, 2005).

Another body of research has investigated how individuals evaluate their social performances and how these evaluations compare to their actual level of performance as determined by observers. In various studies individuals with social phobia rated their own public performance on a social evaluative task (e.g., impromptu speech) as significantly worse than observers, although the observers tended to rate the performance of the highly anxious group as worse than the low socially anxious individuals (e.g., Abbott & Rapee, 2004; Alden & Wallace, 1995; Hirsch & Clark, 2007; Mellings & Alden, 2000; Rapee & Lim, 1992). In their review Heimberg and Becker (2002) concluded that individuals with social phobia do exhibit performance deficits in social evaluative situations but they also evaluate their performance much more negatively than others. We can conclude that research support for Hypothesis 4 is strong, with social phobia characterized by an internal attentional bias and exaggerated negative interpretation of interoceptive cues indicative of anxiety, loss of control, and inadequate public performance.

Clinician Guideline 9.10

Cognitive therapy addresses excessive and deleterious self-evaluative monitoring of one's internal state in social situations by redirecting the socially anxious person's attention outward to encourage increased processing of salient feedback cues in the environment.

Hypothesis 5

Feared social situations will provoke in the socially phobic individual maladaptive compensatory and safety responses aimed at minimizing or suppressing the expression of anxiety.

Although only a few studies have investigated safety behavior in social phobia, there is emerging evidence for its role in the persistence of social anxiety. Alden and Bieling (1998) found that when socially anxious individuals used safety behaviors during a standard conversation (e.g., talked briefly and selected nonrevealing topics) they elicited more negative reactions from others. In a more recent study individuals with social phobia reported greater use of safety behaviors and exhibited larger performance deficits in standard conversation and speech tasks than individuals with other anxiety disorders or nonclinical controls (Stangier et al., 2006). A subsequent path analysis revealed that safety behaviors partially mediated group differences in social performance. In a series of single-case studies, Wells et al. (1995) found that a single session of exposure plus decreased use of safety behaviors was significantly more effective than a single session of exposure alone in reducing within-situation anxiety and catastrophic beliefs. At this point, only a few studies have investigated the role of safety behaviors in social phobia but these initial findings suggest that maladaptive safety seeking may play a role in the persistence of social anxiety. More research is needed, especially on the relation between involuntary inhibitory behavior and production of safety-seeking coping responses.

Clinician Guideline 9.11

Target cognitive and behavioral safety or concealment responses in cognitive therapy of social phobia.

Hypothesis 6

Postevent processing of social situations is characterized by an explicit autobiographical memory bias for past negative social experiences in those with social phobia.

Unlike other disorders in which anxiety declines or ceases after escape from a threatening situation, individuals with social phobia will experience recurrence of anxiety as they recall past social incidents that were embarrassing and associated with perceived negative evaluation. Postevent processing involving repeated biased recall and rumination about past threatening social events will increase anticipatory anxiety for future social situations by providing schema-congruent evidence of social threat and ineptitude.

Researchers have only recently begun to investigate the role of postevent processing in social phobia. In a study by Mellings and Alden (2000), high and low socially anxious students, who participated in a standard social interaction, were assessed for rumination and recall of the interaction 1 day later. The highly anxious group reported significantly more rumination and there was a tendency for postevent rumination to predict recall of negative self-related information about the previous day's interaction with the laboratory confederate (see also Kocovski & Rector, 2008). Abbott and Rapee (2004) found that socially phobic individuals engaged in significantly more negative rumination about a 3-minute impromptu speech given 1 week earlier and this was related to how negatively they appraised their speech performance. In addition 12 weeks of CBT led to a significant reduction in negative postevent rumination.

A questionnaire study of past learning experiences found that individuals with social phobia indicated that they ruminated about their poor performance in past embarrassing social situations significantly more than nonclinical controls (Harvey et al., 2005). In response to vignettes depicting an embarrassing social event, high socially anxious students had more thoughts about the negative aspects of the situation than low anxious individuals, a finding that is consistent with a postevent, ruminative coping style (Kocovski, Endler, Rector, & Flett, 2005). In another study, high socially anxious students tended to recall more negative and shameful memories when asked to recall a past ambiguous social event (Field, Psychol, & Morgan, 2004; see also Morgan & Banerjee, 2008).

Although still preliminary, it is apparent that postevent processing is an important contributing factor to social anxiety. In their review Brozovich and Heimberg (2008) concluded that self-report, diary, and experimental studies indicate that postevent processing is a prominent cognitive process that contributes to social anxiety by reinforcing negative impressions of oneself (i.e., mental representation of self from the assumed perspective of the audience), negative memories of social situations, and negative assumptions about future social encounters (see also Abbott & Rapee, 2004). Moreover, autobiographical memory recall bias for the negative aspects of past social events may be a pivotal cognitive feature of postevent processing that accounts for its effects on anxiety. Overall, there is some empirical support for Hypothesis 6, although a number of issues remain such as whether postevent processing is more likely in performance than social interaction situations, whether it becomes more negative and less positive over time, and the role played by imagery (Brozovich & Heimberg, 2008).

Clinician Guideline 9.12

The cognitive therapist must also target change in postevent processing when treating social anxiety. This is accomplished by reducing negative rumination about past performance and encouraging a more positive reappraisal of past social performance and its consequence.

Anticipatory Phase

Although we have not generated a specific hypothesis about the anticipatory period of social anxiety, this is not to minimize the importance of this phase in the pathogenesis of social phobia. Even though only a few studies have investigated anticipatory processing in social phobia, the preliminary findings are supportive of the cognitive model.

Mellings and Alden (2000) found that only a high social anxiety group became more apprehensive about participating in a second standard social interaction 1 day after completing an initial unstructured 10-minute conversation with a confederate. Based on a semistructured interview that assessed periods of anticipation before social interactions, Hinrichsen and Clark (2003) reported that the high socially anxious group (1) recalled more past perceived social failures; (2) were more aware of negative bodily sensations, thoughts and images; and (3) relied more on problematic cognitive strategies to manage their anticipatory anxiety. In a subsequent study both high and low socially anxious students who were given anticipatory anxiety compared to distraction instructions during 20 minutes of preparation for a speech exhibited significantly higher anxiety ratings (Hinrichsen & Clark, 2003; see also Vassilopoulos, 2008).

Clinician Guideline 9.13

Address biased and maladaptive anticipatory processing by emphasizing the use of planning and rehearsal of anticipatory strategies that focus on how to improve social performance and resist the urge to avoid.

COGNITIVE ASSESSMENT AND CASE FORMULATION

Various critical reviews have been published on the cognitive and symptom measures specifically developed for social anxiety (e.g., D. B. Clark et al., 1997; Heimberg & Turk, 2002; Hofmann & Barlow, 2002; Turk, Heimberg, & Magee, 2008). In this section we focus on a few of the more common symptom measures as well as a couple of specific questionnaires that assess the cognitive profile of social phobia. We begin with a brief consideration of standardized instruments for social phobia and end with a framework for case formulation derived from the current model.

Diagnostic Interview and Clinician Ratings

The ADIS-IV (Brown et al., 1994) is recommended over the SCID-IV (First et al., 1997) when administering a structured diagnostic interview for social phobia. Reliability studies (Brown et al., 2001) indicate that the ADIS-IV Lifetime Version achieved high interrater reliability for diagnosis of social phobia (kappa = .73) and for dimensional ratings of situational fear (r = .86), avoidance (r = .68), and severity of general interference or distress (r = .80). If a clinician rating scale is desired, the Liebowitz Social Anxiety Scale (LSAS; Liebowitz, 1987) is recommended. It has good psychometric properties, with a LSAS Total cutoff score of 30 distinguishing social phobia from nonclinical individuals (Fresco et al., 2001; Heimberg et al., 1999; Mennin et al., 2002). The LSAS is reprinted in the original article as well as in Heimberg and Turk (2002).

Symptom Questionnaires

Social Phobia Scale and Social Interaction Anxiety Scale

The 20-item Social Phobia Scale (SPS) and 20-item Social Interaction Anxiety Scale (SIAS) are companion scales developed by Mattick and Clarke (1998) to assess fear of being observed by others while doing routine tasks and fear of more general social interaction. Both scales have good internal consistency (Cronbach alphas range from .88 to .94), high 12 week test–retest reliability of .92 (SIAS) and .93 (SPS), strong concurrent validity, and adequate convergent validity with interview-based indices of social anxiety as well as measures of negative cognition (Brown, Turovsky, et al., 1997; Cox, Ross, Swinson, & Direnfeld, 1998; Mattick & Clarke, 1998; Osman, Gutierrez, Barrios, Kopper, & Chiros, 1998; Ries et al., 1998). Social phobics score significantly higher than other anxiety disorder groups or nonclinical controls (e.g., Brown et al., 1997; Mattick & Clarke, 1998), and the SPS and SIAS are sensitive to cognitive-behavioral treatment effects (Cox et al., 1998). Peters (2000) reported that a cutoff score of 26 on the SPS and 36 on the SIAS were optimal for discriminating social phobia from panic disorder, whereas Brown et al. (1997) note that cutoff scores of 24 (SPS) and 34 (SIAS) may be useful for screening but not diagnosing social phobia. Copies of the questionnaires can be found in Orsillo (2001, Appendix B) or Mattick and Clarke (1998), where all items are reproduced except SIAS item 5.

Social Phobia and Anxiety Inventory

The Social Phobia and Anxiety Inventory (SPAI) is a 45-item empirically derived questionnaire that assesses physical, cognitive, and behavioral responses to various social interaction, performance, and observation situations (Turner, Beidel, Dancu, & Stanley, 1989). The administration and scoring of the SPAI are more complex and time-consuming than other social anxiety questionnaires. The questionnaire includes a 13-item Agoraphobia subscale that was included to provide a better differentiation of social phobia from agoraphobia (Beidel & Turner, 2007). The SPAI Total score is calculated by subtracting the total score on the Agoraphobia subscale from the Social Anxiety subscale score, which is intended to be a "purer" measure of social phobia (Turner, Stanley, Beidel & Bond, 1989).

The SPAI Social Anxiety and Agoraphobia subscales have acceptable internal consistency (alphas range from .83 to .97; D. B. Clark et al., 1994; Osman et al., 1996), and SPAI Total has a 2-week test–retest reliability of .86 (Turner et al., 1989). In addition the SPAI correlates highly with other measures of social anxiety and related constructs (Beidel, Turner, Stanley, & Dancu, 1989; Cox et al., 1998; Osman et al., 1996; Ries et al., 1998), and discriminates social phobia from other anxiety disorders and nonclinical controls (D. B. Clark et al., 1994; Peters, 2000; Turner, Beidel et al., 1989). In addition individuals with generalized social phobia score significantly higher than those with the circumscribed subtype (Ries et al., 1998). It is also sensitive to treatment effects (Cox et al., 1998) and factor analysis confirms the existence of separate social anxiety and agoraphobic dimensions (Osman et al., 1996; Turner, Stanley, et al., 1989). Peters (2000) recommends a SPAI Total cutoff score of 88 to distinguish social phobia from panic disorder, whereas the manual recommends a cutoff of 60 for distinguishing social phobia in treatment-seeking samples (Turner, Beidel, & Dancu, 1996). However, cutoff scores must be used cautiously and for screening only since 10% of nonclinical individuals score above the cutoff (Gillis, Haaga, & Ford, 1995). An abbreviated 23-item SPAI was recently developed that holds promise as a comparable measure to the original inventory (Robertson-Ny, Strong, Nay, Beidel, & Turner, 2007). The 45–item SPAI can be purchased from Multi-Health Systems Inc. (Turner et al., 1996).

Clinician Guideline 9.14

Assessment for social phobia should include the ADIS-IV (current or lifetime version) and one of the specialized symptom questionnaires. Either the SPAI or the SPS and SIAS companion scales will provide comparable clinical information on social anxiety severity as well as an evaluation of treatment effectiveness.

Cognitive Questionnaires of Social Anxiety

Fear of Negative Evaluation Scale

The Fear of Negative Evaluation Scale (FNE) is the most widely used questionnaire in social anxiety because it assesses a core cognitive feature of the disorder, fear of negative evaluation. The 30-item true/false scale was originally developed by Watson and Friend (1969) to assess expectation, apprehension, distress, and avoidance of social evaluative situations. It was intended to be administered along with its companion scale, the 28-item Social Avoidance and Distress Scale (SAD). Although the FNE demonstrates good reliability and correlates with other measures of social anxiety especially in university student samples, questions have been raised about its divergent validity with depression and general distress as well as its differential sensitivity to diagnosable social phobia (see D. B. Clark et al., 1997; Hope et al., 1996–1997).

Leary (1983) developed a brief 12-item version of the FNE and replaced the dichotomous rating with a 5-point Likert scale ranging from 1 ("not at all characteristic of me") to 5 ("extremely characteristic of me"). The Brief Fear of Negative Evaluation Scale (BFNE) has good internal consistency (a = .90) and correlates highly with the original FNE (r = .96; Leary, 1983). Moreover, it has positive correlations with other measures of social anxiety and individuals with social phobia score significantly higher than those with panic disorder or a community sample (Collins, Westra, Dozois, & Stewart, 2005). However, confirmatory factor analysis revealed problems with the four reverse-scored items (Duke, Krishnan, Faith, & Storch, 2006; Rodebaugh, Woods, et al., 2004). Thus a revised BFNE 8-item (BFNE-II) was produced in which all items are straightforwardly worded and the total score correlated .99 with the 12-item BFNE (Carleton, Collimore, & Asmundson, 2007). At this point either the 8- or 12-item BFNE-II is recommended with all items worded in a straightforward fashion. The BFNE-II items can be found in Carleton et al. (2007).

Social Interaction Self-Statement Test

The Social Interaction Self-Statement Test (SISST) consists of 15 positive (facilitative) and 15 negative (inhibitory) self-statements associated with heterosocial dyadic interactions (Glass, Merluzzi, Biever, & Larsen, 1982). Some researchers have eliminated the role play and instruct individuals to rate frequency of thoughts before, during, or after any interactions with the opposite sex (Dodge, Hope, Heimberg, & Becker, 1988). Various studies have shown that the SISST Positive and Negative scores correlate with other self-report measures of social anxiety (Dodge et al., 1988; Glass et al., 1982) and individuals with social phobia score significantly higher on SISST Negative and lower on SISST Positive than other anxiety disorder groups or nonclinical controls (Becker, Namour, et al., 2001; Beidel et al., 1985; Turner et al., 1986), although SISST Negative subscale may be more sensitive to social anxiety than SISST Positive (Dodge et al., 1988). Unfortunately, the SISST has limited clinical value because of its specific focus on heterosocial interactions. A copy of the questionnaire can be found in an appendix to Glass et al. (1982) as well as in Orsillo (2001, Appendix B).

Other Cognition Measures

A number of new measures have recently been developed to assess thought content in social phobia. One that holds particular promise is the 21-item Social Thoughts and Beliefs Scale (STABS) that assesses negative cognitions of social comparison and ineptitude in social situations (Turner, Johnson, Beidel, Heiser, & Lydiard, 2003). It has high test–retest reliability and significantly differentiates social phobia from other anxiety disorders. A copy of the STABS can be found in the original article. A second cognitive measure is the 20-item Appraisal of Social Concerns (ASC) that assesses degree of perceived threat associated with various experiences relevant to social anxiety (Telch et al., 2004). The measure correlates with other cognition and symptoms measures of social anxiety and is sensitive to treatment effects. A copy of the instrument can be found in the original article.

Clinician Guideline 9.15

Unfortunately, there is no standardized measure of negative cognition in social phobia that has widespread acceptance or validation. The BFNE-II comes closest to being a measure of negative social evaluative thoughts and beliefs that has general applicability. The SISST can be used to assess cognitions relevant to social interactional anxiety. The STABS holds promise as providing the most direct questionnaire assessment of negative cognitions in social phobia but more research is needed before it can be an accepted into clinical practice.

Case Conceptualization

A cognitive case formulation explicates the key cognitive and behavioral processes responsible for heightened anxiety during the anticipatory, exposure, and postevent processing phases of social phobia. The case formulation follows the general format we outlined in Chapter 5 with particular application to the unique cognitive processes proposed in the cognitive model of social phobia (see Figure 9.1). Table 9.6 presents the main elements of the cognitive case conceptualization for social phobia as well as examples of questions that can be used to assess each construct.

Situational Analysis

The cognitive therapist begins by identifying the full range of social situations that the client finds anxiety-provoking and may avoid. It is important to identify mildly anxious situations as well as those that elicit intense anxiety and avoidance. In addition it is often helpful to determine whether there are some social situations that are not anxiety-provoking and what features of these situations make them safe for the individual. In Table 9.6 we listed a number of other characteristics of anxious social situations that should be assessed. The ADIS-IV and symptom measures like the SPAI can be useful in obtaining this information. Furthermore, self-monitoring forms like the Situational Analysis Form (Appendix 5.2) or the Daily Social Anxiety Self-Monitoring Form (Appendix 9.1) will provide valuable information on the social situations that

TABLE 9.6. Elements of the Cognitive Case Formulation for Social Phobia

Elements of case conceptualization	Key questions
Specify range of feared social situations.	• What are the most commonly feared social situations? • How often do they occur (i.e., daily, weekly, rarely)? • Determine average level of anxiety and extent of avoidance associated with each situation. • Are the feared situations primarily performance, social interaction, or a mixture? • Which situations provoke the most anxiety? • Which situations are most important for improving the client's daily functioning?
Determine relative contribution of the three components.	• How often are anticipatory anxiety, exposure, and postevent processing associated with each fear social situation? • What is the usual duration of each phase (i.e., hours, days, or weeks)? • What is the average level of anxiety associated with each phase? • What is the consequence or outcome associated with each phase of anxiety? • What role does each phase play in the persistence of the person's social anxiety?
Assess for explicit threat interpretation bias and anxious thoughts/ images.	• What is the nature of the perceived threat associated with each fear situation? • What external social cues or perceived audience feedback reinforces the social threat? • What is the worst scenario or catastrophe associated with a social threat situation? • What is the client's estimated likelihood of a catastrophe or other negative outcome happening in the social situation? • Obtain examples of the automatic anxious thoughts and images that occur during anticipation, exposure, or postprocessing of a feared social situation. • Is the client able to process any competing or more positive information when feeling anxious about a social situation?
Assess heightened self-focused attention, intolerance of anxiety, and awareness of inhibitory behaviors.	• What is the extent of excessive self-consciousness and self-focused awareness in social situations? • What physical sensations, behaviors, thoughts, or feelings are self-monitored when anxious? • How are these internal cues interpreted negatively? What's so awful or catastrophic about this unwanted internal state? • How important is it to conceal this internal state from others in the social situation? • What aspects of social performance does the individual self-monitor? What is his evaluation of his social performance? How does he think he is seen by others in the social setting (i.e., the "audience")? • What inhibitory behaviors are present during exposure to anxiety-provoking social situations? What is their effect on social performance and their contribution to perceived loss of control?
Determine the role of safety strategies and anxiety suppression.	• What mental or behavioral safety strategies does the individual use to reduce anxiety or prevent a negative evaluation by others? • What is the perceived effectiveness of these safety responses? Is the client able to report any negative consequences of her safety behaviors? • What is the person's tolerance of anxiety in social settings? How important is it to conceal anxiety from others? • What is the discrepancy between a person's desired level of social performance and her perceived actual level of performance?

(cont.)

TABLE 9.6. *(cont.)*

Elements of case conceptualization	Key questions
Assess autobiographical memory recall for past social experiences.	• Does the individual engage in rumination over past "social failures"? Obtain a description of these past negative experiences. • Is there any evidence of biased negative reappraisal of past social performance and its outcome? Is the individual able to recall positive aspects of past social experiences? • How much shame or embarrassment is associated with past social experiences?
Formulate the core social self-schemas that constitute vulnerability for social anxiety.	• What beliefs do individuals hold about how they are seen by others in social situations? What is the "self as social object" or "mental representation of self as seen by the audience"? (See Table 9.5 for other core schemas in social anxiety.)

elicit anxiety and avoidance. The therapist should review the self-monitoring form with the client to obtain ratings on degree of avoidance associated with each recorded situation.

In our case example Gerald identified a host of performance-based and social interaction situations at work and home that elicited significant anxiety. For example, taking a walk alone caused mild anxiety (20/100) because he might meet someone he knew, going to the market caused moderate anxiety (40/100) because there was an increased chance he would have to talk to a familiar person, and presenting a plan at a work meeting caused intense anxiety (100/100) because he anticipated that his anxiety would be so severe that his mind would go blank, he would stutter, and he would really "screw up" in front of people. Gerald identified 27 social situations that caused him mild to intense anxiety, each one associated with moderate to strong urge to avoid.

Three Phases of Social Anxiety

There can be considerable variability across individuals in the relative importance of the three phases of social phobia. For some individuals, like Gerald, anticipatory anxiety was almost constantly elevated whenever he left his house because there was always a chance he might meet someone he knew and would have to carry on a conversation. For others anticipatory anxiety may be less prominent because their social anxiety is confined to a few situations that occur only occasionally (e.g., making a presentation, answering questions in a meeting). Although one might expect exposure to social situations to be invariant across individuals, this is not the case. Avoidance may be so extensive in some individuals that they rarely are confronted with anxious social situations. Moreover, we would expect that some degree of postevent processing would be evident in most individuals with social phobia, but here again some patients are much more ruminative about their past social performance than others. For these individuals, continually reliving their past embarrassment will play a critical role in the persistence of social anxiety. Interestingly, postevent processing was not a major component of Gerald's social anxiety. Instead anticipatory anxiety was very intense and led to a pervasive pattern of avoidance of any potential social interaction.

Explicit Social Threat Bias

An automatic attentional bias for social threat as well as selective evaluation of social threat cues that result in overestimated appraisals of the probability, severity, and consequences of negative evaluation by others is a core proposition in the cognitive model of social phobia. The Apprehensive Thoughts Self-Monitoring Form (Appendix 5.4) and the Anxious Reappraisal Form (Appendix 5.10) can be used to obtain information on the client's social threat bias. In addition the Social Situation Estimation Form (Appendix 9.2) is useful for obtaining online estimates of threat in social situations. There are three critical facets of the social threat bias that the clinician must assess.

1. What is the client's common "social threat theme" that is evident across all anxious social situations? What is the "catastrophe" or worst-case scenario that the individual fears?
2. Estimates of the probability and severity of this dreaded outcome or its variant should be obtained for each anxious situation. Is there evidence of biased probability and severity expectations? If so, what external social information supports the interpretation? Is the client able to access positive information that challenges the social threat evaluation?
3. What automatic anxious thoughts or images does the individual experience when anticipating or participating in an anxious situation? These thoughts and images will provide valuable information on the perceived social threat and the maladaptive social self-schemas activated when socially anxious.

Whenever Gerald was around people, he would search for evidence that people were looking at him, especially at his face. He was particularly self-conscious that they might be looking at the redness of his face and thinking "This guy doesn't look after himself, what's his problem?" Gerald rated the probability that people were looking at him as very high (80/100) and the severity of their negative evaluation as very upsetting (75/100). Some situations, such as talking to the office staff at work, were associated with low probability and severity estimates, whereas other situations, such as carrying on a conversation with an acquaintance at the pub, was associated with high estimates. In the treatment sessions, exposure and cognitive restructuring began with social situations that elicited moderate levels of threat estimation.

Self-Focused Attention and Involuntary Inhibition

Excessive self-monitoring of an anxious internal state, the occurrence of inhibitory behaviors, and poor social performance are critical processes that are assessed in the cognitive case formulation. The cognitive therapist must determine the frequency and extent of self-monitoring that occurs during exposure to anxious social situations. To what extent do individuals become self-conscious in the social situation? How completely self-absorbed do they become? Are they aware of anything in their external environment or is their focus entirely internal? Are there particular physical sensations, symptoms, thoughts, or behaviors that become the object of their self-focus? Are they conscious of being overly inhibited in the social situation? What perceived negative consequence is associated with the self-monitored symptom or inhibition? For example, an individual might become excessively self-aware of blushing, trembling, verbal hesitations, stuttering, mind gone blank, or other involuntary inhibitory behaviors in social situations. The self-monitoring is motivated by a desire to conceal the symptoms and involuntary inhibitions from others in an effort to avoid a negative evaluation such as "What's wrong with her, she's blushing" or "He must be terribly anxious because he is stuttering so bad I can't understand what he's saying." The Self-Consciousness Rating Form (Appendix 9.3) can be used to obtain critical information on the role of heightened self-focused attention in anxiety-provoking social situations. Furthermore, the Physical Sensation Self-Monitoring Form (Appendix 5.3) and the Expanded Physical Sensations Checklist (Appendix 5.5) can be used to determine if certain physical symptoms of anxiety are excessively self-monitored when the person is socially anxious. Assessment of excessive self-awareness should provide the cognitive therapist with an indication of how the person thinks he appears to others when in social settings.

Gerald was very concerned that other people would notice that he was socially awkward or inhibited around other people. When exposed to social interactions he became intensely aware of blushing, his verbal hesitations and difficulty in maintaining a conversation, the tension in his muscles, and a general sense of feeling extremely uncomfortable. Gerald was convinced that he appeared anxious and inept to others, to put it in his words "a real arse," who must have a serious mental illness.

Safety Behaviors

The socially phobic person's reliance on safety-seeking strategies in order to conceal anxiety, counter unwanted inhibitory behavior, and appear more socially competent is another key element in the case formulation. Butler (2007) listed a number of common safety behaviors that are seen in social anxiety such as looking at the floor to avoid eye contact, wearing heavy makeup to hide blushing, rehearsing or mentally checking one's verbal comments, hiding the face or hands, speaking slowly or mumbling, avoiding challenging or controversial comments, being accompanied by a safe person, or the like. It is important to identify the various cognitive and behavioral safety strategies the individual uses to reduce social threat. In particular, does the client think these strategies are effective in reducing anxiety or the social threat and does he perceive any negative consequences associated with the safety strategy? In our case illustration, avoidance of eye contact, slow and hesitant verbal responses (i.e., involuntary inhibitory behaviors), as well as reluctance to initiate conversation, were common coping strategies that Gerald used to minimize social interaction. In fact these response strategies were very prominent even in the therapy sessions. The Behavioral Responses to Anxiety Checklist (Appendix 5.7) and the Cognitive Responses to Anxiety Checklist (Appendix 5.9) can be useful for exploring the client's use of safety-seeking responses.

Autobiographical Recall of Social Threat

Another important element in the cognitive case formulation is to determine whether recall of past social experiences plays any role in the individual's social anxiety. Are there particular past incidents that come to memory when the client anticipates or is exposed to a similar social situation? During postevent processing, does the individual focus on the most recent social event, or does she recall other past experiences? Does the client only recall certain negative aspects of the experience or is she able to recall more positive information as well? What is the negative interpretation or conclusion that the client makes about that social situation? What inference is drawn about herself and about the risk of social interaction?

Individuals will differ in how much they recall past social failures when feeling anxious. For some individuals there may be one or two events of intense embarrassment that come to mind when they interact with others. For others it may be the accumulative effect of many past social encounters which are recalled as very anxiety-provoking, even embarrassing. Whatever the case, the cognitive therapist should assess the client's recollection and interpretation of past social events and determine their impact on current levels of social anxiety. Gerald, for example, could not recall a particularly embarrassing social failure experience. However, it was clear that he had a tendency to recall all the negative and threatening aspects of past social experiences, even though cognitive restructuring revealed that these experiences were not nearly as threatening or disastrous as Gerald remembered. These memories reinforced his beliefs that "he could not handle being with people," "that he was different from others," and "that he would be better off if he socially isolated himself."

Core Social Self-Schemas

Assessment of the previous cognitive constructs of social phobia will allow the therapist to specify individuals' core beliefs about the self in relation to others. These social self-schemas represent the end point of the cognitive case formulation and include how individuals believe they are seen by others. Table 9.5 lists a number of the core beliefs that are found in social phobia. In the course of treatment a number of Gerald's core social self-beliefs became apparent. He believed that "others can see through me," "people tend to be harsh and rejecting," "I become weak and pathetic in social situations," and "I can't stand feeling anxious and uncomfortable around others."

Clinician Guideline 9.16

A cognitive case formulation for social phobia should include (1) contextual analysis of social situations; (2) focus on the anticipatory, exposure, and postevent processing phases of social anxiety; (3) specification of the social threat interpretation bias; (4) assessment of heightened self-consciousness and inhibition; (5) identification of safety-seeking responses; (6) sampling of prominent social threat recall bias; and (7) specification of the core social self-schemas.

DESCRIPTION OF COGNITIVE THERAPY FOR SOCIAL PHOBIA

The primary objective of cognitive therapy for social phobia is to reduce anxiety and eliminate feelings of shame or embarrassment as well as to facilitate improvement in personal functioning in social evaluative situations by correcting the faulty appraisals and beliefs of social threat and personal vulnerability. Table 9.7 presents the specific cognitive treatment goals for social phobia.

TABLE 9.7.   Treatment Goals in Cognitive Therapy for Social Phobia

- *Reduce anticipatory anxiety* by correcting social threat interpretation bias and preventing avoidance of anxiety-provoking social situations.
- *Counter excessive self-consciousness* during social exposure by re-directing information processing toward positive external social cues.
- *Eliminate safety strategies* employed to conceal and reduce anxiety.
- *Strengthen anxiety tolerance* and a more adaptive, coping perspective.
- *Reduce inhibition*, improve social skills, encourage a more realistic standard of performance, and develop a balanced self-evaluation of social performance.
- *Eliminate post-event rumination* and encourage more adaptive reappraisals of past social performance and its effects.
- *Modify core beliefs* about personal vulnerability in social interaction, the threat of negative evaluation by others, and the self as social object.

These goals are achieved by the use of cognitive restructuring and exposure-based behavioral interventions that target the specific maladaptive thought content and interpretative biases specified in the cognitive case formulation (see Table 9.6). There are six treatment elements to cognitive therapy of social phobia (see also Butler & Wells, 1995; D. M. Clark, 2001; Turk et al., 2008; Wells, 1997).

Education, Goal Setting, and Hierarchy Construction

The first couple of treatment sessions focus on educating the client into the cognitive model of social phobia. Information obtained from the diagnostic interview, self-report questionnaires, and the self-monitoring forms assigned for the case formulation are used to develop the client's personal idiosyncratic version of the cognitive model (refer to Figure 9.1).

During the education phase the cognitive therapist uses guided discovery to illustrate important features of the cognitive model by identifying biased cognitive processes associated with recent experiences of social anxiety. It is important that individuals learn about the three phases of social anxiety and the role that overestimated appraisals of the likelihood and consequences of social threat play during anticipation, exposure, and postevent recall of social situations. In addition the deleterious effects of heightened self-focused attention, awareness of inhibitory behaviors, and failure to process external social information should be explained, as well as the maladaptive effects of safety or concealment behaviors. The cognitive therapist will also discuss how an overly negative interpretation and recall of one's social performance as well as assumptions about making a negative impression on others will increase feelings of anxiousness in social settings. It is explained that long-held negative beliefs and assumptions about one's ability and effectiveness in relating to others can increase vulnerability to social anxiety. Finally, a treatment rationale must be included as part of the education phase. Clients are told that practice in identifying and correcting faulty thinking, the adoption of more positive approaches to anxiety, and gradual but repeated exposure to feared social situations are critical elements of treatment. With repeated practice in effortfully processing positive social information the tendency to selectively evaluate social situations in a threatening manner is weakened and social anxiety reduced.

As part of educating the client into the cognitive model, the therapist should elicit specific goals that the individual would like to achieve from therapy. In their self-help manual *The Shyness and Social Anxiety Workbook*, Antony and Swinson (2000b) suggest that individuals write down how social anxiety has affected their relationships, work or education, and daily functioning. This is followed by specifying the costs and benefits of overcoming one's social anxiety and then setting 1-month and 1-year goals for change. We believe this is a critical part of the education process that could improve compliance with the exposure exercises. Many individuals with social phobia are reluctant to commit to treatment because of the heightened anxiety expected from exposure. A firm appreciation of the long-term benefits of exposure-based treatment will increase treatment motivation and compliance. In fact Hope et al. (2006) have adopted the slogan *"Invest anxiety in a calmer future"* to emphasize that facing one's fear today can lead to later long-term payoffs. By specifying the costs of social anxiety and the goals for change, the therapist can encourage clients to "keep their eye on the target" when treatment becomes particularly challenging. Chapter 3 in the client workbook entitled *Managing Social Anxiety: A Cognitive-Behavioral Therapy Approach* contains an excellent discussion on the causes of social anxiety, the role of dysfunctional thinking, and the rationale for CBT of social phobia (Hope et al., 2000).

Before concluding the education phase, a social anxiety hierarchy should be constructed based on a range of anxiety-provoking situations recorded in the Daily Social Anxiety Self-Monitoring Sheet (Appendix 9.1). Furthermore, the Exposure Hierarchy (Appendix 7.1) can be useful for hierarchically arranging social situations from least to most anxiety-provoking. Construction of an exposure hierarchy was discussed in Chapter 7 (see section on graduated vs. intense exposure) and the guidelines outlined in that section will apply to development of a social anxiety hierarchy. It is important to generate a range of 15–20 social situations that occur fairly frequently, with a higher proportion of situations in the moderate to high anxiety range.

Gerald accepted the cognitive explanation for his long-standing and severe social phobia. In particular we focused on the important role played by anticipatory anxiety which led to a strong urge to avoid as much social interaction as possible. We noted that he became excessively self-conscious of his facial appearance and limited conversational skills in social situations, and was convinced that he appeared inadequate and disturbed to others because of his natural social inhibitions. He assumed that others must think negatively about him because they would observe his intense anxiety. Certain core beliefs became apparent such as "other people can see right through me," "people are naturally negative and critical of others," "my anxiety is so intense that it is intolerable and obvious to others," and "I am better off alone, away from other people." However, Gerald also realized that the more socially isolated he became, the more severe his clinical depression. His long-term goal was to gain sufficient confidence in social situations that he could start dating, whereas his more immediate goal was to reestablish connections with past friends and acquaintances. Since calling "old friends" on the telephone and arranging to meet them at a pub was moderately anxiety-provoking, we started exposure to these situations.

Clinician Guideline 9.17

Educating clients into the cognitive model of social phobia emphasizes that reduction in social anxiety is achieved by (1) correcting exaggerated judgments of social threat, (2) shifting attentional focus from internal anxiety cues to positive external social stimuli, (3) engaging in a realistic appraisal of one's social performance and tendency to be inhibited, (4) taking a more constructive perspective on anxiety tolerance, and (5) adopting more realistic assumptions of how the individual appears to others in social settings.

Cognitive Restructuring of Anticipatory Anxiety

After educating the client into the cognitive model, the next couple of sessions focus on teaching cognitive restructuring to counter the biased threat interpretation when anticipating an anxiety-provoking social situation. We believe it is important to start treatment here because (1) most individuals with social phobia experience strong anticipatory anxiety that leads to avoidance, (2) some variant of anticipatory anxiety can be more readily generated in the therapy session, and (3) this part of therapy tends to be less threatening for clients. Also the cognitive restructuring skills will be useful throughout the remaining treatment sessions. Table 9.8 summarizes the elements of cognitive restructuring for social anxiety.

The socially anxious client is asked to describe a recent period of high anticipatory anxiety over an expected social situation. Level of anxiety is rated on the 0–100 scale and the client is asked about any thoughts and images that occurred while thinking about the upcoming event. Pertinent questions include:

- "What were you worried would happen in this situation?"
- "Were you thinking of any negative consequences or outcome in this situation?"
- "Were you thinking about people's reactions to you in that situation?" "How would they react negatively or positively toward you?"

TABLE 9.8. Elements of Cognitive Restructuring for Social Anxiety

1. Identify a recent period of anticipatory anxiety.
2. Rate level of anxiety (0–100).
3. Use guided discovery to identify core social threat interpretation that may include:
   - Perceived intolerance of anxiety
   - Expectation of embarrassment
   - Negative evaluation (impression) by others.
4. Rate perceived likelihood and severity of anticipated social threat.
5. Challenge core social threat using:
   - Evidence of confirming and disconfirming information
   - Short- and long-term consequences (cost–benefit analysis)
   - Decatastrophizing
   - Identification of cognitive errors.
6. Develop a more realistic alternative anticipatory threat interpretation.
7. Rerate likelihood and severity of social threat and its alternative based on evidence.
8. Assign behavioral experiment (i.e., empirical hypothesis-testing task).

- "Were you thinking about how anxious you would feel in the situation?" "Are there any particular ways your anxiety might be evident to others?" "Did you have an image or could you imagine what you would be like in the situation?" "Were you thinking about how hard it would be to conceal your anxiety from others?" "What would happen if people knew you were anxious?"
- "Were you thinking about how you would perform in that situation or that you would be quite inhibited?" "If so, how do you imagine you would come across to others; what behaviors would they focus on?" "How do you think you'd embarrass yourself?" "If so, how would you act in an embarrassing manner?"
- "As you are thinking about this anticipated event, what is the worst outcome you can imagine?" "Has that ever happened to you in the past?" "If so, what was it like?"
- "Are you thinking about the impression you are likely to make on others?" "What do you imagine other people in that situation will end up thinking about you?" "How will you appear to them?"

Socratic questioning about the anticipated social threat will yield information on (1) perceived intolerance of anxiety in the situation, (2) how the client will embarrass or humiliate herself in front of others, and (3) how she thinks she will be perceived by others. Once this information is obtained, the therapist asks for probability and severity ratings on each aspect of the social threat judgments. For example, the client would rate the probability (0–100) as well as the severity that anxiety in the situation will be intense, that she will embarrass herself in the situation, and that others will conclude that she is "stupid" or "incompetent."

Once the core social threat interpretation has been specified, evidence gathering, cost–benefit analysis, and decatastrophizing can be used to challenge the client's faulty anticipatory thinking. These interventions have been discussed thoroughly in Chapter 6. For evidence gathering, the therapist asks for any information that confirms the social threat thinking as well as opposing information that disconfirms or at least questions the veracity of the anxious anticipatory cognitions. The Testing Anxious Appraisals: Looking for Evidence form (Appendix 6.2) can be helpful. A cost–benefit intervention would explore the actual costs (negative consequences) and benefits (both immediate and long term) associated with exposure to the anticipated social event (use Cost–Benefit Form in Appendix 6.3). Finally, decatastrophizing can be employed in which the client is asked to imagine the feared negative outcome. After generating the worst-case scenario, the client can be asked (1) "Would it really be as terrible as you think?", (2) "What is the most likely immediate and long-term impact on you?", (3) "What could you do to minimize the negative impact of embarrassment?", and (4) "How often do people embarrass themselves in front of others and yet somehow survive without life-changing negative effects?" In addition identifying errors in thinking (see discussion in Chapter 6) is an important part of challenging anxious thinking (use Common Errors and Biases in Anxiety handout and Identifying Anxious Thinking Errors Form, Appendix 5.6).

After challenging the faulty social threat thinking, the cognitive therapist works with the client on generating an alternative way of anticipating the forthcoming social situation. Again this has been discussed in Chapter 6. The Alternative Interpretations Form (Appendix 6.4) can be used to strengthen acceptance of a more realistic alternative interpretation. The alternative interpretation will probably acknowledge that the client may feel highly anxious and not perform as well as he likes, but the catastrophic, embarrassing outcome he anticipates is much less likely than expected. Instead "tolerable discomfort" is the most likely outcome.

In addition the therapist challenges the client's biased interpretation that her inhibitory behavior will automatically be evaluated negatively by others. Instead the alternative interpretation is "people are tolerant of a fairly wide range of social behavior. I don't have to make an award-winning performance to be accepted." Once this alternative has been fully described the client is asked to rerate the probability that the initial catastrophic embarrassment will occur versus the alternative of "tolerable discomfort" and others' acceptance of "somewhat inhibited social performance." It must be emphasized that the rating is based not on how the client feels but on the realistic probability based on the weight of the confirming and disconfirming evidence.

Cognitive restructuring normally concludes with the assignment of a behavioral experiment. In most cases this involves some form of exposure to a variant of the anticipated anxious situation in order to collect evidence that disconfirms the exaggerated social threat appraisal. We discuss the use of exposure in cognitive therapy for social phobia more fully in a separate section below. In the meantime, Table 9.9 illustrates use of cognitive restructuring for anticipatory social anxiety.

Clinician Guideline 9.18

Cognitive restructuring in social phobia involves the correction of exaggerated interpretations of the probability and severity of social threat (i.e., negative evaluation by others) through evaluation of confirming and disconfirming evidence, consideration of realistic consequences, preparation for the worst outcome, and reevaluation in light of a more likely alternative interpretation of the social situation and one's inhibited social performance.

Heightened Self-Focused Attention: Use of Role-Play Feedback

After completing a couple of cognitive restructuring thought records in-session and assigning this as homework, the cognitive therapist introduces live or videotaped role-play feedback. This is typically introduced by the third or fourth treatment session. Role plays have long been recognized as a central ingredient in cognitive and behavioral interventions for social anxiety (e.g., Beck et al., 1985; Beidel & Turner, 2007; D. M. Clark, 2001; Heimberg & Juster, 1995; Wells, 1997). They serve a number of therapeutic objectives. Role-play feedback or behavioral rehearsal can be used to highlight the negative effects of excessive self-focused attention, inhibitory behaviors, and safety responses, as well as to learn a more adaptive external focus of attention (D. M. Clark, 2001). Role plays are also a less anxious form of within-session exposure that can be used to correct exaggerated threat appraisals and negative self-evaluations of social performance. Finally, role-play feedback and behavioral rehearsal can be used to help the socially anxious person learn more effective communication and interaction behaviors with others.

Role play was previously discussed in Chapter 7 in the section on "directed behavioral change." In the context of social anxiety, the therapist begins by role-playing with the client moderately anxious social situations from the anxiety hierarchy. The client is

TABLE 9.9. Clinical Example of Cognitive Restructuring of Anticipatory Social Anxiety

Anticipatory situation

Carol is informed by her supervisor that an office meeting is scheduled later that day to discuss the need to upgrade the office computer system. There will be 15 of Carol's coworkers present and the supervisor will be asking each of them to speak about the problems they have encountered with the present computer network.

Level of anticipatory anxiety

Carol rated her anxiety at 90/100, which increases as she approaches the meeting time.

Carol's anticipatory social threat cognitions

- "I can't get out of this meeting; I have to go."
- "We'll be seating around the board table and she'll [supervisor] ask everyone for their opinion."
- "The anxiety will build until finally she gets to me and I have to say something. By that time I'll be in panic mode." [intolerance of anxiety]
- "Everyone will be staring at me. I'll get really blushed, feel hot, my hands will tremble, and my mind will go blank."
- "I'll feel so self-conscious about my anxiety that I won't be able to give a clear answer." [excessive self-focused attention]
- "Everyone will wonder what's wrong with me, how could I be so anxious around my work colleagues. They'll see me as weak, incompetent, and mentally ill." [negative evaluation, appearance to others]
- "I'll feel so embarrassed by this fiasco that I won't be able to face my colleagues for days. Going to work will be a painful experience." [expectation of embarrassment]

Estimation ratings of likelihood and severity

Carol rated the above scenario as 70% likely to happen and the severity as 85% because it involved coworkers who she would see everyday.

Challenging the social threat cognitions

1. *Confirming evidence*—she has become extremely anxious at such meetings in the past; at least one of her closer friends in the office commented that she seemed quite nervous; she recalls feeling embarrassed for days after the meeting.
2. *Disconfirming evidence*—despite feeling like she was inarticulate, others seemed to understand what she was saying at past meetings as indicated by their comments after she spoke; everyone seemed to treat her the same after the meeting; when Carol mentioned to a coworker a couple of weeks later how anxious she felt in the meeting, the coworker didn't recall noticing Carol's anxiety; there are a couple of other coworkers who are shy and appear nervous at these meetings and yet they are well liked and respected; when she is speaking, no one looks embarrassed or disapproving, they seem to be paying attention.
3. *Consequences*—the immediate consequence is an escalation in anxiety and discomfort but there have been no long-term, life-changing consequences to Carol's anxiety at work meetings; people have not changed how they treat her and within a week any embarrassment seems to subside.
4. *Decatastrophizing*—the therapist worked with Carol to write out the worst-case scenario that could be associated with speaking out in a work meeting. She decided that the worst that could happen is that she might have a full-blown panic attack and have to excuse herself from the meeting. Her work colleagues would know something was wrong and then question her after the meeting. Together Carol and her therapist worked on a possible response to how she would handle other people's reactions if she did leave a meeting prematurely because of panic. We also worked on how she could stay in the meeting and ride out the panic attack as an alternative response strategy.

(cont.)

TABLE 9.9. *(cont.)*

5. *Error identification*—going over her thought processes when anticipating the meeting, Carol was able to see that she was catastrophizing (assuming her coworkers will think she is mentally ill), and engaging in tunnel vision (only focused on the negative aspects of the situation) as well as emotional reasoning (assuming that things must be going really bad because of her anxiety level).

Construct alternative interpretation

Carol and her therapist developed the following alternative interpretation: "I will feel uncomfortable in the meeting and others may notice my discomfort. However, it is a tolerable discomfort that does not prevent me from offering an opinion. I may not be as eloquent as some and I may show signs of discomfort but my work colleagues know me well and are most likely to conclude that I'm a shy person who feels uncomfortable expressing myself in a group."

Rerated likelihood and severity

Based on the evidence, Carol rerated the more extreme social threat scenario as 40% likely and the alternative interpretation as 90% likely. Likewise the alternative was rated much less severe than the original threat interpretation.

Assigned behavioral experiment

Carol indicated that a follow-up meeting had been scheduled at work. She agreed to go to that meeting and attend as closely as possible to other people's reactions to her rather than to her own internal feelings of anxiety. She was able to use the Alternative Interpretation Form (Appendix 6.4) to record her observations.

first asked to role-play "how she typically would respond in the situation." Ratings of anxiety are obtained and the cognitive therapist, acting as the observer, elicits the individual's anxious thoughts and interpretations associated with the role-played situation. The therapist then discusses an alternative approach in which the client shifts attention from an internal focus to processing external feedback from others (see D. M. Clark, 2001). Safety or concealment responses are eliminated and attention to positive cues in the external environment is encouraged. Adaptive coping statements that counter automatic social threat interpretations can be constructed. The therapist then models this more adaptive approach in the role play, after which the client repeatedly practices the constructive approach with the therapist providing corrective feedback.

D. M. Clark (2001) considers role play and video feedback critical for modifying the heightened self-focused attention in social phobia. First, clients rate their anxiety after role-playing a social situation in which they self-focus on interoceptive cues and rely on safety behaviors. In a second condition they rate their anxiety after adopting an external focus of attention and drop maladaptive safety responses. D. M. Clark notes that this exercise teaches individuals that intense self-focus and safety behaviors actually increases their anxiety and their assumptions of how well they think they performed are greatly influenced by how they felt during the role play. D. M. Clark found videotape feedback particularly useful in helping socially anxious individuals obtain realistic information on their social performance and how they actually appear to others. Furthermore, videotape role plays provide feedback on clients' inhibitory behaviors and corrects their negative assumptions that their inhibitory behavior has a detrimental effect on how they are received by others.

In order for the videotaped role play to be effective, the socially anxious client must be asked how she thinks she appeared to others in the video before actually viewing the tape and then to view her videotaped performance as though watching a stranger. In this way the client can learn that her evaluation of how she thinks others perceive her is negatively biased. Thus the main purpose of videotaped feedback is to provide corrective information for the client's faulty assumption of making a negative impression on others by being anxious or inhibited.

Live and videotaped role plays provide an excellent introduction to *in vivo* exposure to anxious social situations. The therapist can introduce increasingly more anxious social situations into the role-play sessions. Within-session role plays can be assigned as homework in which a spouse or family member becomes the observer. This will increase the chance that therapeutic effects from role plays will generalize to the actual social situation.

A case illustration of the therapeutic benefits of role plays was Erin, a 32-year-old financial planner. Erin suffered considerable anxiety in her job because she had great difficulty being assertive with customers. When they would make unreasonable demands, she would agree to an early deadline for completing their work even though it would be impossible to meet the deadline given her current workload. Erin was terrified of anger and criticism from her customers, so she quickly agreed to an unreasonable deadline in order to avoid conflict. When Erin first role-played her usual interaction with demanding customers, it was clear she was excessively focused on her own feelings of discomfort and inhibitions such as avoiding eye contact or refraining from asking the customer questions that might suggest possible confrontation. Her automatic thoughts were "I getting very uncomfortable, I need to get this guy out of my office," "He seems to be getting quite angry at me," and "I'll just agree now and figure out what to do later." The therapist worked with Erin on an alternative, more assertive response to demanding customers that helped her set more realistic deadlines while not allowing her anxiety to dictate her response. It took many repeated role plays in session and as homework assignments with her spouse acting as a "demanding customer" before Erin was ready to try this at work.

Clinician Guideline 9.19

Employ role plays or behavioral rehearsal as an integral part of cognitive therapy to reduce heightened self-focused attention, reliance on safety behaviors, negative evaluation of social performance and inhibitory behavior, and long-held assumptions of negative impression on others.

Cognitive Restructuring of Faulty Threat Appraisals during Exposure

Prior to initiating within-session and between-session exposure to socially threatening situations, it is important that the cognitive therapist correct biased threat interpretations, excessive self-focused attention, and emotional reasoning by completing cognitive restructuring thought records on the moderate- and high-anxiety situations in the hierarchy. The same cognitive restructuring protocol as described for anticipatory social anxiety will be used in the present context, except now the focus is on experiences of actual exposure to the anxious situation. Along with role-play feedback, cognitive restructuring of actual social situations is introduced in the fifth and sixth sessions in order to correct biased threat interpretations, redirect attention to external stimuli, and deliberately refocus processing capacity on the positive cues in the social environment. This therapeutic focus will begin to address some of the underlying core beliefs about social threat, personal vulnerability, and inadequacy that are important in social phobia.

Clinician Guideline 9.20

Throughout treatment cognitive restructuring is routinely applied to the biased thoughts, images, and interpretations associated with various situations in the social anxiety hierarchy in an effort to achieve crucial change in the maladaptive social self-schemas that underlie social phobia.

Exposure to Social Threat

By the seventh or eighth session *in vivo* exposure to moderately anxiety-provoking situations in the social anxiety hierarchy should be introduced into treatment. Heimberg and colleagues offer a comprehensive outline for exposure sessions and recommend the integration of within-session and between-session exposure exercises (Heimberg & Becker, 2002; Turk et al., 2008). As with cognitive therapy for other anxiety disorders, exposure to anxious social situations is essential for effective treatment of social phobia. Moreover, the most effective way to correct the maladaptive interpretations and beliefs of social anxiety is through exposure-based behavioral experiments. Exposure exercises also allow clients (1) to practice shifting attention away from internal states toward external social stimuli, (2) to learn better tolerance of moderate anxiety levels, (3) to interpret their social performance and inhibitions more positively, and (4) to gather critical disconfirming evidence of their biased social threat interpretations.

A detailed description of the use of exposure within cognitive therapy can be found in Chapter 7; the guidelines outlined there apply to treatment of social phobia. The therapist should begin exposure with the low to moderately anxious social situations in the social anxiety hierarchy. It is preferable to first role-play the situation in session before assigning it as an *in vivo* between-session homework assignment. Heimberg and Becker (2002) list numerous social situations that might be used for exposure such as initiating a conversation with an acquaintance, talking to a classmate before or after class, introducing yourself to a stranger, making a telephone call to someone you like, making a speech, asking a question in class, eating in front of other people, engaging in a job interview, asking someone out on a date, and the like. The within-session role play identifies any faulty thinking that will undermine the *in vivo* exposure and allows the client opportunity to practice corrective modes of cognition and more adaptive responses to social anxiety. Of course, in cognitive therapy exposure is presented as a behavioral experiment to test whether the client's experience confirms or disconfirms his exaggerated social threat interpretation or its alternative. The Empirical Hypothesis-

Testing Form (Appendix 6.5) can be used to record critical observations from exposure exercises (see also Hope et al., 2000, for suggestions on exposure in social phobia).

The following example illustrates how exposure-based empirical hypothesis testing was incorporated into Gerald's treatment. In his social anxiety hierarchy Gerald rated calling an old friend as moderately anxious (40/100). His automatic anxious thoughts were "I feel guilty for not calling him in such a long time," "He doesn't want to hear from me," "I'll be bothering him," and "I'll feel so anxious, why bother doing it?" After correcting the negative interpretations through a cognitive restructuring exercise, Gerald and the therapist role-played the telephone call to the friend. They brainstormed various conversational topics that Gerald could employ with this friend in order to counter Gerald's verbal inhibitions. Coping statements from the cognitive restructuring exercise were employed to correct negative expectations and encourage tolerance of anxiety. After practicing the social interaction in session, Gerald was able to commit himself to the homework assignment, which involved calling his friend. He returned to the next session exuberant about the assignment. He called his friend and contrary to his expectations his friend was very receptive. In fact he made plans to have dinner together with Gerald the following week. Moreover, Gerald discovered that his anxiety was not as crippling as he had predicted and that his ability to carry on a conversation was better than expected. The exercise proved to be an important turning point in therapy because Gerald experienced disconfirmation of his anxious thinking.

Clinician Guideline 9.21

Repeated exposure to social anxiety situations is critical for providing evidence that disconfirms the faulty appraisals and beliefs of threat and vulnerability that maintain social anxiety.

Cognitive Interventions for Postevent Processing

The prominence of postevent processing will vary across individuals with social phobia. For those who engage in considerable rumination about past social experiences, postevent processing must be targeted early in treatment. Much of the critical information about the client's idiosyncratic form of postevent processing can be obtained from the case formulation (see previous discussion).

After obtaining a clear description of the client's postevent thought content, the therapist should inquire about the perceived costs and benefits of engaging in this repeated reappraisal of past social performances and their outcome (D. M. Clark, 2001). For some clients the disadvantages of reevaluating past social encounters may be obvious, whereas other socially anxious clients believe such reanalysis helps them prepare for similar events in the future. For example, Henry was unsuccessful with a job interview he had with a very prestigious company many years ago. It was quite clear that his anxiety during the interview was so intense that he did not perform well. However, years later he continued to ruminate about the failed interview as proof that he was not smart enough, that "he had been found out." Another client would think back to past difficulties when making reports at quarterly shareholder meetings, trying to figure out how she could improve her public speaking skills. Whatever the case, it is important that the client realizes that in the end postevent rumination is a maladaptive cognitive strategy that contributes to the persistence of social anxiety because it ultimately reinforces the perception that social situations are threatening. The Cost–Benefit Form (Appendix 6.3) is useful in this regard.

Cognitive restructuring is a second intervention for postevent processing. The client is asked to describe in detail his recollection of any past social experiences that continue to come to his mind on a fairly regular basis. The therapist focuses on memories that recur repeatedly or that are interpreted as clear evidence of social threat, embarrassment, or ineptitude. Memory of a specific past social experience is targeted and the therapist determines what the client concludes from this event about social threat, how he appeared to others, his performance in that situation, and the personal consequences of the social encounter. The therapist then evaluates the accuracy of the client's recollection through evidence gathering and inductive reasoning to emphasize the possibility that the client's recall of the past event is marred by biased appraisals of threat and vulnerability. An alternative evaluation of the past experience is formulated that offers a more realistic perspective on the experience. The client is then encouraged to repeatedly challenge the negative memory with the possibility of the more benign alternative whenever he starts ruminating on the past social event—that is, to engage in "cognitive debriefing" in which performance is evaluated in terms of meeting predefined goals rather than evaluated on the basis of one's emotional response (Brozovich & Heimberg, 2008). Cognitive restructuring was employed with Henry to evaluate whether his unsuccessful job interview was due to lack of intelligence. In fact there was considerable evidence that he was a highly intelligent and gifted computer programmer. Gradually he came to believe in the possibility that intense anxiety during the interview caused him to underperform in that situation. This represented a more benign interpretation because anxiety was something he could counter, whereas lack of intelligence meant he was doomed to failure and disappointment.

Cognitive restructuring should be followed up with behavioral assignments that seek out disconfirming evidence for the negative recall of past experiences. For example, the client could be asked to survey friends, family members, or coworkers who were present at a social event to determine their recollection. The client's recollection of the event could be compared to how others recall the experience in order to highlight areas of discrepancy. Another exercise involves videotaping an in-session role play of some social situation. The client provides an evaluation of her anxiety, her social performance, and how inhibited she appears in the role play. Two weeks later the therapist asks the client to recall what she remembers about the role play and to evaluate her anxiety, performance, and appearance based on the memory. The two sets of evaluations are then compared. The objective of this exercise is to highlight how negative biases creep into memory when socially anxious individuals remember their past social experiences.

Finally, cognitive restructuring can be used to encourage the client to shift from an observer perspective on their past social experiences (i.e., seeing oneself as if from an external point of view) to a field perspective (i.e., as if looking out through one's own eyes). D. M. Clark (2001) emphasizes that this shift in perspective is necessary for focusing on information that is inconsistent with a negative self-image. In other words, clients are encouraged to remember past social situations from their own perspective rather than from how they imagine they appeared to others. This will allow the client to focus on the external cues in social situations that contradict the exaggerated threat and failure interpretations.

Clinician Guideline 9.22

Employ cognitive restructuring and behavioral assignments to correct biased recall of past social experiences that characterize the postevent ruminative processing in social phobia. Encourage individuals to take a field perspective when reevaluating their past social experiences.

Efficacy of Cognitive Therapy for Social Phobia

In their original publication of empirically supported treatments, Chambless et al. (1998) concluded that CBT for social phobia was probably an efficacious treatment (see also Chambless & Ollendick, 2001). Since then a number of treatment outcome reviews have concluded that CBT produces immediate and enduring treatment effects for social phobia (e.g., Butler et al., 2006; Hollon et al., 2006; Hofmann & Barlow, 2002). For example, Rodebaugh, Holaway, and Heimberg (2004) concluded that CBT produces moderate to large effect sizes, that group and individual treatment yields similar results, and that combined cognitive restructuring plus exposure might confer a slight advantage over exposure alone, although the difference is nonsignificant. Beidel and Turner (2007) offered a more negative outlook, concluding that group CBT produced higher responder rates for specific (67–79%) than generalized (18–44%) social phobia. However, Turk et al. (2008) were more optimistic, claiming that three out of four individuals with social phobia will realize a clinically significant gain from an intensive trial of exposure and cognitive restructuring.

Cognitive restructuring and exposure are key components of the cognitive therapy for social phobia presented in this chapter. For this reason our brief and highly selective review focuses on a few key studies that include both cognitive restructuring and exposure in their treatment package. In one of the first major outcome studies on CBT for social phobia, 133 patients with DSM-IV social phobia from two sites were randomly assigned to twelve 2½ hour sessions of group CBT, an educational-supportive group (attention control psychotherapy), 15 mg of phenelzine (Nardil) alone, or matching placebo tablets (Heimberg et al., 1998). At 12-week posttreatment the medication and group CBT conditions were significantly more effective than the pill placebo or attention control conditions with 75% of completers in each group classified as responders. At 6-month follow-up 50% of the phenelzine responders relapsed compared to only 17% of the CBT responders (Liebowitz et al., 1999).

D. M. Clark and colleagues conducted a series of outcome studies on their version of CBT for social phobia. In one study 71 patients with social phobia were randomly assigned to group CBT, individual CBT, or a wait list condition (Stangier, Heidenreich, Peitz, Lauterbach, & Clark, 2003). At posttreatment both types of CBT were significantly better than the wait list group but individual CBT proved superior to group CBT at both posttreatment and 6-month follow-up. In a randomized placebo-controlled trial, 61 patients with generalized social phobia were assigned to 16 individual weekly sessions of cognitive therapy, fluoxetine (Prozac) plus self-exposure, or placebo pill plus self-exposure (D. M. Clark et al., 2003). At 8 weeks midtreatment and then 16 weeks posttreatment, cognitive therapy was superior to the fluoxetine and placebo groups. Cognitive therapy produced very large effect sizes whereas medication produced only small effect sizes. At 12-month follow-up cognitive therapy remained superior to fluoxetine. Furthermore, the effects of cognitive therapy were quite specific to social anxiety given that the three groups did not differ at posttreatment on general mood measures.

In another study 62 patients with social phobia (88% had a generalized subtype) were randomly assigned to 14 weeks of individual cognitive therapy, exposure plus applied relaxation training, or a wait list control (D. M. Clark et al., 2006). At posttreatment both interventions were superior to the wait list condition but cognitive therapy was significantly more effective than exposure plus applied relaxation at posttreatment, 3-month, and 6-month follow-up. Other studies have also reported significant treatment effects for CBT of social phobia that includes both cognitive restructuring and exposure (e.g., Davidson et al., 2004; Herbert, Rheingold, Gaudiano, & Myers, 2004; Mörtberg, Karlsson, Fyring, & Sundin, 2006). Overall these studies indicate that cognitive therapy produces clinically significant reductions in social anxiety for the majority of individuals, even those with more severe generalized social phobia, and the gains are maintained after treatment termination (see also Rodebaugh et al., 2004). Moreover, cognitive therapy may produce more enduring effects than medication alone (Hollon et al., 2006), although medication may be slightly more effective in the short term (see Rodebaugh et al., 2004).

A number of studies have examined factors within cognitive therapy that may influence its effectiveness. As noted previously, individual cognitive therapy may be more effective than a group format and it would appear that the therapy has less impact on general psychopathology or mood state. Moreover, there is some evidence that individuals with social phobia who have a comorbid depression may show a poorer response to treatment (Ledley et al., 2005). More recently, Hofmann and colleagues found that sudden gains occurred in 15% of individuals in their group CBT condition, with the fourth and 11th sessions the modal points in which this occurred (Hofmann, Schulz, Meuret, Moscovitch, & Suvak, 2006). However, sudden gains were not associated with better treatment outcome nor were they more likely to be preceded by significant cognitive change.

One question that deserves special mention is the debate over the additive benefits of cognitive restructuring beyond exposure alone in the treatment of social phobia. In one of the first studies to address this question, Mattick and Peters (1988) found that therapist-assisted exposure plus cognitive restructuring was more effective for treatment of severe social phobia than therapist-assisted exposure alone (see Feske & Chambless, 1995, for contrary conclusion). More recently Hofmann (2004b) randomly assigned 90 individuals with social phobia to receive 12 weekly sessions of group CBT, exposure group therapy (EGT) without explicit cognitive interventions, or a wait list control. At posttreatment the CBT and EGT conditions produced similar treatment effects that were significantly greater than the wait list control. However, at 6-month follow-up only the CBT participants showed continued improvement after treatment termination. These findings suggest that interventions aimed at directly changing faulty cognition may produce more enduring treatment benefits for social anxiety. In addressing this topic Rodebaugh et al. (2004) warned that comparing the added benefits of cognitive restructuring over exposure alone will produce misleading results because it is very difficult to ensure external validity of the treatment conditions. They concluded that "both cognitive restructuring and exposure should be considered fundamental and essential aspects of CBT for social anxiety disorder and that they are best considered as interrelated techniques designed to do the same thing: allow the client to experience what the situation is actually like, as opposed to how they fear or think it will be" (Rodebaugh et al., 2004, pp. 890–891). We believe practitioners and clinical researchers alike would be well advised to heed this recommendation before concluding that one interrelated therapeutic ingredient is more effective than another.

Clinician Guideline 9.23

Cognitive therapy that includes both cognitive restructuring and systematic exposure to social anxiety situations produces clinically significant effects for three-quarters of individuals with specific or generalized social phobia. Moreover, cognitive therapy may produce more enduring benefits for social phobia than pharmacotherapy alone, although more research is needed to establish this finding.

SUMMARY AND CONCLUSION

Social phobia is a marked and persistent apprehension and nervousness about social situations due to an exaggerated fear of negative evaluation by others. It is unique among the anxiety disorders in its self-defeating effects. The occurrence of intense social anxiety is associated with involuntary inhibitory behaviors that interfere in social performance, thereby conferring some of the very effects most feared by the individual. The disorder fits most closely to a dimensional conceptualization with milder, more circumscribed forms of social anxiety at one end, more severe generalized social phobia at the upper end, and avoidant personality disorder at the extreme end of severity.

A reformulated cognitive model of social phobia was presented (see Figure 9.1) in which anticipated or actual exposure to anxiety-provoking situations activates enduring maladaptive self-referent social schemas that cause an automatic attentional bias for schema-congruent social threat stimuli and an explicit interpretative bias in which the probability and severity that others have formed a negative impression of the socially anxious person is exaggerated. In addition excessive self-focused attention on an internal anxious state is taken as strong confirmatory evidence that they are viewed by others as weak and ineffective. Socially anxious individuals exhibit involuntary inhibitory behavior when around others and engage in various safety behaviors to conceal their anxiety and perceived ineffectiveness. However, these strategies tend to exacerbate anxiety and individuals' negative evaluation of their social performance. They leave the situation feeling embarrassed and humiliated, with postevent recall of past social experiences biased for retrieving evidence of social threat and personal failure. Empirical evidence that social phobia is characterized by an explicit social threat interpretation bias, a maladaptive social self-schema organization, an automatic attentional bias for social threat cues, a heightened self-focused attention on interoceptive cues, and excessive postevent rumination supports key elements of the cognitive model.

Cognitive therapy for social phobia seeks to reduce social anxiety and avoidance by correcting faulty social threat attention and interpretation biases, reversing the excessive self-focus on internal cues, eliminating reliance on safety strategies to conceal anxiety, increasing tolerance of anxiety and a tendency to be inhibited, and decreasing postevent rumination. A review of the treatment outcome literature indicates that cognitive therapy that includes both cognitive restructuring and repeated exposure to anxious social situations produces clinically significant and enduring improvement in 75% of individuals who complete treatment.

Despite the substantial advances made in our understanding of the cognitive basis of social phobia and its treatment, a number of key issues remain for future investigation. It is unclear whether the information-processing bias apparent when first encountering a social threat situation (i.e., "online inferences") is different from the processing bias that occurs when social phobia individuals reflect back on social interactions (i.e., "offline inferences"). Also, is the main problem in social phobia heightened accessibility of negative social threat or diminished processing of positive social information? Less is known about the role of safety behaviors and inhibitory behaviors, the nature of postevent processing, and the causal status of faulty information processing in social phobia. Finally, the cognitive approach to social phobia would be further advanced by more psychometric research on self-report measures that specifically assess the negative cognitions and beliefs of social phobia, and randomized controlled trials with longer follow-up periods in order to determine the long-term effectiveness of cognitive therapy for social phobia.

Daily Social Anxiety Self-Monitoring Sheet

Name: _____ Date: from _____ to: _____

Instructions: Use the following form to record your daily experiences with anxious or distressing social situations that may involve some performance on your part, an evaluation by others, and/or interpersonal interactions. It is important to complete this form as soon after the social event as possible in order to maintain its accuracy.

Date	Describe Difficult or Anxious Social Situation (what happened, who was involved, where, what was your role?)	Anticipation of Event (duration and average anxiety level; 0–100)	Actual Event Exposure (duration and peak anxiety level; 0–100)	Postevent Remembering (duration and average anxiety level; 0–100)	Long-Term Outcome (rate embarrassment 0–100)

Note. Duration refers to the length of time (i.e., minutes, hours, or days) spent anticipating a social event, being exposed to it, or thinking back on it. Estimate the average (or peak where applicable) level of anxiety on 0 ("no anxiety"), 50 ("moderately intense"), to 100 ("extreme," panic level"). Whenever a panic attack is experienced in the anticipation, exposure, or postevent period, record with initials PA. In last column, rate level of embarrassment that remains associated with the situation from 0 ("none") to 100 ("the most embarrassing, humiliating experience in my life").

From *Cognitive Therapy of Anxiety Disorders: Science and Practice* by David A. Clark and Aaron T. Beck. Copyright 2010 by The Guilford Press. Permission to photocopy this appendix is granted to purchasers of this book for personal use only (see copyright page for details).

Social Situation Estimation Form

Name: _____   Date: from _____ to: _____

Instructions: The following form is used to record your estimates of the likelihood and degree of negative consequence associated with daily social experiences that involve feelings of anxiety or distress. It is important to complete this form as soon after the social event as possible in order to maintain its accuracy.

Date	Describe Difficult or Anxious Social Situation (what happened, who was involved, where, what was your role?)	Anticipation of Event (rate likelihood & expected severity of negative outcome from 0–100)	Actual Event Exposure (rate likelihood & expected severity of negative outcome from 0–100)	Post-Event Outcome (rate likelihood & expected severity of negative outcome from 0–100)
		Likelihood rating = Outcome rating =	Likelihood rating = Outcome rating =	Likelihood rating = Outcome rating =
		Likelihood rating = Outcome rating =	Likelihood rating = Outcome rating =	Likelihood rating = Outcome rating =
		Likelihood rating = Outcome rating =	Likelihood rating = Outcome rating =	Likelihood rating = Outcome rating =
		Likelihood rating = Outcome rating =	Likelihood rating = Outcome rating =	Likelihood rating = Outcome rating =

<u>Note:</u> *For likelihood ratings, 0 = "I think there is no chance the negative consequence that I fear will occur in this situation", to 100 = "I am certain the negative consequence will occur in this situation." For outcome ratings, 0 = "there is no negative consequence to this situation", to 100 = "an intolerable, worst case scenario is expected in this situation"*

Self-Consciousness Rating Form

Name: _____ Date: from _____ to: _____

Instructions: The following form is used to record your estimates of the likelihood and degree of negative consequence associated with daily social experiences that involve feelings of anxiety or distress. It is important to complete this form as soon after the social event as possible in order to maintain its accuracy.

Date	Describe Difficult or Anxious Social Situation (what happened, who was involved, where, what was your role?)	Extent of Self-Focus (rate extent of focus on yourself from 0 = no self-focus to 100 = completely self-absorbed)	Target of Self-Focus (list specific physical sensations, thoughts, images, verbal expressions, or behavioral actions of which you were intensely aware in the social situation)	Negative Consequence (describe any negative impression that you might have made on others)

Chapter 10

Cognitive Therapy
of Generalized Anxiety Disorder

There is nothing that wastes the body like worry....
—MAHATMA GANDHI (Indian philosopher,
humanitarian, and political leader, 1869–1948)

Rebecca is a 38-year-old mother of two children who manages a large retail clothing store with 150 employees and 15 department managers. Although a very successful businesswoman who has risen rapidly through her company, has received numerous work evaluations praising her abilities, and has been promoted over her peers on a number of occasions, Rebecca is plagued by anxiety, feelings of uncertainty, and worries about her personal effectiveness both at work and at home. Although she traced her anxiety back to childhood and has been a chronic worrier since adolescence, in the last 5 years her anxiety has intensified with her job promotion and added work demands.

Numerous issues worried Rebecca including her aging parents' health problems, her own personal health, her children's safety and performance at school, family finances, and whether her marriage can survive the stresses of two highly demanding careers. However, much of her daily worries focused on work and whether she could meet her company's expectations. She worried that the store would miss its monthly productivity targets and she wondered if her superiors perceived that she was less competent than other store managers. She worried that her employees had lost respect for her and that she had been too soft and indecisive when dealing with employee discipline matters. She worried that an employee might lodge a complaint against her to human resources and that she would get entangled in messy litigation over her managerial practices. The regular reports submitted to company headquarters or a visit to the store by the district manager triggered a particularly intense period of anxiety. The underlying core belief that drove Rebecca's work-related anxiety concerned doubts about her own competence. She was fearful that others might perceive her as incompetent or that she would fail and this would reveal her vulnerability to all.

Rebecca experienced anxiety and worried daily, especially at work when the demands were greatest. During stressful work periods she experienced chest tightness, tense muscles, and heart palpitations. Various anxious thoughts automatically intruded into her mind at such times like "This job is too stressful for me," "I'm not 'cut out' to be a store manager," "My incompetence will become obvious to everyone," and "I don't have what it takes to do this job." She felt tense and on edge much of the work day, but unfortunately the anxious symptoms followed her home because she would sit and rehearse all the day's work activities in order to evaluate her performance (e.g., "Did I make the right decision?", "Did I handle that situation well or not?"). She would also think about her agenda for the next day and worried whether she was about to experience an unexpected calamity. Rebecca's sleep was very disrupted by anxiety and worry. She averaged about 5 hours per night, having great difficulty with sleep onset due to "racing thoughts." She found it difficult to relax, and there were signs of some decline in her physical health as indicated by high blood pressure and an irritable bowel syndrome. She also experienced periods of deep dysphoria that met diagnostic criteria for a major depressive episode on at least two occasions, although both episodes went undetected. Rebecca did not abuse alcohol nor was she prescribed anxiolytic medication. However, her anxiety and worry led to procrastination, avoidance, and frequent reassurance seeking from others about her performance.

This chapter presents a modified cognitive model and treatment of generalized anxiety disorder (GAD) that is based on an earlier cognitive formulation for chronic anxiety disorder (Beck et al., 1985). We begin by considering key diagnostic issues and phenomenology of GAD, followed by a presentation of the cognitive model and its empirical status. Cognitive assessment and case conceptualization for GAD is discussed, as well as a disorder-specific treatment approach based on the cognitive model. The chapter concludes with a consideration of treatment efficacy and directions for future research.

DIAGNOSTIC CONSIDERATIONS

DSM-IV Diagnosis

In DSM-IV-TR (American Psychiatric Association [APA], 2000) GAD is considered an anxiety disorder characterized by excessive anxiety and worry that persists for at least 6 months and concerns a number of events or activities. GAD was first recognized as a separate disorder in DSM-III, and since then a number of diagnostic changes were made to improve its reliability and to shift from a focus on "free-floating anxiety" to worry as the central defining feature of the disorder (Mennin, Heimberg, & Turk, 2004). The current DSM-IV-TR conceptualizes GAD as chronic, excessive, and pervasive worry (i.e., occurs more days than not about a number of events or activities for at least 6 months) that is difficult to control. The worry is associated with three or more symptoms of anxiety and some of these symptoms have to occur more days than not for at least 6 months. Moreover, the anxiety and worry must cause clinically significant distress or impairment and it can not be restricted to concerns that characterize another Axis I disorder. Table 10.1 presents the DSM-IV-TR criteria for GAD.

TABLE 10.1. DSM-IV-TR Diagnostic Criteria for Generalized Anxiety Disorder

A. Excessive anxiety and worry (apprehensive expectation), occurring more days than not for at least 6 months, about a number of events or activities (such as work or school performance).

B. The person finds it difficult to control the worry.

C. The anxiety and worry are associated with three (or more) of the following six symptoms (with at least some of the symptoms present for more days than not for the past 6 months).
   (1) restlessness or feeling keyed up or on edge
   (2) being easily fatigued
   (3) difficulty concentrating or mind going blank
   (4) irritability
   (5) muscle tension
   (6) sleep disturbance (difficulty falling or staying asleep, or restless unsatisfying sleep)

D. The focus of the anxiety and worry is not confined to features of an Axis I disorder e.g., the anxiety or worry about having a Panic Attack (as in Panic Disorder), being embarrassed in public (as in Social Phobia), being contaminated (as in Obsessive Compulsive Disorder), etc., and the anxiety and worry do not occur exclusively during Posttraumatic Stress Disorder.

E. The anxiety, worry or physical symptoms cause clinically significant distress or impairments in social, occupational, or other important areas of functioning.

F. The disturbance is not due to the direct physiological effects of a substance (e.g., drug of abuse, medication) or to a general medical condition (e.g., hyperthyroidism), and does not occur exclusively during a Mood Disorder, a Psychotic Disorder or a Pervasive Developmental Disorder.

Note. From American Psychiatric Association (2000). Copyright 2000 by the American Psychiatric Association. Reprinted by permission.

Clinician Guideline 10.1

Generalized anxiety disorder (GAD) is a persistent state of generalized anxiety involving chronic, excessive, and pervasive worry that is accompanied by physical or mental symptoms of anxiety that cause significant distress or impairment in daily functioning. The worry and anxiety must involve multiple life events or activities and they can not be limited to concerns that are characteristic of another Axis I disorder.

GAD: A Diagnostic Enigma?

The origins of GAD can be traced back to the concept of anxiety neurosis, characterized as excessive anxiety over prolonged periods without marked avoidance (Roemer, Orsillo, & Barlow, 2002). DSM-II (APA, 1968) retained the term "anxiety neurosis" but the diagnosis failed to distinguish between chronic, generalized anxiety and acute panic attacks (Mennin et al., 2004). DSM-III (APA, 1980) partially rectified this problem by providing specific diagnostic criteria for GAD but the imposition of hierarchical exclusionary criteria meant that DSM-III GAD was largely a residual category with poor diagnostic reliability that was excluded if the patient met criteria for another anxiety disorder. As a result practitioners were left bewildered over whether individuals met criteria for GAD (Mennin et al., 2004; Roemer et al., 2002). However DSM-III-R (APA, 1987) offered a substantial revision to GAD with most of the hierarchical exclusionary rules lifted, the duration criterion was extended to 6 months, and a more central role was assigned to worry. Now GAD could be diagnosed in the presence of another anxiety disorder as long as the anxiety and worry focused on additional concerns not related to the co-occurring anxiety disorder. Subsequent research based on the DSM-III-R criteria supported the central role of worry but revealed that autonomic hyperactivity is the least reliable and frequently endorsed of the GAD symptoms (Roemer et al., 2002). Thus DSM-IV (APA, 1994) introduced a further revision in which the number of physical symptoms of anxiety needed to meet diagnostic criteria was reduced from six out of 18 to three out of six symptoms. Although this led to an improvement in the reliable diagnosis of GAD, many of these physical symptoms overlap with depression, making differential diagnosis with major depression more difficult (see Roemer et al., 2002, for discussion). For example, we found that two-thirds of our sample with GAD was misclassified as having major depression or panic disorder based on a discriminant function analysis of common symptom and cognition measures of anxiety and depression (D. A. Clark, Beck, & Beck, 1994). Unfortunately, GAD lacks symptom specificity which can make it difficult to differentiate from other disorders.

Generalized Anxiety and Depression

In recent years there has been considerable debate among researchers on whether GAD is an anxiety disorder or whether it fits more closely with the affective disorders, especially major depression. Although it has been argued that GAD may be the basic "anxiety disorder" because worry, its central feature, is common across the anxiety disorders (Roemer et al., 2002), many others have questioned the diagnostic distinctiveness of GAD because none of its features are exclusive or specific to the disorder (Rachman, 2004). Moreover, GAD appears to have a particularly close relationship with depression. High comorbidity rates for GAD and major depression have been reported in the NCS-R (Kessler, Chiu, et al., 2005), as well as in large-scale surveys of primary care practice (Olfson et al., 2000). In a large sample of treatment-seekers, 40% of individuals with GAD had a secondary mood disorder and the rate jumped to 74% for lifetime co-occurrence (Brown, Campbell, et al., 2001; see also Mofitt et al., 2007). Moreover, there was no temporal priority of one disorder over the other.

Research on symptom structure indicates there is a great deal of overlap between GAD and major depression, with GAD having the highest associations of the anxiety disorders with the higher order nonspecific negative affect (NA) dimension and minimal or reverse associations with autonomic arousal (Brown, Chorpita, & Barlow, 1998; McGlinchey & Zimmerman, 2007; see also Krueger, 1999). Mineka et al. (1998) proposed that GAD and major depression are both distress-based disorders that contain a large nonspecific NA component. More recently Watson (2005) concluded that GAD is misplaced within the anxiety disorders because GAD and major depression are indistinguishable phenotypically and genetically. He recommended reconceptualizing DSM-IV anxiety and depression into a quantitative hierarchical organization with major depression, dysthymia, GAD, and PTSD categorized together as distress disorders. In support of this view there is evidence that panic disorder can be distinguished from GAD and major depression by its close association with physiological hyperarousal (e.g., Joiner et al., 1999).

On the other hand, there is a large body of cognitive research showing that GAD is associated with an automatic attentional bias for threat (see Chapter 3 and discussion below) and that worry is distinct but intricately related to anxious apprehension and fear (Barlow, 2002). Thus we contend that strong arguments exist for retaining GAD within the anxiety disorders but we also must recognize that it has a much closer relationship to depression than any of the other anxiety disorders. This juxtaposition of GAD with depression has implications for treatment. For example, cognitive therapy for generalized anxiety draws more directly from standard cognitive therapy for depression than the treatment protocols for the other anxiety disorders. In addition individuals with comorbid GAD and major depression have more severe cognitive biases than individuals who have GAD without comorbid major depression (Dupuy & Ladouceur, 2008).

Clinician Guideline 10.2

GAD is a distress disorder with a similar but distinct diagnostic and symptom structure to major depression. Clinical assessment and treatment of GAD must include the high probability of affective disturbance in the form of a co-occurring depressive disorder or symptoms.

Boundary Issues in GAD

GAD can be difficult to detect because worry is such a common complaint in the general population as well as in all the anxiety disorders and depression. To improve the differentiation of GAD, DSM-IV-TR requires that the worry be chronic, excessive, pervasive, associated with some anxious symptoms, and cause clinically significant distress or impairment. However, is this sufficient? Ruscio (2002) compared non-GAD high worriers and GAD high worriers on various symptom questionnaires. He found that GAD worriers had significantly higher worry frequency or distress and impairment than the non-GAD worriers. However, the difference between the two groups was a matter of degree, with the GAD worriers showing greater severity on most symptom measures (see also Ruscio, Chiu, et al., 2007). Thus GAD clearly fits a dimensional model of psychopathology, making it difficult to determine the optimal diagnostic criteria for differentiating pathological from normal general anxiety.

So, are there symptom features that are distinct to GAD? Barlow and colleagues have argued that GAD may be distinct by the greater frequency and severity of worries about a number of life circumstances, especially minor or miscellaneous tasks, as well as associated muscle tension (Roemer et al., 2002). A variety of constructs have been proposed as unique to GAD such as (1) an unsuccessful search for safety (Rachman, 2004), (2) activation of negative (metacognitive) beliefs about worry and counterproductive attempts at thought suppression (Wells, 2006), (3) intolerance of uncertainty (Dugus, Gagnon, et al., 1998), or (4) deficits in the regulation of emotional experience (Mennin, Turk, Heimberg, & Carmin, 2004). Unfortunately, empirical evidence that these proposed constructs are indeed specific markers of GAD is lacking at this time.

Clinician Guideline 10.3

There are no qualitative symptom features that are specific to GAD. Rather, the disorder varies in terms of the chronicity, severity, and pervasiveness of worry and associated anxiety. For this reason distinguishing GAD from non-GAD high worriers will present special challenges for the clinician.

THE NATURE OF WORRY

Worry is ubiquitous to the human condition. Who among us has not been preoccupied about some important task that we face or worried about an anticipated negative or threatening future situation? Borkovec (1985) noted that because human beings have the cognitive capacity to create mental representations of past events as well as anticipated future events in order to plan and problem solve, we are able to generate internal representations of future aversive events that cause anxiety in the absence of existing threat. It is this capacity to symbolically represent threat that is the basis of worry. The worry experience stems from the production of thoughts and images of exaggerated anticipation of possible negative outcomes. It is an important component of trait anxiety or neuroticism and can be considered the cognitive component of anxiety (Eysenck, 1992), although worry is distinguishable from anxiety (i.e., Brown et al., 1998; Ruscio, 2002; Mathews, 1990; Zinbarg & Barlow, 1996). Nevertheless, since the publication of DSM-III-R (APA, 1987), excessive worry is now considered the cardinal feature of GAD.

Defining Worry

Borkovec and colleagues offered one the earliest definitions of worry that has become widely accepted in research on generalized anxiety: "Worry is a chain of thoughts and images, negatively affect-laden and relatively uncontrollable. The worry process represents an attempt to engage in mental problem-solving on an issue whose outcome is uncertain but contains the possibility of one or more negative outcomes. Consequently, worry relates closely to fear processes" (Borkovec, Robinson, Pruzinsky, & DePree, 1983, p. 10). However, in the intervening years a more complicated picture has emerged on the nature of worry. Worry is predominantly a verbal–linguistic cognitive phenomenon that may serve an avoidant coping function by suppressing somatic and negative emotional responses to internally represented threat cues (Borkovec, 1994; Sibrava & Borkovec, 2006). Mathews (1990) defined worry as a "persistent awareness of possible future danger, which is repeatedly rehearsed without being resolved" (p. 456) and is maintained by an automatic information-processing bias for threat that underlies high trait anxiety and vulnerability to GAD. Wells (1999) argued that worry is an intrusive ideational process that is predominantly ego-syntonic and is perceived as serving an adaptive function.

One of the most important debates about worry as it relates to GAD is whether worry can be constructive and adaptive whereas the excessive worry in GAD is clearly maladaptive and pathological. Some researchers have argued that worry can lead to effective problem solving of stressful life events because it involves problem-focused active coping, information seeking, and task orientation with at most a minimal level of associated anxiety (e.g., Davey, 1994; Wells, 1999; see Watkins, 2008). On the other hand, pathological worry is (1) more pervasive, (2) time-consuming, (3) uncontrollable, (4) focused on more minor matters and more remote but personal future-oriented situations, (5) selectively biased for threat, and (6) associated with greater restricted autonomic variability (Craske et al., 1989; Dugas, Gagnon, et al., 1998; Dupuy et al., 2001; see also Ruscio et al., 2001). However, attempts to delineate adaptive worry from pathological worry will be difficult because of the strong association between worry and heightened anxiety (Roemer et al., 2002) and the dimensional nature of normal and abnormal worry (Ruscio et al., 2001). One solution might be to reserve the term "worry" for the maladaptive forms of repetitive thought associated with heightened anxiety or distress and which serve no particular adaptability for dealing with anticipated future danger. The core distinguishing element of pathological worry is an exaggerated anticipation of future negative outcomes (i.e., "that something bad might happen"). On the other hand, adaptive worry is more constructive, task-oriented repetitive thought that acts as preparatory coping or a problem-solving activity (Mathews, 1990).

The Function of Worry

One of the consequences of worry is its ability to generate and maintain anxiety in the absence of an external threat by perpetutating thoughts and images of nonexistent threats and dangers anticipated in the future (Borkovec, 1985). In this way worry is a contributor in the etiology and maintenance of anxiety. Most clinical researchers now consider worry a maladaptive cognitive avoidant coping strategy. Mathews (1990) suggests that worry contributes to the persistence of heightened anxiety by maintaining high levels of vigilance for personal danger. M. W. Eysenck (1992) proposed that worry has three functions: (1) alarm—introduces threat cues into conscious awareness, (2) prompt—repeatedly represents threat-related thought and images into consciousness, and (3) preparation—permits the worrier to anticipate a future situation by generating a solution to the problem or emotional preparation for the negative consequences. He argued that worry can be constructive (i.e., leading to problem resolution) or it can become excessive and maladaptive if the perceived threat is considered highly probable, imminent, aversive, and unmanageable (i.e., perceived limited access to postevent coping strategies). There is a self-perpetuating quality to worry because its functions as a negative reinforcer by creating the illusion of certainty, predictability, and control of anticipated threat or danger (Barlow, 2002).

Borkovec has developed the most extensive conceptualization of worry as a maladaptive cognitive avoidance response to future threat (Roemer & Borkovec, 1993). Worry is a predominantly conceptual, verbal–linguistic process that is self-perpetuated via negative reinforcement through the nonoccurrence of the predicted negative outcome or catastrophe. In addition worry is thought to suppress (inhibit) autonomic arousal and other disturbing emotional processes (Borkovec, 1994). Worry, as an attempt to problem solve a possible future threat or danger, is therefore an effort to avoid distal dangers (Borkovec et al., 2004). More recently Borkovec suggested that the core problem in GAD may be fear of emotional experience in general, with worry serving as a cognitive avoidance strategy for any emotional experience (Borkovec et al., 2004; Sibrava & Borkovec, 2006).

Beck and Clark (1997) proposed that worry is an elaborative processing strategy triggered by activation of automatic schematic threat processing. It is a deliberate effort to reappraise automatic threat interpretations and establish a sense of safety in an attempt to deactivate the hypervalent threat and vulnerability schemas that characterize generalized anxiety. In our cognitive model of GAD pathological worry functions as an ironic process (i.e., Wegner, 1994) that invariably increases rather than decreases anxiety because it magnifies the schema-congruent automatic thoughts of anticipated negative outcomes. Clinician Guideline 10.4 provides our definition of worry and its function in GAD.

Clinician Guideline 10.4

Chronic and excessive worry is an important characteristic of GAD and its vulnerability. It is a self-perpetuating maladaptive cognitive avoidance strategy that contributes to the persistence of anxiety by (1) magnifying a biased interpretation of anticipated threat; (2) generating a false sense of control, predictability, and certainty; (3) ensuring erroneous attribution of the nonoccurrence of the dreaded outcome to the worry process; and (4) culminating in frustrative attempts to establish a sense of safety.

EPIDEMIOLOGY AND CLINCIAL FEATURES

Prevalence

In the NCS epidemiological study DSM-III-R GAD had a 12-month prevalence of 3.1% and a lifetime prevalence of 5.1% (Kessler et al., 1994). Similar prevalence figures (3.1% for 12 month; 5.7% for lifetime) were recently reported in the NCS-R that was based on DSM-IV diagnostic criteria for GAD (Kessler, Berglund, et al., 2005; Kessler, Chiu, et al., 2005). The prevalence rates for GAD vary considerably across different countries (Holaway, Rodebaugh, & Heimberg, 2006). It is difficult to know whether this reflects cross-national differences in rates of GAD or methodological variations in diagnostic criteria and interview measures. Some of the older studies were based on DSM-III criteria whereas more recent studies utilized DSM-III-R or DSM-IV.

Higher rates of GAD have been found in primary care settings. For example, Olfson et al. (2000) reported a current prevalence of 14.8% in a large urban general practice, making GAD the most prevalent anxiety disorder in this setting. In the NCS-R GAD was second to panic disorder in the 12-month prevalence rates for use of general medical services and similar to social phobia in the use of mental health specialties (Wang, Lane, et al., 2005; see also Deacon et al., 2008). However, unlike panic disorder or PTSD, GAD does not have a strong association with physical disorders except for gastrointestinal illnesses (Rogers et al., 1994; Sareen, Cox, Clara, & Asmundson, 2005). GAD, then, may be almost as common in primary care settings as major depression (Olfson et al., 2000), a finding that is consistent with our previous discussion of GAD as a distress disorder.

Gender and Ethnicity

There is a strong gender difference in GAD, with the disorder twice as common in women. DSM-III-R GAD had a 12-month prevalence of 4.3% for women and 2% for men, and lifetime prevalence of 6.6% for women and 3.6% for men (Kessler et al., 1994). In some countries women had lower rates of GAD, although the most consistent pattern is a female gender bias in prevalence rates (e.g., Gater et al., 1998). Others have found that women with GAD may have a higher lifetime rate for an additional anxiety disorder (Yonkers, Warshaw, Massion, & Keller, 1996) and that comorbid GAD is associated with greater probability of seeking professional help (Wittchen, Zhao, Kessler, & Eaton, 1994). Significant gender differences have not been found in severity of clinical presentation, level of impairment, presence of comorbid depression, or response to pharmacotherapy for GAD (Steiner et al., 2005).

Despite some evidence of cross-national differences in GAD prevalence (e.g., Gater et al., 1998), no ethnic differences emerged in the NCS (Kessler et al., 1994). However, in the NCS-R non-Hispanic black and Hispanic participants had significantly lower rates of all anxiety disorders than non-Hispanic whites (Kessler, Berglund, et al., 2005). Cultural differences may be seen in worry content, with Asian Americans significantly more worried about future goals and African Americans worried significantly less than Asian Americans or Caucasian Americans about relationships, self-confidence, future aims, or work incompetence (Scott, Eng, & Heimberg, 2002).

Onset and Age Differences

In the NCS-R 50% of GAD cases had an onset under 31 years of age and 75% had an onset before 47 years old (Kessler, Berglund, et al., 2005). Compared with the other anxiety disorders assessed in the NCS-R, a higher percentage of GAD cases had a late onset, with approximately 10% having a first occurrence after 60 years of age. However, in their review Holaway, Rodebaugh, and Heimberg (2006) concluded that late teens to late 20s was the most common age range for the onset of GAD.

Given the broader age range for GAD onset, there has been considerable interest in rates of GAD across the lifespan, especially among older adults. In the NCS-R lifetime prevalence was highest in the 45–59 age cohort (Kessler, Berglund, et al., 2005), whereas Holaway, Rodebaugh, and Heimberg (2006) concluded that 25–54 years had the highest prevalence of GAD. For individuals younger than 18 years old, overanxious disorder is diagnosed as the counterpart to GAD. Overanxious disorder in childhood and adolescence is associated with increased risk for GAD and major depression in adulthood (e.g., Mofitt et al., 2007).

A Dutch community survey of 4,051 individuals between 65 and 86 years of age found that 3.2% met criteria for current GAD and 60% of these cases had concurrent depression (Schoevers, Beekman, Deeg, Jonker, & van Tilburg, 2003). Although GAD appears to have the same clinical presentation in older and younger individuals (J. G. Beck, Stanley, & Zebb, 1996), Mohlman (2004) indicated that the disorder may be harder to detect in older adults. She concluded that older adults may worry less than younger age groups, and the content and their response to worry may differ. Older adults worry more about health, death, injury, and work affairs, whereas younger individuals worry about work and relationships, and they rely on different strategies to control their worry (Hunt, Wisocki, & Yanko, 2003). Moreover, CBT may produce more modest treatment effects with older GAD patients (see Mohlman, 2004). Evidence that older adults with major depression and GAD may have more suicidal ideation highlights the clinical importance of GAD symptoms in this segment of the population (Lenze et al., 2000). However, more recent research indicates that GAD is not associated with a higher mortality rate in the elderly (Holwerda et al., 2007).

Clinician Guideline 10.5

GAD is the third most common anxiety disorder with a lifetime prevalence of 5.7%. It is twice as common in women and may be somewhat more prevalent among Caucasians. Higher rates are found in primary care settings. Although GAD is most prevalent in young to middle age adults, GAD and worry are common in older persons who may show less response to cognitive-behavioral interventions.

Course and Impairment

GAD tends to be chronic and unremitting. In the Harvard–Brown Anxiety Research Program (HARP) which followed 558 patients over 8 years, only 46% of women and 56% of men experienced full remission of their GAD, while over the same period 36% of women and 43% of men relapsed (Yonkers et al., 2003). Further analysis of the HARP data set revealed that worsening impairment and presence of comorbid panic disorder significantly increased risk for recurrence of GAD (Rodriguez et al., 2005). In addition early age of onset and presence of a comorbid Axis II disorder are predictive of chronicity and relapse (Massion et al., 2002; Yonkers, Dyck, Warshaw, & Keller, 2000). Individuals with GAD are more likely to seek treatment and have a shorter delay in help seeking than those with social phobia (Wagner et al., 2006). In the NCS-R, GAD was associated with an 86.1% cumulative lifetime probability of treatment contact and a median treatment-seeking delay of 9 years (Wang, Berglund, et al., 2005). In general, individuals with GAD have treatment-seeking rates that are generally similar to the other anxiety disorders (e.g., Wang, Lane, et al., 2005).

GAD is associated with significant impairment in social and occupational functioning as well as quality of life. Various studies have found that individuals with GAD experience significant decrements in work and social relationships as well as quality of life that is even greater in comorbid conditions (e.g., Henning, Turk, Mennin, Fresco, & Heimberg, 2007; Massion et al., 1993; see Hoffman, Dukes, & Wittchen, 2008). Moreover, the impairment due to GAD is equivalent in magnitude to that seen in major depression and is associated with a significant economic burden that may actually be higher than that of the other anxiety disorders (Wittchen, 2002). In their meta-analysis of quality of life studies, Olatunji et al. (2007) concluded that GAD had similar decrements in quality of life to the other anxiety disorders except PTSD. Thus the disorder represents a significant cost to society in terms of diminished work productivity, high primary health care utilization, and substantial economic burden (Wittchen, 2002). Treatment of GAD is costly relative to panic disorder and increases markedly when a comorbid depression is present (Marciniak et al., 2005).

Clinician Guideline 10.6

GAD tends to take a chronic and unremitting course that causes significant social and occupational impairment, leads to a decrement in life satisfaction, and places a significant economic burden on society.

Comorbidity

Like other anxiety disorders GAD is associated with a very high rate of Axis I and Axis II comorbidity, which leads to greater functional impairment and poorer outcome (see Holaway, Rodebaugh, & Heimberg, 2006; Rodriguez et al., 2005; Yonkers et al., 2000). In the NCS-R, 85% of individuals with DSM-IV GAD had a comorbid condition (Kessler, Chui, et al., 2005; see also Carter, Wittchen, et al., 2001; Mofitt et al., 2007). Similar high rates of comorbidity have been found in clinical studies with the most common being major depression, social phobia, and panic disorder (e.g., Brown, Campbell, et al., 2001). Moreover, individuals with GAD or panic disorder with agoraphobic avoidance are more likely to have a substance use disorder than individuals with other mood and anxiety diagnoses (Grant et al., 2004). Finally, between one-third and two-thirds of individuals with GAD will have an Axis II personality disorder, the most frequent being avoidant, obsessive–compulsive, and possibly paranoid and dependent personality disorders (e.g., Dyck et al., 2001; Massion et al., 2002; Grant et al., 2005; Sanderson et al., 1994). GAD is most often the temporal primary disorder, especially in relation to the mood disorders (Kessler, Walters, & Wittchen, 2004).

Clinician Guideline 10.7

Most individuals with GAD will have a current or lifetime history of other psychiatric disorders that will complicate response to treatment. The most common secondary diagnoses are major depression, social phobia, panic disorder, substance abuse, and avoidant personality disorder. Assessment and treatment planning must take into account the presence of these co-occurring conditions.

Personality and Life Events

As noted in Chapter 4, diathesis–stress models have been proposed to explain the etiology and persistence of anxiety in general which, of course, are directly applicable to GAD (e.g., Barlow, 2002; Chorpita & Barlow, 1998). In their earlier cognitive model of generalized anxiety, Beck et al. (1985) proposed a diathesis–stress perspective in which low self-confidence and perceived inadequacy in specific areas of functioning are cognitive-personality diatheses that precipitate a state of chronic anxiety when triggered by an event that represents a threat to the individual's physical or psychological survival.

In Chapter 4 we discussed a number of personality diatheses that have been implicated in the development of anxiety and, by extension, GAD. Negative affectivity (NA) has consistently emerged as the most important latent construct in factor-analytic studies of GAD. Although few studies have focused on the development of GAD specifically (Hudson & Rapee, 2004), retrospective studies and research on anxiety more generally suggests that high NA, neuroticism, or negative emotionality are personality diatheses in GAD (L. A. Clark, Watson, & Mineka, 1994). In support of this contention, a recent large twin study found that neuroticism had a substantially greater impact on increasing risk for GAD than any other psychiatric disorder (Khan, Jacobson, Gardner, Prescott, & Kendler, 2005). High trait anxiety has been considered practically synonymous with GAD to the point where it has been suggested that GAD may be "a relatively pure manifestation of high trait anxiety (Rapee, 1991, p. 422). Barlow

(2002) has argued that a chronic inability to cope with unpredictable and uncontrollable events is a psychological vulnerability in GAD. Behavioral inhibition is a temperamental construct that has been implicated in the development of anxiety but would be expected to have relevance for GAD (Hudson & Rapee, 2004). More recently Rapee proposed an etiological model for GAD in which anxious vulnerability was defined in terms of a temperament of increased emotionality, inhibition, and physiological arousal that causes a tendency to misinterpret situations as threatening and something to avoid (Hudson & Rapee, 2004).

Like the personality research, few studies have focused specifically on life events in GAD. In the ECA stressful life events were associated with the onset of DSM-III GAD (Blazer, Hughes, & George, 1987). Stressful life events were shown to correlate with both major depression and GAD in a large community sample (Newman & Bland, 1994). Moreover, individuals are at higher risk for developing major depression when they experience a severe life event in the presence of GAD (Hettma, Kuhn, Prescott, & Kendler, 2006). In another study, Roemer, Molina, Litz, and Borkovec (1996–1997) found that individuals with GAD reported significantly more potentially traumatizing events than nonanxious individuals. Although the life event research in GAD is not extensive, there is evidence that stressful events contribute to the onset and impact of the disorder.

There has been some interest in whether childhood adversities might play an etiological role in GAD. In one study parental psychopathology (i.e., depression, GAD, drug/alcohol abuse), parental separation/divorce, child physical or sexual abuse, and witnessing a trauma were associated with onset but not persistence of GAD (Kessler et al., 1997). Other studies, however, have not found that GAD was particularly associated with childhood emotional, physical, or sexual abuse (Gibb et al., 2007; Pribor & Dinwiddie, 1992). Although further research is needed on specific GAD samples, the diathesis–stress research on anxious states and symptoms more generally suggests that various personality constructs and life events are probable contributors to the development of generalized anxiety and worry (e.g., Brozina & Abela, 2006).

Clinician Guideline 10.8

Assessment for generalized anxiety should include a thorough investigation of stressful life events and circumstances as well as certain broad personality dimensions like negative affect, trait anxiety, and negative emotionality or neuroticism.

COGNITIVE MODEL OF GAD

Figure 10.1 presents an elaborated cognitive model of GAD that is based on the generic model we discussed in Chapter 2 as well as on theoretical considerations discussed in Beck and D. A. Clark (1997). In addition we are indebted to the advances made by other researchers on the cognitive basis of generalized anxiety and worry (e.g., Borkovec, 1994; Borkovec et al., 1991; Dugas, Gagnon, et al., 1998; M. W. Eysenck, 1992; Wells, 1995, 1999; Woody & Rachman, 1994).

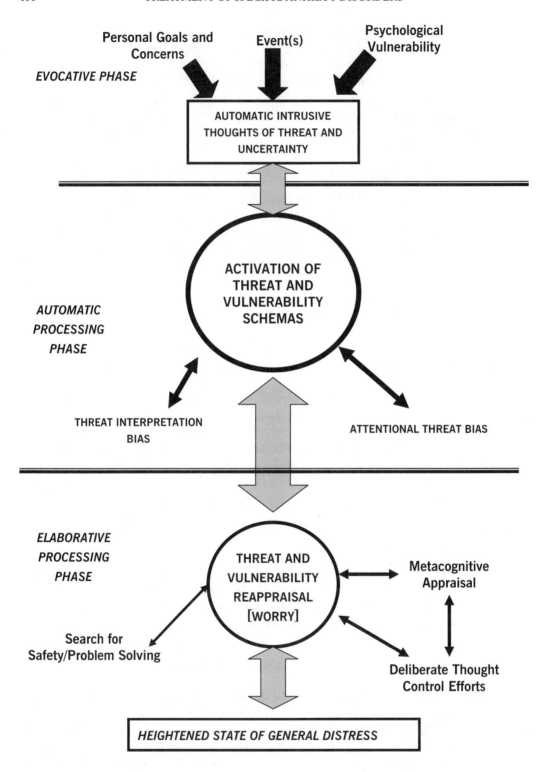

FIGURE 10.1. Cognitive model of generalized anxiety disorder.

Evocative Phase

The cognitive model of GAD begins with the assertion that GAD worry does not occur in a vacuum but rather reflects the life circumstances, goals, and personal concerns of the individual. The cognitive perspective on personality has long recognized that individual behavior is determined by an interaction between daily life experiences or situations, schematic content, and personal goals (Cantor, 1990). These self-articulated goals are the things that people work on and care about in their current lives (Cantor et al., 1991). Cantor (1990) refers to them as *life tasks*, or personal projects that people work on and devote energy toward in a specified time period in order to bring meaning to the basic human pursuits of love, work, and power. For example, university students might share normative life concerns about "academic success," "making new friends," or "romantic commitment," but they would differ in the actual activities and their evaluation relevant to the pursuit of these life concerns. Klinger (1975) introduced the term *current concerns* as being committed to the pursuit of particular goals (e.g., to avoid threats to personal security or to disengage from loss), whereas Emmons (1986) refers to *personal strivings* as "what individuals are characteristically aiming to accomplish through their behavior or the purpose or purposes that a person is trying to carry out" (p. 1059). All of these constructs refer to the influence of goal-directed strivings on human behavior and cognition, especially during periods of life transition (Cantor, 1990).

In the current model we propose that the personal goals, values, or concerns of individuals as well as the context of their daily experience will play an important role in triggering worry. For example, an important life transition for young adults might be accepting their first permanent employment after graduation. A personal goal might be "recognized as achieving success and productivity" and the person might engage in various activities in pursuit of this goal such as working overtime on projects, doing more in order to produce a higher quality of work, getting feedback and reassurance from work colleagues, and the like. In this context a vulnerable individual might begin to worry about the quality of her work, how she is perceived by others, and whether she is succeeding in her new job. Likewise, a person who has just retired and for whom the generation of wealth has been an important life task might be vulnerable to worry about financial loss and insecurity. In this way our life tasks, current concerns, or personal strivings can be an important catalyst for worry in the vulnerable individual. As discussed previously, the individual with high NA or neuroticism would be particularly prone to worry within the context of these important life goals. In addition we proposed that enduring schemas of low self-confidence (i.e., helplessness) and threat would constitute a predisposition for generalized anxiety and chronic worry.

The interaction of these prepotent schemas or personality vulnerability with particular current life tasks could trigger threat-relevant intrusive thoughts or images. *Intrusive thoughts* are "any distinct, identifiable cognitive event that is unwanted, unintended, and recurrent. It interrupts the flow of thought, interferes in task performance, is associated with negative affect, and is difficult to control" (D. A. Clark & Rhyno, 2005, p. 4). In the present context, future-oriented intrusive thoughts involving some uncertain threat about the attainment of one's cherished goals or life tasks (i.e., automatic anxious thoughts) can elicit anxiety and eventually trigger a worry process. Intolerance of uncertainty is readily apparent in GAD (Koerner & Dugas, 2006), and so we would expect uncertainty to be reflected in the automatic anxious intrusive thoughts of

GAD. This can be readily seen during sleep onset, which is commonly associated with a surge in intrusive anxious thoughts and worry, as individuals with insomnia and GAD frequently describe a problem with "racing thoughts" (Harvey, 2005). Obviously the worry-prone individual does not have to intentionally and purposefully try to generate unwanted thoughts of threat and uncertainty when trying to sleep. Instead this thinking is experienced as quite spontaneous, unintended, and automatic. The thoughts literally intrude into conscious awareness against the person's will and are then very difficult to control or dismiss (Rachman, 1981). They have a certain adhesive quality and are associated with a feeling of apprehension or anxiousness. Wells (2005a) noted that negative intrusive thoughts often occur in GAD and can be exacerbated by the worry process. In the current model, we propose that automatic anxious intrusive thoughts involving uncertain threat play a critical role in triggering the worry process by activating the maladaptive schemas of threat and vulnerability that characterize GAD.

Automatic Processing Phase

There is now considerable evidence that automatic information processing of threat occurs in the pathogenesis of GAD. In their review Macleod and Rutherford (2004) concluded that there is compelling evidence that individuals with GAD selectively attend to threatening stimuli at the encoding phase and make biased interpretations of threat when presented with ambiguous information (see discussion below). Thus there is considerable empirical support for an automatic processing phase in GAD.

Schematic Activation

There are three critical elements to the automatic threat processing proposed in Figure 10.1. The first is activation of the cluster of schemas relevant for GAD. In the cognitive model, intrusive thoughts of uncertainty are both a cause and a consequence of threat schema activation. We would expect that these thoughts will become more frequent and salient with sustained activation of the GAD-relevant schemas. The cognitive model proposes four types of schemas that characterize GAD. These are presented in Table 10.2 along with illustrative examples.

Because GAD and depression are closely related in clinical presentation and diagnostic comorbidity, it should be no surprise that the underlying schematic organization is similar in the two disorders (Beck et al., 1985, 2005). The lower self-confidence and increased sense of helplessness represented in the general threat and vulnerability schemas share many similarities to the negative self-referent schemas of depression. However, the schemas in GAD have greater specificity to important personal life goals and vital interests and, of course, they deal with beliefs about future threats, the "what if's." For example, in our case illustration Rebecca believed she would be criticized at any moment for not performing well as store manager and she was convinced she was poor at handling problems with her employees. She did not believe people were generally critical of her outside the work context nor did she believe that she suffered from poor social skills. Rather her threat and vulnerability schemas were specific to the work situation and so she worried excessively about her work performance and whether or not she was perceived as incompetent.

TABLE 10.2. Schemas That Characterize Generalized Anxiety Disorders

Schema categories	Illustrative examples
General threat (beliefs about probability and consequences of threats to one's physical or psychological security)	• Negative outcomes (events) that threaten important life goals are more likely to happen to me. • If I experience a negative event that threatens an important life goal, it will have a serious, long-term effect on me. • The distress and anxiety will be severe if this negative event happens.
Personal vulnerability (beliefs about helplessness, inadequacy, lack of personal resources to cope)	• I would be unable to cope with the negative event if it occurred. • I can't control whether this negative event happens or its effects on me. • I am weak and helpless in the face of this event.
Intolerance of uncertainty[a] (beliefs about the frequency, consequence, avoidance, and unacceptability of uncertain or ambiguous negative events)	• Uncertainty will increase the stress and adverse effects of negative events. • It is important to be ready for any unexpected bad things that could happen to you. • If I can reduce the doubt and ambiguity of a potentially negative situation, I will be better able to cope with it.
Metacognition of worry[b] (beliefs about the positive and negative effects of worry and its controllability)	• Worry helps me solve problems and prepare for the worst. • If I worry, it means that I am taking a situation seriously. • If I were a stronger person, I would be able to control my worries. • I experience a great deal of anxiety and distress because of uncontrollable worry.

[a]See Freeston, Rhéaume, Letarte, Dugas, and Ladouceur (1994).
[b]See Cartwright-Hatton and Wells (1997).

The last two schema categories, uncertainty beliefs and metacognition, may seem more unique to GAD but even these beliefs can be found in other anxiety disorders like OCD. Dugas and his colleagues have proposed a model of pathological worry and GAD in which intolerance of uncertainty is a causal factor (Dugas, Buhr, & Ladouceur, 2004). The construct is defined as "the tendency to react negatively on an emotional, cognitive, and behavioral level to uncertain situations and events" (Dugas et al., 2004, p. 143). Furthermore, intolerance of uncertainty is associated with difficulty in responding to ambiguous or uncertain situations and beliefs that uncertainty is negative and should be avoided. Although initial studies found that intolerance of uncertainty was elevated in individuals with GAD relative to nonanxious controls or individuals with panic disorder (Dugas, Gagnon, et al., 1998; Dugas et al., 2005), it was equally apparent in analogue OCD and GAD (Holaway, Heimberg, & Coles, 2006). Thus the cognitive model does not contend that uncertainty beliefs are necessarily unique to GAD but when activated along with personal threat and vulnerability schemas about important life goals and concerns, the constellation of beliefs will prime excessive worry. Rebecca believed that at any moment a district manager might appear and evaluate her store. She found this uncertainty very troubling because she believed in the importance of being well organized and prepared for even the unexpected. This led to excessive worry that "her incompetence" might be discovered at any moment.

Wells (1995, 1999) proposed a cognitive model for GAD in which maladaptive positive and negative beliefs about worry play a key role in a dysfunctional metacognitive process that leads to excessive worry and GAD. According to Wells (1999), "metacognition" refers to appraisals and beliefs about the nature of cognition and our ability to monitor and regulate our thoughts. The metacognitive beliefs in GAD represent self-knowledge about the importance of attending to one's thoughts, a tendency to appraise self-referent thinking negatively, and the necessity of engaging in thought control efforts that ultimately prove unhelpful (Wells & Matthews, 2006). In GAD these metacognitive beliefs will generate "metaworry," or worry about worry, as well as ineffective efforts to control anxious thinking and worry, attentional biases for threat monitoring, and maladaptive coping strategies such as emotion-focused coping (Wells & Matthews, 2006). Wells (1999, 2004) argues that positive metacognitive beliefs about worry (e.g., "Worry helps me cope") are activated early in the worry process and are central to initiating worry as a coping strategy. This results in Type I worry in which the individual focuses on the potential threat of a situation (e.g., "What if I lose my job?"). The threat and uncertainty involved in Type I worry will activate negative metacognitive beliefs about worry. Beliefs about the uncontrollability and negative consequences of worry lead to Type II worry, or meta-worry, in which the individual becomes focused on trying to suppress or control worry because of the associated rise in anxiety.

Based on Wells's fresh insights into the nature of GAD and worry, the present model proposes that enduring beliefs about the nature of worry, its consequences, and its control are key to the schematic organization of GAD. These beliefs explain why the person with GAD seems drawn to worry as a coping strategy, on the one hand, but then, on the other hand, appears frantic to gain control over the worry process.

Attentional Threat Bias

There is considerable empirical evidence that generalized anxiety and worry are associated with automatic attentional biases for threat (see MacLeod & Rutherford, 2004; Mathews & MacLeod, 1994; Matthews & Funke, 2006). We have discussed this topic in Chapter 3 and in the following section on empirical status we will briefly review selected studies on attentional processing in GAD. In the meantime an important issue is whether the attentional bias in GAD is specific to threat or is it a more general bias for negative emotional information. The latter, of course, would be entirely consistent with the more general distress nature of GAD.

Threat Interpretation Bias

A final automatic process proposed in the cognitive model is the rapid, unintended selective bias to interpret ambiguous personally relevant information in a threatening manner. In their review MacLeod and Rutherford (2004) concluded that individuals with GAD have a tendency to interpret ambiguity in a threatening manner. Given processing priority for schema-congruent information, it would be expected that the schematic activation in GAD would lead to threat interpretations. With the information-rich complexities of daily experience, it is not surprising that an automatic threat interpretation might be rapidly generated by individuals intolerant of ambiguity and uncertainty. Of course, the automatic processing biases associated with GAD schema activation will trigger a much slower, more elaborative processing response that is an attempt to dampen down the hypervalent threat mode.

Elaborative Processing Phase

Elaborative processing is at the heart of the cognitive basis of GAD and is the level at which we intervene in cognitive therapy. Worry is a highly conscious, elaborative cognitive process that is viewed in the current model as a deliberate attempt to reappraise negative possibilities in a less threatening manner. Worry is a deliberate, effortful response intended to suppress or counter schematic threat activation and its associated anxiety by engaging in a reappraisal of a threat and one's level of vulnerability (Beck & Clark, 1997). In this sense worry functions as a cognitive avoidance response intended to inhibit emotional arousal (Borkovec, 1994; Sibrava & Borkovec, 2006). In nonpathological states, worry is adaptive because the individual is able to reappraise the potential threat in a more positive manner. The worry or reappraisal process enables individuals to process benign or positive aspects of the situation as well as their coping resources, and so the impending situation is downgraded in threat level.

In GAD threat reappraisal or worry leads to a much different outcome because it is associated with a number of faulty cognitive processes. As illustrated in Figure 10.1, worry in GAD is characterized by faulty metacognitive appraisal. Because of the beliefs activated in GAD, the vulnerable person evaluates the worry itself as distressing, ineffective, uncontrollable, and self-damaging. As discussed by Wells (2006), this negative evaluation of worry gives rise to "metaworry," or worrying about worrying. It is very common for individuals with GAD to acknowledge the deleterious effects of their worry and start to worry about worrying. Frank, for example, worried about the stock market and the security of his retirement investments. He often laid awake at night fretting about his investment decisions and their outcome. He came to dread the evenings because he worried that he would get caught in another frenzy of worry. This, of course, led to valiant efforts to control or suppress his worries but with little success.

A negative evaluation of worry will lead to efforts to control or suppress worry by direct thought suppression, rationalization, distraction, or cognitive avoidance (Wells, 1999). Attempts to disengage from worry are rarely successful, especially over the long term, and may in fact result in a rebound in worry once suppression efforts cease (Wenzlaff & Wegner, 2000). Although there is considerable debate on the effects of thought suppression (Purdon, 1999), at the very least deliberate efforts at control of worry are rarely successful in GAD. In fact their unintended effect is to increase the salience and threatening nature of worry, magnify anticipated threat cognitions, and heighten the perception of uncontrollability.

Finally, Woody and Rachman (1994) have argued that GAD is characterized by a failure to achieve a sense of safety because of insufficient or ineffective use of safety signals. Even though they seek to maximize safety and avoid even minimal risk by checking and seeking reassurance from others, they are rarely successful. As a result they remain vigilant for threat, apprehensive, and in a persistent search for safety. Although Woody and Rachman (1994) did not directly implicate worry, their formulation has relevance for understanding pathological worry in GAD. The futile efforts to generate solutions to anticipated threatening outcomes can be viewed as an effort to find safety through worry. For example, when Rebecca was worrying about how she would confront an employee who was persistently late for work, she would imagine various scenarios of how she might deal with this problem. She was looking for a "solution" that would relieve her anxiety, a way of dealing with this problem that would bring her relief, a sense of safety. However, each scenario she generated was flawed and so the worry only led to more anxiety and uncertainty rather than to the relief she so desperately desired. Ultimately the failure to find an acceptable solution, to achieve a sense of relief or safety, contributed to the perpetual cycle of worry.

The outcome of the cognitive processes illustrated in Figure 10.1 is a heightened state of general distress. Because the schematic content in GAD deals with general threat and helplessness, we expect the resulting emotional state to be more mixed or generalized than what is seen in panic disorder or social phobia. Naturally this elevated anxiousness or distress will feed back into the cognitive apparatus by contributing to further activation of the GAD schemas. In this way the cognitive basis of GAD is a self-perpetuating vicious cycle that can be terminated only by intervention at the automatic and elaborative reappraisal levels.

EMPIRICAL STATUS OF THE COGNITIVE MODEL

A number of hypotheses have been proposed that are germane to the cognitive perspective on GAD. In the following section we review six hypotheses that are central to the cognitive formulation presented in this chapter.

Hypothesis 1

Intrusive thoughts of uncertainty about significant goals and important life tasks will elicit more worry in vulnerable than nonvulnerable individuals.

Over the years various studies have indicated that both intrusive thoughts and worry are triggered by immediate situations, stressful events, and other current concerns of the individual. In a review of earlier research on worry Borkovec and colleagues (Borkovec et al., 1991) concluded that differences in the worry content of children, students, and the elderly reflect the life circumstances and current concerns of individuals (see also Mathews, 1990). Moreover, worry may result from a problem situation in which a sense of security, safety, or certainty has not been attained (Dugas, Freeston, & Ladouceur, 1997; Segerstrom et al., 2000; Woody & Rachman, 1994). In a study comparing worry in GAD and non-GAD patients, findings indicated that worry about immediate problems may be more adaptable, whereas worry about highly remote events was more pathological, distinguishing the GAD from non-GAD sample (Dugas, Freeston et al., 1998).

In terms of intrusive thoughts, naturalistic and experimental studies indicate that exposure to a stressful situation will increase the number of negative stress-relevant intrusive thoughts, especially if individuals engage in worry about the stressor (e.g., Butler et al., 1995; Parkinson & Rachman, 1981b; Wells & Papageorgiou, 1995). In one of the original studies on cognitive intrusions, Parkinson and Rachman (1981a) found that two-thirds of intrusive thoughts were triggered by an identifiable external stimulus. Thus it is widely recognized that unwanted negative intrusive thoughts and worry are often elicited by the personal goals, life tasks, and current concerns of the individual. Moreover, there is a close relationship between intrusive thoughts and worry, with experimental studies indicating that brief periods of worry induction result in a subsequent increase in negative intrusive thoughts (Borkovec, Robinson, et al., 1983; Pruzinsky & Borkovec, 1990; York et al., 1987; see also Ruscio & Borkovec, 2004; Wells, 2005). However, no studies have directly examined whether worry can arise from unwanted intrusive thoughts, so empirical support for Hypothesis 1 is tentative at this time.

Clinician Guideline 10.9

Individuals' personal goals, prominent life tasks, and significant current concerns will determine the main themes of their worry content. A contextual analysis that takes into account the presence of intrusive thoughts and images is needed to determine the factors that trigger excessive worry.

Hypothesis 2

Maladaptive beliefs about general threat, personal vulnerability, intolerance of uncertainty, and the nature of worry relevant to valued personal goals and vital interests will be more characteristic of GAD than non-GAD individuals.

Many cognitive theories of GAD view maladaptive beliefs about personal threat, vulnerability, risk, and uncertainty as central to the pathogenesis of chronic worry (e.g., Beck et al., 1985, 2005; Dugas, Gagnon, et al., 1998; Freeston et al., 1994; Wells, 1995, 1999). Unfortunately, though, specific GAD self-report measures do not exist for the threat and personal vulnerability schema content described in Table 10.2. However, there is strong evidence that threat schemas play a critical role in GAD. In Chapter 3 studies finding a higher rate of automatic threat cognitions in anxiety often included GAD patients in their samples (see Hypothesis 6) and many studies showing an elaborative threat interpretation bias in anxiety were based on GAD patients (see Hypothesis 8). In their review MacLeod and Rutherford (2004) concluded that GAD is characterized by an automatic attentional bias for threat during the encoding of information and a selective threat interpretation bias in ambiguous situations. However, Coles and Heimberg (2002) concluded that an explicit threat memory bias was not evident in GAD, a conclusion that would appear to run counter to the current hypothesis. They suggest that the lack of findings may be due to difficulty in developing a set of threat stimuli that is specific to the idiosyncratic worry domains of GAD patients.

Cognitive research on GAD has tended to focus on intolerance of uncertainty and metacognitive beliefs because these constructs may be more specific to the disorder. Koerner and Dugas (2006) have argued that intolerance of uncertainty and ambiguity may be the "threat" that is unique to GAD. To assess this important schema construct, a 27-item Intolerance of Uncertainty Scale (IUS; Freeston et al., 1994) was developed that assesses beliefs about the negative consequences and unacceptability of being uncertain. Various studies have shown a specific relationship between the IUS and self-report worry measures in GAD and nonclinical samples, and individuals with

GAD score significantly higher on the measure than nonclinical controls (Dugas et al., 1997; Dugas, Gagnon, et al., 1998; Dugas, Gosselin, & Ladouceur, 2001; Freeston et al., 1994). Furthermore, GAD patients scored significantly higher on the IUS than individuals with panic disorder (Dugas et al., 2005), although Holaway, Heimberg, and Coles (2006) found that intolerance of uncertainty was equally relevant to OCD in a nonclinical analogue study. Although there is considerable empirical evidence for the importance of intolerance of uncertainty beliefs in the pathological worry of GAD (see review by Koerner & Dugas, 2006), it is doubtful that the construct is unique to GAD (e.g., OCCWG, 2003; Tolin, Abramowitz, Brigidi, & Foa, 2003).

Various studies have investigated whether positive and negative metacognitive beliefs about worry are unique cognitive features of GAD. Particular interest has focused on the positive beliefs about worry because these schemas may be particularly instrumental in initiating worry as an avoidant coping response to perceived threat (Koerner & Dugas, 2006; Sibrava & Borkovec, 2006; Wells, 2004). Wells (2006) considers the negative beliefs about worry a unique feature of pathological worry in GAD because a focus on the uncontrollable and dangerous quality of worry leads to meta-worry, or "worrying about worrying," a process that is unique to GAD. Wells and colleagues developed the 65-item Meta-Cognitions Questionnaire (MCQ) to assess beliefs about worry and unwanted intrusive thoughts, with one subscale that assesses positive beliefs about worry and the other subscale negative beliefs about the uncontrollability and dangers of thoughts (Cartwright-Hatton & Wells, 1997). Scores on the positive and negative beliefs subscales have a significant relationship with measures of worry, obsessional symptoms, and trait anxiety, although negative beliefs have a much stronger association with worry than positive beliefs (Cartwright-Hatton & Wells, 1997; Wells & Cartwright-Hatton, 2004; Wells & Papageorgiou, 1998a). Moreover, GAD samples score significantly higher than nonclinical controls and other anxiety disorder groups on negative beliefs (i.e., MCQ Uncontrollability and Danger subscale) but not on the positive beliefs subscale (Cartwright-Hatton & Wells, 1997; Wells & Carter, 2001).

Other measures have been developed to assess beliefs about worry. Positive beliefs about worry as a coping strategy for dealing with difficult situations distinguished clinical and analogue GAD individuals from non-GAD controls and correlated with measures of anxiety and worry (Dugas, Gagnon, et al., 1998; Freeston et al., 1994). Borkovec and Roemer (1995) found that analogue GAD and non-GAD students believed worry (1) motivates them, (2) is effective problem solving, (3) prepares them for bad events, (4) helps avoid or prevent bad outcomes, and (5) superstitiously makes something bad less likely to happen. However, one belief, that worry helps distract from emotional topics, was endorsed significantly more by the GAD students. Davey, Tallis, and Capuzzo (1996), who assessed beliefs about the positive and negative consequences of worry with their own Consequences of Worry Scale, found that negative but not positive beliefs correlated with measures of worry, trait anxiety, and poor problem-solving confidence. They conclude that positive beliefs about worry may be involved in constructive, task-oriented worrying as well as in chronic pathological worry. Finally, negative but not positive beliefs about worry predicted GAD severity in a Spanish community sample of older adults (Montorio, Wetherell, & Nuevo, 2006).

In summary there is considerable empirical evidence that threat, personal vulnerability, intolerance of uncertainty, and metacognitive beliefs about worry are activated in GAD. However, capturing the core fear content that is distinctive to GAD has proven more elusive for researchers. We do not have specific measures of GAD threat and vulnerability beliefs that take into account the current concerns and life tasks of the individual. Negative beliefs about ambiguity and uncertainty feature strongly in GAD but are unlikely to be specific to the disorder. And it is clear that negative beliefs about worry are more pathognomonic to GAD than the positive beliefs. However, research into these constructs is still preliminary, and more experimental research is needed to determine how these beliefs might interact with other cognitive processes that contribute to the persistence of worry.

Clinician Guideline 10.10

Cognitive therapy of GAD must target personal beliefs about the perceived threat and negative consequences associated with ambiguous and uncertain future negative outcomes as well as negative beliefs about the uncontrollable and dangerous nature of worry.

Hypothesis 3

Individuals with GAD will exhibit an automatic attention and interpretation threat bias when processing information relevant to valued goals and personal life concerns.

The proposition that an automatic preferential encoding, interpretation, and retrieval bias for threat is a causal contributor to the development and maintenance of GAD is a central aspect of most cognitive theories of GAD (MacLeod & Rutherford, 2004). Numerous information-processing experiments have been conducted that are supportive of this hypothesis; much of this material is reviewed in Chapter 3. In this section we take a brief look at encoding and interpretation of ambiguity studies that have utilized GAD samples.

There is strong empirical support for an encoding bias for threat in GAD patients and high trait-anxious individuals that occurs both at the automatic and the elaborative processing levels. Various studies using the emotional Stroop task have found that color-naming latencies for threat stimuli were significantly longer for GAD or high trait-anxious individuals than nonanxious groups (e.g., Bradley, Mogg, et al., 1995; Edwards, Burt, & Lipp, 2006; Martin et al., 1991; Mogg, Bradley, et al., 1995; Mogg et al., 1993; Richards et al., 1992; Rutherford, MacLeod, & Campbell, 2004). Moreover, threat bias is apparent at both subliminal and supraliminal levels but exposure to a current stressor may enhance automatic but not elaborative threat bias for high trait-anxious individuals (Edwards et al., 2006). In addition there is evidence that the encoding bias in GAD may not be specific to threat but to negative information more generally (Martin et al., 1991; Mogg, Bradley, et al., 1995; Mogg et al., 1993; Rutherford et al., 2004).

A number of visual and semantic dot probe experiments have found an automatic attentional vigilance for threat in GAD patients (e.g., MacLeod et al., 1986; Mogg, Bradley, & Williams, 1995; Mogg et al., 1992) as well as high trait-anxious individuals (e.g., Koster et al., 2006; Mogg et al., 2000; Wilson & MacLeod, 2003). However, at slower presentation rates, high trait-anxious individuals may show attentional avoidance of threat (Koster et al., 2006) and findings by Wilson and MacLeod (2003) suggest that high trait-anxious individuals may show disproportionate vigilance for threat only at moderate levels of threat intensity (see Chapter 3, Figure 3.3, for further discussion). In addition it has been suggested that the dot probe effects may be partly explained by difficulty disengaging from threat rather than by hypervigilance for threat, at least in nonanxious individuals (Koster, Crombez, Verschuere, & De Houwer, 2004). Recently, inviduals with GAD trained to attend to neutral rather than threat words showed a significant decrease in anxious symptoms (Amir et al., 2009). It should be noted that like the emotional Stroop task, the dot probe bias in GAD is not specific to threat stimuli but to negative information more generally (Mogg, Bradley, & Williams, 1995).

In order to determine whether individuals with GAD have a tendency to impose threatening interpretations in ambiguous situations, researchers have used a variety of ambiguous stimuli. Studies employing homophones (for further discussion, see Chapter 3, Hypothesis 8) have found that patients with GAD and high trait-anxious individuals produced significantly more threatening spellings than nonanxious individuals (Mathews, Richards, & Eysenck, 1989; Mogg et al., 1994). Likewise a threat interpretation bias has been detected when individuals with GAD are presented with ambiguous sentences (Eysenck et al., 1991) or when speed of comprehending ambiguous sentences is measured in high trait-anxious individuals (MacLeod & Cohen, 1993). There was evidence that individuals with GAD exhibited a negative interpretation bias (i.e., facilitation effect) in an emotional priming task in which sentences depicting positive or negative life events preceded positive and negative self-referent trait adjectives (Dalgleish et al., 1995). Furthermore, Ken, Paller, and Zinbarg (2008) found that only high-trait anxious individuals' word-stem completion performance for threat words was affected by a unconscious threat prime, again a finding consistent with presence of an automatic hypervigilance for threat and subsequent facilitative interpretation of threat stimuli. Although, negative results have also been reported in other studies (e.g., Hazlett-Stevens & Borkovec, 2004), recent evidence suggests training in generating benign interpretation to threat can reduce anxious reactivity to a stressor (Hirsch et al., 2009).

In summary there is fairly strong and consistent evidence that GAD and its precursor, high trait anxiety, are characterized by an automatic attentional bias for threat, as predicted by the third hypothesis. Empirical evidence for a threat interpretation bias for ambiguity is also moderately strong, especially in light of recent reports of the causal effects of interpretation threat bias training (see discussion in Chapter 4, Hypothesis 12; also see MacLeod & Rutherford, 2004). However, it would appear that the processing bias in GAD is not specific to threat but is sensitive to negative emotional stimuli in general. Also the bias is not apparent in individuals who have recovered from GAD and may be influenced by stressors that elevate state anxiety. It is also not clear whether hypervigilance for threat or difficulty disengaging from threat is the primary feature of the attentional bias. Finally, although the current model, like most cognitive theories of GAD, argues that presence of threat encoding and interpretation biases are critical processes that characterize worry, little is still known about the information-processing biases that underlie worry per se. One development that might help in this regard would be to use experimental stimuli that more closely resemble the idiosyncratic life concerns of GAD worriers.

Clinician Guideline 10.11

Cognitive interventions must address the anxious person's automatic tendency to assume a more negative and threatening interpretation of ambiguous and uncertain life situations.

Hypothesis 4

Pathological worry is characterized by negative appraisal of worry and the presence of "metaworry" (i.e., worry about worry).

As depicted in Figure 10.1 the cognitive model proposes that metacognitive processes play a critical role in the persistence of worry. A number of researchers have compared how pathological worriers and nonworriers appraise their worrisome thoughts in an effort to specify the faulty metacognitive processing in GAD. Vasey and Borkovec (1992) found that chronic worriers engaged in more catastrophizing during the worry process than nonworriers and on average they believed that the catastrophe was more likely to occur. Others have also found that increased subjective risk bias (i.e., estimated probability that the feared outcome will occur) or catastrophizing is associated with propensity to worry (e.g., Constans, 2001; Molina et al., 1998). Furthermore, GAD worriers experience more negative intrusions as a result of worrying, have less perceived control over their worries, and believe that failure to control worry would lead to greater harm or danger (Ruscio & Borkovec, 2004).

A number of researchers have compared subjective appraisal of worry with other negative thoughts like obsessions or rumination. Langlois, Freeston, and Ladouceur (2000a) used the Cognitive Intrusions Questionnaire to compare individuals' appraisals of their most frequent worry versus obsessional intrusive thought. Worry was considered significantly more difficult to control, more attention grabbing, more unpleasant and interfering, more ego-syntonic, and considered more likely to come true (see also Wells & Morrison, 1994, for similar results). In a similar study D. A. Clark and Claybourn (1997) found that worry was rated as more disturbing and more closely linked to the perceived consequences of real-life negative events. Studies comparing appraisal of worry with depressive rumination found that most of the appraisals are similar in the two types of cognition (e.g., ratings of reduced control, increased disapproval, and negative consequences) but worry was uniquely characterized as more focused on the consequences of the worry topic, more future-oriented, and more disturbing than rumination (Watkins, 2004; Watkins, Moulds, & Mackintosh, 2005).

Another important metacognitive process in the maintenance of pathological worry is Wells's concept of metaworry, or worrying about worrying. Wells and colleagues developed the Anxious Thoughts Inventory (AnTi) to assess various process characteristics of worry (Wells, 1994a). Factor analysis revealed that seven AnTi items formed a coherent dimension of metaworry. Subsequent research reveals that scores on metaworry correlate with trait anxiety and worry measures, and analogue samples of GAD score higher on metaworry than nonanxious controls (Wells, 1994a, 2005b; Wells & Carter, 1999).

The distorted and faulty appraisal evident in pathological worry shares more similarities than differences with how individuals appraise other types of unwanted repetitive thoughts such as obsessions or depressive rumination. However, there is emerging evidence that certain metacognitive processes may be especially critical to the persistence of worry. A tendency to catastrophize, to believe that negative outcomes are likely to occur and will lead to significant negative effects in one's life, and to perceive worry itself as a highly uncontrollable, disturbing, and dangerous process are metacognitive appraisals that are likely to contribute to an escalation of the worry process. Although empirical research relevant to Hypothesis 4 is still preliminary, these early findings are encouraging for further exploration of the role of metacognitive processing in GAD.

Clinician Guideline 10.12

Individuals with GAD will engage in extensive catastrophizing and consider their worrisome thoughts as dangerous and uncontrollable. The cognitive therapist must address this faulty appraisal process in order to achieve the desired therapeutic gains over worry.

Hypothesis 5

Individuals with GAD (1) will expend greater effort toward disengagement from or suppression of worry, (2) are more likely to use faulty control strategies, and (3) will experience less success controlling their worry than nonanxious worriers.

Given that individuals with GAD tend to appraise their worrisome thoughts as disturbing and associated with a greater likelihood of negative outcomes, Hypothesis 5 is a natural extension of the previous hypothesis. According to the cognitive model illustrated in Figure 10.1, we predict unsuccessful and futile efforts to control or suppress worry will paradoxically contribute to its persistence, in accord with Wegner's ironic process theory of suppression (Wegner, 1994; Wenzlaff & Wegner, 2000). As predicted by Hypothesis 5, researchers have consistently found that GAD is characterized by a heightened subjective experience of worry as an uncontrollable process and any efforts at control prove futile and unproductive (Craske et al., 1989; Hoyer et al., 2001; Wells & Morrison, 1994). Despite their acknowledged inability to control worry, it is interesting that individuals with GAD are highly invested in continuing with their efforts toward gaining control over worry (Hoyer et al., 2001).

There is now some evidence that deliberate attempts to suppress worrisome thoughts can have adverse effects on the worry process. For example, we found that university students instructed to suppress thoughts of failing an exam experienced a rebound in worry once suppression efforts ceased (Wang & Clark, 2008). Becker, Rinck, Roth, and Margraf (1998) also found evidence of impaired mental control with GAD patients having less success suppressing their main worry than speech phobic and nonanxious controls. However, other studies have failed to find adverse effects with attempts to suppress worry (e.g., Mathews & Milroy, 1994; McLean & Broomfield, 2007).

It is possible that thought suppression might not directly influence the frequency of worry but instead have other untoward effects on the worry experience. Harvey (2003) reported that individuals with insomnia try to suppress and control their intrusive thoughts and worry during the presleep period more than good sleepers. In addition, individuals instructed to suppress their presleep worrisome thoughts experienced longer sleep-onset latency and poorer quality of sleep but did not report more unwanted worrisome thought intrusions. In a recent study, high trait-anxious students were randomly assigned to suppress previously presented threat and neutral words, concentrate on the words, or just allow the thoughts to wander (Kircanski, Craske, & Bjork, 2008). Analyses revealed that suppression of threat words generated an enhanced explicit memory bias for threat but not increased physiological arousal. Thus it is possible that suppression of worry might negatively influence how unwanted thoughts are appraised or emotionally experienced (see Purdon, 1999, for discussion). There is consistent evidence from questionnaire studies that increased effort at thought control is associated with heightened scores on a broad range of psychopathological measures including various process measures of worry (e.g., de Bruin, Muris, & Rassin, 2007; Sexton & Dugas, 2008).

A few studies have investigated whether high worriers engage in less effective thought control strategies. Langlois et al. (2000b) found that students reported similar coping strategies for worry and obsessional intrusive thoughts, with escape/avoidance and problem-focused strategies associated with both types of repetitive thought. Wells and Davies (1994) developed the Thought Control Questionnaire (TCQ) to assess various mental control strategies associated with worry such as distraction, punishment, reappraisal, worry (e.g., think about more minor worries), and social control (e.g., talk to a friend). Coles and Heimberg (2005) found that GAD patients reported significantly higher levels of TCQ punishment and worry and significantly lower use of social control and distraction than nonanxious controls. Both TCQ worry and punishment were significantly correlated with the PSWQ, indicating that these control strategies have the closest association with psychopathology (see also Fehm & Hoyer, 2004). Although attempts to control worry by worrying about other issues in one's life or being excessively self-critical may contribute to pathological worry in GAD, these maladaptive strategies may also be evident in other anxiety disorders (Coles & Heimberg, 2005; Fehm & Hoyer, 2004).

The perception that worry is uncontrollable is so pervasive in GAD that it is now entrenched as a key diagnostic criterion of the disorder. Moreover, there is some evidence that individuals with GAD may try harder to control their worrisome thinking. However, the experimental research on thought suppression is divided on whether chronic worriers are actually less successful at worry control than nonanxious individuals. In addition it is not at all clear how excessive efforts at suppressing one's worries might influence its course. For example, thought suppression may have less direct influence on the frequency of worry and more effects on biased information processing (Kircanski et al., 2008), faulty appraisal, or emotional response (D. A. Clark, 2004; Purdon, 1999). In addition it is likely that individuals with GAD do rely on less effective thought control strategies but it is unlikely this is unique to the disorder. At this point we must consider the empirical evidence for Hypothesis 5 tentative at best. More research is needed on mental control, especially with GAD clinical samples, in order to explore this important aspect of the worry process.

Clinician Guideline 10.13

Even though the research is still tentative, cognitive therapists must encourage individuals with GAD to abandon their efforts to suppress worry. At the very least, the mental control strategies employed in GAD have not proven effective and are probably counterproductive in the long term.

Hypothesis 6

In GAD worry is associated with a greater loss of perceived safety and poorer problem solving compared to non-GAD worry.

Rachman (2004) made a compelling argument that GAD is the unsuccessful search for safety (see also Lohr et al., 2007; Woody & Rachman, 1994). Individuals with GAD perceive a wide range of threats involving uncertain future possibilities. They search for safety cues that will delimit the range and duration of the threat. Safety strategies such as seeking reassurance from others, repeated checking, avoiding risks, and generally engaging in overprotective behaviors could potentially reduce immediate general anxiety and avoidance if the sense of safety is achieved (Rachman, 2004). But safety signals may be more difficult to detect than danger signals, even at the best of times, and given the abstract future-oriented threat in worry, they may be particularly ill-suited for this type of threat (Lohr et al., 2007; Woody & Rachman, 1994). If safety remains elusive, general anxiety and worry will increase. Thus unsuccessful attempts to attain a sense of safety must be considered a factor that could contribute to the persistence of worry. Unfortunately, very little research has examined safety seeking in worry or GAD. An exception is an experimental study involving a simple detection of threat and safe stimuli, in which high trait-anxious students with good attentional control were better able to disengage from the threat stimulus and shift attention to the safe cue at the later, more strategic stage of information processing (Derryberry & Reed, 2002).

Problem solving could be construed as a type of safety-seeking strategy as worried individuals search for some way to resolve or at least prepare themselves for the possibility of a future negative threat. It is not surprising that researchers have been particularly interested in the relation between problem solving ability and worry given that failed problem-solving is embedded in the very notion of worry (e.g., Borkovec, Robinson, et al., 1983). Two aspects of problem solving have been investigated. The first is whether pathological worry reflects deficiencies in problem-solving abilities such as problem formulation, generating alternative solutions, decision making, solution implementation, and evaluation. The second possibility is that chronic worriers adopt a negative problem orientation which, coupled with intolerance of uncertainty, impedes their ability to solve problems and maintains the worry process (Koerner & Dugas, 2006). Davey and colleagues suggested that pathological worry might result from high-trait anxious individuals not accepting any solutions generated by their constructive, task-oriented worrying because of low problem-solving confidence, lack of perceived control over the problem-solving process, and a tendency to seek further information due to catastrophic thinking (Davey, 1994; Davey et al., 1992). Although Davey (1994) focused mainly on problem-solving confidence, Koerner and Dugas (2006) argued for the broader construct of *negative problem orientation* that includes (1) a tendency to view problems as threats, (2) a lack of self-confidence in one's problem-solving ability, (3) a tendency to become easily frustrated with problem solving, and (4) negative expectation about the problem-solving outcome.

Numerous studies have failed to find any evidence of problem-solving deficiencies in GAD or that poor problem solving is associated with worry (e.g., Davey, 1994; Dugas et al., 1995; Ladouceur et al., 1999). However, there is considerable evidence that negative problem orientation and low problem-solving confidence in particular may be specific to GAD and pathological worry (e.g., Dugas et al., 1995; Dugas et al., 2005; Ladouceur et al., 1999; Robichaud & Dugas, 2005). Moreover, negative problem orientation may interact with intolerance of uncertainty (Dugas et al., 1997) or catastrophizing (Davey, Jubb, & Cameron, 1996) to increase the risk of engaging in pathological worry.

There is qualified support for Hypothesis 6. It is clear that individuals with GAD do not suffer from problem-solving deficits but they do exhibit less confidence in their problem-solving abilities. This negative problem orientation is primarily due to negative problem-solving beliefs rather than to more generalized negative expectations (Robichaud & Dugas, 2005). Moreover, negative problem orientation combined with a tendency to catastrophize and search for more certain solutions to a future negative situation will lead to an endless search for and then rejection of solutions to the anticipated threatening situation. In this way the chronic worrier experiences repeated failures to establish a sense of safety. Although much of this remains conjecture until further research is conducted, at least some aspects of Hypothesis 6 (i.e., low problem-solving confidence) have been partially supported in the empirical literature.

Clinician Guideline 10.14

Target dysfunctional beliefs about effective problem solving and the attainment of safety from imagined future negative outcomes for change in cognitive therapy of GAD.

COGNITIVE ASSESSMENT AND CASE FORMULATION

Diagnostic and Symptom Measures

As with the other anxiety disorders we recommend the ADIS-IV (Brown et al., 1994) as the best diagnostic interview for GAD. The GAD module provides dimensional ratings on excessiveness (i.e., frequency and intensity) and controllability of worry in eight domains of interpersonal, work, health and daily living. In addition to questions on key diagnostic features, the ADIS-IV assesses the context of worry, presence of safety-seeking responses, and degree of interference in daily living. The ADIS-IV (lifetime version) has good interrater reliability with a kappa of .67 for a principal diagnosis of GAD (Brown, Di Nardo, et al., 2001). The main source of disagreement was between GAD and a depressive disorder (60% of disagreements). The SCID-I/NP (First, Spitzer, Gibbon, & Williams, 2002) is an alternative to the ADIS-IV but the reliability of the more recent version of the interview has not been assessed in a large-scale study (Turk et al., 2004).

Generalized Anxiety Disorder Questionnaire–IV

The Generalized Anxiety Disorder Questionnaire–IV (GAD-Q-IV; Newman et al., 2002) is a nine-item questionnaire developed as a screening tool for GAD. The GAD-Q-IV is a refinement of the original GAD-Q (Roemer, Borkovec, Posa, & Borkovec, 1995) intended to make it more compatible with DSM-IV criteria. The GAD-Q and GAD-Q-IV have been used most extensively in analogue research to identify individuals who might meet diagnostic criteria for GAD. Newman et al. (2002) found that a cutoff score of 5.7 was optimal for identifying GAD from other anxiety disorder groups and that the GAD-Q-IV correlated positively with measures of worry. In their review Turk and Wolanin (2006) concluded that the GAD-IV-Q is sensitive to GAD but it may over-diagnose the disorder, especially in more urban, ethnically diverse populations. In clinical practice the GAD-Q-IV is unnecessary if an ADIS-IV or SCID-IV is administered. A copy of the GAD-Q-IV can be found in Newman et al. (2002).

Measures of Worry

Penn State Worry Questionnaire

The 16-item Penn State Worry Questionnaire (PSWQ; Meyer et al., 1990) is the most widely used measure of worry with a cutoff score of 45 recommended to distinguish pathological worry in a treatment-seeking population (see Chapter 5 for further discussion). The PSWQ should be included in the standard assessment for GAD and should be readministered at posttreatment given its sensitivity to treatment effects.

Worry Domains Questionnaire

The Worry Domains Questionnaire (WDQ; Tallis et al., 1992) is a 25-item measure of worry content that assesses extent of worry in five domains: relationships, lack of confidence, aimless future, work, and financial matters. Items are assessed on a 0 ("not at all") to 4 ("extremely") scale, with a total score and subscale scores for each domain calculated by summing across respective items. The questionnaire displays good temporal reliability exhibits convergent validity with the PSWQ and trait anxiety, and GAD samples score substantially higher than nonclinical controls (Tallis, Davey, & Bond, 1994; Stöber, 1998). Moreover the five-factor structure of the WDQ has been replicated (Joorman & Stöber, 1997) and the WDQ correlates significantly with peer and self-ratings of daily worry (Stöber, 1998; Verkuil, Brosschot, & Thayer, 2007). However, the WDQ has some limitations for clinical practice. The questionnaire reflects some aspects of constructive or adaptive worrying and so should not be construed as a "pure" measure of pathological worry like the PSWQ (Tallis et al., 1994; Turk et al., 2004). In addition, only certain subscales may be specific to GAD (Diefenbach et al., 2001) and responses may be influenced by age and ethnicity (Ladouceur, Freeston, Fournier, Dugas, & Doucet, 2002; Scott et al., 2002). A 10-item short form of the WDQ has been published (Stöber & Joorman, 2001) and a copy of the original 25-item WDQ is available in Tallis et al. (1994). The WDQ is primarily a research instrument but can be used clinically as a complementary tool for assessing worry content.

Cognitive Measures of Worry

Anxious Thoughts Inventory

The Anxious Thoughts Inventory (AnTi; Wells, 1994a) is a 22-item questionnaire designed to assess both worry content and negative appraisal about worry (i.e., meta-worry). The AnTi has three subscales: social worry, health worry and metaworry. Although all three subscales correlate with the PSWQ, only the AnTi Meta-Worry subscale shows a unique relationship with pathological worry and significantly discriminates GAD from other anxiety disorders (Wells & Carter, 1999, 2001). Thus AnTi Meta-Worry is the only subscale that is likely to provide clinically useful information since it focuses on negative appraisals of worry. More recently Wells (2005b) published a short seven-item measure of metaworry, the Meta-Worry Questionnaire, that holds considerable promise.

Meta-Cognitions Questionnaire

The Meta-Cognitions Questionnaire (MCQ; Cartwright-Hatton & Wells, 1997) is a 65-item self-report measure that assesses positive and negative beliefs and appraisals about worry and unwanted intrusive thoughts. The questionnaire has five subscales: positive beliefs about worry, negative beliefs about the danger and uncontrollability of worry, cognitive confidence, control of intrusive thoughts, and cognitive self-consciousness. The MCQ Danger and Uncontrollability subscale has the most relevance for pathological worry (Cartwright-Hatton & Wells, 1997; Wells & Carter, 2001; see discussion in Chapter 3, Hypothesis 2) and so can be useful when developing a case formulation. Wells and Cartwright-Hatton (2004) published a brief 30-item version of the MCQ that appears to be psychometrically sound.

Intolerance of Uncertainty Scale

The Intolerance of Uncertainty Scale (IUS; Freeston, Rhéaume, et al., 1994) is a 27-item questionnaire that assesses maladaptive beliefs that uncertainty is unacceptable, that it reflects badly on a person, will lead to frustration and stress, and causes inaction (Dugas et al., 2004). Although the measure is multidimensional, the total score has proven most useful in research studies (Freeston, Rhéaume, Letarte, Dugas, & Ladouceur, 1994; Dugas et al., 2004). Numerous studies have shown that the IUS has a specific association with pathological worry and discriminates GAD (e.g., Dugas, Gagnon, et al., 1998; Dugas et al., 2001; Dugas et al., 2005). Given its strong discriminant validity, the IUS is useful for assessing key pathologic beliefs in GAD.

Thought Control Questionnaire

The Thought Control Questionnaire (TCQ; Wells & Davies, 1994) is a 30-item questionnaire that assesses the extent that individuals use five different thought control strategies: distraction, punishment, reappraisal, social control, and worry. Research suggests that individuals with GAD score significantly higher than nonanxious controls only on the TCQ Punishment and Worry subscales (Coles & Heimberg, 2005; Fehm & Hoyer, 2004) and only these two subscales correlate with the PSWQ (Wells & Davies, 1994).

Clinician Guideline 10.15

Cognitive assessment for GAD should include the ADIS-IV, the PSWQ, and possibly a measure of worry content such as the Worry Domains Questionnaire. In addition the IUS and certain subscales of the MCQ may be helpful when assessing maladaptive beliefs that characterize GAD.

Case Formulation

Cognitive therapy for GAD focuses on the faulty elaborative processing that contributes to the persistence of anxious thinking and pathological worry (see Figure 10.1) as well as the dysfunctional schemas responsible for the state of generalized anxiety. Thus the cognitive case formulation centers on a clear specification of the idiosyncratic schemas and faulty metacognitive processes of worry. Figure 10.2 illustrates the main components of a cognitive case conceptualization for GAD.

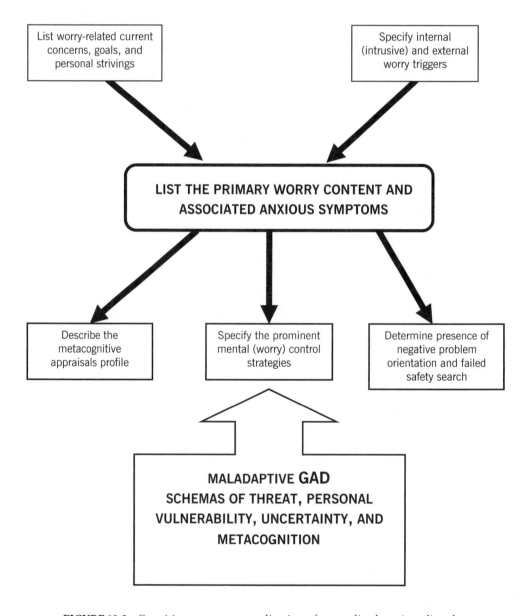

FIGURE 10.2. Cognitive case conceptualization of generalized anxiety disorder.

Primary Worry Content

Although current concerns and internal/external triggers are antecedents to worry, it is more practical to begin by assessing the client's primary worries and associated anxious symptoms. Information from the ADIS-IV as well as any worry content questionnaires that might be administered, such as the WDQ, will provide the first clues about the client's worries. However, daily monitoring of worry activity and a more detailed clinical interview will be needed to obtain a full understanding of the client's worry concerns.

Appendix 10.1 provides a Worry Self-Monitoring Form B that can be used to collect critical information on individuals' primary worry content. Chapter 5 (Appendix 5.8) presents an alternative worry form that can be used if less detailed information is required. We suggest that Appendix 5.8 be used for non-GAD worry and that Appendix 10.1 be used with GAD clients. There are a number of features of worry content that should be assessed from the self-monitoring form and clinical interview.

1. What is the range or extent of the client's worries?
2. What are the frequency, intensity, and duration of the worry episodes?
3. What is the level of anxiety or distress associated with each worry topic? What symptoms of anxiety are experienced during worry?
4. What is the worst outcome or catastrophe that underlies each worry topic? What is the client's estimate of the probability or likelihood of the catastrophic outcome?
5. If the worst outcome is rated as highly unlikely, what does the client perceive as the most likely negative outcome?
6. If more than one primary worry content is present, rank-order the worries from most important/disturbing to least important/disturbing. Determine which worry topic the client would choose for focus of therapy.

In our case illustration Rebecca expressed a number of worry concerns: worries about her parent's health, her own health, her children's safety, family finances, and her work performance. Assessment of worry frequency, duration, and associated distress indicated that her performance at work and her own health were the most distressing worries. She selected her work performance as the most important topic for therapy. When we explored these worries further, she indicated that the catastrophe associated with this worry was of being reprimanded by her supervisors for mishandling an employee problem. This could result in litigation against her, but the greatest consequence is that she would loose the respect of her employees and be seen within the company as a weak and inadequate leader. Interestingly, her worry had a more social focus that subsequently guided cognitive restructuring of this worry issue. It is always important to determine the catastrophizing process associated with each worry.

Personal Goals and Current Concerns

In order to understand the personal context of worry, the cognitive therapist must appreciate the client's immediate and long-term personal goals, strivings, and ambitions. This information should become apparent from the clinical interview but a few direct questions may be needed as well. The therapist can ask the client to indicate her immediate goal in key areas of her life such as work/school, family, health, intimate relationships, finances, leisure, friendships, and the like. For example, in the area of intimacy the therapist could ask "Where would you like to be in 3 years with regards to an intimate relationship?", "What do you see as the greatest barrier to achieving this goal in intimacy?", "How likely is it that you will make this goal?", and "What would be the worst possible outcome for you in 3 years?" This type of questioning will provide the therapist with a better understanding of the motivational features of worry.

One of Rebecca's primary concerns was to maintain a reputation with her employees as a fair, competent, and understanding manager. The problem for her was that any criticism was viewed as a threat to this goal and would trigger a heightened state of anxiety in which she worried that others viewed her as a weak and incompetent leader. It is easy to see how Rebecca's desire to be admired by others (i.e., a major current concern) fed into a vicious cycle of worry about how her employees perceived her managerial style.

Worry Triggers

The Worry Self-Monitoring Form B (Appendix 10.1) will provide an indication of the type of stimuli that trigger worry episodes. Again this information is critical for completing a contextual analysis of worry episodes. A variety of external factors may trigger worry such as when Rebecca received even a slightly negative remark from an employee. Another client had pathological worry about his finances and was plunged into one of these episodes whenever there was even a slight decline in his monthly investment statement (a much too common occurrence, as any investor knows!). Martin, an older client with GAD, would start worrying about mowing his lawn whenever he looked out the front window of his house. Most clients can generate a list of external cues that trigger their worry. Sometimes the list of triggers is broad and other times it is very narrowly focused.

Internal cues such as automatic anxious intrusive thoughts, images, or even physical sensations are important triggers of a worry episode. Martin would have an intrusive thought that tomorrow was garbage day and then he would start worrying about whether he will have enough energy to move his trash to the curb. Sarah would feel a slight nausea that she interpreted as a possible sign of the flu, and then worried that she might be getting sick. Rebecca would remember that she hadn't visited her parents, wonder if they were still well, and then start worrying that they might get terribly ill or soon die before she could spend more time with them. Clients may not be aware of all the internal or external triggers to their worry but within the first few sessions the main worry triggers should be identified.

Metacognitive Appraisals of Worry

How individuals appraise or evaluate their worries is another key component of the case conceptualization. This part of the assessment focuses on how clients evaluate the worry process associated with each of their primary worry concerns. Here we are emphasizing individuals' "online" appraisals of worry episodes rather than the core beliefs about worry that may underlie the faulty appraisals of worry. The following metacognitive appraisals should be specified in the case formulation:

- Tendency to engage in catastrophizing
- Estimates of the probability of threat or catastrophe
- Perceived uncontrollability of worry
- Extent of metaworry (i.e., worry about worry)
- Expected negative consequences of worry
- Expected positive aspects of worry

The client will have already articulated the catastrophic outcome when the primary worry concerns were assessed. A student with GAD, for example, might frequently worry about his performance on a test. The therapist would ask, "When you worry about an exam, how often do you end up convinced you will fail the course and be put on academic probation" (i.e., the student's catastrophic outcome)? "Are there other negative outcomes that you think about more often when you worry about exams?" "On a scale from 0% (no probability of being put on academic probation) to 100% (complete probability of being put on academic probation), what is the likelihood of this catastrophe?" "What is the likelihood of less extreme outcomes such as not passing the exam or failing the course?" "As you look at this now, do you think you are exaggerating the likelihood of a bad outcome?" "What do you think is the most likely outcome?" "How difficult is it to think about the most likely outcome when you are worrying about exams?"

The cognitive therapist also obtains ratings on the perceived controllability associated with each primary worry concern. In the previous example the therapist would ask "how difficult is it for you to stop worrying about the exam once you start the worry process?" "On a scale from 0 (absolutely no control) to 100 (complete control), what is the average amount of control you have over worry about exams? "Does this control vary at all?" "Are there times when you have good control over the worry and other times when your control is terrible?" "Have you noticed what seems to encourage worry control and things that interfere in your level of control?"

It is important to determine the extent that metaworry is associated with each of the primary worry concerns (Wells, 1999, 2006). For example, Rebecca indicated she had difficulty falling asleep each night because of "racing thoughts" (i.e., worry) about how she responded to employee problems that day and also what might lie ahead of her tomorrow. However, she quickly shifted from these "primary worries" to worry about the consequences of not being able to shut down her racing thoughts and fall asleep. A rating from 0 ("no worry about worry") to 100 ("extremely concerned about being worried") was obtained each time Rebecca worried about her managerial performance with employees. What was interesting is that metaworry was sometimes very strong in certain situations (e.g., when trying to fall asleep at night) but less prominent in others (e.g., worrying about how she will handle an employee situation just before the interview). Thus in the case formulation it is important to specify the extent of metaworry associated with each primary worry content, the situations when metaworry is strong and when it is weaker.

The perceived positive and negative consequences of worry are a related aspect of metaworry. Again it is important to determine perceived consequences associated with each worry concern when the individual is engaged in the worry process. It is expected that the perceived consequences are highly idiosyncratic and will vary greatly between worry concerns. Rebecca, for example, perceived mainly negative consequences with her work worries, noting that the worry probably made her less confident and assertive with her employees and more distressed and irritable at home. However, she appraised her worries about her preschool daughter's safety more positively, thinking this worry caused her to be a more cautious mother and so reduced the risk of injury for her child. As discussed below, the perceived consequences of worry are a primary target for change in cognitive therapy of GAD.

Worry Control Strategies

As indicated in the cognitive model of GAD (Figure 10.1), attempts to suppress or control worry will contribute to its persistence because the ineffectiveness of these strategies confirms the individual's belief that the worry is dangerous and uncontrollable. Thus it is critical to assess the frequency, type, and perceived effectiveness of the various thought control strategies employed with each primary worry concern. Table 10.3 presents a list of positive and negative worry control strategies based on the empirical literature.

In addition to interview questions about worry control strategies, the cognitive therapist can use the Cognitive Response to Anxiety Checklist in Chapter 5 (Appendix 5.9) to assess the client's use of thought control strategies. The wording of Appendix 5.9 should be changed from "anxious thinking" to "worrisome thinking." Furthermore, the clinician will want to determine the positive and negative control strategies used with each primary worry concern and obtain information on how frequently it is employed as well as its perceived effectiveness.

Safety Scripts and Problem Orientation

Individuals with GAD should be asked to describe what would give them a sense of peace or safety in a particular worry domain—that is, to write out a script of how a

---

TABLE 10.3. Worry Control Strategies in Generalized Anxiety Disorder

Negative control strategies

- *Directed suppression* (i.e., "Tell myself not to worry")
- *Self-reassurance* (i.e., "Tell myself everything will be okay")
- *Seek reassurance from others* (i.e., ask family/friends if everything will be alright)
- *Checking* (i.e., engage in some repetitive act to relieve doubt)
- *Punishment* (i.e., criticize self for worrying)
- *Emotion suppression* (i.e., try to suppress the distress, anxiety associated with worry)

Positive control strategies

- *Directed expression* (i.e., intentionally allow myself to worry, let it run its course)
- *Distraction* (i.e., get involved in a distracting activity, or replace worry with more positive thinking)
- *Threat reappraisal* (i.e., reappraise the imagined threat of the worry concern)
- *Engage in problem solving* (i.e., develop an action plan for dealing with the worry concern)
- *Relaxation* (i.e., engage in meditation or relaxation)

sense of safety could be achieved with the worry concern. In other words, what would have to happen for worry to cease? Louise was a single woman in her mid-30s who was highly successful in her career and had recently become romantically involved with a man she met over the Internet. However, she was racked with worry over whether he really liked her and whether he would drop her at any moment. Her catastrophic thinking was "This is my last chance at happiness. If this relationship doesn't work, I'll be left alone the rest of my life." When asked what needed to happen for her to feel safe or confident about the relationship, Louise answered that she needed some sign of his undying commitment to her. But the more she thought about this, the more she realized there was nothing he could do to eradicate her uncertainty about the relationship. It is the nature of intimate relationships that a spouse or partner can always leave. It is important for the clinician to determine what constitutes safety for each of the primary worry concerns, what cues would signal the attainment of safety, and whether individuals can recall a time when a sense of peace or safety was attained in this area of their life. It may be that, like Louise, a client will discover that the search for safety is futile, maybe even impossible to achieve.

Worry always involves efforts toward problem solving, often with the goal of achieving a sense of safety and certainty of outcome. It is important to determine the range of problem solutions that the client generated around a particular worry topic. "What solutions have you come up with for this particular problem (i.e., the worry concern)?" "Are you able to generate any good solutions for this problem?" "On a scale from 0 (no confidence) to 100 (extremely confident), how confident are you that a good solution will be found for this problem?" "How frustrated do you feel with your problem-solving efforts?", "Do you expect to eventually resolve this problem or will it continue unresolved indefinitely?"

Pierre was a retired government worker who worried excessively about his retirement income and whether he had enough saved to see him through to old age. He decided that the best solution to his anxiety and worry was to start a small part-time business to supplement his retirement income. Unfortunately, this did little to relieve his anxiety because he now worried about the uncertainties of business and whether he could sustain a steady income over many years. When he eventually decided to seek treatment, he was discouraged and convinced there was no solution to his worry. He had done the most logical thing, which was to earn more money, and yet this only intensified his worry about finances. He adopted a most extreme negative problem orientation, believing there was no solution to his chronic financial worries.

Dysfunctional GAD Schemas

A cognitive assessment should culminate with an identification of the core maladaptive schemas of threat, personal vulnerability, intolerance of uncertainty, and metacognitive beliefs about worry that are responsible for the individual's chronic worry. Table 10.2 provides a summary of the types of beliefs that will be prominent in GAD. Different beliefs may be associated with different primary worry concerns, so it is important in the case formulation to identify the core maladaptive beliefs that underlie each worry concern.

Rebecca's primary worry involved her managerial skills when relating to her employees. Cognitive assessment revealed that a core threat belief was that "her employees thought she was a weak, passive leader—a real pushover." She believed this was part of her personality and something she could not change: "She had always been a shy person, an introvert" (vulnerability belief). When she received no response on how she handled a difficult employee situation, she would seek out feedback from her assistant managers, believing that she could not stand the uncertainty of not knowing whether she was too assertive or too passive (intolerance of uncertainty belief). On the one hand, she believed the worry was detrimental to her work performance because she was always trying to "second guess herself," but on the other hand, she felt that the heightened vigilance prevented her from getting into nasty arguments with employees (metacognitive beliefs). Obviously the primary goal of cognitive therapy for GAD is to modify these core dysfunctional beliefs that underlie the pathological worry process.

Clinician Guideline 10.16

A cognitive case conceptualization of GAD will include the following elements: (1) description of the primary worry concerns, (2) specification of current life goals and personal strivings, (3) list of internal and external triggers of worry, (4) identification of metacognitive appraisals of each worry concern, (5) description of the idiosyncratic worry control profile, (6) extent of safety search and negative problem orientation, and (7) formulation of the underlying schematic organization responsible for chronic worry and generalized anxiety.

DESCRIPTION OF COGNITIVE THERAPY FOR GAD

The overarching goal of cognitive therapy for GAD is reduction in the frequency, intensity, and duration of worry episodes that would lead to an associated decrease in automatic anxious intrusive thoughts and generalized anxiety. This will be achieved by modifying the dysfunctional appraisals and beliefs as well as the maladaptive control strategies that are responsible for chronic worry. A successful trial of cognitive therapy would transform worry from a pathological avoidant coping strategy to a more controlled, problem-oriented constructive process in which the anxious person is more tolerant and accepting of risk and uncertainty. The cognitive perspective is expressed by a number of specific treatment goals that are presented in Table 10.4.

To achieve the stated goals of cognitive therapy for GAD, a typical course of therapy will include a number of intervention strategies that will be variably employed depending on the individual case. Table 10.5 summarizes the treatment components of cognitive therapy.

Education Phase

The objective of the first session is to introduce clients to the cognitive model of GAD as well as the treatment rationale. Most individuals with GAD have suffered with excessive worry for many years. As a result they will enter therapy with their own beliefs about why they struggle with pathological worry and possibly some ideas on how it should be treated. The cognitive therapist should start by asking, "Why do you think you have struggled so with worry?" Individuals with GAD might give a variety of answers such as "It's my personality, I've always been a worrier," "Worry runs in my family," "I have a

TABLE 10.4. Treatment Goals for Cognitive Therapy of Generalized Anxiety Disorder

- Normalize worry
- Correct biased threat beliefs and interpretations of worry concerns
- Modify positive and negative metacognitive beliefs about worry
- Eliminate meta-worry (i.e., worry about worry)
- Reduce reliance on dysfunctional worry control strategies and promote adaptive control responses to worry
- Improve confidence in problem-solving ability
- Increase perceived control over worry
- Enhance a sense of safety and self-confidence to deal with future challenges
- Accept risk and tolerate uncertain outcome of future situations and events
- Increase tolerance of negative emotion

very demanding life, there's a lot to worry about," "I'm a highly anxious person and this causes me to worry," "I have a chemical imbalance that makes me worry too much," and so on. The therapist should follow up by asking, "What do you think is the solution to your worry, the best way to treat worry?" Again the client may generate a number of ideas such as find a way to resolve the worry concerns or situations, learn to relax, take medication to reduce anxiety, reduce stress, and the like. The therapist could also ask, "over the years has your anxiety and worry fluctuated at all? If so, have you noticed what makes the worry better or worse?"

After assessing the client's personal theory of anxiety and worry, the therapist is in a better position to determine whether she will be receptive to socialization into the cognitive model of worry. If the client holds strong beliefs about anxiety and worry that are incompatible with the cognitive perspective, these beliefs must be targeted for change before proceeding with cognitive treatment of worry. There are five main elements of the cognitive model that should be communicated to the client:

TABLE 10.5. Treatment Components in Cognitive Therapy for Generalized Anxiety Disorder

- Educate on the cognitive perspective of worry
- Distinguish between productive and unproductive worry (see Leahy, 2005)
- Cognitive restructuring and empirical hypothesis testing of biased threat appraisals and beliefs about worry
- Worry induction and decatastrophizing (Craske & Barlow, 2006)
- Repeated worry expression with response prevention of ineffective worry control strategies (Borkovec et al., 2004)
- Self-directed effortful processing of safety cues
- Cognitive restructuring of negative metacognitive beliefs about worry (Wells, 2006)
- Risk and uncertainty inoculation
- Constructive problem-solving training
- Elaborative processing of the present (Borkovec et al., 2004)
- Relaxation training (optional)

1. Worry is a normal part of life but there are two types of worry: productive worry and unproductive or pathological worry. It is pathological worry that is associated with high anxiety and distress.
2. Pathological worry is caused by our attitude and the way we try to deal with worry. Research has shown that certain types of negative thoughts and beliefs about risk, uncertainty, and worry itself characterizes excessive or unproductive worry. You can think of these as the psychological causes of a tendency to worry.
3. This negative attitude toward worry causes individuals to adopt ways to control their worry that in the long run make the worry even more persistent and difficult to control.
4. The goal of cognitive therapy is to identify the underlying thoughts and beliefs that cause chronic worry as well as any counterproductive responses that make the worry persistent, and then help the individual adopt a more constructive attitude and response to worry.
5. The ultimate goal of cognitive therapy is to change unproductive worry into productive worry by modifying the underlying psychological causes of chronic worry. The elimination of pathological worry will lead to a reduction in general anxiety level as well.

Wells (1997) noted that the cognitive therapist must shift a client's focus from worry content as the problem (e.g., "I don't have much job security so that's why I worry about losing my job") to the factors that underlie the tendency to worry. To assist in this process the client could be asked, for example, "Even if you had good job security, do you think that would stop you from worrying?" The cognitive therapist can then ask the client why some people worry and yet are not bothered by it, whereas other people are very upset, anxious about their worries. One could also determine if there are some uncertainties in the person's life that are not associated with worry (e.g., a young person who does not worry about being seriously injured in a car accident), whereas other uncertainties lead to great worry (e.g., Will I get into graduate school and be able to pursue my chosen career?). A comparison could be made between the different "cognitive sets" associated with each of these situations and how the different ways of thinking leads to excessive worry or no worry at all. A possible homework assignment might be to survey family or close friends who face issues similar to the client's worry concerns and ask how they think about or deal with the issue (e.g., work insecurity, uncertain medical test, questionable commitment of romantic partner). In the end clients must be socialized to accept that the problem is not *worry per se* but rather *how they worry*.

Clinician Guideline 10.17

Begin the education phase by determining each client's personal theory of worry and then using Socratic questioning and guided discovery to teach individuals that reduction in chronic worry is possible by changing the maladaptive appraisals and beliefs as well as the ineffective mental and behavioral control strategies responsible for the persistence of their pathological worry.

Differentiating Productive and Unproductive Worry

In his self-help manual for worry Leahy (2005) noted that teaching individuals with chronic worry how to distinguish productive from unproductive worry is a critical treatment ingredient (see also Davey, 1994; Davey et al., 1992). Table 10.6 presents the main elements of productive and unproductive worry based on Leahy's discussion.

Clients should be taught early in cognitive therapy how to distinguish productive worry from unproductive (i.e., pathological) worry. Given the intensive assessment of worry, clients should be well aware of their pathological worry even during the first couple of sessions. So the challenge is to make clients more aware of their productive worry. It is likely they have not even considered the possibility that at times they may engage in productive worry. Using guided discovery, the cognitive therapist can ask clients to tell how they coped with various daily concerns or personal strivings that did not elicit excessive worry. A list could be made of productive worry and pathological worry experiences along with a brief description of how the client handled the problem in a productive or unproductive fashion. Learning that they engage in both productive and unproductive worry will reinforce what was learned in the education phase: that chronic, pathological worry is caused by *how you worry* and not the fact of worry. Also more realistic worries imply a different treatment approach than that taken with chronic worry. If the client's primary worries more closely match the profile of productive worry, than the main treatment approach would be problem solving and development of an action plan. Worries that are more pathological will require the full cognitive treatment package described in this chapter.

In our case illustration Rebecca exhibited predominantly pathological worry, with occasional instances of more realistic or productive worry. Despite her worry about her work performance, she rarely worried excessively about making the sales projections

TABLE 10.6. Characteristics of Pathological and Productive Worry

Pathological worry.	Productive worry
• Focused on more distant, abstract problems.	• Focused on more immediate, realistic problems.
• Person has little realistic control or influence over the situation.	• Person could exercise some control or influence over the situation.
• Greater focus on negative emotion associated with worry situation.	• Greater focus on problem solving the worry situation.
• Cannot accept any solution because it can not guarantee success.	• Can try out and evaluate imperfect solutions.
• Relentless pursuit of safety and certainty of outcome.	• Willingness to tolerate reasonable risk and uncertainty.
• Exaggerated and narrowed processing of the potential threats in a situation with a tendency to catastrophize.	• A broader, more balanced processing of the negative, positive, and benign potential outcomes in a situation.
• Perceived helpless to cope with the worry situation.	• Higher level of self-efficacy in coping with worry situation.
• Associated with high levels of anxiety or distress.	• Associated with low anxiety or distress.

Note. Based on Davey, Hampton, Farrell, and Davidson (1992) and Leahy (2005).

for her store. She managed a highly successful store and consistently made her monthly sales goals. However, this could change quickly with fluctuations in the economy and yet Rebecca rarely worried about her sales figures. On the other hand, she did worry excessively about whether her employees considered her a competent and resourceful manager or whether they considered her weak and easy to manipulate. This latter worry met most of the criteria of pathological worry and so became the focus of our therapy sessions.

Clinician Guideline 10.18

Within the first couple of sessions teach individuals with GAD how to distinguish their realistic or productive worry from chronic, excessive, and pathological worry.

Cognitive Restructuring of Threat Appraisals

Cognitive restructuring is an important therapeutic element of cognitive therapy for GAD. The cognitive therapist begins by identifying the threat-related thoughts and beliefs represented in the primary worry concern. Ratings are made on the perceived likelihood that the threat (i.e., worst possible outcome) could actually occur in real life. The therapist uses evidence gathering to determine whether the client's threat estimation is realistic or exaggerated (see Chapter 6). Appendix 6.2, Testing Anxious Appraisals: Looking for Evidence, can be employed to facilitate the evidence-gathering exercise. It is important to focus on gathering evidence that the client is exaggerating threat when she worries rather than on trying to prove that the worry threat could never happen. The latter is a misguided focus on worry content that will only fail to produce therapeutic effects. After completing evidence gathering, the client is asked to generate an alternative view on the worry topic that represents a more realistic probable outcome. The therapist can follow this with a cost–benefit analysis (see Appendix 6.3) to reinforce the advantages of the alternative interpretation.

Naturally, it is important to follow cognitive restructuring with a homework assignment. For example, whenever the client started to worry, he could record his estimate of the worst outcome and the more realistic alternative outcome. He could then generate a list of reasons why thinking the worst is an exaggerated and unrealistic estimate of threat and reasons why the alternative outcome is a more likely outcome. An empirical hypothesis-testing exercise could also be assigned to determine if "thinking the worst" is an exaggeration of threat. The client could be asked to intentionally seek out evidence that refutes his worry-related automatic threat estimate. When treating worry, the focus of cognitive restructuring must be on the threat appraisal and not the worry content. The objective is teach individuals with GAD how to catch themselves exaggerating the threat ("thinking that the worst is likely to happen") and to replace it with a less exaggerated negative outcome that is more realistic.

Cognitive restructuring of worry-related threat estimation was employed with Rebecca. The catastrophic outcome associated with her primary work-related worry was "I haven't been assertive enough with my staff when problems arise. They will loose respect for me and then I will fail as store manager." She rated the likelihood of this outcome as high, 85/100. There was very little evidence for this feared outcome except that a senior assistant manager had complained that she was too soft on the employees. The other main evidence was every time she had to confront a human resource problem she experienced hesitation, self-doubt, and anxiety, which Rebecca thought made her look indecisive. On the hand, there was plenty of evidence that she was exaggerating the likelihood of the worst outcome. She recently had an employee situation that she handled well and it had a good outcome. Ironically, she had to deal with another situation in which some employees complained that the senior assistant manager, who thought she was too soft, was actually too aggressive and unreasonable with the employees under his supervision. Furthermore, she had received positive evaluations from the district manager on her human resource skills. An alternative interpretation was developed, "One can never know for sure what people think of you. Therefore, I need to judge the effectiveness of my human resource skills in terms of more objective outcomes such as whether employees change their behavior after I intervene. My natural tendency to be sympathetic and less intimidating when confronting employees might cause them to have more respect for me rather than if I attacked them in a verbally aggressive manner." A follow-up homework assignment involved Rebecca collecting evidence that her less confrontational style might actually result in more respect from her employees rather than less respect. She learned from this that when she worried about human resource issues, she was exaggerating the probability of the worst outcome and forgetting the more probable, realistic alternative. She was encouraged to repeatedly practice the cognitive restructuring of threat exercise whenever she started to worry about employee issues.

Clinician Guideline 10.19

In cognitive therapy for GAD cognitive restructuring is employed to modify individuals' tendency to engage in automatic exaggerated threat interpretations for future negative events during their worry episodes.

Worry Induction and Decatastrophizing

By the third or fourth session the cognitive therapist should introduce the concept of worry induction. This involves instructing the client to intentionally worry about a particular concern for 5–10 minutes in the therapy session. The individual is encouraged to verbalize the worry process aloud so the therapist is able to assess the quality of the worry. Before beginning the worry induction, the client is asked to provide two ratings on a scale from 0 to 100: "If I asked you to worry about X [a primary worry topic] right now for 10 minutes, how anxious would this make you feel? How uncontrollable would the worry be?" The client is then instructed to start worrying and try to worry as completely as possible. That is, the worry exercise should continue until the client is totally focused on thoughts or images of the worst possible outcome represented in the worry topic. If the client has difficulty initiating a worry episode, the therapist can help start the induction by asking the client "What is it about [the worry situation or concern] that worries you?" If the client has difficulty progressing to his catastrophic outcome, the cognitive therapist can prime this using the downward arrow technique: "What would be so bad or worrying about that outcome?" and so on. This worry induction exercise should be practiced three or four times in the therapy session before it is assigned as a between-session exposure task (see below). The purpose of the within-session worry induction exercise is (1) to teach clients how to engage in worry exposure, (2) to provide empirical evidence that worry is more controllable than assumed by the client, and (3) to help the client learn that worry is less anxiety-provoking and uncontrollable if worry suppression efforts cease.

Before initiating worry induction it is necessary that the catastrophic outcome or "worst-case scenario" associated with the primary worry concern is fully articulated. As a verbal–linguistic phenomenon, worry may function as an avoidance of emotional processing of fearful imagery (Borkovec, 1994). For this reason the catastrophic outcome may take the form of an image. To determine the catastrophic outcome, the cognitive therapist can employ a variant of the catastrophizing interview (Davey, 2006; Vasey & Borkovec, 1992) in which the therapist continues to ask, "What is it that worries you most about [a previously mentioned worry outcome]?" until the client can no longer respond. A full description of the worst-case outcome should be provided so that clients have a *worry catastrophe script* that can be referred to during their worry exposure sessions.

After generating the catastrophizing script, the cognitive therapist and the client work collaboratively in session developing a *decatastrophizing plan* (Craske & Barlow, 2006; Rygh & Sanderson, 2004). This involves writing out a hypothetical response if the worst-case scenario actually came true. The therapist can state "Let's come up with some ideas, a plan on how you would cope with this catastrophic outcome if it actually happened to you." The decatastrophizing plan is written down underneath the catastrophizing script and given to the client for future reference. The client should be asked, "How disturbing does the worst-case scenario seem in light of your potential coping plan?" For further discussion of decatastrophizing see Chapter 6.

Worry induction and decatastrophizing are illustrated in the case of Clare, a middle-aged woman with GAD who worried about her health. Recently she had a consult with her family physician because of worries that she might have breast cancer. Her physician ordered a mammograph which only intensified Clare's worry about cancer. To determine her "most feared outcome," the therapist conducted the following catastrophizing interview:

THERAPIST: Clare, what worries you about having a mammography test?

CLARE: I'm afraid that the result will be positive.

THERAPIST: And what worries you about a positive mammogram result?

CLARE: It will turn out that I have breast cancer.

THERAPIST: And what worries you most about having breast cancer?

CLARE: That I'll need chemotherapy and possibly a mastectomy.

THERAPIST: What worries you most about these treatments for cancer?

CLARE: That I'll get real sick from the chemo, lose my hair, and end up with a disgusting body.

THERAPIST: What worries you most about the effects of the treatment on your body?

CLARE: That my husband will divorce me because I am so ugly, I'll hate myself, and become severely depressed.

THERAPIST: That sounds really terrible, but is there anything beyond this that worries you?

CLARE: No, that's bad enough isn't it?

THERAPIST: Sure is! So for you, Clare, the worst catastrophe you can imagine about cancer is that you will end up alone, depressed, and with a disgusting body. Can you actually imagine yourself in that state, can you form a picture of it in your mind?

CLARE: Yes, I have an actual image of how I would look and feel as a cancer survivor.

The cognitive therapist recorded in detail Clare's image of herself as a cancer survivor. He then developed with her a decatastrophized script: how she might more realistically cope with breast cancer. This was based on the experiences of two women Clare knew who had breast cancer. The therapist then had Clare engage in 10 minutes of worry induction about cancer, ensuring that at least half of the induction time was spent imagining that she had treatment for breast cancer and was looking at herself in the mirror. This also included her husband's negative reaction to the effects of her treatment and her own feelings of despair. This was followed by imagining how she would realistically cope as a breast cancer survivor using the decatastrophizing script as her reference.

Clinician Guideline 10.20

To enhance worry control and to decatastrophize worry threat, a worry induction exercise is employed that utilizes catastrophizing and decatastrophizing scripts to encourage exposure to individuals' most feared outcomes.

Repeated Worry Expression

Worry exposure (or expression) has become an important component of cognitive behavioral treatments for GAD (e.g., Borkovec et al., 2004; Craske & Barlow, 2006; Rygh & Sanderson, 2004; Wells, 1997). The concept is based on a stimulus control treatment procedure first described by Borkovec, Wilkinson, Folenshire, and Lerman (1983). Individuals initially identified their worrisome thoughts and then established a standard 30-minute period each day when they engaged in worry. If individuals caught themselves worrying any other time of the day, they were to postpone their worrying for the worry period by attending to their present-moment experience. During the worry period, individuals were to engage in problem solving to eliminate their worry concerns. Borkovec et al. (2004) viewed stimulus control treatment as a type of response prevention in which worriers learn to gradually restrict their worry to a more limited range of discriminative cues (i.e., to worry only during a specified time and location).

Over the years various modifications and refinements have been introduced to worry exposure. In cognitive therapy repeated worry exposure is a behavioral experiment that (1) challenges metacognitive beliefs that worry is dangerous and uncontrollable, (2) counters avoidance of the worry catastrophe, (3) prevents suppression and other ineffective worry control strategies, and (4) increases clients' confidence in their ability to deal with worry concerns. The goal of worry exposure is for the client to experience worry and its images as hypothetical possibilities rather than as realistic representations of actual threats to well-being (Rygh & Sanderson, 2004). Appendix 10.2 provides a Worry Exposure Form that can be used when individuals engage in worry exposure homework.

Individuals are given instructions in worry expression prior to its assignment as homework. Clients are instructed to set aside the same 30-minute period in a specified location of their home and to engage in a prolonged period of imagining the worst outcome (i.e., catastrophe) to a single primary worry theme. They should keep their attention focused on the catastrophe "and to think about it or imagine it with as much detail and vividness as possible." They should not try to problem-solve or decatastrophize the worry but simply concentrate on it as fully as possible. If their mind wonders off the worry topic, try to pull it back to the worry as quickly as possible. Clients are encouraged to use the catastrophe script to help them focus on the worry. After each worry exposure, the Worry Exposure Form (Appendix 10.2) should be completed. Particular attention should be given to recording the quality of the catastrophe exposure and any anxious thoughts about engaging in the worry exercise. The client should write down challenges to the anxious thoughts that will encourage more repetition of the worry sessions. If worry occurs during some other time of the day, individuals are to postpone the worry until the worry exposure session. This can be accomplished by writing down the worry content on the Worry Self-Monitoring Form B (Appendix 10.1) as a reminder for the worry exposure session and then focus attention on some aspect of their present-moment experience. Individuals with GAD must be told that it will take daily practice sessions of worry exposure over 2 to 3 weeks before the benefits of this intervention may be felt.

Clinician Guideline 10.21

Repeated exposure to the catastrophic worry outcome is an important behavioral experiment in cognitive therapy of GAD. It challenges individuals' maladaptive beliefs about the dangers and uncontrollability of worry and prevents the use of ineffective worry control strategies.

Safety Cue Processing

Chronic worriers become so focused on threat and uncertainty during the worry process that they often fail to process positive, safe, or benign aspects of a worry situation. Thus the cognitive therapist takes every opportunity while assessing aspects of worry or employing cognitive restructuring to explore the positive or safety aspects of situations. Individuals are encouraged to write down aspects of a worry situation that are positive or safe as a counter to their automatic threat and danger interpretations. The purpose of this intervention is to help individuals develop a more balanced, realistic perspective on the worry. Sometimes there may be one or two primary safety cues associated with the worry, whereas at other times there may be multiple indicators of safety that are evident throughout the worry process.

In our previous example Clare had suffered from chronic worry about cancer. After generating the catastrophic scenario, the cognitive therapist helped Clare think about the possible positive or safety aspects of her cancer worry.

THERAPIST: Clare, you have suggested one possible outcome of the mammogram, that it is positive indicating that you have cancer. What do you think is the probability that the test is positive?

CLARE: I think it is probably 50/50.

THERAPIST: That sounds very high but it sounds like you are saying there is a 50% chance the test will be negative.

CLARE: Well, I suppose, but all I can think about is the 50% chance that it is positive.

THERAPIST: I understand. But what if you are overestimating the chance of a positive test result and underestimating the chance of a negative outcome? What effect will that have?

CLARE: I suppose it will make me feel more anxious and worried.

THERAPIST: That's right. This kind of thinking will increase your worry and yet it's not going to change the outcome of the test. It really is a very unproductive way of thinking. So let's see if we can change it.

CLARE: How can I do that?

THERAPIST: Well, one thing would be to very intentionally train yourself to pay closer attention to the positive or safety aspects of this situation. You could begin by getting some information on the real likelihood that the mammogram result will be positive. You could also survey family and friends to see how many have had negative results or false positive results and never had cancer. You could then practice reminding yourself of this information whenever you start to worry about cancer. I'm not saying this will magically reduce your worries, but gradually over time you will get better at thinking about cancer in a more balanced fashion. You can't change the fact there is always uncertainty about cancer for everyone but you could correct how you think about this uncertainty. Would you like to give this a try?

CLARE: Sure, it sounds like a good idea.

Before leaving the issue of safety cue processing, it must be emphasized that the objective of this intervention is to counter the client's tendency to be overly focused on processing the threatening aspects of situations. The therapist does not try to persuade the client that the worst outcome is unlikely to happen. For example, the therapist can not try to persuade Clare that her mammography results will be negative. Instead Clare is being taught to intentionally process safety cues in order to counter her excessive emphasis on thinking that the test will indicate she has cancer. Obviously safety signal processing can not change the fact that a positive test result is a distinct possibility.

Clinician Guideline 10.22

In cognitive therapy chronic worriers are taught to effortfully process the positive or safety cues of a worry situation to correct their tendency to overlook positive aspects of a worry issue.

Cognitive Restructuring of Metacognitive Beliefs

Another important therapeutic component of cognitive therapy for GAD is the identification and modification of positive and negative metacognitive beliefs about worry. Wells (1997, 2006, 2009) has discussed how cognitive restructuring and behavioral experiments can be used to challenge the GAD client's core beliefs about the dangers and uncontrollability of worry as well as any misconceived beliefs about the potential benefits of worry. The therapist is able to identify the individual's main metacognitive worry beliefs from the worry induction exercise and from cognitive restructuring of biased threat interpretations. Moreover, the Worry about Worry Self-Monitoring Form (Appendix 10.3) can be used to collect additional information on the client's core metacognitive beliefs.

Wells (2006) notes that cognitive restructuring of negative metacognitive beliefs involves questioning the evidence that worry is harmful, questioning how worry could be dangerous, reviewing counterevidence, and learning new information. For example, individuals with GAD often believe that worry is stressful and so could cause physical harm such as a heart attack. Wells (2006) suggests that the client can be provided information that worry is not stressful but instead a coping strategy in response to stress. The client could be assigned a homework task of finding information that worry can directly cause heart attacks. A list of individuals the client knows could be generated with one list for all chronic worriers and the other list of all individuals who suffered a heart attack. How many people appear on both lists? Students who are chronic worriers are often convinced that the worry will cause a significant decline in their academic performance. Again a survey could be conducted to determine how many engaged versus disengaged students are worriers. An alternative explanation is that many factors determine a student's level of academic performance and worry can play a small, even insignificant, part of it. Beliefs about the uncontrollability of worry can be challenged by having clients participate in worry induction exercises, paradoxically increase their level of worry during stressful times, or try to lose complete control of worry (Wells, 2006). The point of these behavioral experiments is to provide evidence that in fact worry is a controlled (i.e., strategic) maladaptive coping strategy and the dangers of losing complete control of worry are more imaginal than real.

Cognitive restructuring of the positive beliefs about worry would follow the same format as described for the negative beliefs. For example, the belief that worries lead to problem solving can be tested by examining how often the individual's excessive worry led to problem resolution. Wells (2006) suggests a mismatch intervention in which the client is asked to compare his catastrophic worry script against a reality-based script. How can worry be adaptive if it is a mismatch with reality? Another behavioral experiment for the individual who believes worry improves his work performance is to ask the client to purposely increase his level of worry prior to leaving for work on certain days and then to monitor the level of improvement in work productivity.

Clinician Guideline 10.23

Cognitive restructuring and behavioral experiments that focus directly on the modification of core positive and negative metacognitive beliefs about worry are an important ingredient of treatment for GAD that is introduced midway through a course of therapy.

Risk and Uncertainty Inoculation

Another component of cognitive therapy for GAD that is related to metacognitive beliefs is targeting the chronic worrier's heightened sensitivity or intolerance of risk and uncertainty. In their cognitive-behavioral treatment program for GAD, Robichaud and Dugas (2006) first educate the client on the role of intolerance of uncertainty in the persistence of pathological worry. They explain that chronic worriers have a strong reaction to even small amounts of uncertainty that causes them to ask "what if" questions. These "what if" questions then trigger a cycle of excessive worry. Robichaud and Dugas note there are only two ways to reduce the role of uncertainty in worry: either reduce uncertainty itself or increase one's tolerance of uncertainty. It is explained to clients that the former option is unrealistic because uncertainty is an inescapable part of life.

In our cognitive therapy approach to worry, changing risk and uncertainty beliefs begins with an explanation of intolerance of uncertainty based on Robichaud and Dugas (2006). Next the therapist collects data on the idiosyncratic uncertainty beliefs associated with the client's primary worry concerns. The Risk and Uncertainty Record Form (Appendix 10.4) can be assigned as homework in order to gather the necessary information. The "what if" questions generated during a worry episode will provide insight into the client's risk aversion and intolerance of uncertainty. The column labeled "Responses to Uncertainty" directly assesses intolerance of uncertainty beliefs and the client's attempts to reduce or avoid uncertainty.

Cognitive restructuring of intolerance of uncertainty beliefs examines evidence that uncertainty can be reduced or eliminated, that living with uncertainty is intolerable, and that one has sufficient control over future events to ensure desired outcomes. Leahy (2005) asks clients to examine the costs and benefits of accepting uncertainty versus striving to eliminate uncertainty associated with worry concerns. The objective of cognitive restructuring is to teach the individual with GAD that uncertainty is a natural part of life and that tolerance of uncertainty is the only option because humans have limited ability to determine future events.

One of the most useful interventions for intolerance of uncertainty involves a form of "uncertainty inoculation" in which clients are exposed to ever increasing amounts of uncertainty in their daily experiences (Robichaud & Dugas, 2006). For example, a student worried that she did not understand what she was reading in her anatomy textbook. Her "what if" questions included "What if I don't understand everything?", "What if I forget what I've studied?", "What if I get mixed up on the facts?", and "What if I become so anxious and confused that I blank out on the final exam?" Her catastrophic outcome was "I'll forget everything and fail the final exam and the course." She believed the uncertainty of the exam outcome was intolerable because it interfered with her ability to study and concentrate. She also believed that the only solution was to reread and repeatedly study the same material over and over again until she was certain she would never forget it. After engaging in a cognitive restructuring exercise in which the therapist challenged the client's belief that she could attain certainty in her knowledge of the subject matter, a series of behavioral exercises were introduced in which the client reduced her checking and rereading responses and worked on tolerating increasing amounts of uncertainty about the anatomy material she had just studied. A target was set for what constituted a reasonable study strategy that was not based on eradicating all sense of uncertainty about the outcome of the final anatomy exam.

A decrease occurred in her level of anxiety and worry, and her mark in anatomy also improved significantly.

Clinician Guideline 10.24

Improving tolerance of risk and uncertainty is an important goal of cognitive therapy of GAD. Cognitive restructuring and systematic exposure to increasing amounts of uncertainty will lead to better acceptance of the uncertainty associated with primary worry concerns.

Constructive Problem-Solving Training

As noted previously, a negative problem orientation, low confidence in problem-solving ability, and dissatisfaction with problem-solving outcome is common in GAD. As a result training in problem solving is included in cognitive-behavioral treatment protocols for GAD (e.g., Craske & Barlow, 2006). Robichaud and Dugas (2006), however, have described the most extensive intervention for poor problem solving in GAD. They first address the clients' negative problem orientation by using cognitive restructuring to modify dysfunctional beliefs involving doubts about one's problem-solving ability, a tendency to view problems as threatening, and pessimism about the outcome of problem solving. The goal is to shift the client's perspective from viewing the problem as a threat to seeing it as an "opportunity" or challenge.

The second part of their intervention involves training in effective use of problem-solving steps; (1) problem definition and goal setting, (2) generation of alternative solutions, (3) decision making, and (4) solution implementation and verification (D'Zurilla & Nezu, 2007). Cognitive intervention for negative problem orientation and poor problem-solving skills may be especially useful when the worry concern is more realistic. For example, the student previously mentioned who worried about failing her anatomy exam had a realistic worry. Her dysfunctional study habits would probably result in poor exam performance. Thus part of her treatment involved training in problem solving to develop a more realistic and practical study routine. This also involved dealing with her doubt and pessimism that any changes would be useless because she held to an erroneous belief that adhering to her unrealistic, rigid study regimen would eventually eliminate her feelings of uncertainty.

Clinician Guideline 10.25

Improvement in negative problem orientation and training in problem-solving ability are included in cognitive therapy of GAD when the primary worry concerns a more realistic negative outcome.

Elaborative Processing of the Present

In the final sessions of cognitive therapy individuals with GAD are encouraged to shift their attention from future-oriented threatening thoughts to being more fully attentive to their thoughts, feelings, and sensations in the present moment. Borkovec et al. (2004)

argue that a *present-moment focus of attention* is an effective antidote to worry. Since anxiety is always anticipatory, there can be no anxiety in the present moment.

Learning to live in the present moment is a challenging task for individuals who are chronically stuck in the threatening, hypothetical (i.e., "what if") future. Borkovec et al. (2004) propose a three-stage approach. First, clients are educated that their negative predictions about the future are usually inaccurate and they practice replacing these predictions with more realistic alternatives. Next, individuals are taught that no prediction can accurately predict the future and individuals are encouraged to live an "expectancy-free life." After clients have become more focused on the present, the final stage involves teaching them how to construct meaning of the present moment. This involves focusing on special features of the moment with particular emphasis on how this connects to the client's values and happiness in the moment. This elaborative processing of the present is similar to more recent developments in mindfulness-based cognitive therapy which emphasize meditative focus on a present activity such as the breath, observing one's negative thoughts in a passive, nonjudgmental manner, and developing acceptance of all thoughts as "just thoughts" and not facts or some aspect of reality (Segal et al., 2002; Williams, Teasdale, Segal, & Kabat-Zinn, 2007). Whether interventions for chronic worry place greater emphasis on cognitive restructuring of worry beliefs and appraisals, or mindfulness-based cognitive therapy, the goal of all treatment should be to redirect the individual with GAD from a preoccupation with controlling hypothetical future threats to a greater focus on and appreciation for one's present experience.

Clinician Guideline 10.26

An important outcome in cognitive therapy of GAD is to redirect the client's preoccupation with possible future-oriented threats to greater appreciation of the present moment in daily living.

Relaxation Training (Optional)

Many cognitive-behavioral programs for GAD still emphasize that training in applied relaxation is an important intervention for GAD (e.g., Borkovec et al., 2004; Craske & Barlow, 2006; Rygh & Sanderson, 2004). However, relaxation training is only used occasionally in cognitive therapy of GAD. It might be offered to individuals who experience unusually intense somatic anxiety or those who find it difficult to focus on their cognitions because of heightened anxiety. In this case a course of applied relaxation might be offered before undertaking direct interventions for pathological worry. Chapter 7 provides a detailed description and implementation for progressive muscle relaxation (see Table 7.5) and the applied relaxation treatment protocol (see Table 7.6). Moreover, there is evidence that applied relaxation is an effective treatment for GAD in its own right (e.g., Arntz, 2003; Borkovec et al., 2002; Öst & Breitholtz, 2000), although there is considerable variability across studies (Fisher, 2006). Also, there is little evidence that relaxation therapy is effective because it reduces muscle tension (Conrad & Roth, 2007). Nevertheless, applied relaxation is a credible treatment option available to the cognitive therapist.

Clinician Guideline 10.27

Muscle relaxation training is a treatment option that may be employed when somatic anxiety is so intense that the individual with GAD is unable to collaborate in cognitive interventions for pathological worry.

EFFICACY OF COGNITIVE THERAPY FOR GAD

The effectiveness of treatment for GAD may be lower than the rates reported for other anxiety disorders. In his review Fisher (2006) concluded that cognitive-behavior therapy that combines applied relaxation and cognitive therapy produces a 50% recovery rate based on the PSWQ and a 60% recovery rate on the State–Trait Anxiety Inventory—Trait Scale. In their meta-analysis of CBT, Gould et al. (2004) found that CBT for GAD produced large effect sizes (i.e., 0.73) but only a few individuals attain a "well status." Likewise Hollon et al. (2006) noted that treatment gains for CBT are significant and maintained over time but "there is a general sense that more can be done with the treatment of GAD" (p. 300).

How effective is cognitive therapy for GAD? Several well-designed outcome studies have addressed this question. In one of the earliest outcome studies conducted on a small GAD sample, group CBT and anxiety management showed more consistent and significant improvement in anxiety compared with a benzodiazepine and wait list control group (Lindsay, Gamsu, McLaughlin, Hood, & Espie, 1987). Durham and Turvey (1987) found that cognitive therapy and behavior therapy produced similar posttreatment improvement in 50–60% of patients, but at 6-month follow-up significantly more individuals from the cognitive therapy condition were improved (62%). In a later study 57 individuals with DSM-III-R GAD were randomly assigned to CBT, behavior therapy (progressive muscle relaxation and graded exposure), or a wait list control (Butler et al., 1991). CBT proved superior to behavior therapy, with 32% of individuals achieving clinically significant change at posttreatment and 58% at 18-month follow-up compared with 5% and 21%, respectively, for the behavior therapy group. Fisher and Durham (1999) reviewed recovery rates based on the State–Trait Anxiety Inventory—Trait Scale change scores in six randomized controlled trials and concluded that individual CBT is one of the most efficacious treatments for chronic worry and GAD, with 6-month follow-up improvement rates of 75% and actual recovery rates of 51%.

These positive outcome results for CBT have also been reported in more recent studies. In a version of cognitive therapy that focused specifically on the cognitive features of worry such as correction of erroneous worry beliefs, modification of intolerance of uncertainty beliefs, and correction of a negative problem orientation, cognitive therapy produced statistically and clinically significant change compared to a wait list condition at posttreatment and 12-month follow-up with 77% of patients no longer meeting criteria for GAD (Ladouceur, Dugas, et al., 2000). This finding was later replicated with a group version of cognitive therapy, with 95% of the cognitive therapy group no longer meeting diagnostic criteria for GAD at 2-year follow-up (Dugas et al., 2003). However, there is evidence that older individuals with GAD do not show as good a response to cognitive therapy or CBT for GAD as younger patients (Covin, Ouimet,

Seeds, & Dozois, 2008; Mohlman, 2004), with approximately 45–54% no longer meeting diagnostic criteria for GAD at posttreatment (Wetherell, Gatz, & Craske, 2003; Stanley et al., 2003).

In a large meta-analysis involving 65 studies Mitte (2005) concluded that CBT was a highly effective treatment for GAD (i.e., average effect size = .82 for anxiety when compared to no treatment controls) as indicated by reductions in both primary anxiety symptoms and depression (see also Covin et al., 2008, for similar conclusion). However, there was no consistent evidence that CBT was significantly more effective than pharmacotherapy, leading the author to conclude that CBT is at least equivalent in effectiveness to pharmacotherapy. However, CBT may be better tolerated and may have more enduring effects at least when compared to the benzodiazepines (Gould, Otto, Pollack, & Yap, 1997; Mitte, 2005).

Unfortunately, very few treatment studies have reported follow-up periods greater than 12 months. The one exception is an 8- to 14-year follow-up conducted on two studies in which cognitive behavior therapy was one of the randomly assigned treatment conditions (Durham, Chambers, MacDonald, Power, & Major, 2003). There was a trend for the CBT groups to be more improved than the non-CBT conditions at posttreatment but the differences were not statistically significant. At long-term follow-up the majority of patients were symptomatic although average symptom severity was still lower than the pretreatment level, indicating maintenance of symptom improvement. However, there were no appreciable differences in recovery rates between the CBT and non-CBT conditions. In a later 2- to 14-year follow-up study involving individuals who participated in one of eight randomized clinical trials of CBT for GAD, PTSD, or panic disorder, the authors concluded that "CBT was associated with a better long-term outcome than non-CBT in terms of overall symptom severity but not with regards to diagnostic status" (Durham et al., 2005, p. iii). Overall, then, we cannot say with any degree of certainty that cognitive therapy or CBT produces more enduring treatment gains in GAD, although some of the findings are somewhat promising.

A number of studies have directly compared cognitive therapy and applied relaxation training. Generally both interventions produce equivalent treatment effects at posttreatment and follow-up, with recovery rates in the 53–67% range (e.g., Arntz, 2003; Borkovec & Costello, 1993; Borkovec et al., 2002; Öst & Breitholtz, 2000). Cognitive therapy is significantly more effective than analytic psychotherapy, with approximately twice as many CBT patients reporting clinically significant improvement at posttreatment and follow-up than the psychodynamic group (Durham et al., 1999; Durham et al., 1994). Moreover, cognitive therapy appears to produce more enduring clinically significant change than anxiety management (e.g., Durham et al., 1999; Durham et al., 1994).

There have been some attempts to determine if certain treatment modifications might improve the effectiveness of CBT for GAD. Fisher (2006) concluded from his updated review of recovery rates that the efficacy of cognitive therapy, CBT, and applied relaxation is highly variable across studies and thus rather limited. However, initial outcome studies of more innovative cognitive therapy approaches that focus on specific cognitive factors in pathological worry such as intolerance of uncertainty and metacognitive beliefs produced better recovery rates than more standard cognitive therapy and CBT approaches. According to Fisher (2006), the combination of cognitive therapy plus applied relaxation may be more effective than either treatment alone. However, individuals with GAD who have a poor prognosis (high disorder complexity and symptom severity) do not benefit significantly from more intense CBT (Durham et al., 2004). Finally, the benefits of CBT for GAD may have broader application than amelioration of chronic worry. In a recent study individuals with GAD randomly assigned to CBT plus gradual medication tapering maintained their discontinuation of benzodiazepines at 12-month follow-up (64.5%) significantly better than individuals (30%) who received nonspecific treatment plus gradual tapering (Gosselin, Ladouceur, Morin, Dugas, & Baillargeon, 2006).

Clinician Guideline 10.28

Cognitive therapy and cognitive-behavioral therapy are effective treatments for GAD that achieve a posttreatment recovery rate of 50–60%. The treatments are highly effective in reducing the pathological worry that characterizes GAD. There is evidence of long-term maintenance of treatment effects, although most individuals will continue to experience some symptoms and even meet diagnostic criteria. Older individuals with GAD may not respond as well to cognitive therapy or CBT and the treatments are at least as effective as pharmacotherapy or applied relaxation training. Overall the effectiveness of cognitive therapy for GAD may be more variable and limited than cognitive therapy for other anxiety disorders.

SUMMARY AND CONCLUSION

GAD has been referred to as the "basic anxiety disorder" (Roemer et al., 2002). Its cardinal feature is excessive, pervasive worry or apprehensive expectation about a number of concerns or situations that occurs more days than not for at least 6 months and is difficult to control (DSM-IV-TR; APA, 2000). Over the years the diagnostic focus in GAD has shifted from an emphasis on anxiety and its symptoms to the cognitive component of anxiety (i.e., worry). An elaborated cognitive model of GAD was presented (see Figure 10.1) in which unwanted automatic intrusive thoughts of uncertain threat about future events or situations activate prepotent generalized threat and vulnerability schemas, resulting in hypervigilance and preferential processing of threat that prime elaborative processes involving a reappraisal of threat and personal vulnerability or helplessness. This sustained reappraisal or worry process becomes a self-perpetuating cycle that intensifies schematic threat activation because of associated maladaptive metacognitive processes. Worry itself becomes viewed as a dangerous and uncontrollable process, with deliberate attempts at worry suppression proving unsuccessful. Moreover, the failure to attain problem resolution or a sense of safety further reinforces the loss of control associated with worry. The process degenerates into a maladaptive cognitive avoidance strategy whose only success is the continued activation of dysfunctional schemas and an information-processing system preferentially biased toward threat.

Empirical support for the cognitive model is mixed. There is considerable evidence that GAD is characterized by (1) worry content related to an individual's personal strivings and current concerns; (2) schemas about general threat, vulnerability, uncertainty, and metacognition; (3) automatic attentional and interpretation biases for threat when processing ambiguous stimuli; (4) negative appraisals of worry control and possible reliance on maladaptive mental control strategies; and (5) negative problem orientation and lack of confidence in problem-solving ability. However, less empirical evidence is available on the role of metaworry and positive worry beliefs, the ability of chronic worriers to actually suppress the worry process in the short term, whether individuals with GAD are overly reliant on ineffective thought control strategies, and whether GAD involves a failed search for a sense of safety. Overall there is a moderate level of empirical support for the proposed cognitive model of GAD but numerous gaps remain for further investigation.

Table 10.5 presents a multicomponent cognitive therapy treatment protocol for GAD that focuses on shifting from reliance on a pathological avoidant coping strategy (i.e., worry) to a more controlled, problem-oriented constructive preparatory coping response to an uncertain future. Cognitive therapy uses cognitive restructuring and behavioral experiments to counter the GAD patient's propensity to exaggerate future threat as well as worry induction and exposure exercises to "decatastrophize" the worry process. A review of the clinical outcome research indicates that 50–60% of cognitive therapy/CBT treatment completers will achieve clinically significant recovery at posttreatment.

Despite the tremendous gains that have been made in our understanding and treatment of GAD, many issues remain unresolved. One of the most fundamental questions concerns whether GAD is truly an anxiety disorder or should be conceptualized more broadly as a distress disorder along with depression. Although we understand much more about the processes that maintain worry, many questions still remain about the propensity to worry despite its futility and anxiety-inducing qualities. For the cognitive model, a number of issues require further investigation such as (1) the role of unwanted intrusive thoughts, (2) whether the information-processing bias is specific to threat or more broadly related to emotional cues, (3) the role of metaworry and positive metacognitive beliefs in pathological worry, and (4) the nature of worry suppression and its effects in GAD. In terms of cognitive therapy little is known about the therapeutic ingredients that are most effective or why cognitive therapy is not more efficacious than behavior therapy or pharmacotherapy, given the cognitive nature of the disorder. Consistent with other anxiety disorders, the long-term effectiveness of cognitive therapy/CBT for GAD still remains largely unknown.

Worry Self-Monitoring Form B

Name: _____   Date: from _____ to: _____

Instructions: Please use this form to record daily occurrences of worry episodes that you experienced during the next week. Try to complete the form as close to the worry episode as possible in order to increase the accuracy of your remarks.

Date and Estimated Time of Day	Anxious Intrusive Thoughts and/ or Initial Worry [Briefly indicate your thoughts when you began to worry]	Worry Content [Briefly describe the focus of your worries; what you were worried about]	Duration of worry [minutes or hours]	Average Distress [0–100]	Outcome [What did you do to control the worry, turn it off? How effective was this?]

Worry Exposure Form

Name: _____   Date: from _____ to: _____

Instructions: This form is to be completed immediately after engaging in a worry exposure homework assignment.

Date and Duration of Session	Worry Topic and Its Catastrophic Outcome [Rate quality of exposure to catastrophic outcome on 0–100 scale]*	Anxiety/ Distress During Session [0–100 scale]	Anxious Thoughts about Worrying [Record any negative thoughts about engaging in the worry exercise]	Countering Anxious Thoughts about Worry [Record how negative thoughts in previous column were countered]	Anxiety/ Distress after Session [0–100]

*Quality of exposure refers to the ability to form a vivid and prolonged image of or thinking about the worst outcome on a scale from 0 (did not imagine/think about catastrophe) to 100 (strong, vivid, and prolonged image or thinking of catastrophe)

Worry about Worry Self-Monitoring Form

Name: _____   Date: from _____ to: _____

Instructions: This form should be completed during episodes of daily worry. Try to complete the form as close to the worry episode as possible in order to increase the accuracy of your remarks.

Date and Duration of Worry	**Primary Worry Concern** [Briefly describe your worries including the worst outcome you are thinking about.]	**Negative Thoughts about the Worry Episode** [What are you thinking is so awful or bad for you about having this worry episode?]	**Positive Thoughts about the Worry Episode** [What are you thinking might be positive or beneficial for you about having this worry episode?]	**Extent of Worry about Worrying** [Rate 0–100]*

Note: Rate extent of worry about worrying associated with present episode from 0 ("not at all worried that I am worrying") to 100 ("extremely worried that I had another worry episode")

Risk and Uncertainty Record Form

Name: _____ Date: from _____ to: _____

Instructions: This form should be completed during episodes of daily worry. Try to complete the form as close to the worry episode as possible in order to increase the accuracy of your remarks.

Date and Duration of Worry	Primary Worry Concern [Briefly describe your worries including the worst outcome you are thinking about.]	Sequence of "What If" Questions [List the "what if" questions that are generated during the worry episode.]	Level of Uncertainty [Rate 0–100]*	Responses to Uncertainty [What makes the uncertainty of this worry concern intolerable? How have you tried to reduce the uncertainty?]

*Note: Rate how much this worry makes you feel uncomfortable and uncertain about the future outcome of this worry concern from 0 ("no feeling of uncertainty") to 100 ("I am feeling extremely tentative, uncertain about the outcome")

From *Cognitive Therapy of Anxiety Disorders: Science and Practice* by David A. Clark and Aaron T. Beck. Copyright 2010 by The Guilford Press. Permission to photocopy this appendix is granted to purchasers of this book for personal use only (see copyright page for details).

Chapter 11

Cognitive Therapy
of Obsessive–Compulsive Disorder

*Once you consent to some concession, you can never cancel it
and put things back the way they are.*
    —HOWARD HUGHES (American entrepreneur, 1905–1976)

Richard was a 47-year-old government office clerk who had suffered for more than 20 years with OCD. He had multiple obsessions involving fear of contaminating others with germs that would make them sick, blasphemous thoughts of cursing God, and concern that others would see a red spot on his lower back that would cause disgust and disapproval. He engaged in compulsive hand-washing and took long showers to ensure he was clean. There was no overt compulsion associated with the religious obsession but he would wear long loose shirts and continually check whether he might be exposing his lower back in response to the "red spot" obsession.

Previously Richard had shown a partial response to a trial of behavior therapy (i.e., exposure and response prevention) for his contamination symptoms. He reluctantly agreed to seek further treatment in response to considerable family pressure. Assessment revealed a moderately severe primary diagnosis of OCD (Clark–Beck Obsessive Compulsive Inventory Total Score = 61) with a secondary social phobia. Richard indicated that his preoccupation with the lower back red spot was now his primary obsession and so this became the target for treatment. Self-monitoring revealed a high daily rate of "red spot" obsessions (average daily rate of over 25 occurrences) that occurred primarily in the work environment. He refused to engage in any exposure assignments even though we started at the lowest end of his fear hierarchy. Thus therapy took a primarily cognitive approach consisting of education into the cognitive therapy model, reappraisal of his biased threat estimation of public exposure of the red spot, and beliefs about the need to control the obsession and reduce his anxiety.

In one of our sessions Richard reported an experience that provides an excellent example of the cognitive basis of OCD. After a number of cognitive therapy sessions, Richard wanted to begin the exposure component of treatment by swimming at a public beach without a shirt. He was planning a vacation with his wife to a resort in Mexico and decided this was a great opportunity to challenge his fear of exposing his lower back. Although the therapist expressed concern that the task was too high on his fear hierarchy, Richard was insistent that he was ready. Upon his return from vacation, Richard admitted that he simply could not be seen in public without a shirt. His anxiety was so intense and his fear of others' negative evaluation so great that he avoided completing the exposure exercise. On the other hand, Richard had an intense fear of roller coasters. While on vacation he decided to prove to himself he could overcome his fear of roller coasters and so forced himself to take three or four rides that resulted in a significant decline in the fear. Interestingly, he had to do this alone because his wife was too frightened to accompany him. Why, then, was Richard able (or willing) to challenge his fear of riding a roller coaster, a common fear that most would consider quite rational, and yet was unable (or unwilling) to face his fear of exposing his lower back, a highly improbable and irrational fear? Clearly Richard's appraisals and beliefs about the dangers of riding a roller coaster were far more rational than his cognitive appraisals of his obsessional concern. His attitude toward the roller coaster (i.e., "I can do this, the worst is so unlikely") led to successful exposure, whereas a dysfunctional attitude (i.e., "I can't risk this, the danger is too great and intolerable") resulted in continued avoidance of exposing his back.

In this chapter cognitive theory and therapy is applied to the problem of OCD. We begin with a brief consideration of definitions, diagnostic criteria, and other descriptive information about the disorder. This is followed by a discussion of the core cognitive features of OCD and a review of the empirical support for the cognitive model of OCD. The third section of the chapter reviews assessment of obsessions and compulsions as well as development of a cognitive case formulation. A description of cognitive therapy for OCD is then discussed, with a review of treatment efficacy and areas of future direction concluding the chapter.

DIAGNOSTIC CONSIDERATIONS

OCD is an anxiety disorder in which the main features are the repeated occurrence of obsessions and/or compulsions of sufficient severity that they are time-consuming (> 1 hour per day) and/or cause marked distress or functional impairment (DSM-IV-TR; APA, 2000). Although diagnostic criteria for OCD can be met by the presence of obsessions or compulsions, the vast majority of individuals with OCD (75–91%) have both obsessions and compulsions (Akhtar et al., 1975; Foa & Kozak, 1995). There is a strong functional relationship between these two phenomena, with obsessions normally associated with a significant elevation in anxiety, distress, or guilt, followed by a compulsion that is intended to reduce or eliminate the anxiety or discomfort caused by the obsession (D. A. Clark, 2004).

Definitions

Obsessions can take the form of repetitive, distressing, and intrusive thoughts, images, or impulses, although obsessive thoughts are by far the most common symptom presentation. Obsessional content can be highly idiosyncratic and shaped by the individual's personal experiences, sociocultural influences, and critical life incidents (for further discussion, see D. A. Clark, 2004; de Silva, 2003; Rachman & Hodgson, 1980). However, certain themes are more common than others, such as:

1. A concern about *dirt or contamination* (e.g., "Did I soil this chair, thereby exposing others to my feces and possible contamination?").
2. *Disease and illness* (e.g., "I can't open this door because the doorknob is covered with germs that could inflict me with a deadly disease.").
3. *Doubts* about security (e.g., "Did I lock the door when I left the office this evening?").
4. *Violence and injury* (e.g., "Did I accidentally run over the pedestrian I just passed while driving?").
5. *Personally repulsive sexual acts* (e.g., "Am I sexually attracted to children?").
6. *Immorality and religion* (e.g., "Did I completely confess all of my sins to God?").
7. *Miscellaneous topics* (i.e., persistent concerns about order, symmetry, exactness, routine, and numbers).

Based on a study of more than 1,000 patients with OCD Rasmussen and Eisen (1992, 1998) reported that fear of contamination (50%) and pathological doubt (42%) were the most common obsessions, whereas symmetry (32%), aggression (31%), sex (24%), and religion (10%) were less common. The following is a working definition of obsessions:

Clinician Guideline 11.1

Obsessions are highly repetitive unwanted and unacceptable thoughts, images, or impulses that are associated with subjective resistance, are difficult to control, and generally produce distress even though the individual may recognize that the thought may be highly exaggerated, irrational, or even senseless to varying degrees (Rachman, 1985).

Compulsions are repetitive, stereotyped overt behaviors or mental acts that are associated with a strong subjective urge to perform even though the individual may desire to resist the response to varying degrees (Taylor, Abramowitz, & McKay, 2007). A compulsion usually involves some overt action such as repeated hand washing or checking, but it can also be a covert or cognitive response like a subvocal rehearsal of certain words, phrases, or a prayer. Overt compulsions, however, like repeated checking (61%), washing/cleaning (50%), or reassurance seeking (34%) are most common, whereas symmetry/precision (28%) and hoarding (18%) are least common (Rasmussen & Eisen, 1998). In the DSM-IV field trial for OCD, Foa and Kozak (1995) found that

80% of the OCD sample reported mental compulsions. Compulsive rituals are usually performed in order to reduce distress (e.g., repeated handwashing reduces anxiety evoked by touching an object perceived as possibly contaminated) or to avert some dreaded outcome (e.g., a person repeatedly checks the stove to ensure the knob is off and the possibility of fire is prevented). Often compulsions are followed in accordance with certain rules such as checking seven times that the light switch is turned off before leaving a room. Compulsions perform a neutralization function that is directed at removing, preventing, or weakening an obsession or its associated distress (Freeston & Ladouceur, 1997a). Even so, compulsions are clearly excessive and often are not even realistically connected to the situation they are intended to neutralize or prevent (APA, 2000). With a strong sense of subjective compulsive and unsuccessful attempts to resist the urge, individuals with OCD usually feel a loss of control over their compulsions. The following definition of compulsions is offered:

Clinician Guideline 11.2

Compulsions are repetitive, intentional but stereotypic behaviors or mental responses that involve a strong subjective urge to perform and a diminished sense of voluntary control that is intended to neutralize the distress or dreaded outcome that characterizes an obsessional concern.

Diagnostic Criteria

Table 11.1 presents DSM-IV-TR (APA, 2000) diagnostic criteria for OCD. The necessary diagnostic criteria are the presence of obsessions or compulsions that are recognized as excessive or unreasonable at some point during the course of the disorder, and are time-consuming, cause marked distress, or significantly interfere with functioning. The impairment criterion is important because many individuals in the general population have obsessive or compulsive symptoms. In fact numerous studies have documented a high frequency of unwanted intrusive thoughts in nonclinical samples that involve content very similar to clinical obsessions (e.g., Parkinson & Rachman, 1981a; Purdon & Clark, 1993; Rachman & de Silva, 1978), with ritualistic behavior also reported in these samples (e.g., Muris, Merckelbach, & Clavan, 1997). Clinical obsessions, however, are more frequent, distressing, strongly resisted, uncontrollable, time-consuming, and impairing than their counterpart in the general population (see D. A. Clark, 2004).

When assessing OCD it is also important to distinguish obsessions from other types of negative cognition. Negative automatic thoughts, worry, and delusions are other types of cognitive pathology that can be confused with obsessional thinking. To determine if a recurring distressing cognition should be classified as an obsession, several characteristics should be present such as (1) experienced as recurring, unwanted mental intrusions; (2) strong efforts to suppress, control, or neutralize the thought; (3) recognition that the thought is a product of one's own mind; (4) heightened sense of personal responsibility; (5) involves ego-dystonic, highly implausible content (i.e., the thought tends to focus on material that is uncharacteristic of the self); and (6) tends to be associated with neutralization efforts (D. A. Clark, 2004).

TABLE 11.1. DSM-IV-TR Diagnostic Criteria for Obsessive–Compulsive Disorder

A. Either obsessions or compulsions.

Obsessions are defined by (1), (2), (3), and (4):
  (1) recurrent and persistent thoughts, impulses, or images that are experienced, at some time
       during the disturbance, as intrusive and inappropriate and that cause marked anxiety or
       distress
  (2) the thoughts, impulses or images are not simply excessive worries about real-life problems
  (3) the person attempts to ignore or suppress such thoughts, impulses, or images, or to neutralize
       them with some other thought or action
  (4) the person recognizes that the obsessional thoughts, impulses, or images are a product of his
       or her own mind (not imposed from without as in thought insertion).

Compulsions are defined by (1) and (2):
  (1) repetitive behaviors (e.g., hand washing, ordering, checking) or mental acts (e.g., praying,
       counting, repeating words silently) that the person feels driven to perform in response to an
       obsession, or according to rules that must be applied rigidly
  (2) the behaviors or mental acts are aimed at preventing or reducing distress or preventing some
       dreaded event or situation; however, these behaviors or mental acts either are not connected
       in a realistic way with what they are designed to neutralize or prevent or are clearly excessive

B. At some point during the course of the disorder, the person has recognized that the obsessions or
    compulsions are excessive or unreasonable. **Note:** This does not apply to children.

C. The obsessions or compulsions cause marked distress, are time consuming (take more than
    1 hour a day), or significantly interfere with the person's normal routine, occupational (or
    academic) functioning, or usual social activities or relationships.

D. If another Axis I disorder is present, the content of the obsessions or compulsions is not
    restricted to it (e.g., preoccupation with food in the presence of an Eating Disorder; hair
    pulling in the presence of Trichotillomania; concern with appearance in the presence of Body
    Dysmorphic Disorder; [etc.]).

E. The disturbance is not due to the direct physiological effects of a substance (e.g., a drug of
    abuse, a medication), or a general medical condition.

Specify if:
       With Poor Insight: if, for most of the time during the current episode, the person does not
       recognize that the obsessions and compulsions are excessive or unreasonable.

Note. From American Psychiatric Association (2000). Copyright 2000 by the American Psychiatric Association.
Reprinted by permission.

OCD Subtypes

OCD is well known as the anxiety disorder with the greatest degree of symptom heterogeneity. Individuals seeking treatment for OCD can present with a broad range of
symptoms in which obsessional content can be quite idiosyncratic to the particular concerns of the individual. This unusual degree of symptom heterogeneity along with varied
treatment response has led researchers to consider whether OCD should be considered
a cluster of symptom subtypes rather than a homogeneous diagnostic entity (McKay et
al., 2004). Could treatment effectiveness for OCD be improved if we developed more
specific and refined interventions that targeted particular types of OCD symptom presentation?

   Most of the research on OCD subtypes has been based on classifying individuals
according to their primary obsessive–compulsive (OC) symptom theme. Earlier studies
that relied on clinical interview and tended to emphasize overt behavioral symptoms

reported that washing/contamination, checking/doubt, order/symmetry, and hoarding were the primary OCD subtypes (Rachman & Hodgson, 1980; Rasmussen & Eisen, 1998). However, in the last few years a series of more rigorous, empirical studies have addressed OCD subtypes through factor analytic and cluster analysis of OCD symptom measures like the Yale–Brown Obsessive–Compulsive Scale (Y-BOCS; Goodman et al., 1989a, 1989b). Although there have been considerable inconsistency across studies, it would appear that the symptom presentation of individuals with OCD can be roughly classified into contamination/washing, harm obsessions/checking, pure obsessions without overt compulsions, and hoarding (e.g., Calamari et al., 2004; see McKay et al., 2004). These classifications may have some limited clinical utility in predicting treatment response, with some evidence that those with predominantly hoarding and pure obsessional symptoms may have a poorer response to standard CBT and pharmacotherapy for OCD (e.g., Abramowitz, Franklin, Schwartz, & Furr, 2003; see D. A. Clark & Guyitt, 2008; Steketee & Frost, 2007). Specialized cognitive-behavioral treatment protocols have been proposed for pure obsessions (Rachman, 2003), fear of contamination (Rachman, 2006), and hoarding (Steketee & Frost, 2007).

Caution must be raised before concluding that different types of OC symptom presentation will require their own unique cognitive treatment protocol. Radomsky and Taylor (2005) raise a number of conceptual and methodological problems with OCD subtype research, not the least being the probability that a dimensional approach to symptoms may be more valid than a categorically based perspective (e.g., Haslam, Williams, Kyrios, McKay, & Taylor, 2005). Furthermore, most individuals with OCD have multiple obsessions and compulsions that cut across categories and the majority of OCD patients will show change in their OC symptoms over the course of the illness (e.g., Skoog & Skoog, 1999). Other researchers have investigated whether OCD samples could be categorized according to cognitive variables such as type of OC-related dysfunctional beliefs. However, the initial studies proved somewhat discouraging, with the most robust finding that individuals simply fall into a high and low belief group (Calamari et al., 2006; Taylor et al., 2006). Given that there is substantial overlap in the treatment strategies utilized in these specialized CBT packages, we believe that a thorough, individualized cognitive case conceptualization is the most efficient clinical strategy for dealing with the idiosyncratic and heterogeneous symptom presentation in OCD.

EPIDEMIOLOGY AND CLINICAL FEATURES

Prevalence

OCD has a lifetime prevalence rate of approximately 1–2% in the general population, with 1-year estimates ranging from 0.7 to 2.1% (Andrews et al., 2001; Kessler, Berglund, et al., 2005; Kessler, Chiu, et al., 2005; Regier et al., 1993; Weissman et al., 1994). Moreover, an even larger number of nonclinical individuals experience milder and less frequent obsessional phenomena that would not meet diagnostic criteria (e.g., Bebbington, 1998; Burns, Formea, Keortge, & Sternberger, 1995; see Rasmussan & Eisen, 1998). Slightly more women than men develop OCD, with age of onset typically between midadolescence to late 20s (Rachman & Hodgson, 1980; Rasmussen & Eisen, 1992; Kessler, Berglund, et al., 2005; Weissman et al., 1994). Men typically have an earlier age of onset than women and so tend to begin treatment at a younger age (e.g.,

Lensi et al., 1996; Rasmussen & Eisen, 1992). Rates of OCD appear to be quite consistent across countries, although cultural differences probably affect rates of symptom presentation in different countries. For example, religious obsessions are more prevalent in cultures with strict religiously based moral codes, and washing/cleaning compulsions may be more prevalent in Muslim countries which emphasize the importance of cleanliness (Okasha, Saad, Khalil, El Dawla, & Yehia, 1994; Tek & Ulug, 2001). Recent studies indicate that OCD is not associated with higher educational attainment or significantly higher intelligence, as was previously concluded from earlier studies (Rasmussen & Eisen, 1992).

Life Events

Onset of OCD can be gradual or an acute response often to a life stressor (see Clark, 2004). Stressful life events, whether related or unrelated to the individual's primary obsessional concern, can lead to disorder onset, while important developmental changes like pregnancy or childbirth are also associated with increased risk for OCD (Abramowitz, Schwartz, Moore, & Luenzmann, 2003; McKeon, Roa, & Mann, 1984). In some cases a traumatic event that is directly relevant to the OCD might trigger an episode through the development of faulty appraisals that are considered responsible for OCD (e.g., a person develops a heightened sense of personal responsibility and subsequent harm and injury obsessions after accidentally causing injury to her child; Rhéaume, Freeston, Léger, & Ladouceur, 1998; Tallis, 1994). In their investigation of traumatic life events in OCD, Cromer et al. (2007) concluded that traumatic events might be a vulnerability factor in OCD by influencing the manifestation of the disorder. However, a critical incident that falls more toward the normal range of life experience can also lead to the onset of OCD (Salkovskis, Shafran, Rachman, & Freeston, 1999). For example, a man with a 10-year history of obsessive fear of HIV infection reported that it began after he had a lap dance at a strip club. Many individuals with OCD, however, can not report any precipitants to the disorder (Rasmussen & Tsuang, 1986).

Personality Correlates

Over the years various studies have examined the personality correlates of OCD. Although early psychodynamic writers considered obsessive–compulsive personality disorder (OCPD) or obsessional personality traits a premorbid condition for OCD, empirical research has cast doubt on this connection (e.g., for discussion of the Freudian concept of the anal character, see Kline, 1968; for discussion of Pierre Janet's concept of the psychasthenic state, see Pitman, 1987). In their review Summerfeldt, Huta, and Swinson (1998) concluded that obsessional personality traits are less frequent in OCD than previously expected, with avoidant personality disorder actually more frequent in OCD samples than OCPD. However, they did conclude that the personality dimensions of harm/avoidance or trait anxiety, certain impulsivity constructs like responsibility and indecisiveness, and self-oriented perfectionism might have particular relevance for OCD.

Research on childhood correlates of adult OCD have produced mixed results. Although children and adolescents with diagnostic OCD most often have a chronic course that persists into adulthood (see Geller, 1998; Shafran, 2003) and a large number of adult OCD patients have their first onset in late childhood or adolescence, most children with obsessional symptoms do not progress to OCD in adulthood (Rachman, Shafran, & Riskind, 2006). Thus presence of obsessional symptoms, at least in childhood, may not play a strong etiological role in OCD. As discussed in the next section, a number of specific cognitive factors have been postulated for elevated vulnerability for OCD.

Course and Consequence

Although it is very difficult to determine the natural course of OCD because of treatment effects, it would appear from various long-term follow-up studies that OCD tends to take a chronic course, with waxing and waning of symptoms over a lifetime, often in response to fluctuations in life stress. In a long-term Swedish study that spanned almost 50 years, Skoog and Skoog (1999) found that only 20% of the sample exhibited complete symptom recovery. Steketee and Barlow (2002) concluded that the majority of patients continue to meet diagnostic criteria for OCD or retain significant obsessional symptoms. In fact OCD may have one of the lowest spontaneous remission rates of the anxiety disorders (Foa & Kozak, 1996). OCD, then, is a chronic unremitting anxiety disorder with early onset and a symptom presentation that waxes and wanes in severity over the course of a lifetime.

Given this characterization, it is not surprising that the disorder has a significant negative impact on occupational and social functioning as well as educational attainment, although the personal cost and suffering of OCD is probably equivalent to that of other anxiety disorders (Antony, Downie, & Swinson, 1998; Karno, Golding, Sorenson, & Burnam, 1988). Nevertheless, OCD can have a significant negative impact on family members, marital functioning, and parent–child relationships. Family members are often implicated in patients' rituals either by accommodating to their demands (i.e., engage in excessive washing and cleaning or provision of reassurance) or totally opposing their obsessional concerns (Calvocoressi et al., 1995; de Silva, 2003). Either coping strategy can lead to an increase in distress and depression for both the OCD sufferer and family members as well as severe disruption of family functioning and relationships (Amir, Freshman, & Foa, 2000; de Silva, 2003). Much of the negative effects of OCD on family life depend on the severity of the illness and the individual's current living arrangements.

Clinician Guideline 11.3

Cognitive assessment and treatment should consider the impact of the OCD on family members and the significant role they may play in maintaining the client's symptomatology.

Comorbidity

Like the other anxiety disorders, OCD has a high rate of diagnostic comorbidity. Half to three-quarters of OCD patients have at least one other current disorder (see Antony, Downie, et al., 1998) and fewer than 15% have a sole diagnosis of OCD over a lifetime (Brown, Campbell, et al., 2001). Major depression is one of the most common comorbid disorders, with a lifetime prevalence rate of 65–85% (Brown, Campbell, et al., 2001; Crino & Andrews, 1996). Presence of depression is associated with a worsening of obsessional symptoms (e.g., significant positive correlation between OCD and depression symptom measures; D. A. Clark, 2002). However it is more likely that a preexisting OCD leads to the subsequent development of major depression than the reverse pathway (Demal, Lenz, Mayrhofer, Zapotoczky, & Zirrerl, 1993). Whereas severe major depression can lead to a poorer treatment response in OCD, presence of mild to moderate depression does not appear to interfere in the patient's response to treatment (e.g., Abramowitz, Franklin, Street, Kozak, & Foa, 2000). Other disorders commonly found in OCD include social phobia, specific phobias, body dysmorphic disorder, tic disorders, and various Cluster C personality disorders (see D. A. Clark, 2004).

Clinician Guideline 11.4

A cognitive evaluation of OCD should assess for the presence and severity of depressive symptoms. If a severe major depressive episode is present, treatment might have to focus on the alleviation of depression before targeting OC symptoms.

Treatment Utilization and Response

Although OCD is associated with a high rate of mental health service utilization second only to panic among the anxiety disorders (Karno et al., 1988; Regier et al., 1993), the majority of individuals with OCD never seek treatment (Pollard, Henderson, Frank, & Margolis, 1989). Even among treatment seekers there is usually a delay of 2–7 years from initial onset to the first treatment session (e.g., Rasmussen & Tsuang, 1986). However, even with the demonstrated effectiveness of CBT, only a minority of sufferers with OCD will actually receive this type of treatment (Pollard, 2007). Approximately 30% of individuals with OCD refuse exposure/response prevention treatment and another 22% fail to complete treatment (Kozak, Liebowitz, & Foa, 2000).

Pollard (2007) has suggested a number of characteristics that might affect an individual's readiness to accept CBT for OCD. Individuals who believe they can deal with their obsessional problems on their own or those who are ashamed or embarrassed by their obsessions may be less likely to seek treatment (e.g., person with obsessional doubts about whether he sexually touched a child may try to conceal such thoughts from others; Newth & Rachman, 2001). In addition a person with low motivation or negative expectations about treatment success may be quite ambivalent about treatment.

A number of other factors have been shown to predict a poorer response to treatment. Certain subtypes of OCD show a more difficult treatment response such as those with compulsive hoarding (Cherian & Frost, 2007) or pure obsessions (D. A. Clark & Guyitt, 2008), and individuals with a severe comorbid major depression tend to have a less favorable response to treatment of OCD symptoms (e.g., Abramowitz & Foa, 2000). Lack of insight into the excessive or irrational nature of one's obsessions (i.e., believing that one's obsessional fears are realistic and somewhat probable and so the compulsive ritual is necessary) may predict poor response to treatment (Franklin, Riggs, & Pai, 2005). In the more extreme case where conviction in the reasonableness of one's obsessional concerns becomes rigid and absolute to the point of being an *overvalued idea* or even a delusion, treatment response may be particularly poor (see Veale, 2007). Finally, noncompliance, failure to complete homework and, to a lesser extent, quality of the therapeutic relationship will have some influence on treatment response (D. A. Clark, 2006a; Franklin et al., 2005).

Clinician Guideline 11.5

Evaluation of treatment readiness and degree of insight into the excessive or irrational nature of the obsessional fear should be included in any assessment of OCD. Ambivalence toward treatment or presence of overvalued ideation should lead to a reconsideration of treatment options.

COGNITIVE MODEL OF OCD

Overview of the Model

According to the cognitive perspective, the presence of dysfunctional schemas and faulty appraisals are critical processes in the etiology and persistence of obsessions and compulsions. A cognitive model of OCD can be understood within the framework of our generic model of anxiety presented in Chapter 2 (see Figure 2.1). Although variations on the cognitive-behavioral model of OCD have been proposed that emphasize different types of schemas and appraisals, they all adhere to certain basic propositions. Figure 11.1 illustrates the common elements of the CBT approach to OCD.

In cognitive appraisal models obsessions are derived from unwanted thoughts, images, or impulses that intrude into the stream of consciousness against one's will and often involve content that is personally unacceptable, distressing, and uncharacteristic of the individual. These thoughts or images often involve the same themes of dirt/contamination, doubt, sex, aggression, injury, or religion that are common in clinical obsessions

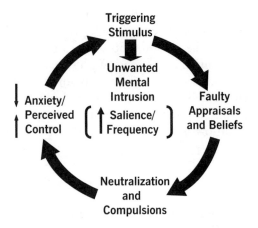

FIGURE 11.1. The cognitive-behavioral appraisal model of obsessive–compulsive disorder. From D. A. Clark (2004, p. 90). Copyright 2004 by The Guilford Press. Reprinted by permission.

(Rachman & de Silva, 1978; Salkovskis & Harrison, 1984; Morillo, Belloch, & Garcia-Soriano, 2007; Purdon & Clark, 1993). However, whether these obsession-relevant intrusive thoughts and images become pathological depends on how the thoughts are appraised (Salkovskis, 1985, 1989; Rachman, 1997, 1998). If an intrusive thought is considered irrelevant, benign, even nonsensical, the person is likely to ignore it. If, on the other hand, the mental intrusion is considered a significant personal threat involving some possible action or outcome that the person could prevent, then some distress will be experienced and the person will feel compelled to engage in responses to relieve the situation. This faulty appraisal of significance will lead to a compulsive ritual or some other type of neutralization strategy that is intended to relieve distress or prevent some dreaded outcome from occurring (Rachman, 1997, 1998). Although neutralization may lead to an immediate reduction in anxiety or distress and a heightened sense of perceived control by diverting attention away from the obsession, in the longer term appraisals of significance and neutralization will lead to an increase in the salience and frequency of the obsession (Salkovskis, 1999). Thus a vicious cycle is established that leads to increasingly more frequent, intense, and distressing obsessions. Figure 11.2 presents four types of clinical obsessions (contact contamination, mental contamination, checking, and pure obsessions) that illustrate the role of faulty appraisals in the persistence of obsessions.

Automatic Processes (Phase I)

The cognitive basis of OCD begins with the occurrence of an unwanted intrusive thought, image, or impulse. O'Connor, Aardema, and Pélissier (2005) note that the intrusion rarely occurs in a vacuum but instead must be understood in a context that might involve a particular mood state, memory, or some current event. Moreover, in their inferential model of OCD, O'Connor and colleagues argue that obsessions are not due to intrusions but instead are a primary inference embedded in a narrative of imagined possibilities (see also O'Connor, 2002; O'Connor & Robillard, 1999). In the current model, an unwanted intrusive thought or image would be the stimulus for the immediate fear response. Particular internal or external cues might provide a context that elicits an unwanted intrusion such as the person with contact contamination who becomes preoccupied with whether he contracted a deadly disease after opening the door to a public washroom, or the person who worries that she may have run over a pedestrian after driving over a bump in the road. With repeated experiences of the intrusive thought, the orienting mode would be primed to automatically detect occurrences of the obsessive intrusive thought. Thus individuals who are prone to OCD are expected to have more frequent unwanted intrusive thoughts and to be more hypervigilant or oriented toward the detection of these intrusions in the stream of consciousness (e.g., Wegner, 1994).

OCD Schemas (Beliefs)

In the last several years considerable progress has been made in characterizing the primary schematic activation in OCD. A number of cognitive themes have been identified that together constitute primal threat mode activation in OCD. Table 11.2 presents

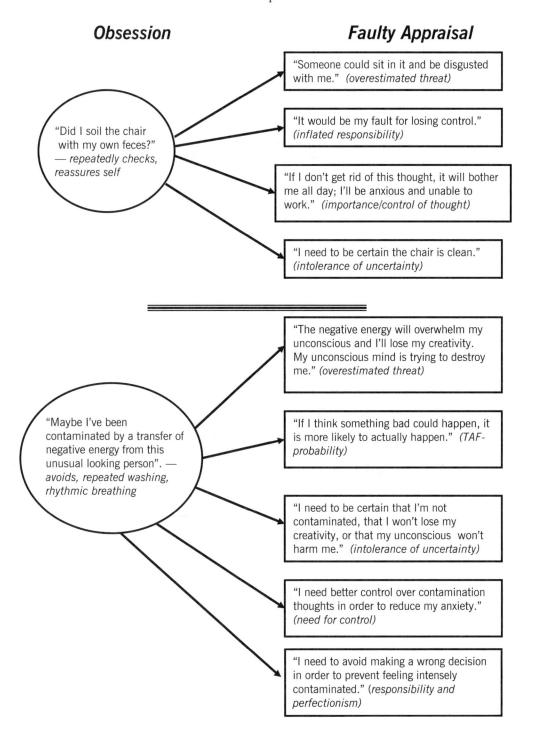

FIGURE 11.2. Clinical illustrations of obsession–faulty appraisal relationship.

(cont.)

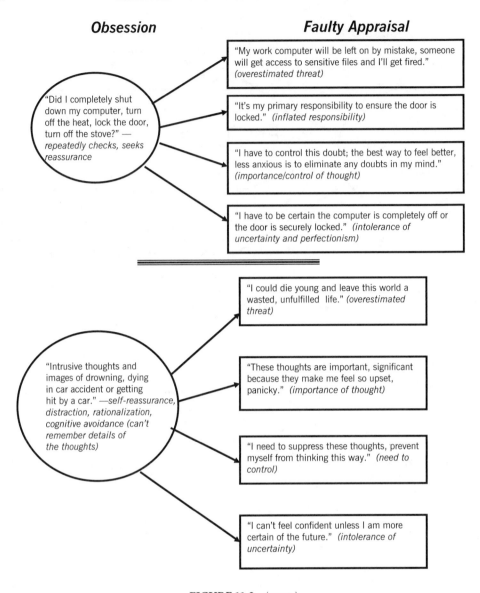

Obsession   **Faulty Appraisal**

"My work computer will be left on by mistake, someone will get access to sensitive files and I'll get fired." *(overestimated threat)*

"It's my primary responsibility to ensure the door is locked." *(inflated responsibility)*

"I have to control this doubt; the best way to feel better, less anxious is to eliminate any doubts in my mind." *(importance/control of thought)*

"I have to be certain the computer is completely off or the door is securely locked." *(intolerance of uncertainty and perfectionism)*

"Did I completely shut down my computer, turn off the heat, lock the door, turn off the stove?" — *repeatedly checks, seeks reassurance*

"I could die young and leave this world a wasted, unfulfilled life." *(overestimated threat)*

"These thoughts are important, significant because they make me feel so upset, panicky." *(importance of thought)*

"I need to suppress these thoughts, prevent myself from thinking this way." *(need to control)*

"I can't feel confident unless I am more certain of the future." *(intolerance of uncertainty)*

"Intrusive thoughts and images of drowning, dying in car accident or getting hit by a car." —*self-reassurance, distraction, rationalization, cognitive avoidance (can't remember details of the thoughts)*

FIGURE 11.2. *(cont.)*

definitions of six belief domains that are thought to characterize the schematic content of OCD.

This schematic organization of OCD was originally proposed by the Obsessive Compulsive Cognitions Working Group (OCCWG) (1997). Although researchers differ on which domains are most critical or specific to the disorder, they do agree that together these beliefs capture the predominant schematic content of OCD. Furthermore, there probably are differences between the OCD subtypes in which of the schema domains is more relevant in conferring maladaptive meaning to the intrusion. In fact schematic differences will be evident even between individuals who have similar obsessional concerns. As discussed below, there is tremendous overlap between these belief

TABLE 11.2. The Six Belief Domains of Obsessive–Compulsive Disorder Proposed by the Obsessive Compulsive Cognitions Working Group

Belief domain	Definition
Inflated responsibility	" ... the belief that one has power which is pivotal to bring about or prevent subjectively crucial negative outcomes" (OCCWG, 1997, p. 677)
Overimportance of thoughts	" ... beliefs that the mere presence of a thought indicates that it is important" (OCCWG, 1997, p. 678)
Overestimation of threat	" ... an exaggeration of the probability or severity of harm" (OCCWG, 1997, p. 678)
Importance of controlling thoughts	" ... the overvaluation of the importance of exerting complete control over intrusive thoughts, images and impulses, and the belief that this is both possible and desirable" (OCCWG, 1997, p. 678)
Intolerance of uncertainty	beliefs about the necessity of being certain, the personal inability to cope with unpredictable change, and difficulty functioning in ambiguous situations
Perfectionism	" ... the tendency to believe there is a perfect solution to every problem, that doing something perfectly (i.e., mistake free) is not only possible but also necessary, and that even minor mistakes will have serious consequences" (OCCWG, 1997, p. 678)

Note. From D.A. Clark (2004, p. 112). Copyright 2004 by The Guilford Press. Reprinted by permission.

domains and there are important individual differences in how strongly persons with OCD will endorse these maladaptive beliefs. Given this heterogeneity even at the schematic level, it is important that a thorough case conceptualization is conducted in order to understand the nature of each patient's schematic activation.

Cognitive Processing Errors

In most cases of OCD maladaptive schema activation involves some belief that the intrusion represents a significant potential harm to self or others that the person is responsible to prevent as indicated by improved control over the obsession and a reduction in anxiety or distress. The activation of these schemas will lead to other automatic processes, the most important being certain cognitive processing errors. O'Connor and his colleagues have argued that the primary cognitive error in OCD is one of *inferential confusion*. An *inference* is "a plausible proposition about a possible state of affairs, itself arrived at by reasoning but which forms the premise for further deductive/inductive reasoning" (O'Connor, Aardema, & Pélissier, 2005, p. 115). The faulty reasoning processes involved in obsessional states leads to the confusion of an imagined possibility (e.g., thinking "Could I have contracted a deadly disease from brushing against this dirty person"?) with actual reality so that the person responds "as if" the obsessional fear was real (O'Connor & Robillard, 1999). O'Connor and colleagues identified a number of inductive reasoning errors that lead to the construction of an idiosyncratic narrative of doubt (i.e., obsessional concern). These include category errors, confusion of comparable events, selective use of out-of-context facts, reliance on purely imaginary sequences, inverse inference, and distrust of normal perception (see D. A. Clark &

O'Connor, 2005; O'Connor, Aardema, & Pélissier, 2005, for further discussion). This faulty inductive reasoning intensifies a state of doubt and confusion which in turn can elevate the threatening nature of the obsessional concern.

Heightened Arousal and Distress

Increased autonomic arousal may play a more prominent role in certain types of OCD such as compulsive cleaning where the obsession has strong phobic elements. Other forms of OCD, such as compulsive checking, may involve different negative emotions like guilt (Rachman & Hodgson, 1980). Thus the extent of physiological hyperarousal associated with schematic fear activation in OCD can vary across individual cases, although autonomic arousal such as elevated heart rate has been well documented when obsessions are provoked (see Rachman & Hodgson, 1980, for review). When heightened physiological arousal is present, the person with OCD is likely to be a motivated to find relief from this negative state like any other individual with an anxiety disorder. Moreover, the most obvious immediate defensive response in OCD is some form of cognitive or behavioral escape/avoidance. Compulsive rituals are a more complex neutralization response that requires considerable elaborative processing and so it is located within the secondary phase of the model. Finally, any automatic thoughts or images that occur during the immediate fear response probably reflect the actual obsessional concerns of the individual.

Secondary Elaborative Processes (Phase II)

Two processes are considered critical to the persistence of OCD at the elaborative phase of anxiety: (1) the appraisal of the obsession and one's ability to cope and (2) the performance of a neutralization response or compulsive ritual in order to reduce anxiety or prevent some anticipated dreaded outcome. The faulty appraisals presented in Figure 11.2 illustrate the evaluations of the obsession that occurs at the secondary phase.

Primary Appraisals of Obsessions

Metacognitive processes, or "thinking about thinking" (Flavell, 1979), are particularly germane to OCD because the appraisal of obsessional thoughts, images, and impulses as well as our ability to control them are key cognitive processes responsible for the persistence of the obsession. Wells and Mathews (1994) presented a metacognitive model of OCD in which beliefs about the significance of intrusive thoughts and a behavioral response to them provide a framework for the etiology and persistence of OCD (see also Wells, 1997, 2000). A number of key metacognitive appraisals have been implicated in the elaboration and persistence of obsessional thinking (see also Table 11.2).

- *Inflated responsibility*—the significance of a thought is evaluated in terms of a perceived personal influence that is pivotal to instigating or preventing a subjectively crucial negative outcome to self or others (Salkovskis, 1999; e.g., "If I think I might have contracted cancer germs, I need to wash myself thoroughly so I don't spread the cancer to others").
- *Thought–action fusion (TAF)*—interpreting the very occurrence of an intrusive

thought as increasing the probability that a dreaded outcome will occur (TAF—Likelihood) or considering a disturbing thought as morally equivalent to a forbidden action (Rachman, 1993; Rachman & Shafran, 1998; e.g., "The more that I have disturbing thoughts of stabbing my children when I use a kitchen knife, the more dangerous I become because I could weaken and actually do it").

- *Threat estimation*—exaggerated estimates of the probability and severity of harm associated with an intrusive thought (Carr, 1974; "I have to check if I left the stove burner on because it could cause a fire").
- *Importance and control*—evaluating the significance of thoughts in terms of their attentional priority and the importance of exerting effective control over the intrusion (Thordarson & Shafran, 2002; Purdon & Clark, 2002; "If I don't get more effective control over these agonizing thoughts of death, I will become overwhelmed with anxiety").
- *Intolerance of uncertainty*—significance of thoughts are evaluated in terms of their deviation from a certain and expected outcome (Sookman & Pinard, 2002; e.g., "If I'm not absolutely certain that I locked the door, this means my obsessive doubt might have some significance").
- *Perfectionism*—evaluating thoughts in terms of an absolute, complete, or perfect criterion (Frost, Novara, & Rhéaume, 2002; e.g., "I need to continue to check this form until I have eliminated any concerns of the possibility of even the slightest error").

According to the cognitive model unwanted intrusive thoughts that are appraised in the above manner will result in an exaggerated evaluation of their personal significance and potential to cause harm or danger to self or others (Rachman, 2003). This metacognitive elaborative faulty appraisal of the intrusion as a personally significant threat is associated with heightened anxiety or distress leading to a sense of urgency to find relief from the distress and neutralize the imagined danger.

Secondary Appraisals of Control

In addition to these primary appraisals of the obsession, D. A. Clark (2004) proposed that obsession-prone individuals also engage in a secondary appraisal of their ability to cope with or control the obsession. Repeated failures to exert effective control over obsessional thinking will also contribute to an increased evaluation of the significance and threatening nature of the obsession as well as a heightened sense of personal vulnerability. Thus both primary appraisals of the obsession and secondary appraisals of one's control efforts are important elaborative processes that contribute to an escalation in the obsessional state.

Neutralization

In OCD cognitive and behavioral responses that seek to reduce distress and neutralize the obsession are an important feature of the elaborative phase that contributes to the persistence of the disorder. Individuals with OCD will engage in a number of neutralization strategies, including compulsive rituals, that are intended to reduce perceived threat and its associated anxiety as well as establish a sense of safety through cessation of the obsession. Neutralization, which often involves covert mental control activities such as reciting a certain phrase to one's self, is mainly directed at undoing or correcting the perceived negative effects of the obsession (Rachman & Shafran, 1998). Even though use of overt and covert compulsive rituals distinguishes individuals with OCD from other anxious and nonanxious comparison groups (Ladouceur, Freeston, et al., 2000), obsession-prone individuals more often use a variety of control strategies in response to their unwanted intrusive thoughts and obsessions including thought stopping, ratio-nalization, distraction, thought replacement, self-punishment, self-reassurance, reassur-ance seeking from others, or more rarely, do nothing (Freeston & Ladouceur, 1997a; Ladouceur, Freeston, et al., 2000; Purdon & Rowa, 2002).

Given the faulty appraisals and beliefs of threat, responsibility, and control that characterize OCD, it is natural that the person with obsessions would turn to compul-sions and other forms of neutralization in a desperate effort to suppress or prevent the obsession, reduce associated distress, absolve one's perceived responsibility, and pre-vent an anticipated negative outcome (Salkovskis, 1989; Salkovskis & Freeston, 2001). Although neutralization efforts may be successful in achieving these aims in the short term, they are nonetheless maladaptive coping strategies that ultimately contribute to an increase in the frequency, salience, and attention given to the obsession (Salkovskis, 1999). The obsessional persons' control efforts are counterproductive because of:

1. *Presence of disconfirmation bias*—a person erroneously believes the neutral-ization was responsible for preventing a feared outcome or for reducing anxi-ety, thus thwarting exposure to any disconfirming evidence (Rachman, 1998, 2003).
2. *Heightened attention*—based on Wegner's (1994) ironic process theory, any deliberate effort to control or suppress an unwanted thought will increase auto-matic attentional search for subsequent reoccurrences of the thought so that the intrusion gains attentional priority.
3. *Elevated personal responsibility*—the temporary success in dealing with the intrusion will elevate its perceived significance and the person's responsibility in preventing the anticipated threat (Salkovskis, 1989).
4. *Excessive control efforts and more ambiguous "stop rules"*—repeated brief suc-cess in terminating the obsessional concern will lead to even more excessive control efforts and increased difficulty knowing when "enough is enough" (e.g., knowing when I have checked enough; Salkovskis & Forrester, 2002).

EMPIRICAL STATUS OF THE COGNITIVE MODEL

The last decade has witnessed an explosion in empirical research investigating various facets of the CBT model of obsessions and compulsions. It is beyond the scope of this chapter to present an extensive review of this burgeoning literature but the interested reader is directed to several extended critical reviews that have been published in recent years (see D. A. Clark, 2004; Frost & Steketee, 2002; Julien, O'Connor, & Aardema, 2007; Rachman et al., 2006; Shafran, 2005; Taylor et al., 2007). Below we examine empirical support for five key hypotheses of the cognitive model.

Hypothesis 1

The unwanted intrusive thoughts, images, or impulses related to the obsessional concerns of individuals with OCD will be more frequent and intense or salient than the unwanted intrusive thoughts with similar obsessive content that occur in individuals without OCD..

Numerous studies have administered either self-report questionnaires or interview checklists and found that the vast majority of nonclinical individuals experience, at least occasionally, unwanted intrusive thoughts, images, or impulses that are similar in content to clinical obsessions (e.g., Freeston, Ladouceur, Thibodeau, & Gagnon, 1991; Parkinson & Rachman, 1981a; Purdon & Clark, 1993; Rachman & de Silva, 1978; for reviews, see Clark & Rhyno, 2005; Julien et al., 2007). This finding has been replicated in countries other than those located in North America such as Korea (Lee & Kwon, 2003), Spain (Belloch, Morillo, Lucero, Cabedo, & Carrió, 2004b), Italy (Clark, Radomsky, Sica, & Simos, 2005), and Turkey (Altin, Clark, & Karanci, 2007).

There is some preliminary evidence that questionnaires may actually underestimate the frequency of obsession-relevant intrusive thoughts in nonclinical samples when more open-ended interviews are employed (D. A. Clark et al., 2005). Although the continuity between nonclinical and clinical intrusive thought content was recently challenged in a content analysis conducted by Rassin and Muris (2006), there is still considerable empirical support for the universality of obsession-relevant intrusive thoughts. As expected, studies that compare individuals with OCD and nonclinical samples have found that nonclinical individuals have significantly less frequent, distressing, unacceptable, and uncontrollable intrusions than their clinical counterparts (e.g., Calamari & Janeck, 1997; Rachman & de Silva, 1978; Morillo et al., 2007). As predicted, the frequency, distress, and uncontrollability of intrusions correlates more highly with measures of OCD symptoms but moderate correlations have also been found with general anxiety, worry, and depression (see reviews by D. A. Clark & Rhyno, 2005; Julien et al., 2007). A recent information-processing experiment involving reaction time in a word recognition task revealed that individuals with OCD showed stronger facilitation (i.e. encoding) and weaker inhibition when processing threat and neutral stimuli (Bannon, Gonsalvez, & Croft, 2008). The authors argued that the combination of strong encoding and weak inhibition might perpetuate obsessionality by making vulnerable individuals more responsive to obsessive-like intrusive thoughts and compulsive behaviors. Overall, then, empirical support for Hypothesis 1 is strong. Even though nonclinical individuals have mental intrusions with similar content to obsessions, those with OCD have more frequent and intense unwanted intrusive thoughts, images, and impulses and they may be cognitively primed to process these internal stimuli more intensely.

Hypothesis 2

Individuals with OCD will have significantly higher endorsement of maladaptive beliefs in personal responsibility, overimportance of thoughts, overestimated threat, need to control thoughts, intolerance of uncertainty, and perfectionism than individuals without OCD.

A number of self-report OCD belief measures have been developed such as (1) the Responsibility Attitudes Scale (RAS) to assess general beliefs about responsibility and the

Responsibility Interpretations Questionnaire (RIQ) to measure responsibility appraisals (Salkovskis et al., 2000); (2) the Thought–Action Fusion Scale (TAF) to assess appraisals and beliefs that distressing thoughts can increase the likelihood of certain negative outcomes (TAF—Likelihood) and that bad thoughts are morally equivalent to bad deeds (TAF—Morality; Shafran, Thordarson, & Rachman, 1996; for copy of scale, see Rachman, 2003); (3) the Meta-Cognitive Beliefs Questionnaire to measure beliefs about the importance and control of intrusive thoughts (D.A. Clark et al., 2003); and (4) the Obsessive Beliefs Questionnaire (OBQ; Obsessive Compulsive Cognitions Working Group [OCCWG], 2003, 2005) which assesses the six belief domains of OCD proposed by this research group (OCCWG, 1997). The OBQ has emerged as the self-report measure with the strongest psychometric properties for the assessment of belief content relevant to OCD. A copy of the OBQ and the Interpretations of Intrusions Inventory can be found in Frost and Steketee (2002).

A number of tentative conclusions can be reached about the beliefs in OCD based on these questionnaire studies. Generally, individuals with OCD endorse the OCCWG beliefs (see Table 11.2), TAF, and responsibility significantly more than nonobsessional anxious and nonclinical comparison groups, and there is a close association between these schematic constructs and OC symptom measures (e.g., Abramowitz, Whiteside, Lynam, & Kalsy, 2003b; Amir, Freshman, Ramsey, Neary, & Brigidi, 2001; OCCWG, 2001, 2003; Sica et al., 2004; Steketee et al., 1998; Tolin et al., 2006). Moreover, cognitive interventions that directly target belief change produce significant decreases in anxiety and other relevant symptoms in OCD patients (e.g., Fisher & Wells, 2005; Rhéaume & Ladouceur, 2000; Wilson & Chambless, 2005).

However, it is apparent that some of the belief domains like TAF—Likelihood and importance/control of thoughts may be more specific to OCD than other beliefs such as threat estimation or inflated responsibility (e.g., Myers & Wells, 2005; Tolin et al., 2006). Most of the belief measures have strong correlations with generalized anxiety, worry, and even depression (e.g., Hazlett-Stevens, Zucker, & Craske, 2002; OCCWG, 2001, 2003) and the distinctiveness of the belief domains has been called into question (OCCWG, 2003, 2005). Furthermore, some of the beliefs may be more relevant for certain OCD subtypes than others (Julien et al., 2006), and there may be a significant number of OCD patients who do not endorse these dysfunctional beliefs (Calamari et al., 2006; Taylor et al., 2006). Inflated responsibility and intolerance of uncertainty beliefs may be more relevant to compulsive checking than to other types of OCD (Foa, Sacks, Tolin, Prezworski, & Amir, 2002; Tolin et al., 2003). Finally, it is apparent that endorsement of OCD-relevant beliefs declines significantly with good response to CBT or exposure and response prevention (ERP) (Emmelkamp, van Oppen, & van Balkom, 2002; O'Connor, Todorov, Robillard, Borgeat, & Brault, 1999; Whittal, Thordarson, & McLean, 2005).

If overestimated threat, inflated responsibility, importance/control of thoughts, perfectionism, intolerance of uncertainty, and TAF schemas are activated in OCD, an information-processing bias should be apparent. In this regard Radomsky and Rachman (1999) found enhanced memory for contaminated (threat) objects in OCD patients, and in a later study Radomsky et al. (2001) determined that this effect was mediated by presence of high perceived responsibility. Muller and Roberts (2005) concluded in their review that several OCD studies have shown selective attentional bias for threat, especially for information relevant to the patients' primary OCD concerns. Overall, then, the questionnaire and information-processing studies support the cognitive theory of schematic threat activation in OCD but the specific characterization of this activation is still a matter of considerable debate.

Hypothesis 3

Individuals with OCD are significantly more likely to engage in exaggerated appraisals that obsession-related mental intrusions represent highly significant personal threats, whereas individuals without OCD are more likely to interpret their intrusions with obsessive-like content as insignificant or benign.

Questionnaires such as the Interpretation of Intrusions Inventory (III; OCCWG, 2001) or the Revised Obsessional Intrusions Inventory (ROII; Purdon & Clark, 1993, 1994a) were developed to assess appraisals of unwanted intrusive thoughts. Ratings of hypothetical scenarios have also been used to assess appraisals relevant to OCD (e.g., Forrester, Wilson, & Salkovskis, 2002; Menzies, Harris, Cumming, & Einstein, 2000). As predicted by the cognitive model, individuals with OCD are more likely to appraise their obsessions in terms of overestimated threat (or distress), personal responsibility, and importance/control (or perceived uncontrollability) compared to nonclinical individuals or when compared to the patient's least upsetting intrusion (Calamari & Janeck, 1997; Morillo et al., 2007; OCCWG, 2001, 2003; Rachman & de Silva, 1978; Rowa et al., 2005).

A number of faulty appraisals such as overestimated threat, inflated responsibility, TAF, and/or importance (or effort) of control have a significant association with frequency of obsessive intrusive thoughts, anxiety or distress, and/or elevated level of OC symptoms (e.g., Belloch, Morillo, Lucero, et al., 2004; Clark, Purdon, & Byers, 2000; Freeston et al., 1991; Menzies et al., 2000; Purdon & Clark, 1994b; Rowa & Purdon, 2003). However, Lee and Kwon (2003) found that importance and control appraisals were more relevant to intrusions that were autogenous in nature (spontaneous occurrence with no identifiable trigger), whereas responsibility appraisals were more relevant for reactive intrusions (those evoked by an external stimulus). Forrester et al. (2002) found that provision of a harm thought intrusion in OC-relevant hypothetical scenarios significantly increased rated anxiety and distress as well as responsibility and TAF—Likelihood appraisals in nonclinical and OCD samples. A greater tendency to reflect on one's cognitive processes, called *cognitive self-consciousness*, characterizes OCD and may be a metacognitive process that contributes to an increased tendency to negatively appraise intrusive thoughts in obsessional states (Cohen & Calamari, 2004; Janeck, Calamari, Riemann, & Heffelfinger, 2003). Overall these studies support the third hypothesis, which posits a close association between how an intrusive thought is appraised (i.e., the meaning of the intrusion) and a person's subjective experience of the unwanted thought.

In order to validate the cognitive model, it is important to demonstrate cause-and-effect relations between faulty appraisals and various parameters of unwanted intrusive thoughts or obsessions. A number of experimental studies have shown that the manipulation of responsibility or TAF causes the predicted increase in frequency and distress of intrusions or other forms of negative thought as well as a greater tendency to engage in neutralization such as checking. For example, individuals randomly assigned to a

high responsibility condition experience more anxiety, greater perceived negative consequences, increased doubt, and more checking behavior or urge to neutralize than those
in a low responsibility condition (Bouchard, Rhéaume, & Ladouceur, 1999; Ladouceur
et al., 1995; Mancini, D'Olimpio, & Cieri, 2004; Shafran, 1997). However, weaker
effects have also been reported, with the main difference attributed to a decrease in
responsibility (Lopatka & Rachman, 1995). In an experiment involving bogus EEG
feedback, nonclinical individuals randomly assigned to a high TAF—Likelihood condition reported more intrusions, discomfort, and resistance than participants in a control
condition (Rassin et al., 1999). Although these results are consistent with the cognitive
view that faulty appraisals may contribute to the transformation of a normal intrusion
into an obsession, there are limitations to this research. There have been inconsistencies
across the studies, most of the focus has been on inflated responsibility to the exclusion
of other appraisal domains, and most fail to control for general distress, which could
account for the observed effects (Julien et al., 2007).

Hypothesis 4

*Individuals with OCD are significantly more likely to engage in neutralization and other
mental control strategies in response to obsession-relevant mental intrusions and this will
increase the frequency and distress of the obsession.*

According to the cognitive model, attempts to neutralize or otherwise control the
occurrence and distress of obsessional intrusions contribute to the persistence of obsessional thinking. Individuals with OCD are more likely to engage in more compulsive
rituals, neutralization, and maladaptive thought control strategies in response to obsessional intrusions than nonclinical individuals but with less perceived effectiveness (Amir,
Cashman, & Foa, 1997; Freeston & Ladouceur, 1997a; Morillo et al., 2007; Rachman
& de Silva, 1978; Wroe, Salkovskis, & Richards, 2000). However, reliance on such
ineffective response strategies can be reduced with treatment (Abramowitz, Whiteside,
Kalsy, & Tolin, 2003a). The negative effects of neutralization were demonstrated in
a 3-day diary study in which individuals with OCD were found to engage in a high
frequency of suppression and neutralization of their obsession and these efforts were
associated with increased discomfort, limited perceived success, and faulty appraisals of
thought control, importance, and responsibility (Purdon, Rowa, & Antony, 2007).

Studies involving the experimental manipulation of neutralization indicate that it
has the same functional characteristics as overt compulsions, as made evident by an
immediate decrease in anxiety and perceived threat but a longer term increase in distress
and urge to neutralize (Rachman, Shafran, Mitchell, Trant, & Teachman, 1996; Salkovskis, Thorpe, Wahl, Wroe, & Forrester, 2003; Salkovskis, Westbrook, Davis, Jeavons,
& Gledhill, 1997). Furthermore, correlational studies indicate that certain maladaptive
thought control strategies like self-punishment and worry may have a particularly close
relationship with OC-relevant appraisals and beliefs as well as OCD symptoms (Larsen
et al., 2006; Moore & Abramowitz, 2007).

Thought suppression experiments indicate that individuals with OCD may not be
as effective in using intentional suppression to prevent the occurrence of unwanted mental intrusions when compared to nonclinical individuals (Janeck & Calamari, 1999;
Tolin, Abramowitz, Przeworski, et al., 2002). However the studies are inconsistent

on the negative consequences of suppression. Some studies failed to find any evidence of immediate enhancement or rebound when OCD samples suppressed their primary obsession (Janeck & Calamari, 1999; Purdon et al., 2005), whereas Tolin, Abramowitz, Przeworski, et al. (2002) found an immediate enhancement effect when individuals with OCD suppressed a neutral thought (i.e., white bears). Based on this finding the authors suggest that OCD might be characterized by a general inhibitory deficit.

Suppression of unwanted obsessional intrusions in nonclinical samples has also failed to produce the expected enhancement or resurgence of unwanted thoughts once suppression efforts cease, although suppression may result in more sustained levels of unwanted target thought occurrence in the postsuppression period (Belloch, Morillo, & Giménez, 2004; Hardy & Brewin, 2005; Purdon, 2001; Purdon & Clark, 2001). In addition failure to completely suppress unwanted target intrusions may have direct or indirect effects on level of distress associated with recurrence of the unwanted mental intrusion (Janeck & Calamari, 1999; Purdon & Clark, 2001; Purdon et al., 2005). Whatever the exact processes involved, the overall findings from the self-report, daily diary, and experimental studies are consistent with Hypothesis 4 that neutralization plays an important role in the persistence of obsessional symptoms with particular effects on the amplification of distress and the misinterpretation of intrusions.

Hypothesis 5

Individuals with OCD are significantly more likely to misinterpret their failure to control obsessional intrusions as a highly significant threat, whereas individuals without OCD are more accepting of failed mental control.

Recent experimental research on the suppression of unwanted intrusive thoughts in both clinical and nonclinical samples indicates that exaggerated misinterpretation of the significance of failed control might be an important contributor to the pathogenesis of obsessions. In a reanalysis of their thought suppression experiment, Tolin and colleagues found that individuals with OCD reported more internal attributions for their thought suppression failures than did nonanxious controls (Tolin, Abramowitz, Hamlin, et al., 2002b). Purdon et al. (2005) also found that misinterpretation of thought failures in a thought suppression experiment was the most important predictor of distress over intrusions and negative mood state. In an earlier nonclinical thought suppression experiment, exaggerated appraisals of the significance of thought control failures was associated with a more negative mood state (Purdon, 2001). Furthermore, individuals who reported a higher need for control exhibited greater thought suppression effort in the experiment. Magee and Teachman (2007) also found that maladaptive attributions of self-blame and importance in controlling thoughts predicted distress and recurrence of unwanted thoughts in a thought suppression experiment. In a recent thought dismissal experiment comparing OCD and panic disorder patients, the OCD group had greater difficulty dismissing their primary obsession than did panic patients their primary panic-related anxious thought (Purdon, Gifford, & Antony, 2007). Moreover, the OCD group interpreted their failures in thought control more negatively than the panic disorder group, but negative appraisals of failed thought control predicted greater difficulty dismissing the target thought and more negative mood state in both groups. The authors concluded that deliberate attempts to suppress unwanted thoughts is ill-advised because failure to control will be appraised negatively and this can lead to further reductions in mental control and increased negative mood. Together these findings are consistent with Hypothesis 5 that faulty appraisals of failed mental control contribute to increased salience of the obsession for individuals with OCD.

Cognitive Vulnerability to OCD

Theory and research on cognitive vulnerability for OCD has lagged far behind development of the descriptive model and cognitive treatment for obsessions and compulsions. A number of possible vulnerability pathways have been described (see Rachman et al., 2006, for discussion). Salkovskis and colleagues argued that inflated responsibility beliefs might constitute an enduring vulnerability for the etiology of obsessions (Salkovskis, Shafran, et al., 1999). They speculated that five different developmental learning pathways could result in the adoption of general inflated responsibility assumptions. A critical incident involving real or perceived blame (i.e., personal responsibility) for causing harm could interact with prior developmental learning history to intensify an inflated sense of personal responsibility. A preexisting generalized sense of inflated responsibility might lead to misinterpretations of certain intrusive thoughts, especially if they are associated with a critical incident of perceived harm (see Shafran, 2005).

Other cognitive constructs have been proposed as possible vulnerability factors in OCD. Rachman (2003) argued that TAF beliefs or proneness to interpret one's value-laden thoughts as highly significant may increase vulnerability to obsessions. High cognitive self-consciousness has also been promoted as a possible cognitive vulnerability for obsessions (Janeck et al., 2003) and the six belief domains proposed by the OCCWG are considered enduring constructs that might predispose to OCD (OCCWG, 1997). Sookman, Pinard, and Beck (2001) described a cognitive vulnerability model of OCD that consisted of enduring beliefs about personal vulnerability, unpredictability, strong affect, and need for control. In his cognitive control model of obsessions, D. A. Clark (2004) suggested that high trait negative affectivity, an ambivalent self-evaluation, and preexisting metacognitive beliefs about the importance and control of thoughts might constitute a vulnerability for obsessions. Finally, Doron and Kyrios (2005) have proposed a most interesting perspective in which vulnerability to OCD is viewed in terms of cognitive-affective structures involving an internal representation of the self that is limited to a few "sensitive" self-domains as well as a representation of the world as dangerous but controllable. Thought intrusions representing failures in these highly valued or sensitive domains of the self (e.g., morality, worthiness, acceptance by others) will be interpreted as highly significant because they involve a threat to the individual's self-worth. The authors trace the origins of these cognitive-affective representations of self and world to certain developmental and early attachment experiences. Doron and Kyrios noted connections between their conceptualization and Bhar and Kyrios's (2000) view that an ambivalent sense of self (i.e., degree of uncertainty about one's self-worth) may be a vulnerability factor in OCD.

Until very recently there was practically no prospective research on cognitive factors in OCD and so the empirical support for cognitive vulnerability was nonexistent. Fortunately, a few studies have begun to appear that address this critical gap in the cognitive literature on OCD. In a 3-month prospective study of 85 new fathers and mothers OC-relevant beliefs as assessed at Time 1 (i.e., prenatal) was a significant predictor of postpartum subclinical OCD but not depressive or anxious symptomatology. Moreover, the majority of parents reported distressing intrusive thoughts of harm to their infant and utilized a variety of neutralization strategies in response to the intrusions (Abramowitz et al., 2006). In a 6-week prospective study involving 377 undergraduates, Coles and Horng (2006) found that Time 1 Obsessive Beliefs Questionnaire (OBQ) and number of negative life events independently predicted Time 2 OCD symptoms as determined by the Obsessive Compulsive Inventory Total Score. However, there was only weak support for these results in a more recent study involving a 6-month follow-up of an undergraduate sample and no evidence of a diathesis–stress interaction between OC beliefs and negative life events (Coles et al., 2008).

Although no prospective studies have yet investigated whether certain self-structure concepts may constitute an enduring vulnerability to OCD, there are some relevant findings that bear on this issue. Bhar and Kyrios (2007) found that self-worth ambivalence (i.e., uncertainty about the self) was significantly associated with self-reported OC symptoms and control, importance, and responsibility beliefs. However, both the OCD and the nonobsessional anxious groups scored significantly higher on self-worth ambivalence than the student control group. In a different study based exclusively on a nonclinical sample Doron, Kyrios, and Moulding (2007) reported that self-worth sensitivity in either the morality or job-competence domains was related to higher levels of OC symptoms. Two studies found that both nonclinical and OCD individuals rated their most upsetting intrusive thought as more meaningful and contradicted important and valued aspects of the self to a greater extent than less upsetting thoughts (Rowa & Purdon, 2003; Rowa et al., 2005). Given their appraised significance for self-concerns, it is little wonder that these upsetting intrusions were associated with appraisals of control and importance of thought. Likewise Ferrier and Brewin (2005) found that individuals with OCD generated more negative self-inferences from their intrusive thoughts than a nonobsessional anxious group and their "feared self" contained more immoral and bad trait attributes. Although only suggestive at this time, these studies indicate that self-worth concerns may play an important role in how individuals evaluate the meaning of intrusive thoughts and so might be a fruitful avenue to explore for vulnerability to OCD.

COGNITIVE ASSESSMENT AND CASE FORMULATION

Diagnostic and Symptom Measures

The SCID-IV (First et al., 1997) or the ADIS-IV (Brown, Di Nardo, & Barlow, 1994) can be used for diagnostic assessment of OCD. The ADIS-IV is more highly recommended because the lifetime version has excellent interrater reliability for OCD (kappa = .85; Brown, Di Nardo, et al., 2001) and it provides a more complete symptom assessment by inquiring into the specific content of obsessions and compulsions, their severity, degree of insight, resistance, and avoidance patterns. The drawback to the ADIS-IV is the length of interview time (2–4 hours) often required for OCD patients to complete the interview (Taylor, 1998; Summerfeldt & Antony, 2002).

Yale–Brown Obsessive–Compulsive Scale

The Yale–Brown Obsessive–Compulsive Scale (YBOCS) is a 10-item semistructured interview rating scale that assesses the severity of obsessions and compulsions independent of the type (content) or number of symptoms (Goodman et al., 1989a, 1989b). It is widely used to assess the effectiveness of pharmacological and behavioral treatments for OCD and has become the "gold standard" for assessment of OC symptom severity in outcome studies. After indicating his past and current obsessions and compulsions on a 64-item checklist, the patient is questioned by the interviewer on five aspects of symptom expression, using a Likert scale to record the severity of each symptom feature. A separate obsessions (sum of items 1–5) and compulsions (sum of items 6–10) severity score is generated based on the same five features of the target symptoms (1) duration/frequency, (2) interference in social or work functioning, (3) associated distress, (4) degree of resistance, and (5) perceived uncontrollability of the obsession or compulsion. A total severity score is most commonly reported by summing over the 10 items.

A number of studies have investigated the psychometric properties of the YBOCS and various reviews of this literature have been published (see D. A. Clark, 2004; Feske & Chambless, 2000; Grabill et al., 2008; St. Clare, 2003; Taylor, 1995b, 1998). The YBOCS Total Score has excellent interrater reliability, good internal consistency, and temporal reliability. It generally has good convergent validity with other OCD symptom measures but discriminant validity is lower given its moderate correlation with anxiety and depression measures. Individuals with OCD score significantly higher on the YBOCS Total Score than nonobsessional patients and nonclinical comparison groups. A cutoff score of 16 on the YBOCS Total Score yields good sensitivity but low specificity (Steketee, Frost, & Bogart, 1996; see also Baer, 2000) and posttreatment scores typically fall by 40–50% in responders (e.g., Abramowitz, Franklin, et al., 2003; Goodman et al., 1989b). A self-report version of the YBOCS is available that correlates highly with the interview format, although Grabill et al. (2007) warned that it may overidentify OCD due to poor specificity (see Baer, 2000, for copy). However, some weaknesses are apparent such as poor validity for the resistance and control items, lack of factorial support for separate Obsessions and Compulsions severity subscales, and omission of an avoidance rating in the standard severity score (Amir, Foa, & Coles, 1997; Deacon & Abramowitz, 2005; Woody, Steketee, & Chambless, 1995). A copy of the YBOCS has been reprinted in Antony (2001b).

Clark–Beck Obsessive Compulsive Inventory

The Clark–Beck Obsessive Compulsive Inventory (CBOCI) is a 25-item self-report questionnaire consisting of 14 items that assess diagnostic and content features of obsessions and 11 items that assess compulsions (D. A. Clark & Beck, 2002; D. A. Clark, Antony, Beck, Swinson, & Steer, 2005). It was developed as a screener for OCD with a structure and response format identical to the BDI-II. The CBOCI items are scored from 0 to 3, with each item consisting of four response option statements. The measure was designed to cover the DSM-IV diagnostic criteria for OCD as well as a number of additional cognitive symptoms. Obsession and Compulsion subscales can be derived as well as a Total Score.

Given the recent development of the CBOCI, investigations into its psychometric properties are limited. The original validation study revealed that the Obsessions, Compulsions, and Total Score have high internal reliability, factorial validity, and moderate to strong convergence with other OCD symptom measures like the YBOCS (D.A. Clark, Antony, et al., 2005). Moreover, criterion validity is strong, with OCD patients scoring significantly higher on all three scales than nonobsessional anxious, depressed, and nonclinical comparison groups.[1] Like all OCD symptom measures, the CBOCI has lower discriminant validity as indicated by its moderate correlations with anxiety and depression measures. The treatment sensitivity of the measure has not yet been investigated and its test–retest reliability has not been determined in an OCD sample. Analysis based on the validation sample indicated that a cutoff score of 22 on the CBOCI Total Score yielded high sensitivity (90%) and specificity (78%) for distinguishing OCD from student controls (D. A. Clark, 2006b). The CBOCI and manual are available from Pearson Assessment at *pearsonassess.com*.

Other OCD Symptom Measures

Three other OCD symptom measures are frequently employed to assess the frequency and severity of obsessive and compulsive symptoms. The 42-item Obsessive–Compulsive Inventory (OCI) was developed by Foa and colleagues to assess the frequency and distress of seven symptom domains of OCD (Foa, Kozak, Salkovskis, Coles, & Amir, 1998). The measure consists of separate frequency and distress scales for washing, checking, doubting, ordering, obsessing, hoarding, and mental neutralizing. Psychometric evidence for the instrument is strong, although the discriminate validity of the hoarding subscale is questionable (Foa et al., 1998). A revised brief version of the OCI was developed that consists of 18 items comprised of six distress scales: washing, checking, ordering, obsessing, hoarding, and neutralizing (Foa, Huppert, et al., 2002). The new OCI-R subscales were highly correlated with the old OCI subscales (r_s = .92) and had sound psychometric characteristics. Two recent clinical studies confirmed a six-factor structure that corresponded to the OCI-R subscales, good convergent validity with other OCD measures (although correlations with the YBOCS are rather weak), more modest discriminant validity (i.e., moderate association with anxiety and depression measures), and consistent ability to discriminant OCD from nonobsessional anxious groups (Abramowitz & Deacon, 2006; Huppert et al., 2007; see similar findings for nonclinical samples reported by Hajcak, Huppert, Simmons, & Foa, 2004). Abramowitz and Deacon (2006) found that the OCI-R obsessions and checking subscales, in particular, had modest relations with OC cognition measures and that an OCI-R Total cutoff score of 14 provided the best differentiation of OCD from other anxiety disorders. A significant limitation of the OCI-R is its underrepresentation of obsessions (only three items) and disproportionate weight toward compulsive symptoms (Grabill et al., 2008). The OCI-R is published as an appendix to Foa et al. (2002).

The Padua Inventory (PI) is a 60-item questionnaire originally developed on an Italian sample to assess the distress associated with common obsessive and compulsive phe-

---

[1] Gabrill et al. (2008) arrived at an erroneous conclusion about the instrument's criterion-related validity based on a misreading of the significant group differences reported in the validation study.

nomena using 5-point Likert scales (Sanavio, 1988). Although possessing good psycho-metric characteristics, a 41-item version of the instrument was developed by van Oppen, Hoekstra, and Emmelkamp (1995) and a 39-item version was developed by research-ers at Washington State University (Burns, Keortge, Formea, & Sternberger, 1996) in order to eliminate items that may have contributed to the high correlation between the PI and measures of worry (Freeston, Ladouceur et al., 1994). The Padua Inventory—Washington State University Revision (PI-WSUR) is the most widely used version of the PI consisting of five rationally determined subscales; (1) obsessional thoughts of harm to self/others (seven items), (2) obsessional impulses to harm self/others (nine items), (3) contamination obsessions and washing compulsions (10 items), (4) checking compulsions (10 items), and (5) dressing/grooming compulsions (three items). The PI-WSUR appears to have improved psychometric properties over the original PI and so it has gained in popularity with OCD researchers (see reviews by Antony, 2001b; Grabill et al., 2008; St. Clare, 2003). However, questions have been raised about the content validity of the measure with some symptoms of OCD not assessed and other items more ambiguous or representing phenomena that may not be germane to OCD. The original PI can be found in Sanavio (1988) whereas the PI-WSUR has been reproduced by Antony (2001b).

The Vancouver Obsessional Compulsive Inventory (VOCI; Thordarson et al., 2004) is a 55-item questionnaire that is the culmination of extensive item development and revision of the Maudsley Obsessive Compulsive Inventory originally developed in the 1970s by Hodgson and Rachman (1977). The VOCI consists of six factorially deter-mined subscales: (1) contamination (12 items), (2) checking (six items), (3) obsessions (12 items), (4) hoarding (seven items), (5) just right (12 items), and (6) indecisiveness (six items). The initial psychometric characteristics of the VOCI are strong as indicated by high convergent validity with other OCD self-report measures, significantly higher scores of OCD samples than nonobsessional anxious or depressed and nonclinical con-trols, and moderate discriminant validity. As the most comprehensive OCD symptom measure with particular relevance to current cognitive-behavioral approaches to OCD, the VOCI is a promising measure. However, more research is needed on its psychomet-ric properties and concerns were raised with the lower criterion validity of the Obses-sions and Hoarding subscales (Thordarson et al, 2004).

Clinician Guideline 11.6

We recommend that the interview version of the YBOCS and the CBOCI be administered as part of the pretreatment assessment to obtain a clinician-based and a self-report evalua-tion of OCD symptom content and severity. The VOCI can also be utilized to obtain a more comprehensive assessment of OC symptom presentation.

Case Conceptualization

In order to formulate an individual case conceptualization of OCD ideographic, process-oriented diaries and ratings forms are needed to determine the individual's spe-cific appraisal and neutralization responses to obsessions. A detailed description of a cognitive case formulation approach to OCD can be found in D. A. Clark (2004) along with numerous clinical record forms and rating scales. Table 11.3 presents a summary

TABLE 11.3. Summary of Idiographic Process-Oriented Assessment of Obsessions and Compulsions

Characteristics of obsessions	Characteristics of compulsions
• List of situations or cues that trigger the obsession • Daily frequency of primary obsession • Type and intensity of emotion associated with obsession • Perceived threat or negative consequences due to obsession • Control effort and its perceived success • Other primary appraisals of obsession • Perceived consequences of failed control of obsession	• Hierarchy of anxious or avoided situations related to obsessions or compulsions • Daily frequency of primary compulsion • Urge to engage in compulsion • Extent and perceived success of resistance to compulsion • Identification of other types of neutralization and control strategies utilized • Level of insight into the excessive or irrational nature of obsessions and compulsions

of the main cognitive and behavioral characteristics of obsessions and compulsions that should be assessed in a cognitive case formulation.

Process-Oriented Assessment of Obsessions

After determining the client's primary obsession from the diagnostic interview and symptom assessment, the therapist obtains a detailed individualized assessment of various features of the obsession and its appraisal that will provide direction for therapy. For clients who have more than one main obsession, the client and therapist should collaboratively select one obsession that will be the initial focus of treatment. The therapist questions the client on all the situations or cues that can trigger the obsession. A list of situations is compiled that includes both frequent (i.e., daily) and less frequent triggers of the obsession. The main focus will be on external situations but it could also include internal cues like certain bodily sensations, emotions, or other thoughts that trigger the obsession. A complete situational analysis should include the average distress associated with each situation or cue, likelihood that the situation will trigger the obsessions, and degree of avoidance associated with the situation. If clients have difficulty reporting on eliciting situations, a situation self-monitoring form can be assigned as homework (for copy of Situational Record Form, see D. A. Clark, 2004).

It is also critical to assign an obsession self-monitoring form as homework in order to collect pretreatment baseline data on frequency, level of distress, effort to control, and urge to engage in neutralization. This information will be useful in estimating the probable length of treatment and for determining the success of the intervention. A copy of a Daily Record of Primary Obsession can be found in Appendix 11.1.

The therapist also determines the type and intensity of emotion associated with the obsession. Although anxiety is the most common emotion associated with obsessions, other emotions like guilt, frustration, shame, and anger can also be present. The therapist also explores with the client the perceived threat or anticipated negative consequences associated with the obsession. For example, a client who compulsively checked that the clothes dryer door was shut was afraid her cat might get locked inside and suffocate. In addition to a few primary threats, clients are often concerned that the obsession will result in overwhelming anxiety or an inability to function at work or school. All threats or negative consequences associated with the obsession should be listed along with ratings of distress associated with the expected consequence, its likelihood of occurrence, and the rated importance of preventing the outcome (see D. A. Clark, 2004, for record form). The cognitive therapist should also assess the level of effort directed at preventing or suppressing the obsessional intrusion as well as the client's perceived success at controlling the obsession. The role played by other primary appraisals in the persistence of the obsession should be determined such as perceived responsibility, TAF, intolerance of uncertainty, perfectionism, importance of the thought, its significance or personal meaning, and need to control the thought. Furthermore, the client's appraisal of his failure to control the obsessions should be assessed to determine the role of secondary appraisals in the pathogenesis of the obsession. It is unlikely that all information can be obtained in the initial assessment session but as treatment progresses a more complete picture of the cognitive basis of the obsession will emerge. Although some of the standardized OCD cognition questionnaires such as the OBQ, III, TAF Scale, or RAS might be useful at this stage, no doubt the most helpful approach is a well-informed interview and self-monitoring records that are assigned as homework (for examples of appraisal recording forms, see D. A. Clark, 2004; Purdon & Clark, 2005; Wilhem & Steketee, 2006).

Process-Oriented Assessment of Compulsions

Table 11.3 also presents various characteristics of compulsions and other forms of neutralization that should be included in a cognitive assessment. As in behavioral treatment of OCD, the development of a hierarchy of anxious situations that are avoided due to obsessional concerns is an important part of the cognitive assessment. The previously discussed situational analysis can be helpful in developing this hierarchy. In addition a number of behavioral treatment manuals present record forms that are useful in constructing an avoidance hierarchy (e.g., Foa & Kozak, 1997; Steketee, 1993). The avoided situations should be arranged hierarchically from the least distressing or avoided situation to the most avoided, distressing situation. Reduction or complete elimination of the avoidance pattern can be incorporated into the treatment goals (Baer, 2000). For example, one of the goals of a client with a cleaning compulsion might be to use public washrooms in a shopping mall with only moderate anxiety, a situation that she currently avoids due to intense anxiety and fear of contamination.

It is also important to obtain self-monitoring data on the daily frequency of the primary compulsion as well as ratings on the subjective urge associated with the compulsion and degree of resistance exerted prior to capitulating to the compulsion. Some individuals with OCD give into the urge almost immediately whereas others can expend a considerable effort at resisting. It is also important to assess the clients' perceived success resisting their compulsions as well as the factors that might contribute to more successful resistance. Given that individuals with OCD engage in neutralization and other forms of mental control even more often than overt compulsive rituals, it is important to assess the type, frequency, and perceived success of various neutralization and mental control strategies. Appendix 11.2 presents a thought control form that can be used for this purpose. Finally, insight into the excessive, unreasonable, or irrational nature of the obsessions and compulsions should be determined. Questions should focus on the extent to which clients believe that the imagined threat or negative consequence associated with the obsessional fear is probable and whether the compulsive ritual or other forms of neutralization are both necessary and effective in preventing the dreaded outcome. For example, a client with poor insight believed that repeated reading and rereading of trivial information in community newspapers and advertisement flyers was necessary to ensure she didn't miss some local news item that was important to her. Perceived consequences and effectiveness of the compulsion may become a primary focus in therapy since clients with poor insight often have a more difficult response to treatment (e.g., Foa, Abramowitz, Franklin, & Kozak, 1999; Neziroglu, Stevens, McKay, & Yaryura-Tobia, 2001).

Clinical Illustration of Cognitive Case Conceptualization

We can return to the case presentation at the beginning of this chapter to illustrate a cognitive case conceptualization of OCD. Recall that Richard had long-standing multiple obsessions (1) of his hands being contaminated and passing on germs to others, (2) that he has disgusting body odor that others can smell, (3) of abhorrent blasphemous and sexual intrusive images that are offensive to God and will send him to hell, (4) of doubt about the accuracy of his work, and (5) that others can see a rash on his lower back and will be disgusted. These obsessions led to a number of compulsive rituals such as repeated hand washing, long shower rituals, excessive checking and rechecking, rigid daily routines, and mental compulsions. However, it was "thoughts of exposing the unsightly red spot" that was the current primary obsession.

Assessment revealed that the body rash obsession occurred at least 25–30 times on bad days and was associated with anxiety levels of 65–70/100. A number of situations were identified that triggered the "body rash obsession" such as being in a public place and sensing people behind him, feeling that his pants are loose, bending over, moving too much in a chair, feeling itchy, and the like. Work was the most common situation associated with the obsession in which getting up from his chair and walking in front of others was particularly anxiety-provoking for fear that his lower back was exposed. Moderate anxiety was the main emotion associated with the obsession. The main primary appraisals were *overestimated threat* ("People will see my lower back, be disgusted by it, and not want to associate with me"), *inflated responsibility* ("I must ensure that no one sees my lower back"), *need to control* ("If I don't get rid of the obsession, I'll become overwhelmed by the anxiety and have to quit work"), *TAF—Likelihood* ("If I think I'm exposing my back hair, I am probably exposing it to others"), *importance of thought* ("The thought about my lower back must be important because it reoccurs over and over again"), and *intolerance of uncertainty* ("I have to be certain that my lower back is completely covered").

Richard developed a number of responses to control his "lower back rash" obsession. His main compulsive ritual involved repeatedly checking on whether his lower back was exposed by pulling down his shirt or sweater. However, he also engaged in safety behaviors such as daily applying large amounts of ointment to his lower back or wearing loose-fitting clothing. He also relied on other neutralization strategies such as reassuring himself that no one can see his bare back, asking his wife if his shirts were well tucked into his pants (reassurance seeking), distracting himself with work, or just trying to ignore the thought. He also avoided any situations associated with a high likelihood of lower back exposure such as beaches, pools, swimming, gymnasiums, and the like. Richard rated the urge to engage in compulsive shirt pulling as very high (90/100) and his level of resistance low. He perceived that his efforts to control the obsession and its associated anxiety were moderately successful. Any failure to immediately reduce anxiety was interpreted as further proof that he was increasing the risk of offending others with exposure of his lower back. Although Richard acknowledged that his obsession was unusual, the intensity of his anxiety convinced him that other people probably would be disgusted by the sight of the red spot on his lower back.

Throughout the course of therapy a number of core beliefs became apparent. Richard believed that "people are easily offended and so it is his responsibility to ensure that this does not happen." He also believed that "anxiety was intolerable" and that "certain thoughts are dangerous and must be controlled or they will lead to a life of misery and torment." As a result he believed that what he needed "was greater control over his thoughts and emotions" in order to achieve stability and calm in his life. Richard's case formulation led to a number of treatment goals.

1. Modify his exaggerated threat appraisal of public exposure of his lower back.
2. Reformulate his control beliefs so that he relinquishes efforts to control the obsession.
3. Increase his tolerance for anxiety.
4. Prevent compulsive rituals associated with the obsession such as checking his lower back and repeatedly pulling at and retucking his shirts and sweaters.
5. Eliminate safety behaviors such as wearing loose clothing or putting ointment on his lower back.
6. Reduce avoidance of "back exposure" situations such as bending, walking in front of people, swimming, and so on.

DESCRIPTION OF COGNITIVE THERAPY FOR OCD

Many clinical researchers now argue that cognitive interventions should be incorporated into the standard behavioral treatment of exposure and response prevention (ERP) in psychotherapy for OCD (e.g., D. A. Clark, 2004; Freeston & Ladouceur, 1997b; Rachman, 1998; Salkovskis & Warwick, 1988; van Oppen & Arntz, 1994). In cognitive therapy improvement in obsessive and compulsive symptoms and alleviation of anxiety is achieved by modifying the faulty appraisals and beliefs of the obsession as well as the individual's efforts to control the obsession. The cognitive model of OCD provides the theoretical framework and guiding principles for the therapy. However, ERP is still a central therapeutic ingredient in cognitive therapy for OCD, with cognitive interventions often utilized to prepare the client for exposure-based homework. Below we present an overview of the eight treatment components of cognitive therapy for obsessions and compulsions. A number of more detailed cognitive-behavioral treatment manuals for OCD are now available (e.g., D. A. Clark, 2004; Purdon & Clark, 2005; Rachman, 2003, 2006; Salkovskis & Wahl, 2004; Wilhelm & Steketee, 2006). Table 11.4 presents a summary of the key therapeutic components of cognitive therapy for OCD.

Education Phase

In Chapter 6 we discussed the central role that education plays in cognitive therapy and how the therapist should inform clients of the nature of anxiety, the cognitive explanation for the persistence of anxiety, and the treatment rationale. Although these issues are

TABLE 11.4. Therapeutic Components of Cognitive Therapy for OCD

Therapy component	Description
Educating Client	Treatment rationale based on the role of appraisals and neutralization in the persistence of obsessions and compulsions.
Distinguishing appraisals and obsessions	Clients are taught how to identify their faulty evaluations that lead to misinterpretations of the personal significance of the obsession.
Cognitive restructuring	Evidence gathering, cost–benefit analysis, decatastrophizing, and cognitive error identification are used to weaken belief in the dangerousness of the obsession and increase willingness to engage in exposure-based behavioral experiments.
Alternative explanation	A more benign, accepting interpretation of the obsession and its control is encouraged.
Response prevention	Strategies are introduced to block or prevent compulsive rituals, safety behaviors, avoidance, neutralization, and other mental control strategies.
Behavioral experimentation	Within- and between-session exposure exercises are employed to modify faulty appraisals and beliefs.
Modify core beliefs	Core beliefs about the dangerousness and control of thoughts and personal vulnerability are addressed later in therapy.
Relapse prevention	Effective response to symptom relapse and recurrence is addressed in the final sessions of therapy.

included in the education component of cognitive therapy for OCD, the therapist also highlights the normalcy of unwanted intrusive thoughts, the role of faulty metacognitive appraisals, and the long-term deleterious effects of neutralization and other attempts at mental control. The objective of educating the client is to facilitate acceptance of the treatment rationale, that is, that reduction in obsessive or compulsive symptoms is best achieved by modifying how the obsession and its control are appraised.

An important part of the education process is to normalize the experience of unwanted intrusive thoughts, images, and impulses so the critical role of exaggerated appraisals of significance is highlighted (Salkovskis & Wahl, 2003). Clients can be shown a list of common unwanted intrusive thoughts that have been collected from nonclinical samples (for lists, see D. A. Clark, 2004; Rachman & de Silva, 1978; Wilhelm & Steketee, 2006). Individuals with OCD are often surprised that nonclinical individuals frequently report thoughts or images that are similar in content to their own obsessions. When demonstrating the role of appraisals the therapist can ask the client to select one or two intrusions that are not problematic and discuss how the thought could be interpreted so it becomes a highly significant threat. This can be contrasted with their own more benign interpretation that reduces the intrusion to an insignificant, even trivial, intrusion into the stream of consciousness. After this the therapist is ready to select the client's primary obsession from the list and explore with the client how she "has turned this intrusion into a highly significant personal threat." The long-term negative effects of neutralization can be demonstrated by the "camel effect" (Freeston & Ladouceur, 1997b). The client is instructed to purposefully hold the thought or image of a camel for 2 minutes and then to suppress the camel thought for 2 minutes. Failures to hold or remove the thought are signaled by the client and recorded by the therapist. This exercise is useful for demonstrating the futility of our efforts to intentional control unwanted thoughts. The potential for rebound effects once suppression efforts cease can also be discussed with clients. Together these exercises, which are introduced early in treatment, emphasize the importance of cognitive change in the client's interpretation and control of obsessional concerns.

Clinician Guideline 11.7

Educating the client into cognitive therapy of OCD requires an acceptance of the normality of unwanted intrusive thoughts, the primary role of faulty appraisals, and the negative effects of neutralization and other mental control efforts.

Distinguishing Appraisals from Obsessions

Educating the client on how to distinguish between the obsession and her appraisal of the obsession can be difficult because individuals with OCD have often spent years preoccupied with their obsessional concerns. Moreover, the concept of metacognition, or "thinking about thinking," will seem rather abstract and esoteric to some clients. However, it is critical to the success of cognitive therapy that clients become aware of the maladaptive meaning that they give to the obsession. In fact it is difficult for therapy to proceed with modification of faulty appraisals if the client is not fully cognizant of her "metacognitive appraisals" of the obsession.

A number of interview questions can be used to ease the client into the concept of metacognitive appraisal. The following are some probes that we have used with OCD clients:

- "What makes this thought [the obsession] important to you?"
- "What's so significant about this thought? Does the thought reflect anything about you—your character or values?"
- "Is there anything frightening or upsetting about the thought? Are you concerned about any possible negative consequences? When you think about your obsessional concerns, what's the worst that could happen?"
- "Is there anything about the thought that draws your attention to it, makes it hard to ignore?"
- "What would happen if you couldn't get the thought out of your mind or you couldn't avoid or complete your compulsive ritual?"

After careful probing with clients about the special meaning or significance of the obsession, the therapist and client together compose a brief narrative about what makes the obsession a highly significant personal threat to the client. Together with a copy of the cognitive appraisal model of obsessions (Figure 11.1) and a sheet that defines the key appraisals and beliefs of OCD (see Table 11.2 or Appendix 10.1 in D. A. Clark, 2004), the therapist and client review the "significance narrative" and pick out various types of specific faulty appraisals (e.g., responsibility, TAF, need for control, perfectionism) that characterize the narrative. This can be followed by a homework assignment in which the client records occurrences of the obsession, what made the obsession significant at the time, and which faulty appraisals were present in that specific instance of evaluating the obsession (see also Purdon, 2007).

Clinician Guideline 11.8

Ensure that clients can distinguish their appraisals of the obsession from their obsessional content before proceeding with cognitive or behavioral interventions aimed at modifying faulty appraisals and beliefs.

Cognitive Restructuring

Chapter 6 provided an extensive discussion of cognitive interventions like evidence gathering, cost–benefit analysis, decatastrophizing, and error identification that are used to challenge anxious thoughts and beliefs. These same strategies can be used to challenge faulty appraisals and beliefs about obsessions and their control with some adaptation for OCD. However, it is important that the cognitive interventions focus on the appraisals of the obsession and not on modifying the obsessional content itself. Salkovskis (1985, 1989) warns that cognitive strategies will not be effective in persuading clients to abandon their obsessional fears. Instead cognitive strategies are used to reeducate clients that their exaggerated evaluation of the significance of the obsession is faulty. For example, in our case example Richard could not be convinced that people would not see "the red spot on his lower back" and be disgusted by it (i.e., his obsessional content). Instead we used evidence gathering, behavioral experimentation, and alternative explanations to challenge his exaggerated threat appraisal about public exposure of the lower back red spot.

Cognitive restructuring should be tailored to target the seven faulty appraisals and beliefs that are crucial to OCD (i.e., overestimated threat, importance of thoughts or TAF, control of thoughts, inflated responsibility, intolerance of uncertainty, perfectionism, and thought control failures). The cognitive therapist will devote more time to appraisals that are particularly important in the individual's OCD. We mention here a few cognitive restructuring strategies that can be used with each of the appraisals (see D. A. Clark, 2004; Purdon, 2007; Purdon & Clark, 2005; Rachman, 2003; Wilhelm & Steketee, 2006, for more detailed descriptions). The downward arrow technique, calculating the probability of harm, and surveys of others' estimates of harm can be used to challenge *overestimated threat appraisals*. A pie chart in which the client assigns percentages of responsibility for an outcome to various factors including the self can be used to *challenge inflated personal responsibility beliefs* (Salkovskis & Wahl, 2003). Socratic questioning is useful in highlighting the circularity and faulty reasoning involved in *importance of thought* appraisals (i.e., "Is the obsession important because it occurs so frequently or is it frequent because we assume it's important?"). Wilhelm and Steketee (2006) discuss the "courtroom technique" in which evidence for and against the "importance of the obsession" can be presented. Purdon and Clark (2005) recommended having clients think about all the times when they had the obsessive thought and it never led to the dreaded deed or outcome, indicating that the obsessive thought may not be as important as assumed. For *intolerance of uncertainty* appraisals, a cost–benefit cognitive intervention can be employed. Clients can be asked to recall a time when they were certain of an action they took or a decision they made and the amount of extra time and effort that was required to attain a "feeling of certainty." Then they can be asked to recall a time when they took an action or decision even in the face of some uncertainty. Compare the outcome of each action or decision and examine the costs and benefits of the extra time expended to reach a higher level of certainty. Was it worth it in the long run? The same type of cognitive intervention can be used with *perfectionism* beliefs in which clients can be asked to rate how perfectly they performed some task, the consequences of their less-than-perfect performance, and whether the extra resources needed to push performance that extra 10 or 20% was worth the effort or not. The negative consequences of striving for perfectionism can also be assigned as homework.

Particular attention should be given to appraisals and beliefs of *need to control* the obsession and *failure to attain complete control*. Clients can be encouraged to experiment with different levels of effort to control the obsession and record the consequences associated with these varying efforts. "What happens to anxiety and frequency of obsession if compulsions, neutralization, or other control strategies are delayed or blocked altogether?" "What are the costs and benefits of expending greater or lesser effort at control of the obsession?" "What's the worst that can happen if you let go of control over the obsession?" One can start with encouraging short periods of "no control" (delay control efforts for a few minutes) and gradually increase the delay periods to hours or even days. To maximize the cognitive impact of these exercises, clients are asked to record the consequences of their efforts. This material is thoroughly examined in subsequent therapy sessions as support for or against the faulty beliefs about control of the obsession. A decatastrophizing intervention can be used for the secondary appraisals of control failure. Clients can be asked to describe the worst possible outcome they could imagine if they lost complete mental control over the obsession. "What would their lives be like?" "How could they cope if the obsession never faded from conscious awareness?" The therapist and client could together develop a contingency plan if she experienced a complete failure in mental control. The client could also survey family and friends on their tolerance of mental control failures. In fact the client could be asked to monitor times of mental control failure with nonobsessional thoughts. Clients may discover that they have less control than they assumed and are more tolerant of imperfect mental control when it involves nonobsessional thoughts.

Evidence gathering and cost–benefit analysis were used to challenge a number of Richard's beliefs about the significant threat posed by the back rash obsession and the need to attain better control over the obsession so its anxiety-provoking properties could be neutralized. For example, Richard was asked to take a photograph of his lower back and then compare it to pictures of other men's lower back to see if he exaggerated the red spot on his back (i.e., overestimated threat appraisal). In another cognitive restructuring exercise we compared Richard's appraisals of threat, importance, and significance for the thought "What if someone sees my lower back rash?" (i.e., the anxious obsession) to the thought "What if someone noticed nasal mucus hanging from my nose?" (i.e., a nonanxious neutral thought). Even though the latter thought was associated with a much higher realistic probability of social disgust and embarrassment, it caused no anxiety because of how it was appraised. Richard was able to see that it was his faulty appraisals of significance that caused his anxiety and preoccupation with the rash. Finally, evidence gathering was used to challenge (1) Richard's imagined danger that exposing his back to others would be dangerous (i.e., "find any known record that someone was horribly disgusted by the sight of a red spot on his lower back"), (2) his insistence that he feel certain that someone is not disgusted when looking at him, and (3) his failure to recognize the negative consequences of trying too hard to control any trace in his mind of the "lower back rash obsession."

Clinician Guideline 11.9

Cognitive restructuring is introduced early in treatment to weaken dysfunctional beliefs in the personal significant threat and importance of the obsession, its need for control, and the perceived negative effects of exposure and response prevention.

Alternative Explanation

Cognitive restructuring interventions should encourage clients with OCD to question their beliefs that obsessions are highly dangerous threats for which they have personal responsibility to control. But cognitive restructuring should also guide clients toward adopting healthier, more adaptive perspectives on the obsession and its control. The goal of cognitive therapy is for clients with OCD to adopt the following perspective on their obsessions and compulsions.

> Obsessions are meaningless, benign intrusions that have no particular personal significance. They are a normal manifestation of an active, creative mind. The thought has become highly frequent and distressing because of "catastrophic misinterpretations of significant threat" and excessive attempts at neutralization and control. Mental control is elusive at the best of times so that the most effective approach is to cease all compulsions, neutralization, or other mental control responses. Efforts to control the obsession and its associated anxiety may lead to immediate relief but it is only temporary. Over time the obsession only grows in frequency and intensity. A passive, accepting approach to the obsession is the best cure for my anxiety.

To facilitate acceptance of this alternative perspective, the cognitive therapist should work collaboratively with clients to write out their own healthy narrative of the obsessions and compulsions. Clients are more likely to accept the alternative explanation if it is expressed in their own words and punctuated with examples from their own experience. The client should be given a copy of the alternative explanation and daily implementation of this perspective would become one of the primary goals of therapy. In the case of Richard, the alternative explanation focused on giving up his efforts to control the obsession and tolerating some initial anxiety in order to achieve long-term reductions in his obsessional concerns and anxiety.

Clinician Guideline 11.10

The alternative explanation normally emphasizes that an obsessional intrusion is a meaningless mental nuisance whose frequency and anxiety-provoking properties will fade if all efforts at control or neutralization cease.

Response Prevention

Response prevention is an important therapeutic element in all cognitive treatment for OCD. In fact continued reliance on compulsive rituals or other forms of neutralization will undermine the effectiveness of cognitive therapy for obsessions. In Chapter 7 we discussed seven steps for implementing response prevention. It is important that therapy focus not only on preventing compulsive rituals but also any neutralization or mental control strategy that functions to reduce anxiety, prevent some dreaded outcome, or divert attention away from the obsession. Naturally, the effectiveness of exposure to the obsessional fear will be diluted if compulsions and other control strategies are not prevented.

It is likely that clients will be reluctant to engage in response prevention when anxiety is very high, so the therapist usually begins with preventing compulsions and neutralization responses to situations that elicit moderate anxiety in the midrange of the exposure hierarchy. It is preferable that the therapist start with in-session exposure and response prevention to ensure that the client blocks all compulsions and other forms of neutralization. This also gives the cognitive therapist an opportunity to discuss appropriate coping responses that can be used during response prevention and to deal with any negative beliefs or appraisals the client may have about exposure and response prevention. Effective ERP sessions are usually 60–90 minutes in duration and the client is always encouraged to daily practice the ERP homework assignments. Clients should record the frequency, duration, and outcome of their ERP homework on self-monitoring forms so the effectiveness of the intervention can be tracked. With Richard, response prevention focused on refraining from pulling down his sweater or checking that his shirt was tucked in or attempting to convince himself that no one was looking at his back (i.e., self-reassurance control strategy).

Clinician Guideline 11.11

Response prevention is one of the main therapeutic ingredients in cognitive therapy of OCD. It directly challenges the secondary appraisals and beliefs about need to control the obsession and its anxiety.

Behavioral Experimentation

Most of the behavioral experiments used in cognitive therapy for OCD involve some form of sustained exposure to the obsession and its associated anxiety. However, the main difference between behavior therapy and cognitive therapy is that in the latter case exposure is used to modify faulty appraisals and beliefs about the perceived significance and dangerousness of the obsession. Exposure-based behavioral experiments are introduced early in treatment, often guided by the fear hierarchy. After educating the client into the cognitive model and various cognitive interventions aimed at highlighting the important role of appraisals and beliefs in the persistence of obsessions, the therapist introduces within-session and between-session exposure exercises as a method of empirically testing the validity of OC-related beliefs. D. A. Clark (2004, Table 11.1) describes a number of specific behavioral exercises that can be used with clients to modify appraisals and beliefs of threat, responsibility, control, intolerance of uncertainty, and the like (see also Purdon, 2007; Purdon & Clark, 2005; Rachman, 2003; Wilhelm & Steketee, 2006; Whittal & McLean, 2002, for descriptions of behavioral experiments for OCD).

Many of these behavioral experiments involve repeated and sustained exposure to the obsession in a variety of avoided situations with response prevention of any form of neutralization. The client is asked to monitor the outcome of these exposure exercises in order to test firmly held beliefs such as anticipated threat, personal responsibility, or need to control the obsession and prevent imagined dire consequences thought to occur if control over the obsession falters. It is important that the cognitive therapist explore with clients the outcome of their behavioral experiments at subsequent sessions in order to consolidate evidence that challenges faulty appraisals and beliefs. For example, clients with a strong belief "that strict control over an obsession is necessary in order to prevent being overwhelmed with anxiety" could be asked to alternate days (or times of the day) when they expend great effort at controlling the thought versus other days when they relinquish control of the thought. The cognitive therapist would then review with clients their self-monitoring records. Some observations or probing questions that would be important in modifying faulty control beliefs might be (1) "I notice from your record form that you didn't have more obsessions or anxiety on 'low versus high control days.' What does this tell you about your concern that the anxiety will get worse if you don't try to suppress the obsession?"; (2) "You predicted that not responding to the obsession would be extremely difficult but what was you actual experience? From the record it looks like you did quite well"; and (3) "I notice that you wrote down that the control days were quite frustrating and exhausting for you compared to the 'no control days.' What does that tell you about the personal costs of repeated neutralization and efforts at mental control?" In cognitive therapy, then, exposure becomes one of the most potent therapeutic tools for directly modifying the faulty appraisals and beliefs that underlie obsessional thinking.

One behavioral experiment employed with Richard was to select periods of time during his work day when he would intentionally bring the obsession to his mind (e.g., "Can other people see my lower back?"), and at the same time refrain from any shirt tucking or self-reassurance. He also placed a Post-it note beside his computer monitor with the words "GO BACK" written on it as a reminder to intentionally think about the lower back rash. The imaginal component of this exposure exercise challenged Richard's belief that the obsession was a significant threat because he would become overwhelmed with anxiety. At the same time the written cue GO BACK was a type of situational exposure because it challenged Richard's belief that any stimulus related to his obsessional concern (i.e., the word "back") would elicit anxiety-provoking queries from his work colleagues. As it turned out Richard found the exercise moderately difficult to complete because of his irrational belief that others would ask about his Post-it message and would somehow find out about his lower back obsession.

Clinician Guideline 11.12

Exposure-based within- and between-session behavioral assignments are used as direct empirical hypothesis-testing exercises to structure experiences that directly challenge obsessional appraisals and beliefs, leading to modification of the cognitive basis of obsessions and compulsions.

The Role of Core Beliefs and Relapse Prevention

The long-term maintenance of treatment effects will be increased if the later phase of cognitive therapy targets individual's maladaptive core beliefs and builds into termination some relapse prevention strategies. Wilhelm and Steketee (2006) suggest that the core beliefs relevant in OCD often revolve around the same themes as noted in the appraisals and beliefs of obsessions. Core beliefs of personal helplessness and vulnerability are related to overestimated threat, beliefs about weakness and lack of control are linked to thought control appraisals, and core assumptions of inferiority and incompetence are related to perfectionism. Over the course of therapy the client can be encouraged to keep a record of experiences that directly challenge these core beliefs about the self. For example, the person who believes she is particularly lacking in "willpower and strong mental control" could keep a record of her experiences of "mental discipline." This information could be used to readjust her core belief to a healthier self-view such as "I obviously have more mental fortitude than I think" and "I am no better or worse than the average person in my ability to direct my thought processes."

The last couple of therapy sessions are devoted to relapse prevention, which has been shown to improve treatment maintenance in CBT for OCD (e.g., Hiss, Foa, & Kozak, 1994). A number of intervention strategies have been described to improve relapse prevention. Tolin and Steketee (2007) suggest that in the latter therapy sessions responsibility for exposure should shift from the therapist to the client (e.g., "What kind of exposure could you now do that would be most helpful?") and individuals should be encouraged to develop permanent life-style changes so they are frequently challenging their fear and avoidance as a natural part of daily living. In addition educating the client about the likelihood of future relapses and identifying high-risk situations are an important part of relapse prevention (D. A. Clark, 2004; Tolin & Steketee, 2007). The client and therapist should develop a written protocol for how to cope with relapse (Freeston & Ladouceur, 1999). The introduction of basic problem-solving skills, support groups, and how to handle changes in medication are also recommended (Wilhelm & Steketee, 2006). Finally, fading treatment sessions and scheduling occasional booster sessions can improve the long-term effects of treatment.

Clinician Guideline 11.13

Given the chronicity of OCD, it is important to focus on modifying core beliefs as well as issues of future relapse during the latter sessions of cognitive therapy. This will help encourage the generalizability and long-term maintenance of treatment effects.

EFFICACY OF COGNITIVE THERAPY OF OCD

A number of well-designed randomized control trials have clearly demonstrated the immediate and long-term effectiveness of exposure and response prevention (ERP) for OCD (for reviews, see Foa & Kozak, 1996; Foa, Franklin, & Kozak, 1998; Kozak & Coles, 2005; Rowa, Antony, & Swinson, 2007). CBT which includes both ERP and cognitive therapy is now recommended as the treatment of choice, either alone or in combination with SRI medication, for all OCD in adults (March, Frances, Carpenter, & Kahn, 1997). In this brief review, we adopt the current custom of referring to ERP as treatment that is primarily behavioral with only a slight emphasis on cognitive processes, cognitive therapy as treatment that consists mainly of cognitive restructuring with no formal ERP, and CBT as treatment with a fairly equal emphasis on ERP and cognitive restructuring.

It is now well established that ERP is an effective treatment for OCD (e.g., Foa, Liebowitz, et al., 2005; Marks, Hodgson, & Rachman, 1975; Rachman et al., 1979) and that it is effective when offered on an outpatient fee-for-service basis (Franklin, Abramowitz, Kozak, Levitt, & Foa, 2000) or when offered to ethnic minority patients (Friedman et al., 2003). In their review of 12 outcome studies involving 330 patients with OCD, Foa and Kozak (1996) concluded that 83% of patients were improved with ERP. Several meta-analytic studies have concluded that ERP is associated with large pre–post treatment effect sizes (Abramowitz, 1996; Abramowitz, Franklin, & Foa, 2002; Eddy, Dutra, Bradley, & Westen, 2004; Kobak, Greist, Jefferson, Katzelnick, & Henk, 1998; van Balkom et al., 1994) and average symptom reduction ranges from 48 to 59% (see Kozak & Coles, 2005). Percentage of patients who reach recovery at post-treatment ranges from 24 to 73% with recovery defined as 25–50% symptom reduction (Eddy et al., 2004; Fisher & Wells, 2005). However, if stricter criteria are utilized, less than 30% of patients are asymptomatic at posttreatment (Fisher & Wells, 2005).

ERP has been shown to be significantly more effective than medication alone (Foa, Liebowitz, et al., 2005), although other studies have found equivalent treatment effects (van Balkom et al., 1998; see comparison review by Christensen, Hadzi-Pavlovic, Andrews, & Mattick, 1987) or a possible advantage of combined ERP and SRI medication (Cottraux et al., 1990; Hohagen et al., 1998). In their meta-analytic study Eddy et al. (2004) reported greater effect sizes for ERP or cognitive therapy than medication alone but the highest effect sizes were found for the combined pharmacotherapy and psychotherapy conditions. Although only a few studies report long-term follow-ups, Foa and Kozak (1996) concluded that 76% of patients maintain their treatment gains for an average 29 months. However, a significant number of individuals with OCD (37%) either refuse ERP, drop out of therapy, or fail to respond (Stanley & Turner, 1995), and only a minority of treatment completers are entirely symptom-free at posttreatment (e.g., Fisher & Wells, 2005). Also, some OCD subtypes may not respond as well to ERP such as individuals with pure obsessions, hoarding, or mental contaminations (Rachman, 2003, 2006; Steketee & Frost, 2007). Thus despite the documented efficacy of ERP, there is still considerable room for improvement.

Recent OCD treatment outcome studies of CBT that place an equal weight on cognitive interventions and ERP are more relevant to the cognitive therapy described in this chapter. Although these studies are fewer in number, the initial results are most encouraging with CBT showing strong treatment effects (e.g., Franklin, Abramowitz, Bux, Zoellner, & Feeny, 2002; Freeston et al., 1997; O'Connor, Aardema, Bouthillier, et al., 2005; McLean et al., 2001; van Oppen, de Haan, et al., 1995; Whittal et al., 2005). Moreover, patients who show a good response to CBT also experience a significant improvement in their quality of life that extends beyond reductions in OCD symptoms (Diefenbach, Abramowitz, Norberg, & Tolin, 2007; Norberg, Calamari, Cohen, & Riemann, 2007). However, a critical question is whether adding cognitive interventions to ERP improves treatment over a strictly behavioral approach to treatment. The findings from these comparison studies are far from clear. Some have found that CBT (cognitive therapy plus ERP) is equivalent to ERP alone (O'Connor, Aardema, Bouthillier, et al., 2005; Whittal et al., 2005), whereas others suggest that more intensive ERP alone might be most effective (McLean et al., 2001) and at least one study reported superiority for CBT (van Oppen, de Haan et al., 1995). It would appear that group CBT for OCD is less effective than individual therapy (Fisher & Wells, 2005; McLean et al., 2001; O'Connor, Freeston, et al., 2005).

Even if CBT versus ERP alone are considered equivalent, this is not an inconsequential finding because it could be argued that the addition of cognitive interventions might detract from the potency of ERP by reducing the amount of exposure patients receive in therapy (see arguments by Kozak, 1999). Kozak and Coles (2005) concluded from their review of the outcome literature that the addition of cognitive therapy interventions to intensive, therapist-supervised exposure and rigorous abstinence from compulsive rituals was not warranted because it might actually detract from the effectiveness of behavior therapy. However, Fama and Wilhelm (2005) point out that an insufficient number of studies have directly compared CBT versus ERP and suboptimal cognitive therapy protocols may have been utilized in some of the studies included in literature reviews. Moreover, Fama and Wilhelm argue that given the recent advent of cognitive therapy for OCD, further refinements and elaboration in cognitive interventions should be encouraged rather than prematurely discarded as ineffective.

A number of studies have shown that cognitive interventions with no explicit instructions to engage in exposure or response prevention can lead to significant improvement in obsessive and compulsive symptoms in their own right. In one study 65 OCD outpatients who were randomly assigned to 20 sessions of cognitive therapy or 20 hours of intensive ERP showed equivalent response at posttreatment and follow-up (Cottraux et al., 2001). Wilson and Chambless (2005) provided cognitive therapy without ERP to six patients with OCD and reported that two out of six recovered at posttreatment. Freeston, Léger, and Ladouceur (2001) employed cognitive therapy that specifically targeted the six appraisals and beliefs of OCD discussed in this chapter and obtained significant posttreatment improvement in four out of six patients with pure obsessions without overt compulsions. Previous multiple case studies indicated that cognitive therapy alone can produce clinically significant change in patients with compulsive checking rituals (Ladouceur, Léger, Rhéaume, & Dubé, 1996; Rhéaume & Ladouceur, 2000). Compared to a wait list control group, Jones and Menzies (1998) reported that patients with compulsive washing rituals who received their DIRT treatment protocol that specifically focuses on cognitive interventions without exposure to anxiety-provoking stimuli showed significant pre– posttreatment symptom reductions. In a later study, four of five patients with intractable OCD who failed to respond to ERP showed significant symptom improvement with DIRT (Krochmalik, Jones, & Menzies, 2001). Together these studies indicate that cognitive interventions alone can have a significant effect on symptom reduction, although the effect sizes may be smaller when compared to intensive ERP (Abramowitz et al., 2002).

Clinician Guideline 11.14

Individual cognitive therapy is an effective treatment for OCD that may eventually prove to be particularly beneficial for certain subtypes of OCD such as individuals with pure obsessions without overt compulsions. Cognitive interventions should be introduced in the early sessions with frequent and intense exposure-based behavioral exercises employed throughout the course of treatment.

SUMMARY AND CONCLUSION

In many respects OCD is one of the most difficult and perplexing of the anxiety disorders given its heterogeneous and idiosyncratic symptom presentation. It is a puzzling condition because individuals report intense anxiety over the most innocuous, even incredulous, thought (e.g., "Might I spread a deadly sickness to others because I am contaminated with radioactivity") while at the same time acknowledging the absurdity and impossibility of the fear. Such an irrational fear requires a refinement of the standard cognitive approach.

This chapter presented a metacognitive theory that explains the persistence of obsessive and compulsive symptoms in terms of faulty appraisals and beliefs that lead to exaggerated evaluations that the obsession represents a significant personal threat that could be associated with catastrophic consequences (Rachman, 1997). Appraisals involving overestimated threat, inflated responsibility, overimportance of thought (i.e., TAF), control of thoughts, intolerance of uncertainty, and perfectionism are implicated as key cognitive processes, along with faulty inductive reasoning, that cause the obsession-prone individual to misinterpret normal unwanted intrusive thoughts. Once the mental intrusion is considered a highly significant personal threat, the individual engages in various overt and covert responses to control or neutralize the obsessional fear. However, repeated neutralization (e.g., compulsive ritual) and misinterpretations of the significance of failed control will also contribute to the persistence of the obsession. This sets in motion an escalating cycle of heightened anxiety with increased frequency and salience of the obsession associated with repeated failure to achieve effective neutralization or a satisfactory state of calm. As reviewed in the chapter, there is mounting empirical evidence for the cognitive model of obsessions, especially overestimated threat, inflated responsibility, TAF, and need for control of thoughts. An eight-component cognitive therapy for OCD was presented in which the main therapeutic ingredients are cognitive restructuring, exposure-based behavioral experimentation, and response prevention that target the faulty appraisals and beliefs specific to OCD.

The last few years have witnessed a burgeoning research on the cognitive basis of OCD. However, we are only beginning to develop a cognitive approach to OCD and many questions remain for future research. Are the faulty appraisals and beliefs specific to OCD, and are they causes or consequences of the disorder? Do individuals with OCD suffer from poor mental control or is the problem with their subjective appraisal of control and its anticipated consequences? Do some individuals have a cognitive vulnerability for OCD? Do cognitive interventions add significant therapeutic value beyond the effects of exposure and response prevention? Is a cognitive approach to treatment more effective for some subtypes of OCD than others? Might the addition of cognitive interventions enhance the prophylactic effects of CBT like that seen in the treatment of depression? Although there are many issues that remain for future investigation, the cognitive perspective is providing fresh insights into our understanding and treatment of obsessions, in particular.

Daily Record of Primary Obsession

Name: _____ Date: _____

Primary obsession: _____

Instructions: In consultation with your therapist, please record the obsessional thought, image, or impulse that is most troubling for you at this time. Record the approximate number of times you experienced the obsession on a particular day. Then complete the rating scales for each day which indicate your most typical experience of the obsession for that day. This form should be completed at bedtime each evening.

Day of Week	Approximate Frequency of Obsession during the Day	Average Distress of Obsession (0 = none to 100 = extreme, panic-like)	Intensity of Effort to Control Obsession (0 = no effort to control to 100 = frantic effort to stop thinking the obsession)	Intensity of Urge to Engage in Compulsion or Neutralization (0 = no urge to 100 = irresistible urge)
Sunday				
Monday				
Tuesday				
Wednesday				
Thursday				
Friday				
Saturday				
Sunday				
Monday				
Tuesday				
Wednesday				
Thursday				
Friday				
Saturday				

Record of Control Strategies Associated with Primary Obsession

Name: _____   Date: _____

Instructions: In consultation with your therapist, please record the obsessional thought, image, or impulse that is most troubling for you at this time. Below you will find a number of ways that people use to try and stop thinking their obsessional thoughts, images, or impulses. Please indicate the frequency and success of each control strategy as it relates to your primary obsession. Use the rating scale provided with each category.

Primary obsession: _____

List of Control Strategies Associated with Primary Obsession	Frequency That Strategy Is Used 0 = never 1 = occasionally 2 = often 3 = frequently 4 = daily 5 = several times a day	How Effective Is This Strategy in Stopping Obsessional Thinking? 0 = never effective 1 = occasionally effective 2 = often effective 3 = frequently effective 4 = always effective	How Effective Is This Strategy in Reducing Distress? 0 = never effective 1 = occasionally effective 2 = often effective 3 = frequently effective 4 = always effective
1. Engage in a behavioral compulsion (e.g., wash, check, repeat). [BC]			
2. Engage in a mental compulsion (e.g., say a particular phrase, repeat a prayer, think certain thoughts). [MC]			
3. Think about reasons why the obsession is senseless, unimportant or irrational. [CR]			
4. Try to reassure myself that everything will be alright. [SR]			
5. Seek reassurance from others that everything will be alright. [OR]			

(cont.)

List of Control Strategies Associated with Primary Obsession (continued)	Frequency That Strategy Is Used 0 = never 1 = occasionally 2 = often 3 = frequently 4 = daily 5 = several times a day	How Effective Is This Strategy in Stopping Obsessional Thinking? 0 = never effective 1 = occasionally effective 2 = often effective 3 = frequently effective 4 = always effective	How Effective Is This Strategy in Reducing Distress? 0 = never effective 1 = occasionally effective 2 = often effective 3 = frequently effective 4 = always effective
6. Distract myself by doing something. [BD]			
7. Distract myself by thinking another, possibly pleasant, thought or image. [CD]			
8. Try to relax myself. [R]			
9. Tell myself to stop thinking the obsession. [TS]			
10. Get angry, down on myself for thinking the obsession. [P]			
11. Try to avoid anything that will trigger the obsession. [A]			
12. Do nothing when I get the obsession. [DN]			

Strategies adapted from Freeston and Ladouceur's *Structured Interview on Neutralization* (see Ladouceur et al., 2000), the *Thought Control Questionnaire* (Wells & Davies, 1994), and the *Revised Obsessional Intrusions Inventory* (Purdon & Clark, 1994b).

Coding Key: BC = behavioral compulsion, MC = mental compulsion, CR = cognitive restructuring, SR = self-reassurance, OR = other reassurance, BD = behavioral distraction, CD = cognitive distraction, R = relaxation, TS = thought stopping, P = punishment, A = avoidance, DN = do nothing.

Chapter 12

Cognitive Therapy
of Posttraumatic Stress Disorder

Vision without action is a daydream.
Action without vision is a nightmare.
—JAPANESE PROVERB

Edward was a 42-year-old man with 20 years of distinguished service in the Canadian infantry. He joined the army after graduating from university with a degree in philosophy. He was full of optimism about his career decision, wanting to "see the world" and make a difference in the lives of people caught in poverty and conflict. Edward's potential was soon recognized by the military and he received many promotions, commendations, and access to special training. He was selected for three United Nations (UN) peacekeeping tours that were viewed by soldiers as highly desired assignments, ones that afforded unprecedented opportunities for advancement. Edward had a close, stable marriage and two beautiful young daughters. They were financially secure and had an active social life with their close military friends. For Edward life was progressing in a predictable and highly fulfilling direction.

But all of this changed in 1994. Two years earlier Edward had accepted a peacekeeping assignment that involved a 4-month tour of duty in the former Yugoslavia. The job was intense with long hours, life-threatening road checks, and witnessing the death of his friend from a landmine. He returned to Canada having increased his level of alcohol consumption, but threw himself back into his work. His next assignment came in 1994 when he volunteered for a 6-month tour of a small African country he barely knew, Rwanda. Unbeknownst to Edward, he was about to step into a country that would experience one of the worst genocides in recorded history—the slaughter of 800,000 people within a 3- to 4-month period. The consequences of the genocide were visible everywhere in Rwanda, and the images of slaughter and suffering became seared into Edward's mind. He remembered the throngs of refugees afraid and hungry walking along the roads or gathering around their trucks seeking food and security. He could still smell the air of rotting and decaying corpses that hung over the countryside and the images of hundreds of women and children hacked to death in churches and village meeting halls. He recalled the scenes of mass graves and dead bodies floating in the river. He could still see the face of a little 5-year-old girl he befriended at an orphanage whom he suspects was later murdered by the Rwandan Patriotic Army (RPA). He relived the fear of approaching checkpoints where he was substantially outnumbered by young intoxicated Rwandan soldiers armed with automatic weapons and machetes. Edward could see the toll that the tour was having on himself and his fellow soldiers. He witnessed the suicide of one of his comrades, who shot himself outside the Kigali stadium.

When Edward returned to Canada, he immediately assumed a normal workload of tasks and duties. In fact, 4 years later he accepted a final 9-month tour of duty in Bosnia in charge of landmine clearance. Though he did not witness any trauma, the work was intense, stressful, and highly dangerous. He returned from that tour with no energy, no interest in life, depressed, hopeless, cynical, feeling angry and out of control, withdrawn and alienated from others. Over the next several years Edward was able to function at work, but his mental and emotional state was deteriorating. He became increasingly depressed, irritable, anxious, easily frustrated, and withdrawn. He frequently had anger outbursts at home that frightened his wife and daughters. He became more and more socially anxious, and finally refused to have any social contact outside his work setting. Most nights and weekends he sat alone, watching TV and drinking until intoxicated. He had great difficulty sleeping, waking frequently with nightmares about Rwanda. In 2002 his wife and daughters finally left him, and several months later his wife filed for divorce. Out of a sense of desperation, and with the encouragement of his family, Edward overcame his stigma about mental health services and initiated a request for psychiatric and psychological treatment.

An initial assessment revealed that Edward met diagnostic criteria for several Axis I disorders: chronic PTSD, as well as alcohol dependence and major depression recurrent. Administration of the SCID module for PTSD revealed that his Rwanda experience qualified as a Criterion A traumatic event. In addition Edward had several reexperiencing symptoms including (1) recurrent, intrusive thoughts and images of Rwandan crowds and the little girl, (2) recurrent nightmares, (3) flashbacks of the Rwandan crowds or intrusive images of the little girl with a gorilla dressed in a RPA uniform, and (4) intense shaking, trembling, and nervousness when exposed to reminders of Rwanda. He developed extensive avoidance of anything that reminded him of Rwanda including a certain stretch of highway close to his community as well as crowded stores and malls. He had little interest in social activities, and felt detached and unable to empathize with others. He also experienced increased arousal symptoms like difficulty falling asleep, anger outbursts, and difficulty concentrating including episodes of dissociation. On the Beck Depression Inventory–II he scored 40 and endorsed the statement of having suicidal thoughts but would not carry them out.

Edward began a lengthy treatment of individual CBT as well as numerous combinations of medications interspersed with a 4-week PTSD recovery program and various alcohol rehabilitation initiatives. CBT targeted various automatic thoughts and beliefs related to trauma, PTSD symptoms and depression, but also included other treatment components such as trauma exposure, applied relaxation, graded exposure, and behavioral activation.

In the remainder of this chapter we will refer back to Edward in order to illustrate the cognitive basis of PTSD and its treatment. But first we begin with a brief consideration of diagnostic issues in PTSD, as well as the nature of trauma and predictors of risk and resiliency. This will be followed by a description of the cognitive model of PTSD and its empirical status. The remainder of the chapter discusses cognitive assessment, case formulation, treatment, and its efficacy.

DIAGNOSTIC CONSIDERATIONS

DSM-IV Diagnostic Criteria

PTSD was first introduced as an official diagnostic construct in DSM-III (American Psychiatric Association [APA], 1980). It is the only anxiety disorder to include an etiologic variable in its diagnostic criteria, that is, PTSD is defined as a person's response to a specific event (McNally, 2003a). To meet diagnostic criteria for PTSD (Criterion A1), DSM-IV requires exposure to an extreme traumatic stressor involving (1) actual or threatened death or serious injury to self or threat to one's physical integrity; (2) witnessing death, serious injury, or threat to the physical integrity of another person; or (c) learning about unexpected death, serious harm, or threat of death or injury to a family member or close friend (APA, 2000). In addition the person's response to the event must involve intense fear, helplessness, or horror (Criterion A2). PTSD, then, can occur in response to a wide range of traumatic events such as war, rape, torture, crime, motor vehicle accidents, industrial accidents, natural disasters, incarceration as a prisoner of war or in a concentration camp, sudden death of a loved one, being diagnosed with a life-threatening illness, and the like (APA, 2000; Keane & Barlow, 2002). Table 12.1 presents the DSM-IV-TR diagnostic criteria for PTSD.

Three other symptom categories must be present in response to the traumatic stressor in order to meet diagnostic criteria for PTSD. Resick, Monson, and Rizvi (2008) made a number of observations about these symptom categories. At least one reexperiencing symptom must be present which represents some form of intrusive recollection or reminder of the trauma that is associated with strong negative affect and is experienced in an uncontrollable fashion. The avoidance and numbing symptoms (Criterion C) may reflect the individual's attempt to gain psychological distance from the trauma and reduce the negative emotions associated with the reexperiencing symptoms. The physiological hyperarousal symptoms (Criterion D) reflect the individual's persistent state of hypervigilance for new threats or dangers but ultimately this will have a detrimental effect on daily functioning. A 1-month duration criterion is included because the majority of individuals (i.e., over 90%) experience symptoms consistent with PTSD immediately after a trauma but these symptoms remit for most individuals by 3 to 6 months (Monson & Friedman, 2006). DSM-IV also introduced a clinically significant distress or functional impairment criterion to PTSD, which along with the addition of

TABLE 12.1. DSM-IV-TR Diagnostic Criteria for Posttraumatic Stress Disorder

Criterion A (*traumatic event*)

The person has been exposed to a traumatic event in which both of the following were present:
(1) the person experienced, witnessed, or was confronted with an event or events that involved actual or threatened death, or serious injury, or a threat to the physical integrity of self or others
(2) the person's response involved intense fear, helplessness, or horror

Criterion B (*reexperiencing symptoms*)

The traumatic event is persistently reexperienced in one (or more) of the following ways:
(1) recurrent and intrusive distressing recollections of the event, including images thoughts, or perceptions
(2) recurrent distressing dreams of the event
(3) acting or feeling as if the traumatic event were recurring (includes a sense of reliving the experience, illusions, hallucinations, and dissociative flashback episodes, including those that occur on awakening or when intoxicated)
(4) intense psychological distress at exposure to internal or external cues that symbolize or resemble an aspect of the traumatic event
(5) physiological reactivity on exposure to internal or external trauma cues that symbolize or resemble an aspect of the traumatic event

Criterion C (*avoidance and numbing symptoms*)

Persistent avoidance of stimuli associated with the trauma and numbing of general responsiveness (not present before the trauma), as indicated by three (or more) of the following:
(1) efforts to avoid thoughts, feelings, or conversations associated with the trauma
(2) efforts to avoid activities, places, or people that arouse recollections of the trauma
(3) inability to recall an important aspect of the trauma
(4) markedly diminished interest or participation in significant activities
(5) feeling detachment or estrangement from others
(6) restricted range of affect (e.g., unable to have loving feelings)
(7) sense of a foreshortened future (e.g., does not expect to have a career, marriage, children, or a normal lifespan)

Criterion D (*increased physiological arousal symptoms*)

Persistent symptoms of increased arousal (not present before the trauma) as indicated by two (or more) of the following:
(1) difficulty falling or staying asleep
(2) irritability or outbursts of anger
(3) difficulty concentrating
(4) hypervigilance
(5) exaggerated startle response

Criterion E (*duration*)

Duration of the disturbance (symptoms in Criteria B, C, and D) is more than 1 month.

Criterion F (*distress or functional impairment*)

The disturbance causes clinically significant distress or impairments in social, occupational, or other important areas of functioning.

Specify if:
        Acute: if duration of symptoms is less than 3 months
        Chronic: if duration of symptoms is 3 months or more
        With Delayed Onset: if onset of symptoms is at least 6 months after the stressor

Note. From American Psychiatric Association (2000). Copyright 2000 by the American Psychiatric Association. Reprinted by permission.

an emotional response to the trauma criterion (A2) was intended to make the diagnosis of PTSD more stringent (Norris & Slone, 2007).

Clinician Guideline 12.1

Posttraumatic stress disorder (PTSD) is a chronic anxiety disorder that occurs in response to one or more traumatic stressors and is characterized by trauma-related intrusive reexperiencing symptoms, avoidance, emotional numbing, and persistent heightened arousal that causes significant clinical distress or functional impairment.

Acute Stress Disorder

Another important development in DSM-IV was the inclusion of acute stress disorder (ASD) in order to account for initial trauma reactions (i.e., peritraumatic responses) and to predict subsequent PTSD. This diagnostic category was developed to cover the 1-month gap imposed by PTSD and to account for individuals' immediate response to a traumatic stressor that often includes significant dissociative symptoms (Friedman, Resick, & Keane, 2007). It was based on the notion that dissociative reactions will impair recovery because they impede access to affect and memories of the traumatic experience (Harvey & Bryant, 2002). Table 12.2 presents the DSM-IV diagnostic criteria for ASD.

There has been considerable controversy over the diagnostic and predictive validity of ASD. The core element of the disorder is the presence of prominent dissociative symptoms (Criterion B). DSM-IV-TR defines dissociation as "a disruption in the usually integrated functions of consciousness, memory, identity, or perception" (APA, 2000), as indicated by derealization, flashbacks, depersonalization, out-of-body experiences, sense of time slowing down or speeding up, emotional numbing, and inability to remember aspects of the traumatic experience. McNally (2003b) argues that defined in this way, the construct of dissociation is too vague, abstract, and global to offer any explanatory power. Furthermore, Panasetis and Bryant (2003) found that persistent or ongoing dissociation may be related to posttraumatic reactions whereas peritraumatic dissociation that occurs during the traumatic event may have a more adaptive function.

ASD occurs in 13–33% of adults and 17–21% of children and adolescents exposed to traumatic events (e.g., Brewin, Andrews, Rose, & Kirk, 1999; Classen, Koopman, Hales, & Spiegel, 1998; Bryant & Harvey, 1998; Harvey & Bryant, 1998b; Kangas, Henry, & Bryant, 2005; Meiser-Stedman, Dalgleish, Smith, Yule, & Glucksman, 2007). Although 75–80% of individuals with ASD will subsequently meet diagnostic criteria for PTSD (Brewin et al., 1999; Bryant & Harvey, 1998; Harvey & Bryant, 1998b), ASD may not be the optimal predictor of PTSD (see review by Harvey & Bryant, 2002) because (1) a diagnosis of ASD does not predict significantly better than preexisting PTSD criteria, (2) many people develop PTSD without an initial ASD, (3) only a subset of ASD symptoms predicts PTSD whereas others do not, and (4) ASD might overpathologize a transient adaptive response to traumatic stress (Bryant, 2003; Harvey & Bryant, 2002; Shalev, 2002). Despite these doubts about its predictive validity, CBT is an effective treatment for ASD in terms of reducing the subsequent development of PTSD (Bryant, Moulds, & Nixon, 2003; Bryant et al., 2006).

TABLE 12.2. DSM-IV-TR Diagnostic Criteria for Acute Stress Disorder

Criterion A. (*traumatic event*)

The person has been exposed to a traumatic event in which both of the following were present:

(1) the person experienced, witnessed, or was confronted with an event or events that involved actual or threatened death, or serious injury, or a threat to the physical integrity of self or others

(2) the person's response involved intense fear, helplessness, or horror.

Criterion B. (*dissociative symptoms*)

Either while experiencing or after experiencing the distressing event, the individual has three (or more) of the following symptoms:

(1) a subjective sense of numbing, detachment, or absence of emotional responsiveness
(2) a reduction in awareness of his or her surroundings (e.g., "being in a daze")
(3) derealization
(4) depersonalization
(5) dissociative amnesia (i.e., inability to recall an important aspect of the trauma)

Criterion C. (*reexperiencing symptoms*)

The traumatic event is persistently reexperienced in at least one of the following ways: recurrent images, thoughts, dreams, illusions, flashback episodes, or a sense of reliving the experience; or distress on exposure to reminders of the traumatic event.

Criterion D. (*avoidance symptoms*)

Marked avoidance of stimuli that arouse recollections of the trauma (e.g., thoughts, feelings, conversations, activities, places, people).

Criterion E. (*arousal symptoms*)

Marked symptoms of anxiety or increased arousal (e.g., difficulty sleeping, irritability, poor concentration, hypervigilance, exaggerated startle response, motor restlessness).

Criterion F. (*distress or functional impairment*)

The disturbance causes clinically significant distress or impairment in social, occupational, or other important areas of functioning or impairs the individual's ability to pursue some necessary task, such as obtaining necessary assistance or mobilizing personal resources by telling family members about the traumatic experience.

Criterion G. (*duration*)

The disturbance lasts for a minimum of 2 days and a maximum of 4 weeks and occurs within 4 weeks of the traumatic event.

Criterion H. (*exclusion*)

The disturbance is not due to the direct physiological effects of a substance (e.g., a drug of abuse, a medication) or a general medical condition, is not better accounted for by a Brief Psychotic Disorder, and is not merely an exacerbation of a preexisting Axis I or Axis II disorder.

Note. From American Psychiatric Association (2000). Copyright 2000 by the American Psychiatric Association. Reprinted by permission.

Clinician Guideline 12.2

Acute stress disorder (ASD) is an immediate anxiety state in response to a traumatic event in which acute dissociative symptoms predominate along with some trauma-related reexperiencing, avoidance, and heightened arousal symptoms that together cause significant distress or functional impairment. The majority of individuals with ASD will eventually meet criteria for PTSD.

Diagnostic Controversy

There has been much debate on the conceptual and practical problems associated with the diagnosis of PTSD (Rosen, Spitzer, & McHugh, 2008; Spitzer, First, & Wakefield, 2007). First, it is apparent that occurrence of a traumatic stressor (i.e., Criterion A) is neither necessary nor sufficient for PTSD (Rosen et al., 2008). Individuals can meet PTSD symptom criteria following non-Criterion A events such as marital disruption, divorce, bereavement, breaking up with a best friend, and the like (Rosen & Lilienfeld, 2008) and support for a dose–response assumption (i.e., the most severe PTSD is not necessarily associated with the most severe trauma) has been inconsistent (McNally, 2003a; Rosen & Lilienfeld, 2008). McNally (2003a) has been critical of the expanded number of events that qualify as Criterion A stressors under DSM-IV, noting that this "bracket creep" may be medicalizing expected human reactions to trauma.

Second, there is weak and inconsistent support from factor-analytic studies for the three core DSM-IV symptom clusters (reexperiencing, avoidance/numbing, and physiological arousal) (e.g., Palmieri, Weathers, Difede, & King, 2007; Simms, Watson, & Doebbeling, 2002; see also Resick et al., 2008, for review). Moreover, taxometric analysis suggests that PTSD is not a discrete syndrome but rather a dimensional condition that represents the more severe end of a continuum with milder reactions to traumatic experiences (Ruscio et al., 2002).

Third, there are other negative emotional responses to trauma such as guilt and shame that are evident in PTSD but not included in DSM-IV (see Resick et al., 2008). Other diagnostic problems include (1) the presence of PTSD symptoms in other disorders like major depression (Bodkin, Pope, Detke, & Hudson, 2007), (2) a marked variability in symptom presentation across PTSD cases, (3) a high rate of comorbidity, and (4) failed attempts to find a distinct biological or psychological marker for the disorder (Rosen & Lilienfeld, 2008). These diagnostic issues may have important implications in terms of making it difficult for clinicians to reliably diagnosis PTSD without the use of structured diagnostic interviews (Nielssen & Large, 2008). Furthermore, concerns about diagnostic validity could lead to a high false positive rate (McNally, 2007b). In light of these diagnostic problems, many researchers are again calling for a reconsideration of the nosology of PTSD with major revisions suggested for DSM-V (Rosen et al., 2008; Spitzer et al., 2007).

Clinician Guideline 12.3

The defining diagnostic features of PTSD continue to be debated, including the nature and severity of the traumatic experience required for the diagnosis.

EPIDEMIOLOGY AND CLINICAL FEATURES

Prevalence of Trauma Exposure

A large discrepancy exists between the number of people exposed to traumatic events that meet DSM-IV-TR Criterion A and the much smaller minority who eventually develop PTSD. In fact by the beginning of adulthood 25% of individuals have experienced at least one traumatic event and by age 45 the majority of adults will have experienced trauma, with a significant number of individuals experiencing multiple traumatic events (Norris & Slone, 2007). Of course prevalence rates of traumatic stress increase dramatically in populations exposed to war, community violence, natural disasters, and the like.

Analysis of the NCS data set indicated that 60.7% of men and 51.2% of women experienced at least one DSM-III-R traumatic event, the most common being witnessing someone being badly injured or killed, being involved in a fire or natural disaster, and being involved in a life-threatening accident (Kessler, Sonnega, Bromet, Hughes & Nelson, 1995). Other large epidemiological or community studies have confirmed that two-thirds to 90% of adults have experienced at least one traumatic event in their lifetime (e.g., Breslau et al., 1998; Creamer, Burgess, & McFarlane, 2001; Elliot, 1997).

The frequency and type of trauma exposure is not evenly distributed across the population. Although it is not clear whether some ethnic groups experience more or less trauma than others, it may be that inner-city residents are exposed to more community violence (see Norris & Slone, 2007). Furthermore, certain occupations are associated with higher rates of traumatic exposure such as military personnel, paramedics, urban firefighters, and the like (e.g., Corneil, Beaton, Murphy, Johnson, & Pike, 1999; U.S. Department of Veteran Affairs, 2003). Moreover, countries that are war-torn, politically unstable, or have low living standards have higher rates of trauma exposure in their population (e.g., Sachs, Rosenfeld, Lhewa, Rasmussen, & Keller, 2008; Seedat, Njenga, Vythilingum, & Stein, 2004; Turner, Bowie, Dunn, Shapo, & Yule, 2003).

Gender is another important factor in prevalence of trauma. Although men are exposed to more traumatic events than women (e.g., Breslau et al., 1998; Vrana & Lauterbach, 1994), women are more likely to experience interpersonal trauma such as physical or sexual assault, rape, and child abuse and men more often report criminal victimization, fire/disasters, life-threatening accidents, combat, and being held captive (Breslau et al., 1998; Creamer, Burgess, & McFarlane, 2001; Kessler, Sonnega, et al., 1995; Williams, Williams, et al., 2007). In fact approximately one-third of women experience sexual or physical assault (Resnick, Kilpatrick, Dansky, Saunders, & Best, 1993). Physical and sexual assault are associated with the highest rates of PTSD, with rape being particularly toxic for posttraumatic disorder (Norris, 1992; Resnick et al., 1993). In a well-known study by Rothbaum, Foa, Riggs, Murdock, and Walsh (1992), rape victims were prospectively assessed 9 months after the assault. At initial assessment 94% met symptom criteria for PTSD, at 1 month 65% met criteria, at 3 months 47% had PTSD, and at 9 months 47.1% met PTSD diagnostic criteria. Thus, interpersonal traumatic events involving a direct threat to an individual's life or safety are associated with the highest rates of PTSD. This trend is also seen in military samples in which there is a significant relationship between amount of combat exposure and rates of PTSD (e.g., Hoge, Auchterlonie, & Milliken, 2006).

Clinician Guideline 12.4

Most adults will experience at least one Criterion A traumatic stressor, with the prevalence higher in men than in women. Although the majority of individuals experience PTSD symptoms as an immediate response to trauma, only a small fraction will subsequently develop DSM-IV PTSD.

Vulnerability and the Development of PTSD

Given the discrepancy between the high prevalence of trauma and the much lower rate of PTSD, a considerable amount of research has focused on potential vulnerability factors in the disorder. Vulnerability constructs fall into three categories: (1) the enduring vulnerability factors that are present prior to a trauma, (2) the characteristics of the traumatic experience, and (3) features of the posttrauma context and the individual's coping responses.

Pretrauma Vulnerability Factors

A large meta-analysis was conducted on 77 studies that investigated a variety of risk factors that predicted PTSD in military and civilian samples exposed to trauma (Brewin, Andrews, & Valentine, 2000). They found different risk factors for each group. In civilian samples the following pretrauma variables had small effect sizes for PTSD: (1) being female; (2) low socioeconomic status; (3) a positive psychiatric history; (4) reported history of abuse, other traumatic experiences, or childhood adversity; and (5) family psychiatric history. For the military studies, younger age, lack of education, and minority status emerged as additional pretrauma variables but gender was no longer a significant predictor. However, these pretrauma variables were much weaker predictors of risk than trauma severity or posttrauma variables like lack of social support and more subsequent life stress.

A more recent meta-analysis of 476 studies confirmed that pretrauma variables like history of prior trauma, previous psychological or psychiatric problems, and family history of psychopathology had small but significant effect sizes in predicting PTSD (Ozer, Best, Lipsey, & Weiss, 2003). Other studies have shown that number of stressful events prior to the trauma (Galea et al., 2002; Vrana & Lauterbach, 1994) and history of child sexual abuse in women survivors of sexual assault predicted severity of PTSD symptoms (Ullman, Filipas, Townsend, & Starzynski, 2007). Breslau (2002) concluded that previous psychiatric disorders, history of childhood trauma, and family history of psychiatric disorders were the pretrauma risk factors most consistently associated with PTSD.

Trauma Characteristics

The type of trauma, its severity, and the individual's emotional response are more potent predictors of subsequent PTSD than any of the pretrauma variables. Personal involvement in a traumatic event is associated with increased risk for PTSD compared to witnessing the event or hearing (i.e., vicarious exposure) about a family member's traumatic experience (Breslau et al., 1998; Eriksson, Vande Kemp, Gorsuch, Hoke, & Foy, 2001; see Vogt, King, & King, 2007). Furthermore, closer geographic proximity to a traumatic community event, such as the 9/11 terrorist attack or proximity to the epicenter of an earthquake, is associated with higher rates of PTSD (e.g., Galea et al., 2002; Pynoos et al., 1993).

There is some evidence that PTSD increases with the severity of the traumatic event (Brewin et al., 2000; Lauterbach & Vrana, 2001; Pynoos et al., 1993), although others have concluded that evidence for a dose–response relationship is inconsistent (McNally, 2003a; Rosen & Lilienfeld, 2008). Trauma severity, defined in terms of combat expo-sure, is the most significant predictor for risk of developing PTSD or its symptoms in military samples (e.g., Hoge et al., 2006; Kulka et al., 1990; Lee, Vaillant, Torrey, & Elder, 1995; Vogt, Samper, King, King, & Martin, 2008). In addition the perception that one's life was in danger during the traumatic event or being threatened by others (Hollifield et al., 2008; Jeon et al., 2007; Ozer et al., 2003; Ullman et al., 2007) as well as events that cause injury are related to higher rates of PTSD (Rasmussen, Rosenfeld, Reeves, & Keller, 2007). Finally, certain types of trauma that involve severe interper-sonal threat and danger, such as rape, sexual and physical assault, and childhood abuse, are particularly toxic for PTSD and its symptoms (e.g., Breslau et al., 1998; Creamer et al., 2001; Norris, 1992; Resnick et al., 1993; Seedat et al., 2004; Vrana & Lauterbach, 1994). On the other hand, traumatic stressors like motor vehicle accidents, natural disas-ters, and witnessing or learning about traumas to others appear to be associated with a lower prevalence of PTSD (Creamer et al., 2001; Jeon et al., 2007; Norris, 1992).

Certain emotional responses at the time of the trauma predict subsequent develop-ment of PTSD. As discussed previously, the presence of ASD increases risk for PTSD or posttrauma symptoms (Brewin et al., 1999; Bryant & Harvey, 1998; Harvey & Bryant, 1998b), as does presence and severity of early PTSD-related symptoms (e.g., avoidance and numbing symptoms) or combat stress reactions (e.g., Koren, Arnon, & Klein, 1999; North et al., 1999; Solomon & Mikulincer, 2007). Individuals who report intense nega-tive emotional responses such as fear, helplessness, horror, guilt, or shame during or immediately after the trauma have the higher levels of PTSD (Ozer at al., 2003). Finally, occurrence of dissociative symptoms or panic attacks around the time of the trauma may be a significant predictor of subsequent PTSD (Galea et al., 2002; Ozer et al., 2003; see Bryant, 2007, for contrary view).

Posttrauma Risk Factors

A low level of perceived social support including negative social reactions from others is a strong predictor of subsequent PTSD symptoms and disorder (Brewin et al., 2000; Galea et al., 2002; Ozer et al., 2003; Ullman et al. 2007). On the other hand, a high level of social support might mitigate the negative effects of exposure to life-threatening events (Corneil et al., 1999; Eriksson et al., 2001). In addition certain coping responses have been associated with higher PTSD including denial, self-blame, seeking social sup-port, delayed disclosure, and disengagement from coping efforts (Silver et al., 2002; Ullman et al., 2007). Long-term negative consequences resulting from the trauma such as losing one's job might increase risk for PTSD (Galea et al. 2002). And finally certain cognitive variables have been predictive of PTSD such as overestimated threat apprais-als, lower perceived safety, absence of optimism, detachment, mental defeat, and negative beliefs and appraisals of the trauma, its consequences, and PTSD symptoms (for further discussion, see section below on empirical research of the cognitive model).

Clinical Implications

The research findings on vulnerability and risk for PTSD provide useful information to incorporate into the education phase of cognitive therapy and can be used in cognitive restructuring to modify negative beliefs and appraisals of initial PTSD symptoms. Many individuals with PTSD blame themselves for the disorder. Edward, for example, believed that it was his fault that he suffered from chronic PTSD. He believed there must be a weakness in his character or some predisposition for mental illness that caused him to have PTSD while other soldiers returned from deployment without apparent mental health difficulties. The therapist was able to discuss with Edward the latest research on risk factors in PTSD, emphasizing that pretrauma variables were only weak predictors of who develops PTSD in military samples and that variables related to severity of trauma exposure like experiencing threats to one's life and extent of combat exposure were the most important predictors of the disorder. We also noted that posttrauma responses such as coping strategies and ways of thinking about the trauma, oneself, and the future are important contributors to the persistence of PTSD and these are variables that can be changed with therapy.

Clinician Guideline 12.5

Peritraumatic and posttraumatic variables are stronger predictors of the development of PTSD than pretrauma risk factors. This finding can be used to counter maladaptive beliefs of self-blame that are common in PTSD.

CLINICAL FEATURES

Prevalence and Course

Epidemiological research on PTSD draws a distinction between prevalence of the disorder in the population and conditional prevalence, which examines rates in populations exposed to trauma (Norris & Slone, 2007). Incidence of PTSD has also been reported for specific occupations associated with high rates of trauma exposure such as the military, police, and emergency rescue workers as well as in response to single community traumas like a natural disaster (e.g., earthquake) or terrorist attack. Rates of PTSD have also been examined over time, with the highest rates occurring immediately after a trauma and then declining steadily over the next 3–6 months.

Population and Occupational Rates of PTSD

The lifetime prevalence for PTSD in the U.S. population was 7.8% in the NCS (10.4% women, 5.0% men; Kessler et al., 1995) and 6.8% in the NCS-R (Kessler, Berglund, et al., 2005). An earlier study based on a representative national sample of women (N = 4,008) reported a lifetime prevalence rate of 12.3% (Resnick et al., 1993). However, lower rates have been reported in other countries such as Australia (Creamer et al., 2001), Chile (Zlotnick et al., 2006), and Korea (Jeon et al., 2007). Based on the American studies, PTSD would be second only to specific and social phobia in terms of higher prevalence in the general population.

Conditional Probability of PTSD

Since presence of trauma is a necessary criterion for PTSD, it is more meaningful to determine rates of the disorder among individuals exposed to trauma. Numerous studies have been conducted on military samples in which risk of PTSD is directly related to amount of combat exposure (e.g., Hoge et al., 2006; Ikin et al., 2007; Lee et al., 1995; Tanielian & Jaycox, 2008). According to the National Vietnam Veterans Readjustment Study (Kulka et al., 1990), 30.9% of men who served in Vietnam developed PTSD and another 22.5% had partial PTSD, an extraordinarily high statistic that has come under criticism (McNally, 2007b). A 50-year follow-up of Australian Korean veterans yielded an estimated lifetime prevalence rate of 25.6% which was substantially higher than the nonveteran comparison group (4.6%; Ikin et al., 2007). And a recent RAND study of randomized telephone interviews with 1,965 veterans of Afghanistan and Iraq deployments concluded that 13.8% have a probable diagnosis of PTSD (Tanielian & Jaycox, 2008). Higher rates of PTSD have also been reported in firefighters (Corneil et al., 1999) and international relief and development workers (Eriksson et al., 2001; see also Whalley & Brewin, 2007). Clearly PTSD is an occupational hazard for those exposed to higher rates of life-threatening experiences.

Numerous studies have also documented elevated rates of PTSD for individuals in the general population exposed to trauma. In the NCS 20.4% of women exposed to trauma had a lifetime probability of PTSD compared to 8.1% of trauma-exposed men (Kessler et al., 1995). Approximately 20–25% of individuals exposed to serious injury, motor vehicle accidents, or natural disasters like Hurricane Katrina (Galea et al., 2007) or the 2004 tsunami in Sri Lanka (Hollifield et al., 2008) develop PTSD (e.g., Koren et al., 1999; Mayou et al., 2001; Zatzick et al., 2007).

Trauma due to terrorism such as the 9/11 attacks on the World Trade Center or the July 5, 2005, bombing in the London subway can cause an immediate increase in distress and stress-related symptoms even in those not directly exposed to the trauma, and these symptoms can persist for months, although at a significantly reduced level (Rubin et al., 2007; Rubin, Brewin, Greenberg, Simpson, & Wessely, 2005; Silver et al., 2002). However, individuals directly exposed to terrorists attacks will have especially high rates of PTSD (30–40%) with 20% of exposed individuals continuing to experience symptoms 2 years later (Galea et al., 2002; North et al., 1999; see Whalley & Brewin, 2007). Thus high rates of PTSD and its symptoms are evident immediately after exposure to a life-threatening event, but 6 months later one-half to two-thirds of these cases will remit, often without treatment (e.g., Foa & Rothbaum, 1998; Mayou et al., 2001; Milliken, Auchterlonie, & Hoge, 2007; see Whalley & Brewin, 2007). And yet a substantial number of individuals (i.e., one-third) who exhibited PTSD symptoms during the acute phase of trauma exposure continue to experience a persistent and chronic form of the disorder that is evident several months or years after exposure to trauma (Kessler et al., 1995; see also Norris & Slone, 2007, for review).

Clinician Guideline 12.6

Even though PTSD is a transient reaction to trauma exposure that remits in two-thirds of individuals in 3–6 months, nevertheless as many as one-third of individuals exposed to trauma will develop a chronic form of the disorder that can persist for many years. Segments of the population with greater exposure to life-threatening traumas have a higher rate of the disorder.

Gender and Ethnicity

Both population-based and conditional risk studies have found that stress-related symptoms and PTSD are evident in more women than men (e.g., Breslau et al., 1998; Jeon et al., 2007; Galea et al., 2002; Galea et al., 2007; Kessler et al., 1995; Silver et al., 2002). Various explanations have been proposed for this gender effect on PTSD such as (1) women's higher rate of exposure to particularly toxic traumas like rape and sexual assault (Creamer et al., 2001; Kessler et al., 1995), (2) an elevated psychiatric history for other anxiety disorders and depression, (3) a greater tendency to endorse an emotional response of fear, helplessness, or horror to trauma (Breslau & Kessler, 2001), or (4) a differential endorsement rate to a small subset of symptoms (Peters, Issakidis, Slade, & Andrews, 2006). There are, then, a number of possible reasons why women exhibit a higher rate of PTSD than men.

There has been considerable debate over ethnic and cultural differences in response to trauma and PTSD. Although there have been cross-national differences in rates of PTSD, no ethnic differences in lifetime prevalence of PTSD were found in the NCS (Kessler et al., 1995) or in the Australian National Survey of Mental Health and Well-Being (Creamer et al., 2001). There was some indication that a higher rate of PTSD after 9/11 was associated with Hispanic ethnicity (Galea et al., 2002) and PTSD prevalence was higher in black and Hispanic male veterans compared to white male Vietnam veterans (e.g., Koenen, Stellman, Stellman, & Sommer, 2003; Kulka et al., 1990; see also Tanielian & Jaycox, 2008, for similar results among Afghanistan and Iraq deployments), although this could be due to differences in severity of combat exposure or pretrauma variables such as younger age, lower education, and aptitude test scores (Dohrenwand, Turner, Turse, Lewis-Fernandez, & Yager, 2008).

Clinician Guideline 12.7

Although PTSD is more prevalent in women than men, this gender difference may be due to a higher rate of interpersonal trauma. Ethnic and cultural diversity may play a weaker role in stress-related responses and development of PTSD after traumatic exposure.

Onset and Age Differences

PTSD has a swift onset with prevalence rates for PTSD symptoms and disorder peaking within the first month of traumatic exposure, followed by steep remission rate in

40–60% of cases within 6–12 months posttrauma (e.g., Breslau et al., 1998; Kessler et al., 1995; Galea et al., 2003). Kessler et al. (1995) reported that remission was shorter in those who obtained treatment (i.e., mean of 36 months) compared with those who did not seek treatment (i.e., mean of 64 months), although this finding has not always been replicated in other studies (e.g., Milliken et al., 2007). DSM-IV-TR (APA, 2000) allows for a specifier indicating that PTSD can have a delayed onset of at least 6 months after a traumatic stressor. However, delayed-onset appears to be rare, especially in nonmilitary samples, occurring in 5% or less of cases (e.g., Mayou et al., 2001; North et al., 1999; see Andrews, Brewin, Philpott, & Stewart, 2007).

Trauma occurs in all ages and so PTSD symptoms are also prevalent across the lifespan, although 23 years was the median onset age in the NCS-R (Kessler, Berglund, et al., 2005). The majority of children and adolescents, especially in urban centers, are exposed to traumatic events (e.g., Breslau, Lucia, & Alvarado, 2006; Seedat et al., 2004). Breslau et al. (2006) determined that 8.3% of 17-year-olds who experienced a traumatic event met criteria for PTSD, whereas Pynoos et al. (1993) reported an astonishing 93% of children exposed to the 1988 Armenian earthquake had severe chronic PTSD 18 months after trauma exposure. As noted previously childhood physical and sexual abuse as well as other childhood adversities may be especially likely to lead to PTSD in adults (see also Norris & Slone, 2007, for discussion). However, new cases of PTSD are rare after the early 50s and the prevalence of PTSD even with trauma exposure may decline with increasing age (Kessler et al., 1995; Kessler, Berglund et al., 2005).

Clinician Guideline 12.8

PTSD is a disorder that is particularly prevalent in adolescence to midadulthood, with exposure to traumatic events during the early years having a cumulative negative effect that can persist well into adulthood.

Quality of Life and Functional Impairment

Chronic PTSD is associated with significant decrements in social, occupational, and educational attainment as well as in quality of life. Compared to the other anxiety disorders, individuals with PTSD have some of the highest rates of physical disorder (e.g., Sareen et al., 2005; Zatzick et al., 1997). In addition chronic PTSD is associated with significant work or school functional impairment (Stein, Walker, Hazen, & Forde, 1997; Zatzick et al., 1997) and significantly worse social functioning in marital and family relationships, parenting, and sexual satisfaction (e.g., Koenen, Stellman, Sommer, & Stellman, 2008). In addition PTSD is associated with a number of negative health behaviors such as increased nicotine and drug use (Breslau, Davis, & Schultz, 2003; Koenen et al., 2008; Vlahov et al., 2002). A meta-analysis of quality-of-life studies revealed that PTSD and panic disorder were associated with the greatest impairments across quality-of-life domains (Olatunji et al., 2007; see also Hansson, 2002).

In the NCS-R 34.4% of individuals with PTSD made contact with a mental health professional in a 12-month period, which is one of the higher utilization rates among the anxiety disorders, although the median delay in initial treatment contact was 12 years (Wang, Berglund, et al., 2005; Wang, Lane, et al., 2005). With an increased utilization of primary health and mental health services coupled with significant functional impairment, PTSD is associated with higher health costs than the other anxiety disorders (Marciniak et al., 2005; Walker et al., 2003). Tanielian and Jaycox (2008), for example, concluded that the 2-year costs resulting from PTSD and major depression for the 1.6 million service members deployed since 2001 could range from $4.0 to $6.2 billion but the provision of evidence-based treatment could reduce this cost by 27%. Clearly, the elevated disability and economic burden caused by chronic PTSD makes this disorder a serious societal health concern.

Clinician Guideline 12.9

Chronic PTSD is associated with some of the highest rates of disability, poor physical health, and reduced social functioning among the anxiety disorders. The disorder takes a heavy toll in human suffering and places a significant economic burden on the health care system.

Comorbidity

Like the other anxiety disorders, PTSD is associated with a high comorbidity rate with other Axis I disorders. In the NCS 88% of men with lifetime occurrence of PTSD and 79% of women had at least one other Axis I diagnosis (Kessler et al., 1995). Half of the men with PTSD had a comorbid major depression or alcohol abuse/dependence, with conduct disorder (43%), drug abuse/dependence (35%), simple phobia (31%), social phobia (28%), and dysthymia (21%) also showing high rates of co-occurrence. For women with PTSD, major depression (49%), simple phobia (29%), social phobia (28%), alcohol abuse/dependence (28%), drug abuse/dependence (27%), dysthymia (23%), and agoraphobia (22%) were common secondary diagnoses (see also Zlotnick et al., 2006, for similar comorbidity rates). The temporal relationship among diagnoses is complex, with many comorbid disorders occurring as a consequence of PTSD, and yet most people with PTSD have at least one preexisting diagnostic disorder (Kessler et al., 1995). Even higher comorbidity may be evident in clinical samples with PTSD. In their large outpatient sample, Brown, Campbell, et al. (2001) reported that 98% of individuals with an index diagnosis of PTSD had at least one comorbid disorder. The most common co-occurring diagnoses were major depression (65%), panic disorder (55%), GAD (45%), and social phobia (41%). Rates of substance abuse/dependence were not reported.

The relationship of major depression and PTSD to traumatic events is especially important because both disorders are highly comorbid and they both can occur concurrently as distinct disorders in traumatized individuals (Blanchard, Buckley, Hickling, & Taylor, 1998; Kilpatrick et al., 2003). Moreover, individuals with PTSD and comorbid major depression are more distressed, more impaired on major role functions, more likely to attempt suicide, and less likely to remit than individuals with PTSD alone (Blanchard et al., 1998; Oquendo et al., 2003).

A high comorbidity rate is also evident between substance abuse/dependence disorders and PTSD. A review of the relevant literature indicates that PTSD usually precedes alcohol or drug abuse/dependence, and is probably an attempt to medicate the symptoms of PTSD (Jacobsen, Southwick, & Kosten, 2001). Moreover, the change in alcohol consumption or increased reliance on drug usage is due to presence of PTSD and not exposure to trauma (Breslau et al., 2003; Chilcoat & Breslau, 1998; McFarlane, 1998). Furthermore, comorbid PTSD and substance use disorders are associated with poorer treatment outcome (Ouimette, Brown, & Najavitis, 1998).

Some individuals with PTSD, especially those suffering from the long-term impact of childhood sexual abuse, present with symptoms of PTSD and borderline personality disorder (McLean & Gallop, 2003). Several investigators have proposed a new nosologic concept called *complex PTSD* (Roth, Newman, Pelcovitz, van der Kolk, & Mandel, 1997) which involves a constellation of symptoms characterized by:

1. Alterations in self-regulation (e.g., affect regulation, anger control, self-destructive behaviors, suicidal preoccupation).
2. Alterations in attention or consciousness (e.g., amnesia, transient dissociative episodes).
3. Alterations in self-perception (e.g., ineffectiveness, guilt and responsibility, shame, minimizing).
4. Alterations in perception of the perpetrator (e.g., idealizing the perpetrator, although this criteria is not required).
5. Alterations in relationships with others (e.g., inability to trust, victimizing others).
6. Somatization (e.g., chronic pain, conversion symptoms, sexual symptoms).
7. Alterations in systems of meaning (e.g., despair and helplessness, loss of previously sustaining beliefs).

There is evidence that complex PTSD is associated with physical and sexual abuse, especially in women (Roth et al., 1997) and it may be even more prevalent in women reporting early-onset childhood sexual abuse (McLean & Gallop, 2003). Furthermore, cluster analysis revealed that an empirically derived symptom subtype of PTSD can be derived that corresponds to complex PTSD (Taylor, Asmundson, & Carleton, 2006). At this point the diagnostic homogeneity of the construct has been questioned and there may be multiple forms of complex PTSD (see Taylor, 2006, for discussion). Nevertheless, individuals with a symptom presentation like complex PTSD will require a longer course of psychotherapy that will have to address core issues of self-definition, affect regulation, and interpersonal relations that are not part of the standard PTSD cognitive-behavioral treatment protocol (e.g., Pearlman, 2001).

Clinician Guideline 12.10

Individuals with PTSD often present with concurrent major depression, substance use disorder or, to a lesser extent, other anxiety disorders like GAD, specific phobia, or social phobia. A more chronic and debilitating condition, called complex PTSD, consists of both posttrauma symptoms and personality pathology that requires a more multifaceted and extended treatment approach.

COGNITIVE MODEL OF PTSD

The cognitive model presented in this chapter is based on the important advances made in the development of a cognitive perspective on PTSD by Ehlers and Clark (2000), Brewin, Dalgleish, and Joseph (1996), and Foa and colleagues (Foa & Rothbaum, 1998; Hembree & Foa, 2004). Key dysfunctional cognitive processes and structures have been identified that are responsible for the persistence of the posttraumatic symptoms even in the absence of current threat. Although these cognitive models offer a full account of PTSD in their own right, each has proposed certain critical constructs that have played an important role in the development of our perspective on the disorder.

Ehlers and Clark (2000) contend that two cognitive processes are critical for producing a sense of a serious current threat in PTSD: (1) excessively negative appraisals of the traumatic event and its sequelae, and (2) poor elaboration and contextual integration of autobiographical memory of the trauma. Negative appraisals and beliefs about the traumatic event and its consequences, a faulty threat interpretation of one's acute stress reaction, a fragmented trauma memory that is biased toward retrieving information congruent with the individual's negative appraisals, and reliance on dysfunctional coping strategies together contribute to the perception of current threat and the symptoms of PTSD (see also D. M. Clark & Ehlers, 2004). From Brewin's dual representation model we find that the negative appraisals of trauma are a complex product of consciously perceived aspects of the trauma stored as *verbally accessible memories* (VAM) and intrusive flashbacks that reflect activation of automatic, involuntary, and sensory-rich *situationally accessible memories* (SAM) of the trauma (Brewin et al., 1996; Brewin & Holmes, 2003). The mental representation of trauma in working memory, then, involves both conceptually based and sensory-rich information encoding that together are responsible for the generation of PTSD symptoms (see also Dalgleish, 2004). Finally Foa and Rothbaum (1998) argue that trauma memory in PTSD is a pathological but highly accessible memory structure involving erroneous stimulus, response, and meaning associations as well as faulty evaluation of danger. Two important stimulus elements of the fear structure associated with the meaning of "danger" are perceptions that the *world is an extremely dangerous place* and views of *oneself* as *extremely incompetent* (Hembree & Foa, 2004). Activation of the trauma memory gives rise to the symptoms of PTSD that are interpreted as aversive and possibly dangerous. As a consequence the individual tries to avoid any cues that might activate the trauma memory. Although each of these cognitive theories offers a distinct perspective on PTSD, they share a common underlying assumption that PTSD symptoms are a result of faulty beliefs and appraisals of trauma-related threat as well as dysfunctional encoding and retrieval of trauma memory.

Figure 12.1 and the following sections present a proposed model of persistent PTSD that organizes the cognitive basis of the disorder around three interrelated levels of conceptualization.

Etiological Level

Since only a minority of individuals exposed to trauma will develop PTSD, all theories of the disorder recognize there must be preexisting individual differences that increase vulnerability to PTSD. In addition to certain background and psychiatric pretrauma

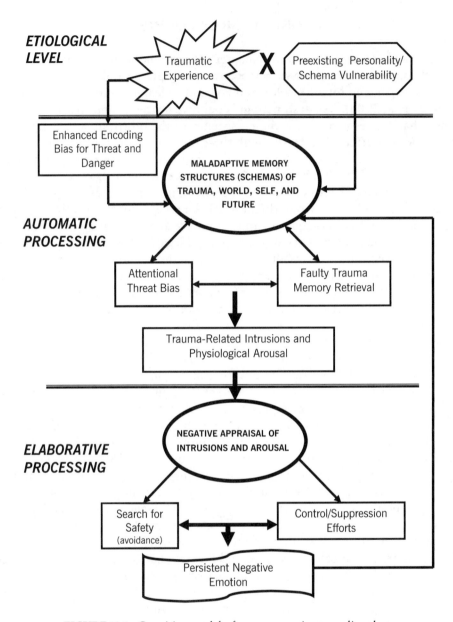

FIGURE 12.1. Cognitive model of posttraumatic stress disorder.

variables discussed above, the cognitive model proposes that particular enduring beliefs about personal threat, vulnerability, and the world might predispose to the persistence of PTSD symptoms in response to a traumatic experience. Rigid beliefs that the world is extremely dangerous or the opposite, extremely safe, and self-schemas representing ideas of extreme competence or incompetence may be predisposing factors for PTSD (Foa & Rothbaum, 1998). Ehlers and Clark (2000) suggested that beliefs about the importance of maintaining control over thoughts and emotions might cause one to appraise reexperiencing symptoms in a more negative and threatening manner.

The cognitive-personality constructs of sociotropy and autonomy, which Beck (1983) originally proposed as vulnerability factors for depression, might have relevance for the development of PTSD. Depending on the type of trauma, a person whose self-worth is excessively dependent on receiving love and approval from others (i.e., high sociotropy) might be more negatively affected by an interpersonal trauma, whereas a person who values mastery and achievement (i.e., high autonomy) might be more affected by trauma that threatens personal safety, being in control, and assumptions about the parameters of achievement. A nonclinical study found that sociotropy and autonomy were significantly related to self-reported PTSD symptoms, although there was no attempt to assess congruence between personality and type of trauma (Kolts, Robinson, & Tracy, 2004). Although speculative at this time, the close association between PTSD and major depression in response to trauma is consistent with the possibility that a common underlying cognitive vulnerability could be evident in the two disorders.

Like other models of PTSD, occurrence of a traumatic event plays a key role in the etiology of PTSD. *Trauma* has been defined as "any experience that by its occurrence has threatened the health or well-being of the individual" (Brewin et al., 1996, p. 675). This indicates that a broad range of events could be traumatic provided they violated the individual's core schemas about oneself, the world, and/or other people. As illustrated in Figure 12.1, the cognitive model proposes an interaction between trauma and predisposing schemas that result in activation of the maladaptive schematic structures of PTSD. A type of diathesis–stress relationship is suggested in which the nature and severity of the trauma interacts with schematic vulnerability. For individuals who are extreme on a vulnerability factor (i.e., beliefs that the world is dangerous), possibly fewer and less severe experiences of a certain type will elicit PTSD symptoms, whereas an individual who exhibits a mild form of the vulnerability will require a much more intense or multiple threatening experiences in order to trigger persistent PTSD. Edward, for example, had a strong belief in the importance of the rule of law, respect for human life, and the effectiveness of control. The chaos and butchery he witnessed in Rwanda shattered his assumptions about the world, human nature, and his ability to control life-threatening events. These core schemas that characterize an autonomous personality orientation may have interacted with the brutality he witnessed to increase his vulnerability to PTSD.

Clinician Guideline 12.11

Cognitive theory proposes a diathesis–stress model of vulnerability for PTSD in which risk is defined in terms of a match between the traumatic experience and preexisting cognitive-personality factors such as high sociotropic or autonomous concerns.

Automatic Processing

Enhanced Encoding during Trauma

The way in which a traumatic event is processed at the time of its occurrence will influence how the event is represented in working memory. An automatic, preconscious selective encoding bias for highly salient threat and danger elements of the trauma with a corresponding inability to process positive or more benign features of the situation will contribute to activation of the maladaptive PTSD schema structure. In addition Ehlers and Clark (2000) noted that if primarily data-driven processing (i.e., processing sensory impressions) occurs during encoding rather than a contextualized, more organized conceptual-driven processing (i.e., processing the meaning of the event), than trauma memories will be more unorganized, fragmented, and susceptible to strong perceptual priming. They also suggested that an inability to adopt a self-referential perspective during the trauma will contribute to difficulty integrating trauma memory with the person's other autobiographical memories. In the cognitive model represented in Figure 12.1, this maladaptive processing during trauma contributes directly to activation of the dysfunctional schematic structure of PTSD, whereas the poorly elaborated, unorganized, or fragmented trauma memory is primarily responsible for the occurrence of trauma-related reexperiencing intrusions (see D. M. Clark & Ehlers, 2004, for further discussion).

Core Schematic Structure and Trauma Memory

A central argument in social-cognitive theories of PTSD is that traumatic events dramatically alter basic assumptions about the self, world, and other people because they can not be readily assimilated into existing schemas (Shipherd et al., 2006). Brewin et al. (1996) indicated that the trauma involves a violation of basic assumptions about (1) personal invulnerability from death or disease, (2) one's status in a social hierarchy, (3) a person's ability to meet personal moral standards and achieve life goals, (4) the availability and reliability of significant others, and (5) the existence of order between actions and outcomes. Brewin and colleagues suggest that the violation of these assumptions causes the individual with PTSD to perceive that the world is an uncontrollable, unpredictable, and more dangerous place (see also Foa & Rothbaum, 1998). Janoff-Bulman (1992) argued that trauma shatters the individual's assumptions about personal invulnerability, the world as meaningful and benevolent, and the self as positive or worthy. On the other hand, a traumatic experience can confirm or strengthen previously held negative beliefs about the self and the world (D. M. Clark & Ehlers, 2004). Horowitz (2001) emphasized that emotional alarms occur when internal representations of the trauma do not match preexisting schemas of self and others. This incongruity will evoke unpleasant emotions such as anxiety, panic, or guilt, which leads to overcontrol processes designed to avoid the dreaded emotional states.

Researchers have proposed a number of negative schemas that are characteristic of PTSD (see Ehlers & Clark, 2000; Foa & Rothbaum, 1998; Janoff-Bulman, 1992; McCann, Sakheim, & Abrahamson, 1988; Taylor, 2006). These are summarized in Table 12.3.

There are three classes of maladaptive schemas that define the schematic structure of PTSD; (1) negative beliefs about the self, (2) negative schemas about the world including other people, and (3) negative beliefs about the trauma and PTSD symptoms. Depending on the nature and frequency of trauma, individuals believe they are vulnerable, scarred by the traumatic experience, and likely to face more harm and danger in the future. They see the world as a dangerous, selfish, and cruel environment in which people are callous, critical, and untrustworthy. They may hold themselves partly responsible for the trauma and believe they have been forever damaged by the terrible

TABLE 12.3. Core Maladaptive Schemas That Characterize Posttraumatic Stress Disorder

Maladaptive beliefs	Clinical example
Beliefs about the self	
• Of being weak and vulnerable to future harm	"Because I am such a weak person, I am more likely to be harmed in the future."
• Cannot trust one's perceptions or judgments	"I can't trust myself anymore because I make such poor judgments."
• Of being inferior to others	"I am not as strong and resourceful as other people."
• Of being a bad person for letting this happen	"I should be punished for letting this happen to me."
• Of lacking control or being effective	"I am unable to control what happens to me so I am incapable of protecting myself."
• Loss of autonomy or sense of being human (i.e., mental defeat)	"I have been defiled; I have lost all dignity and respect as a human being. I am just an object."
Beliefs about others	
• Of being alone	"I feel so empty and alone."
• That no one really cares	"No one really understands or cares about me."
• That others blame the victim for what happened or for not getting over it	"People blame me for what happened. They think I am exaggerating and should be able to put this all behind me."
• People are basically bad, evil, or malicious	"Human nature is basically evil and so capable of great cruelty."
• People will harm you and so can't be trusted	"People are cruel and will hurt you so you can't trust them."
• Human life is worthless, expendable	"There is no value or special meaning to a human life."
Beliefs about the world and future	
• The world is a dangerous place	"I can never be safe in such a dangerous world."
• There is little benevolence or good in the world	"In this world cruelty and selfishness are far more common than kindness or caring."
• Expectation of future harm and danger	"In the future bad things are likely to happen to me again."
Beliefs about the trauma	
• Harm is random and unpredictable	"You are in the greatest danger when you least expect it."
• Negative interpretation of responses during the trauma	"I should not have frozen during the attack."
• Failure to be more effective in protecting oneself.	"I should have fought off the attacker. If I had, I wouldn't be suffering as much as I am now."
• About causing the trauma	"I should have known better than to walk alone."
• About the long-term negative effects of trauma	"I will never be the same after what happened to me."

(cont.)

TABLE 12.3. *(cont.)*

Maladaptive beliefs	Clinical example
Beliefs about the Posttraumatic Stress Disorder	
• That the disorder has enduring negative consequences	"I will never get over PTSD. It has ruined my life."
• The catastrophic misinterpretation of particular symptoms of posttraumatic stress disorder	"I must be going crazy because I keep having these uncontrollable flashbacks."
• The need to exercise greater self-control over trauma-related symptoms	"I will never get better as long as I keep thinking about the trauma."
• Self-blame for having posttraumatic stress disorder	"I have PTSD because I am a weak, helpless person."
• Thwarted life goals and purpose	"I will never achieve my life goals or live a productive, fulfilling life."
• About the importance of controlling negative emotions	"I need to keep tight control over my emotions or I will become overwhelmed by them."
• The beneficial effects of avoidance	"It is better to avoid anything that is potentially upsetting or reminds me of the trauma."

event(s) in their life. They believe that PTSD will continue to have an enduring negative effect and this negative interpretation of PTSD symptoms, especially intrusive recollections of the trauma, will cause the individual to engage in maladaptive control strategies that have the unintended effect of contributing to the persistence of the disorder (D. M. Clark & Ehlers, 2004). In cognitive therapy of PTSD a great deal of effort is focused on modification of these three types of core maladaptive schemas and their associated appraisals.

How trauma is represented in working memory is an important aspect of the maladaptive schema constellation in PTSD. There is general agreement among researchers that trauma is stored differently in those with PTSD compared to those who experienced trauma without persistent PTSD (see previous discussion of Brewin et al., 1996; Dalgleish, 2004). Ehlers and Clark (2000) argue that the intrusive characteristics of PTSD are due to poor elaboration (i.e., fragmentation) and integration of the trauma memory into its context in time, place, and other informational sources as well as with other autobiographical memories. In addition strong stimulus–stimulus and stimulus–response associations as well as reduced perceptual threshold for trauma-related stimuli causes unintended, cue-driven retrieval so that the individual has reexperiencing symptoms caused by exposure to triggers and activation of trauma memory that is outside awareness (D. M. Clark & Ehlers, 2004; Ehlers & Clark, 2000). Ehlers and D. M. Clark concluded that the disorganized, fragmented representation of trauma contributes to a sense of current threat by creating selective recall of trauma details and forming strong associations between certain trauma stimuli and appraisals of severe danger to self.

Faulty Trauma Memory Retrieval

In the current cognitive model, we propose that a sensory-rich, fragmented or poorly elaborated memory of trauma that cannot be accommodated with other autobiographical memories will maintain a low activation threshold so that it provides recurring confirmatory evidence for the negative beliefs about the self, world, future, and trauma. In turn these negative core beliefs will bias memory recall so that individuals will recall aspects of the trauma that are congruent with the dysfunctional PTSD schemas. Because the memory structure for trauma is fragmented and poorly elaborated, the individual experiences recurring intrusive recollections of the trauma that confirm the negative core schemas of PTSD. Thus a reciprocal relationship exists between the way trauma is represented in memory and the dysfunctional core schemas about the self, world, and future. Aspects of the trauma will be recalled that confirm negative beliefs about a dangerous world, a vulnerable self, and the enduring negative consequences of PTSD. Information inconsistent with the posttrauma schemas will be inaccessible for retrieval because it is not represented in the trauma memory.

An example of biased and fragmented trauma recall emerged during cognitive therapy sessions with Edward. One of the traumatic events Edward experienced while in Rwanda was the apparent murder of a 5-year-old orphaned girl and her friends by the RPA. Edward assumed the children had been murdered because they were no longer at the orphanage at his last visit and an RPA soldier was present, with a smile on his face, and gesturing by sliding his hand across his throat toward the Canadian soldiers. Edward interpreted this to mean that the soldiers had slaughtered the children. However, when we explored this memory in depth, it was clear there was other information inconsistent with this assumption such as no indication from the nuns who cared for the children that some of the children had been taken away and murdered. Also this incident occurred after the genocide had ceased when many children were being returned to their villages. Edward was shocked to realize that all these years he had not remembered other information that was incompatible with his immediate interpretation of the event. It was clear that all he had encoded was the ominous presence of the RPA soldier and the disappearance of the children. In cognitive therapy of PTSD, a great deal of effort is directed toward evaluating and restructuring the trauma memory so that it ceases to be a source of confirmatory evidence for the core negative schemas of self, world, and future.

Attentional Threat Bias

Like other anxiety disorders, dominance of the maladaptive schematic constellation of threat and vulnerability will lead to an automatic attentional bias for threat. Since the traumatic experience has violated basic positive self-referent schemas about personal safety and security, we expect that the attentional bias in PTSD is for generalized threat and danger and not just information specific to the trauma. Trauma-related information should have the greatest pull on attention but any information that represents a personal danger is expected to have processing priority.

Traumatic Intrusions and Physiological Arousal

In the cognitive model (see Figure 12.1), the reexperiencing symptoms and physiological hyperarousal in PTSD are products of maladaptive schema activation and fragmented, sensory-rich trauma memory, as well as consequent selective attention and recall of trauma-relevant threat information. Researchers have proposed that Criterion C symptoms (i.e., avoidance and numbing) are maladaptive responses to the symptoms of Criteria B (reexperiencing) and D (physiological/emotional arousal) (Ehlers & Steil, 1995; Wilson, 2004; see Resick et al., 2008, for discussion). Thus automatic faulty information processing of trauma is the basis for the persistence of reexperiencing intrusions and physiological/emotional arousal, whereas avoidance and numbing are maladaptive coping responses that are a product of more conscious, elaborative processing efforts.

Clinician Guideline 12.12

Intrusive recollections of trauma and physiological/emotional hyperarousal symptoms are due to automatic information processing involving (1) activation of maladaptive schematic structures about self, vulnerability, world, others, and future; (2) fragmented mental representation of the traumatic experience; (3) selective retrieval of trauma information; and (4) attentional bias for personal threat. Consequently cognitive restructuring of negative beliefs about self, world, future, trauma, and PTSD symptoms as well as promotion of a more elaborated, integrated, and conceptually based trauma memory are key elements in cognitive therapy for PTSD.

Elaborative Processing

Negative Appraisals of Trauma-Related Intrusions and Arousal

The frequent intrusion of trauma-related thoughts and images as well as heightened physiological arousal will lead to a conscious, deliberate reappraisal of current threat, personal vulnerability, and the enduring negative effects of the trauma. In fact it is this deliberate reappraisal of the trauma intrusions that produces the sense of a serious current threat (Ehlers & Clark, 2000). Because trauma-related intrusions are usually inaccurate recollections of what happened that are highly distressing, uncontrollable, and more reflective of data-driven processing (i.e., processing of sensory perceptions more than the meaning of the event), the individual with PTSD will misinterpret the intrusive symptoms in a threatening, even catastrophic manner (see Falsetti, Monnier, & Resnick, 2005, for discussion). For example, Edward experienced intrusive memories of Rwanda as well as flashbacks about the little orphan girl many times throughout the day and as terrifying nightmares during the night. He interpreted these symptoms as an indication that he was not getting better and that his life was ruined by PTSD. He wondered if the flashbacks in particular might eventually "drive him crazy." His heightened state of arousal was perceived as highly aversive and a sign of losing control. He concluded that he must be weak and incompetent for losing control of his thoughts and emotions, and considered his future bleak, characterized by persistent distress and an inability to achieve anything worthwhile or satisfying in his life.

Ehlers and Steil (1995) proposed that the negative appraisal of intrusive symptoms was an important contributor to the persistence of PTSD. Negative idiosyncratic meanings of intrusive symptoms will cause an associated level of distress that confirms their threatening nature. In addition negative interpretations of the intrusive symptoms will motivate the person to employ cognitive and behavioral avoidance strategies that inadvertently lead to an increase in intrusion frequency and associated distress. Likewise, in the current cognitive model (see Figure 12.1), the negative appraisal of trauma-related intrusions will lead to a variety of control efforts that might reduce reexperiencing symptoms and emotional arousal, but in the long term they contribute to the persistence of PTSD.

Cognitive Control and Suppression Efforts

The activation of maladaptive posttrauma schemas, the dominance of threat-biased information processing, the repeated occurrence of intrusive recollections, and the negative appraisal of these trauma-related intrusions will cause the individual with PTSD to be strongly motivated to immediately terminate the intrusions and reduce their associated distress. A variety of cognitive and behavioral strategies will be employed that lead to quick relief of PTSD symptoms even though they contribute to the persistence of the disorder over the longer term. Ehlers and Clark (2000) note that maladaptive control strategies contribute to the maintenance of PTSD by directly producing symptoms, preventing change in the negative appraisals of the trauma, and preventing change in the trauma memory itself.

Thought suppression is a common maladaptive coping strategy found in PTSD. In his review Rassin (2005) concluded that trying not to think about a trauma can lead to the same paradoxical increase in the frequency of trauma-related intrusions as seen in the suppression of more neutral thoughts like white bears. However, it is unclear what effects suppression may have on the quality of the recollection. Furthermore, active attempts to dismiss an intrusive image of the trauma, for example, may increase its salience by confirming the individual's misinterpretation of threat. Failure to effectively gain control over the intrusion would confirm the individual's belief that these trauma-related thoughts or images really are a threat to personal well-being that will lead to long-term negative consequences (i.e., Ehlers & Steil, 1995; Ehlers & Clark, 2000). Other untoward effects of thought suppression might be an increase in the individual's level of distress as well as cognitive load, which would make it harder to concentrate on daily tasks and activities. Thus attempts to suppress trauma-related intrusions might paradoxically increase the extent of their interference in daily functioning, which would reinforce the patient's belief that PTSD symptoms are having significant and enduring negative consequences.

Two other response strategies associated with trauma-related intrusions are *rumination* and *dissociation* (Ehlers & Clark, 2000). *Rumination* is a persistent, recyclic, and passive form of thinking about the trauma and its consequences that leaves individuals with PTSD stuck in their current emotional state (i.e., Ehlers & Clark, 2000; Papageorgiou & Wells, 2004). Ehlers and Clark suggested that rumination is a cognitive avoidance strategy that strengthens negative appraisals of the trauma and might interfere with the formation of more complete trauma memories. Dissociative symptoms such as derealization, depersonalization, and emotional numbing may be automatic or deliberate cognitive coping strategies intended to avoid awareness of distressing recollections of the trauma or to suppress hyperarousal symptoms (Taylor, 2006). Ehlers and Clark (2000) suggested that dissociative symptoms might impede elaboration of the trauma memory and its integration with other autobiographical memories.

Search for Safety and Avoidance

Avoidance is so pervasive in PTSD that it is included as an important diagnostic criterion. Behavioral (i.e., avoiding people, places, or other cues that are reminders of the
trauma), cognitive (i.e., avoiding thinking about aspects of the trauma), and experiential
(i.e., avoiding negative emotions associated with the trauma) avoidance are included in
Criterion C. As in the other anxiety disorders, avoidance is a maladaptive strategy that
prevents disconfirmation of the dysfunctional beliefs and appraisals of current threat. In
this way avoidance will contribute to the persistence of PTSD. In addition, other behaviors may be initiated in order to provide a sense of safety. Edward, for example, avoided
large crowds because they reminded him of the throngs of hungry and frightened Rwandans in overcrowded refugee camps. Moreover, hypervigilance in public places was a
safety behavior he used to anticipate any cue that might remind him of Rwanda. Despite
his reliance on avoidance and safety behaviors, the person with PTSD rarely achieves
the "sense of safety" that he so desperately seeks.

Clinician Guideline 12.13

Deliberate attempts to manage the unwanted reexperiencing symptoms and hyperarousal
of PTSD significantly contribute to a persistence of the disorder. Threat misinterpretations
of trauma-related intrusions, ineffective thought control efforts, emotional and behavioral
avoidance, and reliance on safety-seeking responses each contribute to the persistence of a
negative emotional state and the disorder itself. Modification or replacement of these maladaptive response strategies is an important component of cognitive therapy for PTSD.

Persistence of Distress

The end result of the maladaptive automatic and elaborative posttrauma processes
described in the cognitive model is the persistence of a negative emotional state. It is well
known that anxiety is not the only negative emotion experienced in PTSD. Individuals
also experience other strong emotions such as shame, guilt, anger, and sadness (Resick,
Monson, & Rizvi, 2008). From the cognitive perspective, a more generalized negative
emotional state is expected given the broad range of dysfunctional schemas involved in
PTSD such as threat to safety and well-being, heightened personal vulnerability, and
negative worldview. As noted in Figure 12.1 the relationship between faulty information processing and negative emotional state is bidirectional, with a persistent negative
affective state feeding back to ensure the continued activation of the PTSD schematic
constellation.

EMPIRICAL STATUS OF THE COGNITIVE MODEL

In this section we review the empirical support for the cognitive model of PTSD. Seven
hypotheses are proposed that are critical to the cognitive model, although this does not
preclude other predictions that can be derived from the model. However, we consider
these seven hypotheses most important for evaluating the empirical status of the model.

Hypothesis 1

In PTSD encoding of trauma information is characterized by a data-driven processing mode that results in enhanced processing of threat and danger features of the trauma.

Studies employing semistructured interviews or questionnaires have investigated whether individuals with PTSD differed from those without PTSD in how they processed the trauma. In a study of 92 individuals who were assaulted, those with PTSD reported significantly more mental defeat, mental confusion, and detachment during the assault than those without PTSD (Dunmore et al., 1999). In a prospective study these same cognitive variables predicted PTSD symptom severity at 6- and 9-month follow-up (Dunmore et al., 2001). In another study individuals with PTSD following an assault reported more trauma memory dissociation, data-driven processing, and lack of self-referent processing than those without PTSD, and these variables predicted PTSD symptoms at 6-month follow-up (Halligan et al., 2003). However, these cognitive processing variables and the memory disorganization associated with trauma encoding may not be specific to PTSD when compared to other emotional sequela of trauma such as depression and phobias (Ehring, Ehlers, & Glucksman, 2006).

Item-cued directed forgetting is an information-processing paradigm that can be used to investigate the differential encoding of trauma information. Individuals are instructed to either remember or to forget a series of words, with subsequent recall usually worse for "to-be-forgotten" words than "to-be-remembered" items. In a study of adult survivors of childhood sexual abuse, those with PTSD showed no recall deficits or enhanced processing of trauma words, indicating that they did not exhibit an avoidant encoding style for trauma words (McNally, Metzger, Lasko, Clancy, & Pitman, 1998; see also Zoellner, Sacks, & Foa, 2003, for similar findings). In an analogue study in which students watched real-life footage of a hospital emergency room case, those instructed to focus on medical procedures reported significantly fewer intrusive recollections of the film in the subsequent week although there was no difference in self-reported memory disorganization (Laposa & Alden, 2006). A focus on medical procedures is consistent with reliance on a more organized, contextual processing of stressful situations. Overall there is consistent support for Hypothesis 1, that individuals with PTSD evidence a problematic encoding of trauma information, when specialized self-report measures are employed. Experimental support for this hypothesis has been less consistent and clearly requires further research.

Clinician Guideline 12.14

Individuals with PTSD encode traumatic information in a manner that results in a disorganized, fragmented memory of the trauma. However, the exact nature of the problematic encoding style remains uncertain, although perceptual or data-driven processing may predominate over conceptually based processing. For the cognitive therapist, assessment of the trauma memory should include processing variables like mental defeat, lack of self-referent perspective, extent of data-driven versus conceptual-based processing, mental confusion, and detachment.

Hypothesis 2

Negative beliefs about a vulnerable self, a dangerous world, the threatening effects of trauma, and the adverse consequences of PTSD symptoms are more characteristic of individuals with persistent PTSD than traumatized victims without persistent PTSD.

There are two ways that dysfunctional beliefs in PTSD can be investigated. At the most basic level, cross-sectional studies have compared endorsement of negative beliefs following trauma exposure in PTSD versus non-PTSD groups. However, one can also examine the issue longitudinally and ask whether trauma has had a greater negative impact on the core beliefs of individuals with PTSD. This latter question is more difficult to answer but is probably more germane to the cognitive model.

A number of cross-sectional studies have compared endorsement of dysfunctional beliefs using self-report questionnaires. Dunmore and colleagues found that negative beliefs about the effects of the trauma were significantly higher in the PTSD group compared to non-PTSD individuals and were related to PTSD severity at 6- and 9-month follow-up (Dunmore et al., 1999, 2001). Belief that future assaults are less likely was associated with lower distress in female sexual assault survivors assessed 2 weeks, 2 months, 6 months, and 12 months after the assault (Frazier, 2003). In a study of 124 New York municipal workers 6 months after the 9/11 terrorist attacks, beliefs reflecting increased expectation of future terrorist attacks and lost confidence in oneself were associated with greater PTSD symptoms (Piotrkowski & Brannen, 2002).

The Posttraumatic Cognitions Inventory (PTCI), which was developed to assess appraisals of trauma and its sequelae, contain many items that actually assess more enduring negative beliefs (e.g., "People can't be trusted," "If I think about the event, I will not be able to handle it," "The world is a dangerous place"). Traumatized individuals with PTSD score significantly higher on the PTCI than individuals without PTSD (Foa, Ehlers, Clark, Tolin, & Orsillo, 1999), although less consistent results have been obtained for the Self-Blame subscale (Startup, Makgekgenene, & Webster, 2007). Also elevated scores on Negative Cognitions about the Self and the World subscales but not PTCI Self-Blame were significantly correlated with PTSD symptoms assessed 3 months after the initial assessment (Field, Norman, & Barton, 2008). In a group of firefighter trainees, Bryant and Guthrie (2007) found that negative self-appraisals (i.e., PTCI Self subscale) during training predicted severity of posttraumatic stress after at least 3 years of active duty that involved multiple exposure to trauma. In addition to evidence that presence of pretrauma dysfunctional beliefs (e.g., negative self-appraisals) predicts tendency to develop PTSD after trauma exposure, optimistic pretrauma beliefs might buffer the effects of trauma (see Taylor, 2006, for discussion). On the other hand, Dunmore et al. (2001) found that change in negative beliefs due to trauma exposure was not a significant predictor of PTSD symptom severity (Dunmore et al., 2001).

Overall there is consistent evidence that individuals with PTSD hold negative beliefs about a vulnerable self, a dangerous world, and the threat of future trauma. The theme of continuing threat and a vulnerable self appear to capture the essence of the negative schematic organization in PTSD. Negative beliefs about the self may be a particularly potent predictor of subsequent posttrauma symptoms. However, it is not entirely clear whether these maladaptive beliefs reflect enduring pretrauma schemas or a change in perspective brought about by trauma exposure.

Clinician Guideline 12.15

Modification of dysfunctional beliefs about a vulnerable self, dangerous world, expectation of future threat, and alienation from others is the primary emphasis in cognitive therapy of PTSD.

Hypothesis 3

Individuals with PTSD will exhibit an automatic attentional bias for information representing a threat to personal safety.

An early review of information-processing studies of PTSD concluded that evidence for an automatic processing bias for threat cues was mixed but the findings were more consistent for a strategic or elaborative attentional bias for trauma-relevant stimuli (Buckley, Blanchard, & Neill, 2000). Most studies have employed the modified Stroop task and investigated attentional bias only at the elaborative stage of information processing. In one of the first studies, Vietnam combat veterans with PTSD showed a significant interference effect that was specific to combat-relevant words but not OCD, positive, or neutral words (McNally, Kaspi, et al., 1990). This supraliminal Stroop interference effect for trauma information has been replicated with motor vehicle accident survivors with PTSD (e.g., J. G. Beck et al., 2001; Bryant & Harvey, 1995), rape victims with PTSD (e.g., Cassiday, McNally, & Zeitlin, 1992), and crime victims with acute PTSD (Paunovic, Lundh, & Öst, 2002) . However, some studies have found that color-naming interference may not be specific to trauma stimuli but sensitive to all emotional stimuli (Vrana et al., 1995; see also Paunovic et al., 2002) and that the attentional bias may be evident only at the elaborative processing stage (Buckley et al., 2002; McNally, Amir, & Lipke, 1996; Paunovic et al., 2002). Finally, attentional bias for trauma may be related to severity of reexperiencing intrusions but not avoidance symptoms (Cassiday et al., 1992).

Findings from other studies also suggest that the attentional bias for threat in PTSD may not be as straightforward as predicted by the cognitive model. Employing a dot probe detection task, individuals with PTSD did not evidence an attentional bias for trauma-relevant pictures compared to nonclinical controls even though they had accelerated heart rate to the trauma-related stimuli (Elsesser, Sartory, & Tackenberg, 2004). Based on a visual search task involving threat and nonthreat target words and distractors, Vietnam veterans with high PTSD symptoms showed attentional interference but not facilitation for threat words (Pineles, Shipherd, Welch, & Yovel, 2007). This finding is consistent with the Stroop interference studies and suggests that the attentional bias in PTSD reflects difficulty disengaging from threat-relevant cues. It is also apparent that the attentional bias for trauma is more transient than enduring as the effect appears to wane with repetition (McNally et al., 1996) or can be suppressed when individuals with PTSD anticipate exposure to a mildly threatening situation (Constans et al., 2004).

In summary there is considerable empirical support for attentional bias for trauma-related information in PTSD. However, there has been little support for a preconscious (but probably involuntary) attentional bias and it is unclear whether the bias is content-specific to trauma. More research is needed using experimental tasks other than the emotional Stroop task in order to determine the robustness of the attentional bias. Like other anxiety disorders, however, the attentional bias in PTSD more likely reflects difficulty disengaging from threat rather than the facilitation of threat cues.

Clinician Guideline 12.16

Avoidance of trauma-relevant situations may be a coping strategy used to curb an attentional bias for threat in PTSD. Graded *in vivo* exposure that is often used in cognitive therapy to decrease avoidance may also address faulty attentional processing bias of trauma-related stimuli.

Hypothesis 4

PTSD is characterized by a selective and distorted recall of trauma-related threat and danger information.

Given the prominence of trauma-related intrusions and other reexperiencing symptoms in PTSD, the cognitive model predicts that selective recall of traumatic events is an important contributor to the persistence of PTSD. In fact most cognitive theories of PTSD consider fragmented representation of trauma in memory a central cognitive process in the disorder (e.g., Brewin et al., 1996; Ehlers & Clark, 2000; Horowitz, 2001). If trauma representation in PTSD is problematic, we might expect enhanced recall of trauma cues and more disorganized, unelaborated autobiographical memory for trauma.

In their review Buckley et al. (2000) concluded there is evidence that PTSD is characterized by an implicit and explicit memory recall bias for trauma stimuli. The most consistent finding is that individuals with PTSD show enhanced recall of trauma or emotion words generally compared to non-PTSD trauma individuals or healthy controls (e.g., Kaspi, McNally, & Amir, 1995; Paunovic et al., 2002; Vrana et al., 1995). However, support for an implicit memory bias has been more inconsistent, with Amir, McNally, and Wiegartz (1996) finding an implicit memory bias for trauma-specific sentences in a high but not medium or low noise condition, whereas others have failed to find disorder-specific effects (e.g., McNally & Amir, 1996; Paunovic et al., 2002). These findings, then, indicate that individuals with PTSD have enhanced explicit recall of trauma information that could contribute to the persistence of intrusive reexperiencing symptoms. However, there is less evidence that this memory bias is evident at a more automatic, preconscious level of processing.

More studies have investigated the organization of traumatic memory, especially whether trauma memories in PTSD involve more data-driven (i.e., greater processing of sensory impressions and perceptual characteristics of the trauma) than conceptual-driven (i.e., processing that focuses on the meaning of a trauma) processing. In a questionnaire study Halligan, Michael, Clark, and Ehlers (2003) found that compared to assault victims without PTSD, those with PTSD had more disorganized trauma memories, more dissociation, and more data-driven encoding of the trauma. These findings have been replicated in children with ASD following assaults or motor vehicle accidents (Meiser-Stedman et al., 2007). Furthermore, McKinnon, Nixon, and Brewer (2008) found that perceptions of trauma memory quality mediated the relationship between data-driven processing and intrusive reexperiencing symptoms in 75 children who had an injury that led to hospital treatment. In two analogue studies Halligan, Clark, and Ehlers (2002) found that data-driven processing of a road accident videotape was associated with poor subsequent intentional recall of the videotape, more disorganized memory, and that students, who scored high on a trait data-driven processing questionnaire, reported more memory disorganization and PTSD symptoms. However, memory disorganization may not be as specific to PTSD as data-driven processing or lack of self-referential processing (Ehring, Ehlers, & Glucksman, 2006). In other studies individuals with PTSD showed significant forgetting of the 9/11 terrorist attacks across a 9-month interval (Qin et al., 2003) and individuals with PTSD retrieve fewer specific autobiographical memories (Sutherland & Bryant, 2008).

Evidence of memory impairment for traumatic events in PTSD is fairly robust. Most studies have found enhanced explicit recall of trauma-related cues and a consistent relationship has emerged between data-driven encoding of the trauma, a more fragmented or disorganized memory of the trauma, and PTSD reexperiencing symptoms. However, it is possible that PTSD has negative effects on memory more generally. A recent meta-analysis found a small to moderate association between PTSD and visual memory impairment of episodic, emotionally neutral material (Brewin, Kleiner, Vasterling, & Field, 2007). Moreover, Taylor (2006) concluded in his review that evidence for fragmented trauma memories is inconsistent at best. Despite lingering questions about the exact nature of poor memory in PTSD, there is considerable empirical evidence that individuals with PTSD have a selective, enhanced memory for the trauma that appears to be a contributor to the persistence of their symptomatology.

Clinician Guideline 12.17

Because individuals with PTSD have an enhanced, selective recall of trauma-related information, an important part of cognitive therapy is improvement of conceptual processing so that a more complete, organized adaptive memory of past traumatic experiences is constructed.

Hypothesis 5

Individuals with persistent PTSD are more likely to misinterpret their trauma-related intrusive thoughts and images in a negative, threatening manner than individuals without persistent PTSD.

This hypothesis proposes that the conscious, deliberate appraisal of intrusive recollections of the trauma in a negative or threatening manner is an important factor in the persistence of PTSD (Ehlers & Clark, 2000). Two sources of information are relevant to this hypothesis: (1) negative appraisals of the trauma, and (2) negative appraisals of reexperiencing symptoms.

A number of studies based on self-report measures have shown that negative appraisal of the trauma and its sequelae are more prominent in traumatized individuals with PTSD. The PTCI has been used most often to assess negative appraisals of trauma and its consequences (Foa, Ehlers, et al., 1999). In these studies perceptions that the trauma had a more negative effect on the self and more pervasive and enduring negative consequences correlated with severity of PTSD symptoms as well as specific symptoms such as severity of intrusions and extent of avoidance (e.g., Ehring et al., 2006; Laposa & Alden, 2003; Steil & Ehlers, 2000).

In addition negative appraisal of intrusive memories and other reexperiencing symptoms is more evident in traumatized individuals with PTSD and is positively correlated with PTSD symptom severity (Dunmore et al., 1999; Halligan et al., 2003; Steil & Ehlers, 2000). Moreover, negative appraisal of initial intrusive symptoms predicts persistence and severity of PTSD symptoms at 6- and 9-month follow-up (e.g., Dunmore et al., 2001; Halligan et al., 2003). These findings, then, are consistent with Hypothesis 5 and indicate that an explicit negative evaluation of trauma-related consequences, especially intrusive reexperiencing symptoms, plays an important role in the persistence of PTSD symptoms. However, this research is limited by an overreliance on retrospective self-report questionnaires. Future studies should consider expanding the assessment of appraisals beyond self-report questionnaires toward adopting more "online" and experimentally based methods of inquiry.

Clinician Guideline 12.18

Negative, maladaptive cognitions and beliefs about PTSD, especially trauma-related intrusions and their symptoms, is a major focus in cognitive therapy given the importance of explicit negative symptom appraisal in the persistence of PTSD.

Hypothesis 6

Maladaptive cognitive strategies like thought suppression, rumination, and dissociation will be significantly more prevalent in those with persistent PTSD compared with their non-PTSD counterparts.

Like other cognitive theories (e.g., Ehlers & Clark, 2000), the current cognitive model posits that presence of deliberate, effortful but maladaptive cognitive strategies like thought suppression, rumination, and dissociation are key contributors to the persistence of PTSD. These strategies are intended to prevent or terminate intrusive recollections and other reminders of the trauma. Although they may momentarily appear effective, in the long term they contribute to a heightened sense of anxiety and increased salience of trauma-related intrusions.

It is well known that individuals with PTSD engage in more peritraumatic dissociation than non-PTSD or recovered trauma survivors, and persistent dissociation is associated with the development of PTSD (Halligan et al., 2003; Ozer et al., 2003). However, it may that ongoing or persistent dissociation is more germane to chronic PTSD than state dissociation at the time of trauma (Ehring et al., 2006). In addition there is evidence that individuals with PTSD engage in ruminative thinking about the trauma and its consequences. Taylor (2006) noted that rumination in PTSD involves repeatedly asking oneself questions about why the trauma happened, whether it could have been prevented, and self-blame. Various studies have found that rumination is positively associated with PTSD symptoms (Meiser-Stedman et al., 2007; Steil & Ehlers, 2000), but this may not be disorder-specific since presence of rumination about trauma and its consequences may also be evident in traumatized individuals who suffer from depression or specific fears (Ehring et al., 2006).

There has been a great deal of research interest in the prevalence and impact of deliberate efforts to suppress trauma-related intrusions in PTSD. Self-report studies have found significantly higher rates of thought suppression in traumatized individuals with PTSD compared with non-PTSD controls (Ehring et al., 2006), and suppression was associated with increased symptom severity especially higher levels of intrusive thoughts (Laposa & Alden, 2003; Morgan et al., 1995). Nonclinical individuals who were shown a 3-minute film clip of a traumatic fire and who reported a stronger tendency to suppress unpleasant thoughts recorded more intrusions in a diary of intrusions kept over the subsequent week (Davies & Clark, 1998b). In a study of women who experienced pregnancy loss, thought suppression was 1 of 4 variables that mediated the relationship between peritraumatic dissociation and PTSD symptoms assessed at one and four months after the pregnancy loss (Engelhard et al., 2003). These correlational studies, then, indicate that deliberate thought suppression may be a maladaptive coping strategy that is associated with the persistence of PTSD.

A number of experimental studies have shown that active efforts to suppress trauma-relevant thoughts paradoxically lead to a significant increase in the unwanted intrusions, especially when suppression efforts cease. In an early thought suppression study, Harvey and Bryant (1998a) found that ASD participants who were instructed to suppress their trauma-related thoughts had significantly more trauma-related intrusions after suppression efforts ceased than those instructed not to suppress. However, Guthrie and Bryant (2000) failed to replicate this finding in a group of civilian trauma survivors with or without ASD. A more direct investigation of the role of thought suppression in PTSD was conducted by Shipherd and Beck (1999). Female sexual assault survivors with PTSD evidenced a significant rebound of rape-related thoughts after suppression efforts ceased, whereas assault survivors without PTSD did not show this rebound effect. Likewise, Amstadter and Vernon (2006) found that individuals with and without PTSD experienced immediate enhancement of trauma and neutral thoughts during suppression, but only the PTSD group had a postsuppression rebound effect that was specific to the trauma thoughts. Furthermore, individuals with a repressive coping style may be more successful suppressing negative target thoughts in the short term but over longer time intervals (i.e., 1 week) their repressive style leads to more unwanted negative thoughts (Geraerts et al., 2006). Although the findings are by no means robust, there is sufficient evidence to indicate that deliberate suppression of trauma-related intrusive thoughts is counterproductive in the long run and probably contributes to a higher frequency of intrusive reexperiencing symptoms.

Clinician Guideline 12.19

Reduction in maladaptive cognitive strategies such as thought suppression, rumination, and even dissociation is an important focus in cognitive therapy because these strategies contribute to the persistence of trauma-related reexperiencing symptoms.

Hypothesis 7

Avoidance of trauma-related cues and safety seeking will be more frequent in persistent PTSD compared to non-PTSD states.

As in the other anxiety disorders, avoidance and reliance on safety seeking are considered important contributors to the persistence of PTSD symptoms. This last hypothesis proposes a direct relationship such that greater avoidance and safety seeking contributes to a more persistent, severe, and adverse posttraumatic state.

There is empirical evidence in support of this contention. Dunmore et al. (1999) found that assault victims with persistent PTSD were significantly more likely to engage in avoidance and safety seeking in the month after the assault than those without PTSD. In a 9-month follow-up study, use of avoidance and safety seeking 1 month after an assault predicted severity of PTSD at 9 months even after controlling for severity of the assault (Dunmore et al., 2001). However, emotional numbing, which is a type of avoidance common in PTSD, has had stronger support from self-report than experimental studies. For example, in a study of autonomic and facial muscle response to emotionally evocative pictures, Vietnam veterans with PTSD did not show augmented or suppressed emotional response to pleasant or unpleasant picture stimuli, although they did show reduced response to pleasant emotional stimuli after being primed with trauma-related pictures (Litz et al., 2000). This latter effect would be consistent with reduced response and possibly poorer cognitive processing of safety cues after exposure to trauma-relevant information.

Clinician Guideline 12.20

In vivo exposure that targets reduction in avoidance and safety-seeking behaviors in trauma-relevant situations and improvement in processing positive safety cues is an important therapeutic ingredient of cognitive therapy of PTSD.

COGNITIVE ASSESSMENT AND CASE FORMULATION

Diagnostic Interview and Symptom Measures

The SCID-IV (First et al., 1997) and ADIS-IV (Brown et al., 1994) both have PTSD modules that closely adhere to the DSM-IV diagnostic criteria. The SCID-IV PTSD module (or earlier SCID for DSM-III) has sound psychometric properties with (1) an interrater reliability kappa of .66 and 78% diagnostic agreement (Keane et al., 1998), (2) high convergent validity with other PTSD symptom measures, and (3) substantial sensitivity (.81) and specificity (.98) (see Keane, Brief, Pratt, & Miller, 2007, for discussion). However, the SCID-IV has been criticized for assessing symptoms based only on the "worst event" experienced as well as relying on a trauma screen that may be inaccurate (Keane et al., 2007).

The psychometric properties of the ADIS-IV PTSD module are promising but less well established. Blanchard, Gerardi, Kolb, and Barlow (1986) reported an interrater kappa of .86 (93% agreement) for the DSM-III version of the interview schedule. However, limitations of the ADIS-IV have been noted such as the failure to provide a total score cutoff for caseness or to recommend whether symptom item endorsements in the rare or mild range should count toward meeting diagnostic criteria (Litz, Miller, Ruef, & McTeague, 2002). Thus the ADIS-IV may not be as strong in diagnosing PTSD as it is with other anxiety disorders.

Clinician-Administered PTSD Scale

The Clinician-Administered PTSD Scale (CAPS) is the most widely used and best researched of the diagnostic interview schedules for PTSD. Developed by the National Center for PTSD (Blake et al., 1998), the CAPS is a structured interview that assesses current and lifetime DSM-IV diagnostic status and symptom severity of PTSD and ASD. It consists of a 17-item life event checklist that patients complete over their entire life according to whether the event "happened to me," "witnessed it," "learned about it," "not sure," or "doesn't apply." From items endorsed on the checklist, the clinician selects up to three events that were the worst or most recent and then asks for a description of the event and the client's emotional response to each event to determine exposure to trauma (i.e., DSM-IV Criterion A1 and A2). This is followed by 17 questions on the frequency and severity of each of the core DSM-IV symptoms of PTSD which are rated on four-point Likert scales that can be summed to create a severity score for each symptom category. Five additional questions determine the onset and duration of symptoms (Criterion E), as well as subjective distress and social and occupational impairment (Criterion F). Three global ratings are made on validity of the patient's responses, overall severity of PTSD symptoms, and degree of symptom change or improvement in past 6 months. Finally, 5 additional questions may be administered to assess the associated features of guilt over actions, survivor guilt, reduction in awareness, derealization, and depersonalization.

It includes a summary sheet in which a subscale score is calculated for each criterion and it is determined whether the patient meets current and lifetime diagnosis of PTSD. A total severity score can be determined by summing over the 17 core symptoms and interpreted with respect to five severity scores ranging from asymptomatic to extreme, with a 15-point change indicating clinically significant change (Weathers, Keane, & Davidson, 2001). Nine different scoring rules can be used to derive PTSD diagnoses from the CAPS frequency and intensity scores and will yield different prevalence rates of PTSD depending on whether they are relatively lenient or stringent (Weathers, Ruscio, & Keane, 1999). Administration of the complete CAPS takes approximately 1 hour (Keane et al., 2007).

The CAPS has sound psychometric properties. Based on five samples of Vietnam veterans, Weathers et al. (1999) found high interrater reliability for the three symptom clusters (r's = .86 to .91) and kappas of .89 and 1.00 for test–retest reliability for a CAPS PTSD diagnosis (see Weathers et al., 2001, for discussion). The 17 symptom items also had high internal consistency and close agreement with a SCID-based diagnosis of PTSD (sensitivity = .91; specificity = .84, efficiency = .88, kappa = .75). Weathers et al. (1999) also found that the CAPS total severity score correlated highly with self-report symptom measures of PTSD (r's = .77 to .94) and moderately with depression and anxiety symptoms (see Weathers et al., 2001, for discussion). In their review of 10 years of research on the CAPS, Weathers et al. (2001) concluded that the CAPS has high interrater reliability, excellent diagnostic utility, strong convergent validity, and sensitivity to clinical change when used by trained and calibrated interviewers, although less is known about its discriminant validity. Clearly, the CAPS is the recommended diagnostic interview protocol for PTSD. The CAPS is available from the National Center for PTSD (*www.ncptsd.va.gov/ncmain/assessment*).

Impact of Event Scale

The Impact of Event Scale (IES) is a 15-item questionnaire developed by Horowitz, Wilner, and Alvarez (1979) to assess intrusion and avoidance symptoms of trauma exposure. After the publication of DSM-IV a revised 22-item version (IES-R) was developed that includes six new items on hyperarousal and one item concerning dissociative reexperiencing symptoms or flashbacks (Weiss & Marmar, 1997). More psychometric research is needed on the IES-R before it can be used in clinical practice (Keane et al., 2007).

Mississippi Scale for Combat-Related PTSD

The Mississippi Scale for Combat-Related PTSD (MPTSD) is a 35-item questionnaire designed to assess combat-related PTSD symptoms (Keane, Caddell, & Taylor, 1988) that has been updated to reflect DSM-IV criteria. Respondents rate the severity of symptoms on a Likert scale in the time interval after experiencing trauma. The MPTSD has excellent psychometric properties including high internal consistency (a = .94), one week test-retest reliability (r = .97), diagnostic utility and convergent validity (Keane et al., 1988; McFall, Smith, Roszell, Tarver, & Malas, 1990). A cutoff score of 106 or above may be optimal for determining a diagnosis of PTSD (Keane et al., 2007). The MPTSD is recommended when assessing combat-related PTSD.

Posttraumatic Stress Diagnostic Scale

The Posttraumatic Stress Diagnostic Scale (PDS) is a self-report questionnaire that provides a diagnosis of DSM-IV PTSD and assesses symptom severity (Foa, Cashman, Jaycox, & Perry, 1997). It has a checklist of 12 traumatic events from which respondents select the one that disturbed them most in the past month. Individuals then use a four-point rating scale to indicate the frequency over the past month of the 17 core symptoms of DSM-IV PTSD. An additional nine items assess impairment in different areas of daily function. A score of 1 or higher is required on symptoms in order to count toward a diagnosis of PTSD and the 17 symptom items can be summed to produce a severity score. In the validation study PDS Total Symptom Severity differentiated those who met a SCID diagnosis of PTSD from a non-PTSD group, had high internal consistency (alpha = .92), good 2 week test–retest reliability (r = .83), and high agreement (82%) with a SCID diagnosis. PDS Total Symptom Severity also correlates highly with CAPS Total (r = .71) and the recommended cutoff score of 15 shows high sensitivity (i.e., 89% of PTSD correctly identified) but poor specificity (Griffin, Uhlmansiek, Resick, & Mechanic, 2004). Griffin and colleagues concluded that the PDS is a good proxy to a full CAPS interview but tends to overestimate the prevalence of PTSD. The PDS is available from National Computer Systems (1-800-627-7271).

PTSD Checklist

The PTSD Checklist (PCL) is a 17-item questionnaire developed at the National Center for PTSD to assess severity of PTSD symptoms (see review by Norris & Hamblen, 2004). Revised for DSM-IV, symptoms are rated on five-point scales for the past month with two versions of the questionnaire available: one that assesses how much you are bothered by symptoms from stressful experiences in the past (PCL-C) or how much you are bothered by symptoms in reaction to a specific event (PCL-S). In addition there is a military version of the PCL (PCL-M). The PCL possesses sound psychometric properties. In the original validation study conducted on the PCL-M, the Total Score (summed over the 17 items) had high internal consistency (alpha = .97), test–retest reliability (r = .96), and strong convergent validity with other measures of PTSD (see Norris & Hamblen, 2004, for discussion). The reliability, convergent validity, and diagnostic efficiency of the PCL have been well supported (e.g., Blanchard, Jones-Alexander, Buckley, & Forneris, 1996; Bliese et al., 2008; Ruggiero, Del Ben, Scotti, & Rabalais, 2003). However, studies of the factorial validity of the PCL failed to confirm a three-factor model that corresponds to the DSM-IV three-factor structure (DuHamel et al., 2004; Palmieri et al., 2007). Even though a suggested cutoff score of 60 yielded good diagnostic utility when compared with the CAPS, different PCL scoring options tend to produce differences in sensitivity, specificity, and diagnostic efficiency (Pratt, Brief, & Keane, 2006). A lower cutoff value between 30 and 34 is recommended for primary care settings and 50 has been suggested for military samples (Bliese et al., 2008). The PCL, then, appears to be a strong measure of PTSD symptoms but suffers from the same limitations that are apparent in most self-report measures of the disorder. A copy of the PCL is available from the National Center for PTSD (*www.ncptsd.va.gov/ncmain/assessment*).

Measures of Cognition

Taylor (2006) noted that several measures have been developed to assess beliefs in trauma survivors but most are research instruments with little psychometric evaluation. For example, the World Assumptions Scale was developed by Janoff-Bulman (1989) to assess beliefs about the world that may be challenged by traumatic events. Although often cited in the PTSD literature, the measure appears to have some psychometric limitations (Kaler et al., 2008) and fails to assess the full range of beliefs described in current CBT models of PTSD.

Posttraumatic Cognitions Inventory

The Posttraumatic Cognitions Inventory (PTCI) is a 33-item questionnaire that assesses trauma-related thoughts and beliefs across three factorially derived cognitive domains: negative cognitions about self, negative cognitions about world, and self-blame for the trauma (Foa, Ehlers, et al., 1999). The factorial structure of the PTCI was supported in a confirmatory factor analysis of motor vehicle survivors (J. G. Beck et al., 2004). In the validation study the internal consistency coefficients of all three subscales were high (*a*'s of .86 to .97) and 1-week test–retest reliability indicated temporal stability (*r*'s of .75 to .89). The PTCI subscales and total score correlate highly with PTSD symptom severity (*r*'s of .57 to .79), depression, and general anxiety, and traumatized individuals with PTSD score significantly higher than traumatized non-PTSD or nontrauma comparison groups (Foa, Ehlers, et al., 1999).

The validity of the PTCI subscales have not been equally supported in subsequent studies. J. G. Beck et al. (2004) found that the PTCI Self-Blame subscale did not correlate with PTSD symptom severity nor did it distinguish between those with and without PTSD. The other two subscales and total score did show the expected convergent and discriminant validity. In a 12-month prospective study of injury survivors, path analysis revealed that the PTCI Negative Self was the most influential subscale in determining later PTSD symptoms whereas higher levels of PTCI Self-Blame in the acute phase were actually associated with improved psychological functioning (O'Donnell, Elliott, Wolfgang, & Creamer, 2007). All the PTCI subscales are sensitive to treatment effects, although Foa and Rauch (2004) found in their regression analyses that only the Negative Cognitions about Self subscale emerged as a significant predictor of change in PTSD symptoms. Samples with PTSD have a median score of 3.60 (*SD* = 1.48) and 5.00 (*SD* = 1.25) on the PTCI Negative Self and Negative World subscales, respectively, compared to 1.08 (*SD* = 0.76) and 2.07 (*SD* = 1.43), respectively, for nontrauma groups (Foa, Ehlers, Clark, Tolin, & Orsillo, 1999). Given the questionable validity of the Self-Blame items, clinicians should only use the Negative Self and Negative World subscales of the PTCI. The PTCI has been reprinted in Foa, Ehlers, et al. (1999).

Clinician Guideline 12.21

Cognitive assessment of PTSD should include (1) a diagnostic interview, preferably the CAPS; (2) a measure of PTSD symptom severity such as the PCL or PDS; and (3) the PTCI as a measure of appraisals and beliefs relevant to PTSD. Only the PTCI Negative Cognition about Self and Negative Cognition about World subscales should be interpreted given the questionable validity of the Self-Blame subscale.

Case Conceptualization

The cognitive case conceptualization follows from the cognitive model of PTSD proposed in this chapter (see Figure 12.1). Table 12.4 presents an outline of the various components of a case conceptualization for PTSD (see also Taylor, 2006). Although much of the information needed to develop a case formulation will be available from the diagnostic interview and standardized questionnaires, it is likely that additional questioning will be necessary to complete the cognitive case formulation described in Table 12.4.

Pretrauma Assumptions and Beliefs

An important objective of the case formulation is understanding how trauma has changed the client's beliefs and assumptions about the world, self, and other people. This requires an assessment of pretrauma beliefs, which in the clinical context requires one to rely on retrospective self-report. If the client is a poor historian, a spouse or family member can be interviewed to provide this crucial information.

TABLE 12.4. Cognitive Case Conceptualization for Posttraumatic Stress Disorder

Components	Specific elements
Pretrauma assumptions and beliefs	• Beliefs about world • Beliefs about self • Beliefs about other people
Nature of trauma	• Description of trauma, its severity, and interpersonal implications • Level of personal involvement in trauma • Negative effects of trauma on self and others • Emotional reactions at time of trauma • Level of social support and response of others to the trauma
Characteristics of trauma memory	• Selective recall of trauma with some elements showing enhancement whereas other features are poorly recalled • Degree of organization, coherence, and elaboration of trauma memory • Relative presence of data-driven versus conceptual-driven processing • Range of cues that trigger trauma recollection • Emotional reaction to trauma memory
Appraisals and beliefs associated with the trauma and its consequences	• Causal attributions and beliefs about the trauma • Negative self-referent thoughts and beliefs associated with the trauma • Perceived enduring consequences of the trauma (i.e., danger, safety, controllability) • Expectancy about the future (i.e., pessimism, hopeless, helpless) • Dysfunctional beliefs about the world and others
Interpretations of trauma-related intrusions and other reexperiencing symptoms	• Perceived enduring negative effects of intrusions and other symptoms of posttraumatic stress disorder • Presence of catastrophic thinking about posttraumatic stress disorder and its symptoms • Causal attributions of intrusive symptoms • Perceived controllability of symptoms • Personal meaning or significance of symptoms of posttraumatic stress disorder
Adaptive and maladaptive coping strategies	• Attempts to suppress trauma recollections • Presence of rumination • Extent of dissociation, emotional numbing, or deliberate suppression of expressive emotion • Ability to engage in adaptive coping
Avoidance and safety-seeking	• Nature and extent of avoidance • Types of safety-seeking behaviors • Perceived efficacy of safety seeking

It is important to determine if the trauma shattered preexisting, rigid beliefs that the world is generally a peaceful and safe place, or whether it reinforced extreme assumptions of the world as dangerous or violent. The following is an example of how clients could be questioned:

"I would be interested to know how you viewed the world, that is your personal world, before the trauma. Based on our experiences in childhood and adolescence, we all develop ideas or assumptions about the world we live in. What were your beliefs, your assumptions about the world before you had this traumatic experience? Did you believe and expect that the world was a safe, secure place for you, your family, and friends? Or the opposite, did you see the world as a dangerous place where you expected harm or physical injury to yourself or others? How strongly did you hold to these assumptions about the world? Did you ever question them? Were there important experiences in your past that confirmed or challenged your assumptions about the world?"

Given the central role of negative self-referent cognitions in PTSD, the clinician must assess the patient's preexisting self-schemas. The clinical interview should include questions about self-evaluation involving competence/incompetence, success/failure, acceptance/rejection, active/passive, loved/abandoned, liked/disliked, confident/unsure, weak/strong, and so on. Again it is important to determine the degree of rigidity and significance of the belief to the individual's self-view. From this the clinician should be able to conclude whether the trauma affected a person with a strong positive self-view or an individual with a weak and vulnerable sense of self.

Preexisting beliefs and assumptions about other people are also an important part of the assessment. Before the traumatic experience, did the client assume that people tended to be kind, caring, compassionate, and gentle? Or were opposite beliefs held, that people were basically selfish, cruel, manipulative, disinterested in others or hurtful? Was the client open and accepting toward others or suspicious and avoidant? Was the individual highly dependent on others (i.e., sociotropic) or more autonomous? From these questions the clinician should be able to determine individuals' level of acceptance of others, their expectations of others, and how much they depend on family and friends for emotional support.

Nature of Trauma

Like any assessment for PTSD, it is important that the cognitive therapist obtain a full and complete account of the trauma(s), their severity, and consequences. Some of this information is available from the diagnostic interview (e.g., CAPS) but this will have to be supplemented with more specific and detailed questions. As discussed in the first part of this chapter, there are many features of the trauma that are important to determine because of their impact on the development of PTSD. The following are some suggested questions that can be asked about the trauma.

- "What was the most recent traumatic experience? How many times have you experienced a serious threat to your safety, health, or well-being? How severe were these threats? Were they somehow related or quite different experiences? Which one was most disturbing for you?"
- "Did the event cause you physical harm, injury, or threat of death? Did you think you were going to die during the trauma? If the trauma did not happen to you, did you witness a tragedy happening to others or were you involved in helping victims of trauma? Or have you been mainly disturbed by hearing of an unexpected tragedy to a loved one?"
- "What effect has the trauma had on you? How has it changed the way you think, feel, and behave? Has it changed how you relate to others? How has it affected you in your daily living, in your work, family, and leisure time?"

- "How would you describe your emotional response after the trauma? How have you been feeling more generally (e.g., depressed, anxious, irritable)? What is your emotional response when reminded of the trauma or when you have intrusive memories of the trauma?"
- "What happened in the hours or days after you experienced the traumatic event? How did your family and friends react? What did they think about what happened to you? Did the trauma change how people related to you? If so, how? Was there any formal help offered to you such as medical or mental health services, or crisis intervention?"

Characteristics of Trauma Memory

Cognitive therapy for PTSD places considerable emphasis on modifying trauma-related intrusive thoughts, images, or memories and their interpretation. Consequently, a careful evaluation of the trauma memory is an important element of the case formulation. It is recommended that the therapist begin by having clients write down what they remember of the traumatic event. If this is too disturbing to complete as a homework assignment, the process could be started collaboratively in the therapy session. It should be explained that this task is important because trauma memories play an important role in the persistence of PTSD and being able to talk about the trauma is a critical step in the therapeutic process. Naturally the cognitive therapist needs to be supportive, caring, and understanding. For many clients this will be a very difficult process and they may have to work on their Trauma Memory Narrative over a number of sessions. Constructing a Trauma Memory Narrative has some similarities to the Impact Statement utilized in cognitive processing therapy (Resick & Schnicke, 1992; Resick, Monson, & Rizvi, 2008) or the trauma imaginal exposure scripts described in Foa and Rothbaum (1998).

Table 12.4 lists a number of factors that the clinician should look for in the Trauma Memory Narrative. What aspects of the trauma are especially well remembered? Are there gaps in memory or aspects of the event that are poorly recalled? How selective is the patient's recall of the trauma? How well does the patient respond to probing questions in order to obtain a more complete account of trauma? Is the Trauma Memory Narrative well elaborated or sketchy? Does it have coherence and organization, or is it quite fragmented? Is there evidence that the memory is primarily data-driven? To what extent are there attempts to derive some meaning or understanding of the trauma? How does the patient interpret the trauma memory? What does it mean or what implication does it have about the self, world, and future? What types of cues trigger or elicit the trauma memory? What is the client's emotional reaction when remembering the trauma? How intense or severe is the felt emotion? By the end of the third or fourth session, the cognitive therapist should have a fairly complete Trauma Memory Narrative as well as a profile of the client's interpretation and emotional response to the memory.

Trauma Beliefs and Appraisals

An in-depth account of the personal meaning of the trauma and its consequences is a central component of the cognitive case formulation. It will be a primary focus for cognitive intervention later in therapy. Trauma-related beliefs and interpretations fall within a number of thematic categories. It is important to determine the client's causal attributions for the trauma. Why does she think the trauma happened? What factors contributed to its occurrence? Does she engage in self-blame for the trauma or how she reacted during the trauma? Is there evidence of maladaptive personal responsibility beliefs? The clinician should also identify maladaptive beliefs associated with feelings of guilt, regret, or remorse that might be associated with the trauma.

Other types of negative self-referent thoughts and beliefs about the trauma and its consequences may also be present. Does the client hold unrealistic probability estimates of traumatic experiences happening to him in the future? Does he hold maladaptive beliefs about the unpredictability and uncontrollability of trauma? In what way are beliefs about the probability and severity of threat or danger exaggerated and those dealing with safety minimized? What is the client's thinking about the consequences of the trauma? Does he believe that it has led to enduring or permanent damaging changes to self or personal world? Does he believe it has changed how others relate to him? The clinician should identify how the client believes others now perceive him as a result of being a trauma victim.

The clinician also needs to identify beliefs and appraisals about future expectancies. How has the trauma changed individuals' attitudes and beliefs about their future? Have they become much more pessimistic and cynical about life and the world more generally? Does their future look bleak, empty, or meaningless? Do they believe they are now helpless, a victim of circumstances that will continue to dictate their life in an unpredictable and uncontrollable manner? Do they hold any ideas for change or for improving their life in the foreseeable future?

Beliefs and Interpretations of Intrusions

Another core element of the cognitive case formulation involves a description of how the person with PTSD interprets the unwanted intrusive thoughts, images, or memories of the trauma as well as the other prominent symptoms of PTSD. Ehlers, Clark, and colleagues have written extensively about the importance of appraisals of trauma sequelae in the persistence and severity of PTSD (D. M. Clark & Ehlers, 2004; Ehlers & Clark, 2000; Ehlers & Steil, 1995). These appraisals and beliefs focus on the personal meaning or significance of having PTSD. For each individual the clinician should determine what it is about having PTSD that is so personally distressing. What symptoms are most distressing or interfere most in the person's daily functioning? What negative effects are caused by intrusive symptoms? Are these effects considered enduring or permanent?

The cognitive therapist should also determine the individual's causal attributions for PTSD and assess for the presence of catastrophizing thinking. Why does the client think she has PTSD? How does she explain the presence of trauma-related intrusive memories or flashbacks? Does the patient believe that all symptoms of PTSD or recollections of the trauma must be eliminated before she can live a satisfying and productive life? Does she believe her life has been ruined by PTSD? What is the perceived significance or personal interpretation given to reexperiencing trauma memories, flashbacks, nightmares, and the like? How does she explain her apparent inability to control these symptoms or overcome the negative effects of the trauma? This in-depth assessment of negative appraisals and beliefs associated with intrusive reexperiencing symptoms plays an important role in shaping the treatment plan for cognitive therapy of PTSD.

Coping Strategies Profile

The cognitive case formulation should also include an assessment of individuals' attempts to minimize the presence of PTSD symptoms and their consequences. How prominent is active and intentional thought suppression in clients' response to unwanted trauma-related intrusions? Are there other types of maladaptive cognitive strategies used to prevent or terminate exposure to trauma-related intrusions? The checklist of cognitive coping strategies presented in Chapter 5 (see Appendix 5.9) can be used to identify maladaptive cognitive coping responses and their perceived effectiveness. Appendix 5.7 can also be utilized to assess for the presence of maladaptive behavioral coping responses associated with PTSD symptoms. Furthermore, the clinician should determine if rumination about PTSD and its effects or preoccupation with having frequent, unwanted trauma-related intrusions is prominent in the client's experience of the disorder.

Dissociation, emotional numbing, and deliberate suppression of emotion are often present in PTSD. Are these maladaptive coping responses frequent and what is their perceived effectiveness? How tolerant or accepting is the client of negative emotion? Can the client engage in healthy expression of negative emotion? How does the individual evaluate or interpret (i.e., understand) his episodes of anxiousness, anger, dysphoria, or guilt? Finally, are there adaptive strategies in the client's coping repertoire? How often are these strategies used, under what circumstances, and to what effect? The presence of some capacity to engage in adaptive coping can be an important starting point in therapy.

Avoidance and Safety Seeking

The final component of the cognitive case formulation involves a specification of the range of situations or trauma-related cues that are avoided as well as the types of safety-seeking behaviors employed and their perceived effectiveness. Foa and Rothbaum (1998) discuss how to construct a hierarchy of avoided situations in their exposure-based therapy for rape trauma. In Chapter 7 the Exposure Hierarchy (see Appendix 7.1) can be used to identify the avoided situations and cues in preparation for *in vivo* exposure which is an important part of cognitive therapy for PTSD. Clients should also be questioned about their use of safety seeking to minimize or prevent PTSD symptoms. Do they rely on being accompanied by a partner, family member, or close friend to confront avoided situations? Do they use medication or other substances to control PTSD symptoms? What other subtle cognitive or behavioral strategies are used to minimize anxiety? It is important to obtain a profile of the client's safety-seeking responses because this will be a focus for change in subsequent CT sessions.

Case Illustration

A cognitive case formulation is illustrated by referring to the clinical example presented at the beginning of this chapter. Edward developed PTSD after returning from a 6-month tour of Rwanda, having witnessed the unspeakable horrors of genocide. Assessment revealed that the genocide had shattered many of Edward's preexisting beliefs about the world, humanity, and himself. Edward expressed long-held beliefs in justice and the rule of law. He believed that personal threat or danger could be minimized through caution, discipline, and resourcefulness. He held to a personal code of morality and believed in the dignity and fairness of humanity. Edward's self-view was of a strong, confident, hard-working individual who treated others fairly and expected the same in return. All of these fundamental beliefs about himself, the world, and the inherent good and dignity of humanity were shattered in Rwanda.

There was no single, specific traumatic event that elicited Edward's PTSD. Rather it was multiple experiences of threat to personal safety such as clearing land mines in Bosnia or being threatened at gun point when passing through road checks in Rwanda. It was witnessing the tragedy of war such as being confronted with masses of starving and frightened Rwandans, coming across mass graves, churches crowded with dead civilians, and rivers filled with dead floating bodies. However, one of the most prominent experiences was the disappearance of children from an orphanage he had visited, especially a 5-year-old Rwandan girl who had befriended him. At the time of these experiences, Edward suppressed his emotions, using humor and a superficial bravado to distance himself from the circumstances. Though feeling shock and disgust by what he witnessed, he soon became numb and dissociated himself from these repeated experiences. He treated threats to his personal safety as "just doing my job" and when he returned home there was no acknowledgment of what he had seen or experienced. He was expected to slip back into his normal life and work routine as if nothing had happened.

Edward's Trauma Memory Narrative focused on what he remembered about the day his convoy arrived at the orphanage and the little girl's absence along with that of dozens of other sick and injured children. Edward could only remember aspects of that day that confirmed his assumption that she had been murdered. He was unable to recall aspects of the experience that would suggest other reasons for the little girl's absence from the orphanage. His recall was mainly driven by strong feelings of rage, sadness, and guilt for what he assumed was the brutal death of the little girl. He experienced fragments of the memory in which he had intrusive images of the little girl and a gorilla dressed in an RPA uniform. These images could occur spontaneously or be triggered by certain external reminders of Rwanda such as being in a crowded store or on a certain section of highway on his way to work. His main emotional response to the intrusions was anxiety, anger, and guilt.

Edward had a strong sense of self-blame for Rwanda. He believed that as a UN peacekeeper he did not do enough to stop the genocide and he blamed himself for not protecting the little girl. He believed that the genocide had permanently changed his beliefs and attitudes about himself, the world, and other people. He concluded that he would never be able to get over its effects, that it had permanently scarred him. Edward believed that danger to himself and his loved ones was much more likely and that he was left a weak, vulnerable person. He must remain vigilant and onguard, especially when around other people. He believed he had utterly failed himself and that his future looked bleak and unfulfilling as he tried to struggle with the guilt and anger of his war-related experiences. He stated, "I cannot plan ahead; I have lost all control of my life." His predominant view of himself was that of a guilty, worthless, and empty individual with no interest, no energy, very limited ability, and no future. In other words he suffered from what Ehlers and Clark (2000) called "mental defeat."

Edward was particularly bothered by the reexperiencing symptoms of PTSD. He believed that the intrusive images were a sign that the PTSD was getting worse. He expressed concern that the intrusive images and memories might eventually drive him crazy. Their persistence as well as his sudden anger outbursts was proof that he had lost all self-control. He was convinced that the PTSD meant he was a psychologically weak or inferior person and that he was now "damaged goods" and of little use to the military or any other potential employer. He blamed himself for being a victim of PTSD and believed he would never get over its effects. He concluded he must have some preexisting flaw to explain why he developed PTSD and others did not. He did not believe he could ever overcome PTSD but with long-term therapy he might learn to manage its effects a little better. He stated, "You [PTSD] have destroyed my life, quality of life, my normal life and future."

Edward tried his best to prevent or suppress the intrusive thoughts and memories of Rwanda. He avoided any movies, books, or media presentations on Africa, and any situations or people that reminded him of Rwanda. He isolated himself from social settings and turned to alcohol abuse to drown his memories. In fact Edward developed a comorbid alcohol dependence disorder because it suppressed the intrusive images and memories and calmed his feelings of being overwhelmed and angry. In addition Edward avoided public places and social interaction outside the work setting. He frequently thought of suicide as the final solution to his pain. He experienced frequent dissociative episodes where he could not account for periods of time while at work and he ruminated on how he could have prevented the little girl's disappearance. He tried to suppress trauma memories by distracting himself and he tried hard to prevent the expression of any strong emotion when talking about Rwanda. Ironically, of course, he did experience strong negative emotions such as anger, anxiety attacks, and deep dysphoria which seemed to occur spontaneously and beyond his control. One of his adaptive responses that became apparent in therapy was his ability to write about his thoughts and feelings. He also read everything he could find about combat-related PTSD and trauma exposure in order to better understand his own emotional state and he started a daily physical exercise and well-being program.

Escape and avoidance were Edward's main safety-seeking behaviors. When he experienced anxious symptoms or an intrusive trauma-related image, he left the situation immediately. He spent much of his time outside of work, alone at home, drinking and watching movies late into the night in order to distract himself and avoid sleep which brought on nightmares. Later in therapy, Edward tried to use various relaxation and meditation techniques to reduce anxiety and the reexperiencing symptoms, which had limited success because they served a safety-seeking function.

Clinician Guideline 12.22

A cognitive case formulation for PTSD specifies (1) how the individual's beliefs about self, world, and others have been changed by the trauma; (2) how the trauma is remembered; (3) the dysfunctional appraisals and beliefs about the trauma and its consequences; (4) the negative interpretations of intrusive trauma-related thoughts, images, and memories; and (5) the maladaptive coping strategies used to suppress intrusive symptoms and minimize anxiety.

DESCRIPTION OF COGNITIVE THERAPY FOR PTSD

The overarching goals of cognitive therapy for PTSD are to reduce the posttrauma reexperiencing symptoms, achieve significant reduction in anxiety and depression, and improve level of social and occupational functioning (see Table 12.5 for a list of goals; see also D. M. Clark & Ehlers, 2004).

It is important that the case formulation culminate in an individualized treatment plan that will guide therapy (see Taylor, 2006). The treatment plan consists of the immediate and long-term goals of therapy. These goals are established in a collaborative manner by referring to the case formulation. The client should be given a copy of the therapy goals and treatment progress should be periodically evaluated throughout therapy by referring to the client's specified goals. Edward's treatment plan focused on a number of specific goals.

- Reduce the frequency and intensity of intrusive images of the "little girl and gorilla."
- Eliminate the use of alcohol as a maladaptive coping strategy.
- Reduce avoidance and subjective anxiety when exposed to situations that trigger reminders of Rwanda (e.g., crowded Wal-Mart store, certain stretch of highway between home and work).
- Increase social contact and leisure activities.
- Reduce anger outbursts and low frustration tolerance.
- Reduce the level of generalized anxiety.
- Eliminate feelings of guilt, blame, and anger over the genocide.
- Improve a sense of confidence and hope for the future.
- Reduce hypervigiliance for threat.
- Recapture his past attitude of optimism and trust of others.

TABLE 12.5. Goals and Objectives of Cognitive Therapy for Posttraumatic Stress Disorder

- Accept the cognitive rationale for the persistence of symptoms of posttraumatic stress disorder
- Improve the organization, coherence, integration, and elaboration of the trauma memory by emphasizing conceptually based processing of the trauma (D.M. Clark & Ehlers, 2004; Ehlers & Clark, 2000).
- Modify dysfunctional beliefs and appraisals of the trauma, its causes, and negative effects on self, world, and future.
- Shift from a negative, threatening interpretation of unwanted trauma-related intrusive thoughts, images, and memories to a more adaptive, accepting, and accommodating perspective of trauma-relevant mental intrusions (i.e., a normalization process).
- Deactivate maladaptive beliefs of a weak and vulnerable self, a threatening or dangerous world, and abandonment or insensitivity of others that have been reinforced by trauma; instead promote the adoption of more constructive, alternative views of a strong self, primarily safe world, caring people, and hopeful future.
- Eliminate maladaptive cognitive strategies such as thought suppression and rumination as well as related processes such as emotional numbing or blunting and dissociation.
- Reduce escape, avoidance, and other safety-seeking behaviors employed to suppress reexperiencing symptoms or minimize heightened anxiety.

- Eliminate an overwhelming conviction of failure, of having been a profound disappointment to himself and others.
- Regain his interest in life and minimize the effects of PTSD on daily living.

There are a number of therapeutic ingredients in cognitive therapy of PTSD that together serve to meet treatment goals and objectives. These are summarized in Table 12.6 and are discussed in greater detail below.

Education Phase

The initial sessions of cognitive therapy focus on educating the client about PTSD, providing the cognitive explanation for the persistence of posttrauma symptoms, presenting the treatment rationale, and clarifying the goals of therapy. As in cognitive therapy for other anxiety disorders, the education phase is critical for the success of treatment for PTSD. The objectives are threefold: (1) to gain the client's acceptance of the cognitive model of PTSD and its treatment so that a collaborative therapeutic relationship can be established, (2) to correct any faulty beliefs about PTSD and its treatment that might interfere with cognitive therapy, and (3) to ensure treatment adherence and increase compliance with homework exercises.

TABLE 12.6. Therapeutic Components of Cognitive Therapy of Posttraumatic Stress Disorder

Therapeutic component	Treatment objective
Education phase	To provide information on posttraumatic stress disorder, correct any misunderstandings about the disorder, gain patients' acceptance of the cognitive model and collaboration in the treatment process.
Trauma-focused cognitive restructuring	To identify and then modify negative beliefs and appraisals about the personal meaning of the trauma in terms of its cause, nature, and consequences for the self, world, others, and future.
Elaboration of and repeated imaginal exposure to the trauma memory	To construct a more elaborated, organized, coherent, and contextualized recollection of the trauma with a greater emphasis on its meaning so that with repeated exposure the trauma memory eventually becomes more conceptually based and better integrated with other autobiographical memories.
Disorder-focused cognitive restructuring	To shift the client's negative, threat-oriented interpretations and beliefs about the symptoms of posttraumatic stress disorder and their consequences, especially the reexperiencing symptoms of the disorder, toward a more adaptive, functional coping perspective.
In vivo exposure to reexperiencing cues	To reduce avoidance and reliance on safety-seeking behaviors as well as decrease anxiety in situations that elicit reexperiencing symptoms.
Modify maladaptive cognitive avoidance and control strategies	To reduce or eliminate worry, rumination, dissociation, and difficulty concentrating by targeting maladaptive cognitive strategies such as thought suppression and overcontrol of unwanted thoughts and emotions, and replace with more adaptive attentional control and acceptance of unwanted thoughts and emotions.
Emotion reduction (supplemental)	To reduce general anxiety, hypervigilance, sleep disturbance, and anger/irritability by developing a more relaxed, benign response style.

Often individuals with PTSD explain the disorder solely in terms of a "brain chemistry imbalance" or the result of an inherent psychological or emotional predisposition. Both explanations could undermine their acceptance of cognitive therapy. Alternatively the cognitive therapist explains that PTSD is a natural psychological response to traumatic events. Foa and Rothbaum (1998) provide a client handout entitled "Common Reactions to Assault" that explains fear/anxiety, reexperiencing the trauma, increased arousal, avoidance, anger, guilt/shame, depression, and negative self-image as immediate reactions to trauma experienced by the majority of survivors. Although the handout deals with physical and sexual assault, slight modifications can be made to include all traumatic experiences. Of course, the therapist's account for PTSD must include an explanation of why PTSD symptoms persist in only a minority of individuals exposed to trauma. The client handout developed by Taylor (2006) is especially helpful in this regard. Persistent PTSD is explained as a "hypersensitivity of the brain's stress response system" which is determined by a person's genetic makeup and the nature and severity of the traumatic experiences. It is explained that everyone has a "breaking point" for the development of PTSD. A person with a strong genetic predisposition for PTSD will develop the disorder in response to less intense trauma, whereas a severe trauma or multiple traumatic experiences may be required to push someone with minimal genetic predisposition over his "breaking point." It is important to emphasize with clients that everyone has a breaking point; it is only a question of how much trauma is needed for the occurrence of PTSD. A copy of Taylor's (2006) handout can be purchased from the Anxiety Disorders Association of Canada (*www.anxietycanada.ca*).

The cognitive account for PTSD must also include an explanation of the role of negative thoughts and beliefs, trauma memory, negative emotion, and avoidance in the persistence of posttrauma symptoms. The therapist explains that whether the initial posttrauma symptoms persist or eventually disappear after a few weeks depends on our response. The following is a possible cognitive explanation for the persistence of PTSD:

> "If many of the PTSD symptoms you experience are a common response to trauma and everyone has a 'breaking point' in their stress response system, you might be wondering why your PTSD symptoms have persisted whereas for others the symptoms disappear within a few weeks. In the last few years researchers have discovered a number of factors that appear to contribute to the persistence of PTSD. First, traumatic experiences often cause people to view themselves, their world, future, and other people in a very negative and threatening manner. During the assessment interview you described a number of ways in which you believe you are weaker and more vulnerable and the world is a more dangerous place. [Therapist lists some of the client's dysfunctional thoughts and beliefs.] The problem with this thinking is that it becomes more highly selective over time so that it increases one's sensitivity to threat and perpetuates a sense of fear and anxiety, which are the main negative emotions of PTSD. A second contributor is how the trauma is remembered. When some aspects of a trauma are remembered too clearly, other aspects are forgotten, and when one can not arrive at a satisfactory meaning or understanding of the trauma, an individual is more likely to have repeated unwanted vivid and intrusive recollections of the trauma that are highly distressing. In some cases it may feel as if

you are reliving the traumatic experience all over again. [Therapist should refer to the client's description of reexperiencing symptoms.] A third contributor to persistent PTSD concerns one's evaluation or interpretation of the reexperiencing symptoms of PTSD. For example, if a person considers the recurrent thoughts, images, memories, or dreams of the trauma as having a substantial and enduring negative effect on himself, then the reexperiencing will be considered a serious threat to his ability to function that must be contained at all costs. Giving the symptoms of PTSD, this serious negative evaluation will have the paradoxical effect of increasing their persistence and salience or intensity. One's life becomes more focused, more dominated by the symptoms. [Therapist refers back to client's interpretation of reexperiencing symptoms to reinforce this point.] And finally, certain strategies that are designed to reduce reexperiencing symptoms, such as the avoidance of trauma cues, attempts to suppress thoughts of the trauma, failure to express natural emotions, and reliance on safety-seeking behaviors, all contribute to the persistence of PTSD symptoms. [Therapist questions client about the effects of avoidance and safety-seeking.]"

After presenting the cognitive explanation for PTSD, the therapist provides a rationale for treatment. Foa and Rothbaum (1998) use the metaphor "psychological digestion" in which it is explained that the goal of treatment is to help clients work through what has happened so their brain can "psychologically digest" the trauma. Taylor (2006) describes cognitive-behavioral therapy as a means of helping individuals make sense of a traumatic experience and to desensitize them to distressing but harmless reminders of the trauma. Resick, Monson, and Rizvi (2008) explain that therapy focuses on modifying thoughts and beliefs that cause the individual to "get stuck," and on helping the person accept what happened, feel natural emotions, and develop more balanced beliefs that will contribute to more helpful emotions. Smyth (1999) discusses treatment of traumatic memories in terms of changing "hot" memories to "bad" memories, whereas Najavitis (2002) presents the goal of treatment as learning to manage PTSD and achieving a sense of safety. Although the cognitive therapist may find reference to these ideas helpful in providing a treatment rationale, it is important to emphasize that cognitive therapy focuses on the reduction of anxiety and PTSD symptoms by (1) modifying negative and threatening appraisals and beliefs about self, world, future, other people, and the reexperiencing symptoms of PTSD; (2) reconstructing a more organized, meaningful, and complete memory of trauma that is associated with less threat and distress; and (3) replacing maladaptive avoidance and other safety-seeking practices with more effective trauma-related coping responses. In addition, cognitive therapy focuses on eliminating substance abuse, dealing with negative thoughts and behaviors that may underlie major depression or suicidality, and improving interpersonal functioning when these are associated clinical problems. Although the education phase "formally ends" with a clear statement of the goals for treatment by referring back to the case formulation, later in therapy a more specific rationale will be provided when each of the therapeutic ingredients of cognitive therapy are first introduced. Also the first session of therapy ends with the client assigned to self-monitor her trauma-related thoughts, images, or memories. The self-monitoring form presented in Appendix 12.1 can be used for this purpose.

Clinician Guideline 12.23

The educational component of cognitive therapy for PTSD focuses on (1) correcting any misconceptions about PTSD and its consequences, (2) explaining the role of negative trauma-related and disorder-focused appraisals and beliefs in the persistence of PTSD symptoms, (3) elucidating the problem of poorly elaborated trauma memories, and (4) highlighting the effects of maladaptive cognitive and behavioral avoidance and safety-seeking strategies. Client collaboration with treatment is determined by acceptance of the therapy rationale which is based on the cognitive model of PTSD.

Trauma-Focused Cognitive Restructuring

After educating the client into the cognitive model of PTSD, the next phase of treatment involves the identification and modification of the client's negative beliefs and appraisals about the trauma and its consequences. We believe it is important to focus on these beliefs before engaging in any trauma-related exposure in order to correct any biases that might undermine the acceptance of exposure. Also, for most people, dealing with trauma-related beliefs will be less threatening than *in vivo* or imaginal exposure.

In cognitive processing therapy developed by Patricia Resick and colleagues, clients with PTSD are first asked to write an Impact Statement about the meaning of the traumatic event(s) (Resick & Schnicke, 1992; Resick, Monson, & Rizvi, 2008; Shipherd et al., 2006). We have found this an excellent exercise for identifying negative appraisals and beliefs about the trauma and its consequences. It should be given as a homework assignment at the end of the first session. The following are instructions for writing an Impact Statement (Resick, Monson, & Rizvi, 2008, p. 90):

> "Please write at least one page on what it means to you that this traumatic experience happened. Please consider the effects that the event has had in your beliefs about yourself, your beliefs about others, and your beliefs about the world. Also consider the following topics while writing your answer: safety, trust, power/competence, esteem, and intimacy. Bring this with you to the next session."

Most of session two will be spent on the Impact Statement in which the therapist highlights, clarifies, and elaborates aspects of the client's account that indicate negative appraisals and beliefs about the trauma. These beliefs will tend to revolve around the causes and consequences of the trauma as they relate to the self, world, other people, and future. Resick and Schnicke (1992) suggest that beliefs about safety, trust, power, self-esteem, and intimacy should be targeted because these are often disrupted by a trauma. For example, a university student who was raped after leaving the bar with a man she had just met believed that "it was my fault for drinking too much and putting myself in a dangerous situation" and "I'll never be able to trust or be intimate with another man."

Various cognitive restructuring strategies discussed in Chapter 6 can be used to modify the negative trauma-related appraisals and beliefs. Evidence gathering will be particularly useful in which clients can be asked, "Is there anything that happened at the time of the trauma or afterward that supports or reinforces the negative interpretation or belief?" On the other hand, "Is there anything that happened during the trauma or afterward that is inconsistent with the negative interpretation or belief?" Cost–benefit analysis is another useful cognitive restructuring in which the client is encouraged to consider the immediate and long-term costs of continuing to put the most negative construction on the trauma and its consequences. The therapist should also teach individuals how to identify thinking errors in their trauma-related beliefs and appraisals. The cognitive therapist can also educate clients on how beliefs can affect trauma memories and vice versa through the processes of accommodation and assimilation (Shipherd et al., 2006). There are two goals to cognitive restructuring. First, the therapist collaborates with the client in the adoption of an alternative, more helpful understanding of the trauma and its enduring impact. And second, cognitive restructuring should help patients develop a more distant or detached mindful attitude toward the trauma-related intrusions (Taylor, 2006; Wells & Sembi, 2004). Individuals are encouraged to observe their thoughts in a detached manner without interpreting, analyzing, or trying to control them in any way. The thoughts can be viewed simply as symptoms that can be allowed "to occupy their own space and time without engaging with them" (Wells & Sembi, 2004, p. 373) or the client can shift perspective by viewing the trauma from another person's perspective or from the distant future (Taylor, 2006). Although cognitive restructuring of trauma-related intrusions is most intense during the early sessions of cognitive therapy, this work will continue intermittently throughout treatment. Appendix 12.2 can be used to help clients consolidate their cognitive restructuring skills through homework assignments.

Taylor (2006) mentions a number of problems that can be encountered with cognitive restructuring in PTSD. One is *invalidation* in which the individual believes the therapist trivializes or does not appreciate the significance and amount of personal suffering caused by the trauma. This can be avoided by giving clients the opportunity to fully discuss their experiences, expressing appropriate levels of empathy, and directly validating their feelings (see Leahy, 2001). Also Taylor (2006) recommends that therapists avoid labeling thoughts/beliefs as "distorted," "wrong," "irrational," or "dysfunctional" but instead frame them in terms of what is "unhelpful" and "helpful" ways of thinking. Another problem occurs when clients hold *unyielding beliefs* and so are resistant to cognitive restructuring. Empirical hypothesis-testing exercises can be most helpful when the client refuses to accept the therapist's verbal disputations. In addition, the individual can be encouraged to temporarily "try out the alternative interpretation or belief" and record any positive or negative effects (see Chapter 6 for further discussion). These experiences may help sow some doubt concerning the veracity of the negative trauma interpretation.

The following is a verbatim account of Edward's Impact Statement:

"In Yugoslavia we were there to keep the peace [United Nations peacekeeping tour] and de-mine and as a result I lost some good friends. I saw the remains of mass burials and murders, vast destruction and I saw the effects of rape and the famous Serbian Necktie [tire placed around victim's neck and set ablaze]. We were constantly being mortared on and in Sarajevo the snipers were everywhere and targets were picked for no reason. I was kept at gunpoint at a UN checkpoint and threatened by a Chechen with an AK-47. When I look back I see the family problems in a lot of the soldiers and the drinking and drugs started. We were on the road to Hell."

"In the fall of 1993 I was in the coffee room when I heard of the possibility of a UN Tour to a place in Africa called Rwanda. Never heard of it but a 7-month tour sounded good. When we got to Kigali we knew we had hit rock bottom and the feeling got very tense. Since the tour I have believed I have no future, I am a loser, I am never going to achieve anything. I believe the world is on a tailspin downward to self-destruction. We are going to run out of natural resources by 2015 and with overpopulation there will be a depression all over the world which will make the crash of 1929 look like child's play. The Rwandans had the answer GENOCIDE (original emphasis). Just kill everyone off—it worked. The people left are going to be well off."

"While you are overseas you are constantly on the lookout for snipers, the enemy, and mines. For the longest time I would not walk on grass or dirt; I stayed on pavement. You are constantly looking all around you and you never let your guard down and to this day I still have problems with safety and fear. I trust no one since Rwanda and I mean no one. You do this to survive. I have no self-esteem. You have the power to choose who lives and dies overseas—it is a hard feeling to live with. Did you make the right decision? I've had a lot of problems with intimacy—I feel as though my heart is split wide open. I am a failure so why try. I failed in Rwanda, my career, my marriage, my family, my future. I have no future; nothing to live for, so why go on. My life has been one major disappointment."

As evident from Edward's Impact Statement, many of the negative beliefs and appraisals were related to having witnessed the effects of genocide and other horrific acts of murder, rape, torture, and intimidation as well as experiencing multiple life-threatening situations during his UN peacekeeping deployments. Numerous cognitive therapy sessions were devoted to evidence gathering, cost–benefit analysis, and generating alternative perspectives on his negative beliefs about himself, his future, and the world. Edward had an unyielding belief that he had failed in Rwanda and now he had completely failed in life. He believed he was a disappointment to himself and to others. He was convinced that his life was meaningless, he had achieved nothing, and that he had been permanently damaged by his war-related experiences (i.e., a state of mental defeat). He believed his future was bleak and contained only disillusionment and misery. He held a particularly cynical view of the world which was doomed to be dominated by evil, greed, and exploitation. It deserved the most severe punishment for its evil. He now rejected his previous religious beliefs in a loving, caring God. He distrusted everyone because he believed people were basically selfish, uncaring, and disinterested in others.

Our work on two of Edward's most prominent negative beliefs, "I have been an utter failure in life" and "I am partly to blame for failing to stop the genocide," will illustrate trauma-focused cognitive restructuring. In both cases we examined whether these beliefs were accurate statements of reality by examining evidence that he achieved nothing in his life, especially his military career. We used an imagery exercise to work through what he could have done differently as one soldier to stop the genocide and we listed all of the possible contributors to the Rwandan genocide. We examined the personal cost associated with continuing to believe he was "an utter failure" and that he should be held responsible for the genocide of innocent women and children. Alternative interpretations were constructed such as "Although I will now end my military career with a medical discharge, I still achieved far more than I ever dreamed possible when I first enlisted" and "I was powerless to prevent the genocide; officers with access to more resources and authority than me could do nothing to stop it so I can not be held responsible in any way." Finally, Edward was taught to take a more detached, distancing perspective on his negative thoughts and beliefs. He learned to counter the emotional negative beliefs with more reality-based alternatives, and he also learned that is was safe to let the unhelpful thoughts float through conscious awareness because they were not true. As a result of cognitive restructuring, Edward experienced an improvement in his level of depression and almost complete elimination of suicidal ideation.

Clinician Guideline 12.24

Identification of unhelpful thoughts and beliefs related to trauma, its cause, and consequence on perspectives about the self, world, future, and other people are obtained through Socratic questioning and guided discovery. Asking clients to write an Impact Statement can be helpful in identifying trauma-related maladaptive thinking, while evidence gathering, cost–benefit analysis, cognitive error identification, empirical hypothesis testing, and generating alternative interpretations are used to modify negative appraisals and beliefs.

Imaginal Exposure to Trauma Memory

Modification of the trauma memory through repeated imaginal exposure, verbal discussion and Socratic questioning is an important component of cognitive therapy for PTSD that should begin within the fifth or sixth session. Most individuals with PTSD will be very reluctant to engage in imaginal exposure to the trauma because they believe this will make their anxiety and distress worse and increase the frequency of reexperiencing symptoms. Also imaginal exposure is completely contrary to common sense, which is that avoidance of painful memories is the best way to reduce anxiety and distress. Thus effective imaginal exposure to the trauma must begin with a rationale for the procedure and opportunity to address any of the client's misconceptions about intentional trauma exposure.

Foa and Rothbaum (1998) begin their rationale by acknowledging that although individuals who experience traumatic events believe that avoiding thoughts or memories about the trauma is the best coping strategy, in reality it is never successful because "no matter how hard you try to push away thoughts about the assault, the experience comes back to haunt you through nightmares, flashbacks, phobias, and distressing thoughts and feelings" (p. 159). The authors explain that the goal of repeatedly reliving the trauma in imagination is to process the memories, to stay with the memories until the anxiety and distress associated with them decreases. They state that their aim "is to help you gain control over the memories rather than having the memories control you" (p. 160). In addition, the cognitive therapist can explain that by repeatedly imagining the trauma and probing the memories through extended verbal discussion and questioning in therapy, the client will begin to think differently about the trauma. The memory will become less emotional, turning it from a "hot" memory to a "bad" memory (Smyth, 1999). This new way of remembering the trauma will reduce the frequency and distress of the reexperiencing symptoms of PTSD (e.g., intrusive thoughts, images, memories of the trauma, nightmares, flashbacks).

In cognitive therapy clients are asked to complete a Trauma Narrative as a homework assignment for the first phase of imaginal exposure. Individuals write an account of the worst traumatic incident in as much detail as can be remembered (see Foa & Rothbaum, 1998; Resick, Monson, & Rizvi, 2008; Shipherd et al., 2006; Taylor, 2006). The following instructions can be given for writing the Trauma Narrative:

"In order to begin our work on your distressing memories of the trauma, I would like to assign homework that asks you to write an account of the worst trauma you have experienced. The account should be written in the present tense, as if you were experiencing the trauma at that moment. Please try to include as much detail of the experience as you can remember. In particular include all the thoughts, feelings, sensations, and responses that you experienced during the trauma. Allow yourself to fully experience the emotions of the trauma. If you come to a difficult spot in the narrative where you can't remember very clearly or have doubts about the experience, place a question mark (?). It is expected that you will find this exercise distressing because you are reliving the events in your mind's eye. You should work on the account over several days and probably limit yourself to 30–45 minutes on each occasion. If you have any concerns about the homework assignment or experience a sustained worsening of your symptoms over several hours, please contact my office immediately and wait for further directions before resuming your work on the narrative. Do not be concerned about the grammar, completeness, or accuracy of your narrative. We will be working on it together in the next session. At this point I would like you to do as much as you can on your own so that we can get a start on your Trauma Narrative."

At the following session the client is asked to read aloud the Trauma Narrative. Individuals are asked to rate their anxiety/distress level on a 0–100 scale before and after reading the narrative. The therapist asks about any automatic thoughts experienced while reading the narrative. Particular attention is paid to the most distressing points in the trauma (i.e., hot spots) and the automatic thoughts or appraisals associated with them (Ehlers, Clark, Hackmann, McManus, & Fennell, 2005). After a complete first reading of the narrative without interruption, the client is asked to read the account several more times. The cognitive therapist may interrupt successive readings with Socratic questioning designed to clarify and elaborate on details about the account and help the client fully explore associated thoughts and feelings. If anxiety/distress ratings decline over repeated readings of the narrative, this should be noted as empirical evidence for the positive benefits of repeated exposure. Also any unhelpful automatic thoughts or beliefs associated with the narrative, especially appraisals that occur during the "hot spots" in the trauma, are dealt with by cognitive restructuring.

The Trauma Narrative can be used as the basis for developing an imaginal trauma script that can be used for within-session and between-session imaginal exposure. An audiotape of the script can be made and the client can be asked to engage in 45–60 minutes of imaginal exposure to the script each day until distress is reduced (Taylor, 2006). The imaginal script should be rewritten periodically to reflect new details and insights. The Exposure Practice Record (see Appendix 7.2) can be used to record between-session imaginal exposures. For further discussion on how to implement imaginal exposure and to troubleshoot various problems associated with this intervention, see Chapter 7 as well as Foa and Rothbaum (1998) and Taylor (2006).

The imaginal exposure component of cognitive therapy ends with production of a reformulated Trauma Narrative. This second account of the trauma should be a closer approximation to the actual traumatic experience including important contextual information and aspects of the trauma that may have been forgotten or minimized in the original account. It should also incorporate more helpful interpretations of the client's role and responses during the trauma. The goal of this reformulated narrative is not to "normalize the trauma" (this would be entirely inappropriate and insensitive), but rather to help the client remember the traumatic experience in a way that brings new meaning and acceptance so it can be assimilated into general autobiographical memory. Producing a more elaborated account of the trauma as well as repeated imaginal exposure play a critical role in constructing a more integrated, conceptually based memory of the trauma.

Edward wrote down the following Trauma Narrative that became the basis for the imaginal exposure component of his treatment:

"I remember going to an orphanage and we were tasked with providing supplies. One day I am sitting having lunch and suddenly felt shocked; I felt something touch me and beside me is a little girl in a pretty dress. She is 5 years old. She is badly burned with no nose or fingers. She seems curious at what we are eating. After overcoming my initial shock, I feel more composed and show her my lunch. She loves the peaches I give her and then follows me the rest of the day. The other children make fun of her but she ignores their brutal harassment. The little girl and I are in our own world delivering supplies to the orphanage. Frequently she looks up at me and smiles. I ask one of the nuns what happened to her and she says that the little girl's family and entire village was murdered or burned by soldiers. She hid under the bed and saw everything. I told my family about the little girl and they mailed me toys, cookies, and some clothes to give to her. The next week I return to the orphanage but she is gone! I search for her, feeling tense, frantic, a terrible sick feeling in my stomach. A lot of the children are missing. I ask a nun about the kids and she tells me the Rwandan soldiers took all the children who were sick, damaged, or showed signs of weakness. They were hacked alive. I feel a rage building inside, I become tense all over and start to shake. I see a Rwandan soldier standing off to one side, laughing at me as I am talking to the nun. The anger is so intense, I start yelling and cursing the soldier. I lunge toward him with my knife, wanting desperately to kill him. My fellow soldiers hold me back. He knows I can't hurt him and so he just keeps laughing at me. I am crying, screaming at him. God, I want to kill that guy; I want to slit open his throat just like he butchered the little girl."

Clinician Guideline 12.25

Ask clients to generate a Trauma Narrative which then becomes the basis for repeated imaginal exposure to the worst trauma aimed at disconfirming misinterpretations about the dangerousness of trauma memories and reconstruction of a more organized, elaborated memory of trauma that can be integrated into general autobiographical memory.

Disorder-Focused Cognitive Restructuring

As noted earlier in this chapter, many of the symptoms of PTSD are common reactions in the immediate aftermath of trauma. However, if these initial symptoms such as intrusive recollections, flashbacks, nightmares, anger, poor concentration, anxiety, numbing, and the like are interpreted negatively as signs of weakness, sickness, mental disturbance, loss of control, and so on. rather than a normal part of the recovery process, these appraisals can contribute to the persistence of the symptoms (Ehlers & Clark, 2000). Taylor (2006) noted that disorder-focused negative appraisals and beliefs fall under three categories: (1) beliefs about specific PTSD symptoms (e.g., "Having frequent flashbacks means that the PTSD is getting worse"), (2) beliefs about arousal-related symptoms (e.g., "If my chest tightens too much and I become short of breath, I might faint"), and (3) beliefs about general psychological functioning (e.g., "PTSD has robbed me of a meaningful life", "I will never achieve anything because PTSD has ruined my memory or ability to concentrate"). We would add that the clients' perceptions of how other people evaluate and respond to them because of the trauma or suffering from PTSD are another important type of disorder-related thinking targeted in treatment.

Cognitive restructuring, empirical hypothesis testing, generating alternative interpretations, and mindful detachment/acceptance will be the primary interventions for modifying disorder-focused appraisals and beliefs. Work on these beliefs will occur throughout the course of cognitive therapy and may become particularly evident when conducting imaginal or *in vivo* exposure sessions. Once a disorder-specific belief is identified, the therapist should focus on modifying that belief before continuing further with exposure or trauma memory reconstruction. If left unchecked, the disorder-specific negative beliefs will interfere in treatment progress. The following evaluation forms may be assigned Testing Anxious Appraisals: Looking for Evidence (Appendix 6.2), Empirical Hypothesis-Testing Form (Appendix 6.5), or Symptom Reappraisal Form (Appendix 8.2).

A number of disorder-related negative beliefs and appraisals were identified in the course of Edward's treatment. For example, he believed that the occurrence of sudden intrusive images of "the little girl and gorilla in an RPA uniform" meant that his PTSD was getting worse and that he could eventually "go crazy" if he did not stop the images. Cognitive restructuring focused on gathering personal evidence that the unwanted images really were associated with deterioration and testing out an alternative perspective where the images were viewed as an annoyance in which the best response was benign acceptance and detached observation. Edward also believed that he could have a heart attack if he experienced heart palpitations, tension, and trembling because of heightened anxiety (he was receiving medical treatment for hypertension and elevated cholesterol). Cognitive restructuring and *in vivo* exposure to anxiety-provoking situations were used to disconfirm Edward's threat interpretations of anxious symptoms. Edward also believed that he no longer had any personal value because of PTSD (i.e., mental defeat) and that he could no longer achieve anything worthwhile or attain any degree of satisfaction in life. His life was one big disappointment because of PTSD. Cognitive restructuring focused on (1) reassessing his personal value based on forgotten past achievements, (2) correcting the overgeneralization error associated with the trauma and its effects, (3) and developing a "management perspective" on PTSD (i.e., "PTSD is like diabetes, people can live productive and fulfilling lives if it is managed properly").

Empirical hypothesis testing involved collecting evidence that Edward could engage in specific pleasure or mastery activities (e.g., having a friend over for dinner, golfing with friends) despite experiencing PTSD symptoms.

Clinician Guideline 12.26

Unhelpful thoughts and beliefs about PTSD and its symptoms are identified and subjected to cognitive restructuring in order to help clients view PTSD as a manageable condition in which acceptance and detached mindfulness may be the optimal response style to symptom occurrence.

In Vivo *Exposure*

Escape and avoidance are common maladaptive coping responses in PTSD so *in vivo* exposure to situations that trigger anxiety and PTSD-related reexperiencing and arousal symptoms is a major focus in cognitive therapy. The purpose of prolonged exposure to PTSD and anxiety-eliciting situations is to (1) provide disconfirming evidence of negative trauma- and disorder-related beliefs; (2) reduce escape, avoidance, and safety-seeking behaviors; (3) increase self-efficacy and perceived ability to cope; and (4) reduce negative emotional responses like anxiety. *In vivo* exposure may also involve revisiting the site of a traumatic event in order to help in the reconstruction of a more elaborated trauma memory so that the intrusive recollections become less responsive to cue-driven retrieval (Ehlers et al., 2005).

Chapter 7 provides a detailed description of how to conduct *in vivo* exposure. The steps for implementing this type of exposure in PTSD will be similar to the procedure in other anxiety disorders with the exception that concerns about re-experiencing symptoms during exposure exercises may require additional attention by the therapist. A graded fear hierarchy should be constructed and exposure sessions often begin with therapist assistance. Prolonged, repeated, and daily exposure continues with each situation until the client experiences a clinically significant decline in anxiety and reexperiencing symptoms. For the cognitive therapist, *in vivo* exposure often provides opportunity to modify negative trauma- and disorder-related beliefs and appraisals. For further description of *in vivo* exposure in PTSD, see Foa and Rothbaum (1998) and Taylor (2006).

Clinician Guideline 12.27

Graded *in vivo* exposure to avoided situations that elicit anxiety and reexperiencing symptoms is an important therapeutic element of cognitive therapy of PTSD used to provide disconfirming evidence for maladaptive thoughts and beliefs, increase perceived coping ability, and reduce heigthened situationally induced anxiety.

Modify Maladaptive Cognitive and Behavioral Control

Reduction of maladaptive cognitive and behavioral safety-seeking and avoidant coping strategies is another important goal of cognitive therapy (Ehlers & Clark, 2000; Ehlers et al., 2005). First the cognitive therapist must determine how the client tries to reduce anxiety or reexperiencing symptoms. The Behavioral Responses to Anxiety Checklist (Appendix 5.7) and the Cognitive Responses to Anxiety Checklist (Appendix 5.9) from Chapter 5 can be assigned to obtain this information. These forms should be expanded to include responses to reexperiencing symptoms as well as anxiety for individuals with PTSD.

The next step in this phase of treatment is educating the client on the negative consequences of the maladaptive coping response. Although safety-seeking and avoidant responses may lead to an immediate decrease in anxiety or termination of reexperiencing symptoms, in the long term they significantly contribute to the persistence of PTSD. Reliance on alcohol or other drugs to avoid trauma-related thoughts and feelings, intentional suppression of intrusive thoughts or memories, avoidance of situations that elicit PTSD symptoms, and dependency on safety-seeking cues are all maladaptive avoidant strategies. Evidence gathering and behavioral experiments can be used to demonstrate the adverse effects of avoidance. Within-session demonstrations such as the "camel effect for thought suppression" (see Chapter 11) can also be used to highlight the negative effects of cognitive avoidance. Response prevention is used to reduce or eliminate escape responses (see Chapter 7). Many individuals with PTSD have substance abuse or dependence which may require referral for addictions rehabilitation and treatment.

The final step in this phase of treatment is teaching clients to adopt a passive, nonjudgmental, and accepting attitude to their episodes of anxiety and trauma-related intrusions. Often this involves teaching individuals to engage in a response that is opposite to their automatic avoidant response (Ehlers et al., 2005). For example, individuals with PTSD often try to suppress thoughts or memories of the trauma because they believe this is the best way to reduce anxiety. As an alternative the client is encouraged to allow the trauma intrusions to enter conscious awareness and to intentionally direct attention to the intrusion until it subsides naturally. Prolonged attention to the trauma intrusion provides disconfirming evidence against the belief "if I don't stop thinking about the trauma, I will become overwhelmed with anxiety" and it also teaches a detached, mindful acceptance of the anxiety-provoking thoughts and images.

Edward engaged in a number of avoidant strategies in an effort to control his anxiety and reexperiencing symptoms. He became severely dependent on alcohol to blunt unwanted thoughts and feelings, he avoided any situations or stimuli that triggered memories of Rwanda, and he desperately tried to suppress intrusive images of the "little orphan girl." He joined Alcoholics Anonymous (AA) and completed a substance abuse rehab program sponsored by the military. *In vivo* and imaginal exposure exercises were used to reduce Edward's cognitive and behavioral avoidance of trauma-related intrusions. In addition Edward practiced allowing (i.e., accepting) intrusive images and memories of Rwanda to occupy his mind and to attend to these thoughts until they decayed naturally. Much to his surprise, Edward learned that the frequency, intensity, and heightened anxiety associated with the unwanted intrusions declined significantly when he adopted a more benign, accepting attitude toward the thoughts and images.

Worry and rumination are often evident in PTSD. Individuals may worry about the negative consequences of chronic PTSD or they might ruminate over various ways in which they could have prevented the trauma. Many of the interventions for generalized worry discussed in Chapter 10 can be applied to the worry manifested in PTSD (e.g., worry induction, decatastrophizing, worry postponement and intentional expression, cognitive restructuring of worry beliefs). Further discussion of treatment approaches for PTSD worry can be found in Taylor (2006) and Wells and Sembi (2004).

Clinician Guideline 12.28

Elimination of dysfunctional cognitive and behavioral avoidant responses and their replacement with a more passive accepting attitude of unwanted thoughts and feelings is a critical component of cognitive therapy of PTSD.

Emotion Reduction (Supplementary)

In some cases it may be necessary to introduce emotion reduction strategies in order to help individuals with PTSD deal with exceptionally high levels of distressing emotions during daily living or when anxiety becomes intolerable during imaginal or *in vivo* exposure (Taylor, 2006). Instruction in progressive muscle relaxation, applied relaxation, or breathing retraining can be used to reduce anxiety (see Chapters 7 and 8). Grounding exercises, in which individuals are taught to turn their attention from their thoughts and feelings toward fully attending to specific stimuli in the external world, are useful for reducing severe dissociative states and flashbacks (see Najavits, 2002; Taylor, 2006). Clients are asked to fully attend to the external world by describing the properties of physical objects such as the furniture in a room, the weather outside, how the floor feels against their feet, and so on. One purpose of grounding is to remind clients that the current environment is safe even though their imagined perception is one of threat. From a cognitive perspective, grounding can be used as a "data-gathering exercise" to challenge the individual's exaggerated threat appraisals associated with reexperiencing symptoms.

Emotion reduction strategies are not an integral part of cognitive therapy for PTSD. One drawback, previously discussed in Chapter 8, is that anxiety-reduction strategies can take on avoidant properties, which is counterproductive for therapy. Individuals with PTSD may become reliant on these strategies to avoid unwanted thoughts and feelings. For this reason caution should be exercised when employing emotion regulation strategies in PTSD. In our case example, Edward received instruction in progressive muscle relaxation and he joined a yoga group. Both interventions had minimal enduring effect in reducing his generalized anxiety and practically no effect on his reexperiencing symptoms. Edward did find grounding and attention refocusing (Wells & Sembi, 2004) helpful in dealing with dissociation and flashbacks.

Clinician Guideline 12.29

Although considered an auxiliary intervention in cognitive therapy of PTSD, emotion reduction strategies are useful for coping with excessively high states of distressing emotions and reluctance to tolerate the heightened anxiety associated with exposure. However, caution must be exercised because emotional reduction can become an avoidant strategy that undermines the effectiveness of treatment.

EFFICACY OF COGNITIVE THERAPY FOR PTSD

In recent years the heightened interest in PTSD and its treatment have led to a strong empirical base for cognitive and cognitive-behavioral therapy for PTSD. Expert consensus guidelines for treatment of PTSD consider cognitive therapy one of the most effective, first-line treatments for PTSD either alone or in combination with medication (Foa, Davidson, & Frances, 1999). The treatment guidelines issued by the National Institute for Clinical Excellence (NICE), which is sponsored by the British National Health System (NHS), recommends trauma-focused cognitive-behavioral therapy or eye movement desensitization and reprocessing as preferred treatments for PTSD (NICE, 2005). DeRubeis and Crits-Christoph (1998) concluded that systematic exposure to trauma stimuli was an efficacious empirically supported treatment for PTSD, while Chambless et al. (1998) considered it a probably efficacious intervention. More recently Harvey, Bryant, and Tarrier (2003) concluded in their review of outcome studies that CBT was clearly an efficacious treatment for a range of traumas, while Hollon et al. (2006) reviewed CBT outcome studies that demonstrated enduring treatment effects.

A sufficient number of randomized control trials (RCTs) have been conducted to enable meta-analyses of the effectiveness of cognitive therapy alone or cognitive therapy plus trauma-focused exposure (CBT) in PTSD. A well-known meta-analysis conducted on 26 outcome studies revealed that exposure plus cognitive restructuring yielded a mean pre- versus posttreatment effect size of 1.66 and 70% of treatment completers no longer met diagnostic criteria for PTSD at posttreatment compared with 39.3% of patients receiving a supportive therapy condition (Bradley, Greene, Russ, Dutra, & Westen, 2005). There were no significant differences in effectiveness between exposure only, cognitive therapy plus exposure, and eye movement desensitization and reprocessing (EMDR), although this conclusion was based on a small number of comparison studies. Treatment for combat-related PTSD had the lowest effect size. In a more recent meta-analysis of 38 RCTs, trauma-focused CBT, which is most like the cognitive therapy protocol described in this chapter, was clinically superior to wait list and treatment-as-usual conditions (Bisson et al., 2007). Moreover, CBT tended to have beneficial effects on depression and anxiety as well as on PTSD symptoms, and both CBT and EMDR may be slightly more effective than stress management or other therapies such as medication alone, although there was no evidence that CBT was significantly better than EMDR. Once again both treatments produced more modest results with combat-related PTSD.

A number of studies have shown that trauma-focused cognitive therapy or CBT produces significantly greater improvement on symptom measures of PTSD, generalized anxiety, depression, and functional impairment than wait list control, treatment-as-usual, or relaxation alone conditions, and these gains are maintained over 6-, 9-, or 12-month follow-up periods (e.g., Ehlers et al., 2005; Ehlers et al., 2003; Foa, Hembree, et al., 2005; Marks, Lovell, Noshirvani, Livanou, & Thrasher, 1998; McDonagh et al., 2005; Mueser et al., 2008; Resick, Nishith, Weaver, Astin, & Feuer, 2002). In a 5-year follow-up Tarrier and Sommerfield (2004) found that no patients who received cognitive therapy relapsed into a full episode of PTSD whereas 29% of the imaginal exposure only group relapsed. This suggests that cognitive therapy for PTSD may have more enduring effects than trauma-focused imaginal exposure alone. However, cognitive therapy may be less effective when PTSD is associated with a severe mental illness like major depression, bipolar disorder, or schizophrenia (Mueser et al., 2008).

Cognitive therapy and CBT have been compared against attention placebo conditions as well as other psychotherapies. Cognitive therapy and/or prolonged exposure are significantly more effective than credible attention placebo conditions such as use of a CBT self-help book (Ehlers et al., 2003), as well as progressive muscle relaxation (Marks et al., 1998), and supportive counseling (Bryant, Moulds, Guthrie, Dang, & Nixon, 2003; Foa, Rothbaum, Riggs, & Murdock, 1991). However, cognitive therapy was not significantly more effective than present-centered therapy (a problem-solving therapy that focuses on the impact of trauma history on present coping style) in the treatment of women with PTSD due to childhood sexual abuse (McDonagh et al., 2005).

A particular controversy in the PTSD treatment literature is whether EMDR is an effective treatment, especially when compared to cognitive therapy. Although most studies have failed to find a significant difference between EMDR and exposure alone or exposure combined with cognitive restructuring or coping skills training (e.g., Lee, Gavriel, Drummond, Richards, & Greenwald, 2002; Power et al., 2002), a more recent comparison found that trauma-focused exposure tended to be more effective and to produce more rapid change than EMDR, with the latter treatment equivalent to relaxation training (Taylor et al., 2003). The full EMDR treatment package contains a strong focus on cognitive reprocessing of traumatic events and restructuring of trauma-related thoughts. Lateral eye movement desensitization is the single therapeutic ingredient that distinguishes the intervention most from cognitive therapy, and yet findings are mixed on the efficacy of this key ingredient of EMDR (see Resick, Monson, & Rizvi, 2008, for discussion). In their meta-analysis Davidson and Parker (2001) concluded that EMDR was no more effective than exposure therapies and that eye movements or other alternating movement is unnecessary because they show no incremental clinical benefit. Until such controversies are resolved, we contend that the outcome literature for cognitive therapy and CBT of PTSD is somewhat stronger and more consistent than it is for EMDR.

Numerous psychotherapy dismantling studies have investigated various components of cognitive therapy in order to isolate its effectiveness. In support of a basic proposition of the cognitive model, cognitive therapy does produce significant reductions on symptom-related cognition measures, which suggests that change in trauma-related appraisals and beliefs might mediate the effectiveness of cognitive therapy for PTSD (e.g., Ehlers et al., 2005; Mueser et al., 2008). However, Foa and Rauch (2004) found that prolonged exposure also led to significant reductions in trauma-related cognitions and the addition of cognitive restructuring did not enhance change in negative cognitions. Another important assumption of cognitive therapy is that focusing on the traumatic experiences that caused PTSD is critical for achieving significant reduction in PTSD severity. However, a randomized comparison involving 360 Vietnam veterans failed to find a significant difference between trauma-focused group psychotherapy and present-centered therapy that avoided any focus on trauma (Schnurr et al., 2003). Also, the cognitive restructuring component of cognitive processing therapy proved to be as effective as the full treatment protocol that included writing about the trauma (Resick, Galovski, et al., 2008). It is unclear from these findings whether a concerted focus on trauma is necessary for the effectiveness of cognitive therapy for PTSD.

Given that cognitive restructuring and exposure are the two primary components of cognitive therapy for PTSD, a comparison of their relative contributions is an important empirical question for understanding treatment effectiveness. Studies comparing trauma-focused imaginal and situational exposure versus CBT (exposure plus cognitive restructuring of trauma appraisals and beliefs) have found both treatments equally effective in reducing PTSD severity (Foa, Hembree, et al., 2005; Foa & Rauch, 2004; Marks et al., 1998; Paunovic & Öst, 2001). Some have questioned whether cognitive restructuring is necessary since it does not appear to enhance the treatment effectiveness of trauma exposure. However, in other studies cognitive therapy without systematic trauma exposure was equally effective to prolonged exposure (Marks et al., 1998; Resick et al., 2002; Tarrier et al., 1999), and in one case imaginal exposure plus cognitive restructuring was superior to imaginal exposure alone (Bryant, Moulds, Guthrie, et al., 2003). We conclude from these studies that exposure and cognitive restructuring are both effective therapeutic ingredients for treatment of PTSD but an incremental clinical improvement from combining them has not yet been demonstrated.

Clinician Guideline 12.30

Cognitive restructuring of trauma-related appraisals and beliefs as well as systematic and repeated trauma-focused *in vivo* and imaginal exposure are effective therapeutic ingredients of cognitive therapy that produce significant and enduring reductions in PTSD symptoms, generalized anxiety, and depression as well as improved daily functioning for chronic PTSD caused by a wide range of traumas.

SUMMARY AND CONCLUSION

PTSD is an anxiety disorder that occurs in response to a traumatic stressor and consists of trauma-related reexperiencing symptoms, avoidance or emotional numbing, and increased physiological arousal. It has a swift onset, with the majority of cases occurring within 1 month of a trauma, followed by a steep remission rate of 40–60% over a 6–12 month period.

Recognizing that only a minority of individuals exposed to trauma develop PTSD, the cognitive theory presented in Figure 12.1 proposes a diathesis–stress perspective in which certain enduring dysfunctional beliefs about personal vulnerability and danger interact with particular features of a traumatic experience to elevate the probable onset of PTSD. Once the threshold for onset is exceeded, cognitive processes at the automatic and elaborative levels of information processing ensure the persistence of PTSD symptoms. At the automatic level, the person with PTSD exhibits selective attentional priority for any trauma-related threat or danger cues, has a poorly elaborated and fragmented autobiographical memory of the trauma, and selective recall of the past trauma experience, which together reinforce negative beliefs about self, world, and future. At the elaborative, or strategic, level of information processing, the person with PTSD engages in deliberate threat appraisal of the trauma and its consequences, as well as the deleterious effects of PTSD symptoms, and relies on various cognitive and behavioral control strategies such as thought suppression, rumination, avoidance, and safety seeking to extinguish reexperiencing symptoms and negative affect. Although these maladaptive coping responses may lead to an immediate sense of relief, in the long term they contribute to the persistence of the disorder by contributing to the activation of maladaptive trauma-related schemas and associated trauma-related intrusive thoughts, images, and recollections.

There was fairly consistent research support that PTSD is characterized by (1) maladaptive, biased encoding of the trauma experience; (2) greater endorsement of negative beliefs about threat, vulnerability, and danger for self, world, future, and other people; (3) a strategic but not preconscious attentional bias for threat; (4) enhanced explicit recall of trauma-related information as well as a more fragmented, poorly elaborated trauma memory; (5) an explicit negative appraisal of trauma, its consequences, and the impact of reexperiencing symptoms; (6) reliance on cognitive avoidant coping strategies like thought suppression to quell unwanted intrusive thoughts, images, or memories of trauma; and (7) presence of avoidance and safety-seeking behaviors. However, a number of issues remain for further investigation. Much of the support for a cognitive basis to PTSD was found at the elaborative phase, with less evidence of a bias in preconscious automatic processes. Most of the research on negative beliefs, appraisals, and coping strategies relied on retrospective self-report questionnaires. More experimental studies utilizing "online" assessment of appraisals are clearly needed. Further research is also needed to determine whether the threat bias in PTSD is due to facilitated processing of threat, difficulty with threat disengagement, and/or failure to process safety cues. Finally, more prospective research is needed to determine the mediational role of these cognitive variables in the persistence of PTSD.

The objectives of cognitive therapy for PTSD are (1) to improve memory of the trauma so it can be integrated with other autobiographical memories; (2) deactivate hypervalent schemas of threat, danger, and vulnerability; (3) increase acceptance of the intrusive thoughts, images, and memories of trauma; (4) eliminate maladaptive cognitive strategies like thought suppression and rumination; and (5) reduce avoidance of PTSD or anxiety-eliciting situations and reliance on safety-seeking cues. These goals are accomplished by psychoeducation into the cognitive model, cognitive restructuring of negative appraisals and beliefs about the trauma and its consequences as well as the adverse effects of PTSD, *in vivo* exposure to avoided situations, modification of dysfunctional cognitive control strategies (e.g., thought suppression), and repeated imaginal exposure to the trauma memory. A number of randomized control trials have shown that cognitive therapy or CBT has immediate and enduring efficacy in the treatment of PTSD. As a result CBT is now recognized as a first-line choice of treatment for the disorder and can be considered an empirically supported treatment for PTSD. Although many fundamental issues are unresolved about the etiology, maintenance, and treatment of PTSD, tremendous progress has been made since the disorder was first introduced into the diagnostic nomenclature in 1980.

APPENDIX 12.1

Trauma Intrusion Self-Monitoring Form

Name: _____   Date: from _____ to: _____

Instructions: Please use this form to record any intrusive thoughts, images, or memories related to the trauma and its consequences that you experienced in the past week. Try to complete the form around the same time that you reexperienced symptoms related to the trauma in order to increase the accuracy of your remarks.

Date, Time, and Duration of Intrusion	Situations or Cues That Triggered the Intrusion	Briefly Describe the Intrusive Thought, Image, or Memory[1]	Label and Rate Severity of Associated Emotions (0–100)	Personal Significance of the Intrusion[2]	Coping Responses and Effectiveness[3]

[1]Indicate by marking an asterisk (*) beside each intrusion that occurred as a "flashback" (i.e., a momentarily reliving of some aspect of the trauma).

[2]In a few words indicate what was so distressing about this particular intrusive thought or memory of the trauma for you. What was so personally significant about the intrusive experience?

[3]What did you do to get rid of the intrusive thought, image, or memory? How effective was it?

Cognitive Restructuring Form for Trauma Intrusions

Name: _____   Date: from _____ to: _____

Instructions: Please use this form to work on challenging unhelpful thoughts and beliefs about the personal significance of intrusive thoughts, images, or memories related to the trauma and its consequences. Try to complete the form around the same time that you re-experienced symptoms related to the trauma in order to increase the effectiveness of therapy.

Date and Time	Briefly Describe the Intrusive Thought, Image, or Memory	Label and Rate Severity of Associated Emotions (0–100)	Initial Evaluation of the Intrusion [What makes this thought/memory threatening, upsetting for you? What makes it personally significant or important to you?]	Reevaluating Initial Thoughts and Beliefs about the Intrusion [What's the evidence, what are the consequences of this evaluation, am I catastrophizing the intrusion?]	Alternative More Helpful Evaluation [What's a more helpful way to think about these trauma-related intrusions?]

References

Abbott, M. J., & Rapee, R. M. (2004). Post-event rumination and negative self-appraisal in social phobia before and after treatment. *Journal of Abnormal Psychology, 113*, 136–144.

Abramowtiz, J. S. (1996). Variants of exposure and response prevention in the treatment of obsessive–compulsive disorder: A meta-analysis. *Behavior Therapy, 27*, 583–600.

Abramowitz, J. S. (2009). *Getting over OCD: A 10–step workbook for taking back your life.* New York: Guilford Press.

Abramowitz, J. S., & Deacon, B. J. (2006). Psychometric properties and construct validity of the Obsessive–Compulsive Inventory—Revised: Replication and extension with a clinical sample. *Journal of Anxiety Disorders, 20*, 1016–1035.

Abramowitz, J. S., & Foa, E. B. (2000). Does comorbid major depression influence outcome of exposure and response prevention for OCD? *Behavior Therapy, 31*, 795–800.

Abramowitz, J. S., Franklin, M. E., & Foa, E. B. (2002). Empirical status of cognitive-behavioral therapy for obsessive–compulsive disorder: A meta-analytic review. *Romanian Journal of Cognitive and Behavioral Psychotherapies, 2*, 89–104.

Abramowitz, J. S., Franklin, M. E., Schwartz, S. A., & Furr, J. M. (2003). Symptom presentation and outcome of cognitive-behavioral therapy for obsessive–compulsive disorder. *Journal of Consulting and Clinical Psychology, 71*, 1049–1057.

Abramowitz, J. S., Franklin, M. E., Street, G. P., Kozak, M. J., & Foa, E. B. (2000). Effects of comorbid depression on response to treatment for obsessive–compulsive disorder. *Behavior Therapy, 31*, 517–528.

Abramowitz, J. S., Khandker, M., Nelson, C. A., Deacon, B. J., & Rygwall, R. (2006). The role of cognitive factors in the pathogenesis of obsessive–compulsive symptoms: A prospective study. *Behaviour Research and Therapy, 44*, 1361–1374.

Abramowitz, J. S., Schwartz, S. A., Moore, K. M., & Luenzmann, K. R. (2003). Obsessive–compulsive symptoms in pregnancy and the puerperium: A review of the literature. *Journal of Anxiety Disorders, 17*, 461–478.

Abramowitz, J. S., Tolin, D. F., & Street, G. P. (2001). Paradoxical effects of thought suppression: A meta-analysis of controlled studies. *Clinical Psychology Review, 21*, 683–703.

Abramowitz, J. S., Whiteside, S., Kalsy, S. A., & Tolin, D. F. (2003). Thought control strategies in obsessive–compulsive disorder: A replication and extension. *Behaviour Research and Therapy, 41*, 529–540.

Abramowitz, J. S., Whiteside, S., Lynam, D., & Kalsy, S. (2003). Is thought-action fusion specific to obsessive–compulsive disorder?: A mediating role of negative affect. *Behaviour Research and Therapy, 41*, 1069–1079.

Abramson, L. Y., Alloy, L. B., & Metalsky, G. I. (1988). The cognitive diathesis–stress theories of depression: Toward an adequate evaluation of the theories' validities. In L. B. Alloy (Ed.), *Cognitive processes in depression* (pp. 3–30). New York: Guilford Press.

Abramson, L. Y., Metalsky, G. L., & Alloy, L. B. (1989). Hopelessness depression: A theory-based subtype of depression. *Psychological Review, 96*, 358–372.

Abramson, L. Y., Seligman, M. E. P., & Teasdale, J. D. (1978). Learned helplessness in humans: Critique and reformulation. *Journal of Abnormal Psychology, 87*, 49–74.

Adolphs, R., Tranel, D., & Damasio, A. (1998). The human amygdala in social judgment. *Nature, 393*, 470–474.

Aikins, D. E., & Craske, M. G. (2008). Sleep-based heart period variability in panic disorder with and without nocturnal panic attacks. *Journal of Anxiety Disorders, 22*, 453–463.

Akhtar, S., Wig, N. N., Varma, V. K., Peershad, D., & Verma, S.

K. (1975). A phenomenological analysis of symptoms in obsessive–compulsive neurosis. *British Journal of Psychiatry, 127*, 342–348.

Alden, L. E., & Bieling, P. (1998). Interpersonal consequences of the pursuit of safety. *Behaviour Research and Therapy, 36*, 53–64.

Alden, L. E., & Philips, N. (1990). An interpersonal analysis of social anxiety and depression. *Cognitive Therapy and Research, 14*, 499–513.

Alden, L. E., & Taylor, C. T. (2004). Interpersonal processes in social phobia. *Clinical Psychology Review, 24*, 857–882.

Alden, L. E., & Wallace, S. T. (1995). Social phobia and social appraisal in successful and unsuccessful social interactions. *Behaviour Research and Therapy, 33*, 497–505.

Alloy, L. B., Abramson, L. Y., Safford, S. M., & Gibb, B. E. (2006). The Cognitive Vulnerability to Depression (CVD) Project: Current findings and future directions. In L. B. Alloy & J. H. Riskind (Eds.), *Cognitive vulnerability to emotional disorders* (pp. 33–61). Mahwah, NJ: Erlbaum.

Alloy, L. B., Kelly, K. A., Mineka, S., & Clements, C. M. (1990). Comorbidity of anxiety and depressive disorders: A helplessness–hopelessness perspective. In J. D. Maser & C. R. Cloninger (Eds.), *Comorbidity of mood and anxiety disorders* (pp. 499–543). Washington, DC: American Psychiatric Press.

Altin, M., Clark, D. A., & Karanci, A. N. (2007). *The impact of religiosity on obsessive–compulsive cognitions and symptoms in Christian and Muslim students.* Paper presented at the World Congress of Behavioural and Cognitive Therapies, Barcelona, Spain.

Ambrose, B., & Rholes, W. S. (1993). Automatic cognitions and the symptoms of depression and anxiety in children and adolescents: An examination of the content specificity hypothesis. *Cognitive Therapy and Research, 17*, 289–308.

American Psychiatric Association (APA). (1968). *Diagnostic and statistical manula of mental disorders* (2nd ed.). Washington, DC: Author.

American Psychiatric Association (APA). (1980). *Diagnostic and statistical manual of mental disorders* (3rd ed.). Washington, DC: Author.

American Psychiatric Association (APA). (1987). *Diagnostic and statistical manual of mental disorders* (3rd ed., rev.). Washington, DC: Author.

American Psychiatric Association (APA). (1994). *Diagnostic and statistical manual of mental disorders* (4th ed.). Washington, DC: Author.

American Psychiatric Association (APA). (1998). Practice guidelines for the treatment of patients with panic disorder. *American Journal of Psychiatry, 155*(Suppl.), 1–34.

American Psychiatric Association (APA). (2000). *Diagnostic and statistical manual of mental disorders* (4th ed., text rev.). Washington, DC: Author.

Amies, P. L., Gelder, M. G., & Shaw, P. M. (1983). Social phobia: A comparative clinical study. *British Journal of Psychiatry, 142*, 174–179.

Amir, N., Beard, C., Burns, M., & Bomyea, J. (2009). Attention modification program in individuals with generalized anxiety disorder. *Journal of Abnormal Psychology, 118*, 28–33.

Amir, N., Beard, C., & Przeworski, A. (2005). Resolving ambiguity: The effect of experience on interpretation of ambiguous events in generalized social phobia. *Journal of Abnormal Psychology, 114*, 402–408.

Amir, N., Bower, E., Briks, J., & Freshman, M. (2003). Implicit memory for negative and positive social information in individuals with and without social anxiety. *Cognition and Emotion, 17*, 567–583.

Amir, N., Cashman, L., & Foa, E. B. (1997). Strategies of thought control in obsessive–compulsive disorder. *Behaviour Research and Therapy, 35*, 775–777.

Amir, N., Foa, E. B., & Coles, M. E. (1997). Factor structure of the Yale–Brown Obsessive Compulsive Scale. *Psychological Assessment, 9*, 312–316.

Amir, N., Foa, E. B., & Coles, M. E. (1998a). Automatic activation and strategic avoidance of threat-relevant information in social phobia. *Journal of Abnormal Psychology, 107*, 285–290.

Amir, N., Foa, E. B., & Coles, M. E. (1998b). Negative interpretation bias in social phobia. *Behaviour Research and Therapy, 36*, 945–957.

Amir, N., Foa, E. B., & Coles, M. E. (2000). Implicit memory bias for threat-relevant information in individuals with generalized social phobia. *Journal of Abnormal Psychology, 109*, 713–720.

Amir, N., Freshman, M., & Foa, E. B. (2000). Family distress and involvement in relatives of obsessive–compulsive patients. *Journal of Anxiety Disorders, 14*, 209–217.

Amir, N., Freshman, M., Ramsey, B., Neary, E., & Brigidi, B. (2001). Thought–action fusion in individuals with OCD symptoms. *Behaviour Research and Therapy, 39*, 765–776.

Amir, N., McNally, R. J., & Wiegartz, P. S. (1996). Implicit memory bias for threat in posttraumatic stress disorder. *Cognitive Therapy and Research, 20*, 625–635.

Amrhein, C., Pauli, P., Dengler, W., & Wiedemann, G. (2005). Covariation bias and its physiological correlates in panic disorder patients. *Journal of Anxiety Disorders, 19*, 177–191.

Amstadter, A. B., & Vernon, L. L. (2006). Suppression of neutral and trauma targets: Implications for posttraumatic stress disorder. *Journal of Traumatic Stress, 19*, 517–526.

Ancoli-Israel, S., & Roth, T. (1999). Characteristics of insomnia in the United States: Results of the 1991 National Sleep Foundation Survey. *Sleep, 22*(Suppl. 2), S347–S353.

Anderson, A. K., & Phelps, E. A. (2000). Expression without recognition: Contributions of the human amygdala to emotional communication. *Psychological Science, 11*, 106–111.

Andrews, B., Brewin, C. R., Philpott, R., & Stewart, L. (2007). Delayed-onset posttraumatic stress disorder: A systematic review of the evidence. *American Journal of Psychiatry, 164*, 1319–1326.

Andrews, G., Henderson, S., & Hall, W. (2001). Prevalence, comorbidity, disability and service utilization: Overview of the Australian National Mental Health Survey. *British Journal of Psychiatry, 178*, 145–153.

Andrews, G., Slade, T., & Issakidis, C. (2002). Deconstructing current comorbidity: Data from the Australian National Survey of Mental Health and Well-Being. *British Journal of Psychiatry, 179*, 306–314.

Andrews, V. H., & Borkovec, T. D. (1988). The differential effects of inductions of worry, somatic anxiety, and depression on emotional experience. *Journal of Behavior Therapy and Experimental Psychiatry, 19,* 21–26.

Anholt, G. E., Cath, D. C., Emmelkamp, P. M. G., van Oppen, P., Smit, J. H., & van Balkom, A. J. L. M. (2006). Do obsessional beliefs discriminate OCD without tic patients from OCD with tic and Tourette's syndrome patients? *Behaviour Research and Therapy, 44,* 1537–1543.

Ansseau, M., Dierick, M., Buntinkx, F., Cnockaert, P., De Smedt, J., Van Den Haute, M., et al. (2004). High prevalence of mental disorders in primary care. *Journal of Affective Disorders, 78,* 49–55.

Antony, M. M. (2001a). Measures for panic disorder and agoraphobia. In M. M. Antony, S. M. Orsillo, & L. Roemer (Eds.), *Practitioner's guide to empirically based measures of anxiety* (pp. 95–125). New York: Kluwer Academic/Plenum.

Antony, M. M. (2001b). Measures for obsessive–compulsive disorder. In M. M. Antony, S. M. Orsillo, & L. Roemer (Eds.), *Practitioner's guide to empirically based measures of anxiety* (pp. 219–243). New York: Kluwer Academic/Plenum.

Antony, M. M., Bieling, P. J., Cox, B. J., Enns, M. W., & Swinson, R. P. (1998). Psychometric properties of the 42-item and 21-item versions of the Depression Anxiety Stress Scales in clinical groups and a community sample. *Psychological Assessment, 10,* 176–181.

Antony, M. M., Coons, M. J., McCabe, R. E., Ashbaugh, A., & Swinson, R. P. (2006). Psychometric properties of the Social Phobia Inventory: Further evaluation. *Behaviour Research and Therapy, 44,* 1177–1185.

Antony, M. M., Downie, F., & Swinson, R. P. (1998). Diagnostic issues and epidemiology in obsessive-compulsive disorder. In R. P. Swinson, M. M. Antony, S. Rachman, & M. A. Richter (Eds.), *Obsessive-compulsive disorder: Theory, research and treatment* (pp. 3–32). New York: Guilford Press.

Antony, M. M., Ledley, D. R., Liss, A., & Swinson, R. P. (2006). Responses to symptom induction exercises in panic disorder. *Behav-iour Research and Therapy, 44,* 85–98.

Antony, M. M., & McCabe, R. E. (2004). *10 simple solutions to panic: How to overcome panic attacks, calm physical symptoms and reclaim your life.* Oakland, CA: New Harbinger.

Antony, M. M., & Norton, P. J. (2008). *The anti-anxiety workbook: Proven strategies to overcome worry, phobias, panic and obsessions.* New York: Guilford Press.

Antony, M. M., Orsillo, S. M., & Roemer, L. (Eds.). (2001). *Practitioner's guide to empirically based measures of anxiety.* New York: Kluwer Academic/Plenum.

Antony, M. M., & Rowa, K. (2005). Evidence-based assessment of anxiety disorders in adults. *Psychological Assessment, 17,* 256–266.

Antony, M. M., Rowa, K., Liss, A., Swallow, S. R., & Swinson, R. P. (2005). Social comparison processes in social phobia. *Behavior Therapy, 36,* 65–75.

Antony, M. M., & Swinson, R. P. (2000a). *Phobic disorders and panic in adults: A guide to assessment and treatment.* Washington, DC: American Psychological Association.

Antony, M. M., & Swinson, R. P. (2000b). *The shyness and social anxiety workbook: Proven techniques for overcoming your fears.* Oakland, CA: New Harbinger.

Argyle, N. (1988). The nature of cognitions in panic disorder. *Behaviour Research and Therapy, 26,* 261–264.

Arntz, A. (2003). Cognitive therapy versus applied relaxation as treatment of generalized anxiety disorder. *Behaviour Research and Therapy, 41,* 633–646.

Arntz, A., Rauer, M., & van den Hout, M. (1995). "If I feel anxious, there must be a danger": Ex-consequentia reasoning in inferring danger in anxiety disorders. *Behaviour Research and Therapy, 33,* 917–925.

Asmundson, G. J. G., & Stein, M. B. (1994). Selective processing of social threat in patients with generalized social phobia: Evaluation using a dot-probe paradigm. *Journal of Anxiety Disorders, 8,* 107–117.

Austenfeld, J. L., & Stanton, A. L. (2004). Coping through emotional approach: A new look at emotion, coping, and health-related outcomes. *Journal of Personality, 72,* 1335–1364.

Austin, D. W., & Richards, J. C. (2001). The catastrophic misinterpretation model of panic disorder. *Behaviour Research and Therapy, 39,* 1277–1291.

Austin, D. W., Richards, J. C., & Klein, B. (2006). Modification of the Body Sensations Interpretation Questionnaire (BSIQ-M): Validity and reliability. *Journal of Anxiety Disorders, 20,* 237–251.

Baer, L. (2000). *Getting control: Overcoming your obsessions and compulsions* (2nd ed.). New York: Plume.

Ball, S. G., Otto, M. W., Pollack, M. H., Uccello, R., & Rosenbaum, J. F. (1995). Differentiating social phobia and panic disorders: A test of core beliefs. *Cognitive Therapy and Research, 19,* 473–482.

Bandura, A. (1977). Self-efficacy: Toward a unifying theory of behavioral change. *Psychological Review, 84,* 191–215.

Bandura, A. (1989). Human agency in social cognitive theory. *American Psychologist, 44,* 1175–1184.

Bandura, A. (1991). Self-efficacy conception of anxiety. In R. Schwartz & R. A. Wicklund (Eds.), *Anxiety and self-focused attention* (pp. 89–110). London: Harwood Academic.

Bannon, S., Gonsalvez, C. J., & Croft, R. J. (2008). Processing impairments in OCD: It is more than inhibition! *Behaviour Research and Therapy, 46,* 689–700.

Baños, R. M., Medina, P. M., & Pascual, J. (2001). Explicit and implicit memory biases in depression and panic disorder. *Behaviour Research and Therapy, 39,* 61–74.

Barlow, D. H. (2000). Unraveling the mysteries of anxiety and its disorders from the perspective of emotion theory. *American Psychologist, 55,* 1247–1263.

Barlow, D. H. (2002). *Anxiety and its disorders: The nature and treatment of anxiety and panic* (2nd ed.). New York: Guilford Press.

Barlow, D. H., Allen, L. B., & Choate, M. L. (2004). Toward a unified treatment of emotional disorders. *Behavior Therapy, 35,* 205–230.

Barlow, D. H., & Craske, M. G. (2007). *Mastery of your anxiety and panic. Workbook* (4th ed.). Oxford, UK: Oxford University Press.

Barlow, D. H., Gorman, J. M., Shear, M. K., & Woods, S. W. (2000). Cognitive-behavioral therapy, imipramine, or their combination for panic disorder: A randomized controlled trial. *Journal of the American Medical Association, 283,* 2529–2536.

Baron, R. M., & Kenny, D. A. (1986). The moderatory–mediator variable distinction in social psychological research: Conceptual, strategic, and statistical considerations. *Journal of Personality and Social Psychology, 51,* 1173–1182.

Barsky, A. J., Cleary, P. D., Sarnie, M. K., & Ruskin, J. N. (1994). Panic disorder, palpitations, and the awareness of cardiac activity. *Journal of Nervous and Mental Disease, 182,* 63–71.

Bebbington, P. E. (1998). Epidemiology of obsessive–compulsive disorder. *British Journal of Psychiatry, 173*(Suppl. 35), 2–6.

Beck, A. T. (1963). Thinking and depression: 1. Idiosyncratic content and cognitive distortions. *Archives of General Psychiatry, 9,* 324–333.

Beck, A. T. (1964). Thinking and depression: 2. Theory and therapy. *Archives of General Psychiatry, 10,* 561–571.

Beck, A. T. (1967). *Depression: Causes and treatment.* Philadelphia: University of Pennsylvania Press.

Beck, A. T. (1970). Cognitive therapy: Nature and relation to behavior therapy. *Behavior Therapy, 1,* 184–200.

Beck, A. T. (1976). *Cognitive therapy of the emotional disorders.* New York: New American Library.

Beck, A. T. (1983). Cognitive therapy of depression: New perspectives. In P. J. Clayton & J. E. Barrett (Eds.), *Treatment of depression: Old controversies and new approaches* (pp. 265–290). New York: Raven Press.

Beck, A. T. (1985). Theoretical perspectives on clinical anxiety. In A. H. Tuma & J. Maser (Eds.), *Anxiety and the anxiety disorders* (pp. 183–196). Hillsdale, NJ: Erlbaum.

Beck, A. T. (1987). Cognitive approaches to panic disorder: Theory and therapy. In S. Rachman & J. Maser (Eds.), *Panic: Psychological perspectives* (pp. 91–109). Hillsdale, NJ: Erlbaum.

Beck, A. T. (1988). Cognitive approaches to panic: Theory and therapy. In S. Rachman & J. Maser (Eds.), *Panic: Psychological perspectives* (pp. 91–109). Hillsdale, NJ: Erlbaum.

Beck, A. T. (1996). Beyond belief: A theory of modes, personality, and psychopathology. In P. M. Salkovskis (Ed.), *Frontiers of cognitive therapy* (pp. 1–25). New York: Guilford Press.

Beck, A. T., Brown, G., Steer, R. A., Eidelson, J. I., & Riskind, J. H. (1987). Differentiating anxiety and depression: A test of the cognitive content-specificity hypothesis. *Journal of Abnormal Psychology, 96,* 179–183.

Beck, A. T., & Clark, D. A. (1997). An information processing model of anxiety: Automatic and strategic processes. *Behaviour Research and Therapy, 35,* 49–58.

Beck, A. T., & Emery, G. (with Greenberg, R. L.). (1985). *Anxiety disorders and phobias: A cognitive perspective.* New York: Basic Books.

Beck, A. T., & Emery, G. (with Greenberg, R. L.). (2005). *Anxiety disorders and phobias: A cognitive perspective* (rev. paperback ed.). New York: Basic Books.

Beck, A. T., Epstein, N., Brown, G., & Steer, R. A. (1988). An inventory for measuring clinical anxiety: Psychometric properties. *Journal of Consulting and Clinical Psychology, 56,* 893–897.

Beck, A. T., & Greenberg, R. L. (1988). Cognitive therapy of panic disorder. In R. E. Hales & A. J. Frances (Eds.), *Review of psychiatry* (Vol. 7, pp. 571–583). Washington, DC: American Psychiatric Press.

Beck, A. T., Laude, R., & Bohnert, M. (1974). Ideational components of anxiety neurosis. *Archives of General Psychiatry, 31,* 319–325.

Beck, A. T., Rush, A. J., Shaw, B. F., & Emery, G. (1979). *Cognitive therapy of depression.* New York: Guilford Press.

Beck, A. T., Sokol, L., Clark, D. A., Berchick, R., & Wright, F. (1992). A crossover study of focused cognitive therapy for panic disorder. *American Journal of Psychiatry, 149,* 778–783.

Beck, A. T., & Steer, R. A. (1990). *Manual for the Beck Anxiety Inventory.* San Antonio, TX: Psychological Corporation.

Beck, A. T., & Steer, R. A. (1993). *Manual for the Beck Depression Inventory.* San Antonio, TX: Psychological Corporation.

Beck, A. T., Steer, R. A., & Brown, G. K. (1996). *Manual for Beck Depression Inventory* (2nd ed.). San Antonio, TX: Harcourt Assessment.

Beck, A. T., Steer, R. A., & Garbin, M. G. (1988). Psychometric properties of the Beck Depression Inventory: Twenty-five years of evaluation. *Clinical Psychology Review, 8,* 77–100.

Beck, A. T., Steer, R. A., Sanderson, W. C., & Skeie, T. M. (1991). Panic disorder and suicidal ideation and behavior: Discrepant findings in psychiatric outpatients. *American Journal of Psychiatry, 148,* 1195–1199.

Beck, A. T., Ward, C. H., Mendelson, M., Mock, J., & Erbaugh, J. (1961). An inventory for measuring depression. *Archives of General Psychiatry, 4,* 561–571.

Beck, A. T., Wenzel, A., Riskind, J., Brown, G., & Steer, R. A. (2006). *Specificity of hopelessness about resolving life problems: Another test of the cognitive model of depression.* Unpublished manuscript, University of Pennsylvania Medical Center, Philadelphia.

Beck, J. G., Coffey, S. F., Palyo, S. A., Gudmundsdottir, B., Miller, L. M., & Colder, C. R. (2004). Psychometric properties of the Posttraumatic Cognitions Inventory (PTCI): A replication with motor vehicle accident survivors. *Psychological Assessment, 16,* 289–298.

Beck, J. G., Freeman, J. B., Shipherd, J. C., Hamblen, J. L., & Lackner, J. M. (2001). Specificity of Stroop interference in patients with pain and PTSD. *Journal of Abnormal Psychology, 110,* 536–543.

Beck, J. G., Ohtake, P. J., & Shipherd, J. C. (1999). Exaggerated anxiety is not unique to CO_2 in panic disorder: A comparison of hypercapnic and hypoxic challenges. *Journal of Abnormal Psychology, 108,* 473–482.

Beck, J. G., Stanley, M. A., & Zebb, B. J. (1996). Characteristics of generalized anxiety disorders in older adults: A descriptive study. *Behaviour Research and Therapy, 34,* 225–234.

Beck, J. S. (1995). *Cognitive therapy: Basics and beyond.* New York: Guilford Press.

Beck, J. S. (2005). *Cognitive therapy*

for challenging problems: What to do when the basics don't work. New York: Guilford Press.

Beck, R., Benedict, B., & Winkler, A. (2003). Depression and anxiety: Integrating the tripartite and cognitive content-specificity assessment models. Journal of Psychopathology and Behavioral Assessment, 25, 251–256.

Beck, R., & Perkins, T. S. (2001). Cognitive content-specificity for anxiety and depression: A meta-analysis. Cognitive Therapy and Research, 25, 651–663.

Beck, R., Perkins, T. S., Holder, R., Robbins, M., Gray, M., & Allison, S. H. (2001). The cognitive and emotional phenomenology of depression and anxiety: Are worry and hopelessness the cognitive correlates of NA and PA? Cognitive Therapy and Research, 25, 829–838.

Becker, C. B., Namour, N., Zayfert, C., & Hegel, M. T. (2001). Specificity of the Social Interaction Self-Statement Test in social phobia. Cognitive Therapy and Research, 25, 227–233.

Becker, E. S., Rinck, M., & Margraf, J. (1994). Memory bias in panic disorder. Journal of Abnormal Psychology, 103, 396–399.

Becker, E. S., Rinck, M., Margraf, J., & Roth, W. T. (2001). The emotional Stroop effect in anxiety disorders: General emotionality or disorder specificity? Journal of Anxiety Disorders, 15, 147–159.

Becker, E. S., Rinck, M., Roth, W. T., & Margraf, J. (1998). Don't worry and beware of white bears: Thought suppression in anxiety patients. Journal of Anxiety Disorders, 12, 39–55.

Behar, E., Alcaine, O., Zuellig, A. R., & Borkovec, T. D. (2003). Screening for generalized anxiety disorder using the Penn State Worry Questionnaire: A receiver operating characteristics analysis. Journal of Behavior Therapy and Experimental Psychiatry, 34, 25–43.

Beidel, D. C., & Turner, S. M. (2007). Shy children, phobic adults: Nature and treatment of social anxiety disorder (2nd ed.). Washington, DC: American Psychological Association.

Beidel, D. C., Turner, S. M., & Dancu, C. V. (1985). Physiological, cognition and behavioral aspects of social anxiety. Behaviour Research and Therapy, 23, 109–117.

Beidel, D. C., Turner, S. M., Stanley, M. A., & Dancu, C. V. (1989). The Social Phobia and Anxiety Inventory: Concurrent and external validity. Behavior Therapy, 20, 417–427.

Belloch, A., Morillo, C., & Giménez, A. (2004). Effects of suppressing neutral and obsession-like thoughts in normal subjects: Beyond frequency. Behaviour Research and Therapy, 42, 841–857.

Belloch, A., Morillo, C., Lucero, M., Cabedo, E., & Carrió, C. (2004). Intrusive thoughts in non-clinical subjects: The role of frequency and unpleasantness on appraisal ratings and control strategies. Clinical Psychology and Psychotherapy, 11, 100–110.

Bennett-Levy, J., Westbrook, D., Fennell, M., Cooper, M., Rouf, K., & Hackmann, A. (2004). Behavioural experiments: Historical and conceptual underpinnings. In J. Bennett-Levy, G. Butler, M. Fennell, A. Hackmann, M. Mueller, & D. Westbrook (Eds.), Oxford guide to behavioural experiments in cognitive therapy (pp. 1–20). Oxford, UK: Oxford University Press.

Bernstein, A., Zvolensky, M. J., Kotov, R., Arrindell, W. A., Taylor, S., Sandin, B., et al. (2006). Taxonicity of anxiety sensitivity: A multi-national analysis. Journal of Anxiety Disorders, 20, 1–22.

Bernstein, D. A., & Borkovec, T. D. (1973). Progressive relaxation training: A manual for the helping professions. Champaign, IL: Research Press.

Bhar, S. S., & Kyrios, M. (2000). Ambivalent self-esteem as meta-vulnerability for obsessive–compulsive disorder. Self-Concept Theory, Research and Practice: Advances from the New Millennium (pp. 143–156). Sydney, Australia: Self Research Centre.

Bhar, S. S., & Kyrios, M. (2007). An investigation of self-ambivalence in obsessive–compulsive disorder. Behaviour Research and Therapy, 45, 1845–1857.

Bienvenu, O. J., Samuels, J. F., Costa, P. T., Reti, I. M., Eaton, W. W., & Nestadt, G. (2004). Anxiety and depressive disorders and the five-factor model of personality: A higher- and lower-order personality trait investigation in a community sample. Depression and Anxiety, 20, 92–97.

Bisson, J. I., Ehlers, A., Matthews, R.,

Pilling, S., Richards, D., & Turner, S. (2007). Psychological treatments for chronic post-traumatic stress disorder: Systematic review and meta-analysis. British Journal of Psychiatry, 190, 97–104.

Blake, D. D., Weathers, F. W., Nagy, L. M., Kaloupek, G. D., Charney, D. S., & Keane, T. M. (1998). The Clinician-Administered PTSD Scale for DSM-IV. Boston: National Center for PTSD, Behavioral Science Division.

Blanchard, E. B., Buckley, T. C., Hickling, E. J., & Taylor, A. E. (1998). Posttraumatic stress disorder and comorbid major depression: Is the correlation an illusion? Journal of Anxiety Disorders, 12, 21–37.

Blanchard, E. B., Gerardi, R. J., Kolb, L. C., & Barlow, D. H. (1986). The utility of the Anxiety Disorders Interview Schedule (ADIS) in the diagnosis of post-traumatic stress disorder (PTSD) in Vietnam veterans. Behaviour Research and Therapy, 24, 577–580.

Blanchard, E. B., Jones-Alexander, J., Buckley, T. C., & Forneris, C. A. (1996). Psychometric properties of the PTSD Checklist (PCL). Behaviour Research and Therapy, 34, 669–673.

Blazer, D. G., Hughes, D., & George, L. K. (1987). Stressful life events and the onset of a generalized anxiety syndrome. American Journal of Psychiatry, 144, 1178–1183.

Bliese, P. D., Wright, K. M., Adler, A. B., Castro, C. A., Hoge, C. W., & Cabrera, O. (2008). Validating the Primary Care Posttraumatic Stress Disorder Screen and the Posttraumatic Stress Disorder Checklist with soldiers returning from combat. Journal of Consulting and Clinical Psychology, 76, 272–281.

Bodkin, J. A., Pope, H. G., Detke, M. J., & Hudson, J. I. (2007). Is PTSD caused by traumatic stress? Journal of Anxiety Disorders, 21, 176–182.

Bögels, S. M., & Lamers, C. T. J. (2002). The causal role of self-awareness in blushing-anxious, socially-anxious and social phobic individuals. Behaviour Research and Therapy, 40, 1367–1384.

Bögels, S. M., & Mansell, W. (2004). Attention processes in the maintenance and treatment of social phobia: Hypervigilance, avoidance and self-focused attention. Clinical Psychology Review, 24, 827–856.

Bögels, S. M., Rijsemus, W., & de Jong, P. J. (2002). Self-focused attention and social anxiety : The effects of experimentally heightened self-awareness on fear, blushing, cognitions, and social skills. *Cognitive Therapy and Research, 26,* 461–472.

Borkovec, T. D. (1985). The role of cognitive and somatic cues in anxiety and anxiety disorders: Worry and relaxation-induced anxiety. In A. H. Tuma & J. Maser (Eds.), *Anxiety and the anxiety disorders* (pp. 463–478). Hillsdale, NJ: Erlbaum.

Borkovec, T. D. (1994). The nature, functions, and origins of worry. In G. C. I. Davey & F. Tallis (Eds.), *Worrying: Perspectives on theory, assessment and treatment* (pp. 5–33). Chichester, UK: Wiley.

Borkovec, T. D., Alcaine, O. M., & Behar, E. (2004). Avoidance theory of worry and generalized anxiety disorder. In R. G. Heimberg, C. L. Turk, & D. S. Mennin (Eds.), *Generalized anxiety disorder: Advances in research and practice* (pp. 77–108). New York: Guilford Press.

Borkovec, T. D., & Costello, E. (1993). Efficacy of applied relaxation and cognitive-behavioral therapy in the treatment of generalized anxiety disorder. *Journal of Consulting and Clinical Psychology, 61,* 611–619.

Borkovec, T. D., & Hu, S. (1990). The effect of worry on cardiovascular response to phobic imagery. *Behaviour Research and Therapy, 28,* 69–73.

Borkovec, T. D., Newman, M. G., Lytle, R., & Pincus, A. L. (2002). A component analysis of cognitive-behavioral therapy for generalized anxiety disorder and the role of interpersonal problems. *Journal of Consulting and Clinical Psychology, 70,* 288–298.

Borkovec, T. D., Robinson, E., Pruzinsky, T., & DePree, J. A. (1983). Preliminary exploration of worry: Some characteristics and processes. *Behaviour Research and Therapy, 21,* 9–16.

Borkovec, T. D., & Roemer, L. (1995). Perceived functions of worry among generalized anxiety disorder subjects: Distraction from more emotionally distressing topics? *Journal of Behavior Therapy and Experimental Psychiatry, 26,* 25–30.

Borkovec, T. D., Shadick, R. N., & Hopkins, M. (1991). The nature of normal and pathological worry. In R. M. Rapee & D. H. Barlow (Eds.), *Chronic anxiety: Generalized anxiety disorder and mixed anxiety-depression* (pp. 29–51). New York: Guilford Press.

Borkovec, T. D., Wilkinson, L., Folenshire, R., & Lerman, C. (1983). Stimulus control applications to the treatment of worry. *Behaviour Research and Therapy, 21,* 247–251.

Bouchard, C., Rhéaume, J., & Ladouceur, R. (1999). Responsibility and perfectionism in OCD : An experimental study. *Behaviour Research and Therapy, 37,* 239–248.

Bouchard, S., Gauthier, J., Laberge, B., French, D., Pelletier, M. H., & Godbout, C. (1996). Exposure versus cognitive restructuring in the treatment of panic disorder with agoraphobia. *Behaviour Research and Therapy, 34,* 213–224.

Bouchard, S., Gauthier, J., Nouwen, A., Ivers, H., Vallieres, A., Simard, S., et al. (2007). Temporal relationship between dysfunctional beliefs, self-efficacy and panic apprehension in the treatment of panic disorder with agoraphobia. *Journal of Behavior Therapy and Experimental Psychiatry, 38,* 275–292.

Bouknight, D. P., & O'Rourke, R. A. (2000). Current management of mitral valve prolapse. *American Family Physician, 61,* 3343–3350.

Bourdon, K. H., Boyd, J. H., Rae, D. S., Burns, B. J., Thompson, J. W., & Locke, B. Z. (1988). Gender differences in phobias: Results of the ECA Community Survey. *Journal of Anxiety Disorders, 2,* 227–241.

Bourne, E. J. (2000). *The anxiety and phobia workbook* (3rd ed.). Oakland, CA: New Harbinger.

Bouton, M. E., Mineka, S., & Barlow, D. H. (2001). A modern learning theory perspective on the etiology of panic disorder. *Psychological Review, 108,* 4–22.

Bradley, B. P., Mogg, K., Falla, S. J., & Hamilton, L. R. (1998). Attentional bias for threatening facial expressions in anxiety: Manipulation of stimulus duration. *Cognition and Emotion, 12,* 737–753.

Bradley, B. P., Mogg, K., & Millar, N. H. (2000). Covert and overt orienting of attention to emotional faces in anxiety. *Cognition and Emotion, 14,* 789–808.

Bradley, B. P., Mogg, K., White, J.,

& Millar, N. (1995). Selective processing of negative information: Effects of clinical anxiety, concurrent depression, and awareness. *Journal of Abnormal Psychology, 104,* 532–536.

Bradley, B. P., Mogg, K., & Williams, R. (1994). Implicit and explicit memory for emotional information in non-clinical subjects. *Behaviour Research and Therapy, 32,* 65–78.

Bradley, B. P., Mogg, K., & Williams, R. (1995). Implicit and explicit memory for emotion-congruent information in clinical depression and anxiety. *Behaviour Research and Therapy, 33,* 755–770.

Bradley, R., Greene, J., Russ, E., Dutra, L., & Westen, D. (2005). A multidimensional meta-analysis of psychotherapy for PTSD. *American Journal of Psychiatry, 162,* 214–227.

Bradley, S. J. (2000). *Affect regulation and the development of psychopathology.* New York: Guilford Press.

Breier, A., Charney, D. S., & Heninger, G. R. (1984). Major depression in patients with agoraphobia and panic disorder. *Archives of General Psychiatry, 41,* 1129–1135.

Brendle, J. R., & Wenzel, A. (2004). Differentiating between memory and interpretative biases in socially anxious and nonanxious individuals. *Behaviour Research and Therapy, 42,* 155–171.

Breslau, N. (2002). Epidemiologic studies of trauma, posttraumatic stress disorder, and other psychiatric disorders. *Canadian Journal of Psychiatry, 47,* 923–929.

Breslau, N., Davis, G. C., & Schultz, L. R. (2003). Posttraumatic stress disorder and the incidence of nicotine, alcohol, and other drug disorders in person who have experienced trauma. *Archives of General Psychiatry, 60,* 289–294.

Breslau, N., & Kessler, R. C. (2001). The stressor criterion in DSM-IV posttraumatic stress disorder: An empirical investigation. *Biological Psychiatry, 50,* 699–704.

Breslau, N., Kessler, R. C., Chilcoat, H. D., Schultz, L. R., Davis, G. C., & Andreski, P. (1998). Trauma and posttraumatic stress disorder in the community: The 1996 Detroit Area Survey of Trauma. *Archives of General Psychiatry, 55,* 626–632.

Breslau, N., Lucia, V. C., & Alvarado, G. F. (2006). Intelligence and other predisposing factors in exposure to trauma and posttraumatic stress disorder. *Archives of General Psychiatry, 63,* 1238–1245.

Breton, J.-J., Bergeron, L., Valla, J.-P., Berthiaume, C., Gaudet, N., Lambert, J., et al. (1999). Quebec Child Mental Health Survey: Prevalence of DSM-III-R mental health disorders. *Journal of Child Psychology and Psychiatry, 40,* 375–384.

Brewin, C. R. (1988). *Cognitive foundations of clinical psychology.* Hove, UK: Erlbaum.

Brewin, C. R., Andrews, B., Rose, S., & Kirk, M. (1999). Acute stress disorder and posttraumatic stress disorder in victims of violent crime. *American Journal of Psychiatry, 156,* 360–366.

Brewin, C. R., Andrews, B., & Valentine, J. D. (2000). Meta-analysis of risk factors for posttraumatic stress disorder in trauma-exposed adults. *Journal of Consulting and Clinical Psychology, 68,* 748–766.

Brewin, C. R., Dalgleish, T., & Joseph, S. (1996). A dual representation theory of posttraumatic stress disorder. *Psychological Review, 103,* 670–686.

Brewin, C. R., & Holmes, E. A. (2003). Psychological theories of posttraumatic stress disorder. *Clinical Psychology Review, 23,* 339–376.

Brewin, C. R., Kleiner, J. S., Vasterling, J. J., & Field, A. P. (2007). Memory for emotionally neutral information in posttraumatic stress disorder: A meta-analytic investigation. *Journal of Abnormal Psychology, 116,* 448–463.

Brown, E. J., Heimberg, R. G., & Juster, H. R. (1995). Social phobia subtype and avoidant personality disorder: Effect on severity of social phobia, impairment and outcome of cognitive-behavioral treatment. *Behavior Therapy, 26,* 467–486.

Brown, E. J., Turovsky, J., Heimberg, R. G., Juster, H. R., Brown, T. A., & Barlow, D. H. (1997). Validation of the Social Interaction Anxiety Scale and the Social Phobia Scale across the anxiety disorders. *Psychological Assessment, 9,* 21–27.

Brown, G. K., Beck, A. T., Newman, C. F., Beck, J. S., & Tran, G. Q. (1997). A comparison of focused and standard cognitive therapy for panic disorder. *Journal of Anxiety Disorders, 11,* 329–345.

Brown, G. W., Harris, T. O., & Eales, M. J. (1996). Social factors and comorbidity of depressive and anxiety disorders. *British Journal of Psychiatry, 168*(Suppl. 30), 50–57.

Brown, M., Smits, J. A. J., Powers, M. B., & Telch, M. J. (2003). Differential sensitivity of the three ASI factors in predicting panic disorder patients' subjective and behavioral response to hyperventilation challenge. *Journal of Anxiety Disorders, 17,* 583–591.

Brown, M. A., & Stopa, L. (2007). The spotlight effect and the illusion of transparency in social anxiety. *Journal of Anxiety Disorders, 21,* 804–819.

Brown, T. A. (2003). Confirmatory factor analysis of the Penn State Worry Questionnaire: Multiple factors or method effects? *Behaviour Research and Therapy, 41,* 1411–1426.

Brown. T. A., Antony, M. M., & Barlow, D. H. (1992). Psychometric properties of the Penn State Worry Questionnaire in a clinical anxiety disorders sample. *Behaviour Research and Therapy, 30,* 33–37.

Brown, T. A., & Barlow, D. H. (2002). Classification of anxiety and mood disorders. In D. H. Barlow (Ed.), *Anxiety and its disorders: The nature and treatment of anxiety and panic* (2nd ed., pp. 292–327). New York: Guilford Press.

Brown, T. A., Campbell, L. A., Lehman, C. L. Grisham, J. R., & Mancill, R. B. (2001). Current and lifetime comorbidity of the DSM-IV anxiety and mood disorders in a large clinical sample. *Journal of Abnormal Psychology, 110,* 585–599.

Brown, T. A., Chorpita, B. F., & Barlow, D. H. (1998). Structural relationships among dimensions of the DSM-IV anxiety and mood disorders and dimensions of negative affect, positive affect, and autonomic arousal. *Journal of Abnormal Psychology, 107,* 179–192.

Brown, T. A., Chorpita, B. F., Korotitsch, W., & Barlow, D. H. (1997). Psychometric properties of the Depression Anxiety Stress Scales (DASS) in clinical samples. *Behaviour Research and Therapy, 35,* 79–89.

Brown, T. A., & Deagle, E. A. (1992). Structured interview assessment of nonclinical panic. *Behavior Therapy, 23,* 75–85.

Brown, T. A., Di Nardo, P. A., & Barlow, D. H. (1994). *Anxiety Disorders Interview Schedule for DSM-IV Adult Version.* Oxford, UK: Oxford University Press/Graywind.

Brown, T. A., Di Nardo, P. A., Lehman, C. L., & Campbell, L. A. (2001). Reliability of DSM-IV anxiety and mood disorders: Implications for the classification of emotional disorders. *Journal of Abnormal Psychology, 110,* 49–58.

Brown, T. A., O'Leary, T. A., & Barlow, D. H. (2001). Generalized anxiety disorder. In D. H. Barlow (Ed.), *Clinical handbook of psychological disorders: A step-by-step treatment manual* (3rd ed., pp. 154–208). New York: Guilford Press.

Brown, T. A., White, K. S., & Barlow, D. H. (2005). A psychometric reanalysis of the Albany Panic and Phobia Questionnaire. *Behaviour Research and Therapy, 43,* 337–355.

Brozina, K., & Abela, J. R. Z. (2006). Behavioural inhibition, anxious symptoms, and depressive symptoms: A short-term prospective examination of a diathesis–stress model. *Behaviour Research and Therapy, 44,* 1337–1346.

Brozovich, F., & Heimberg, R. G. (2008). An analysis of post-event processing in social anxiety disorder. *Clinical Psychology Review, 28,* 891–903.

Bruch, M. A., & Cheek, J. M. (1995). Developmental factors in childhood and adolescent shyness. In R. G. Heimberg, M. R. Liebowitz, D. A. Hope, & F. R. Schneier (Eds.), *Social phobia: Diagnosis, assessment, and treatment* (pp. 163–182). New York: Guilford Press.

Bryant, R. A. (2003). Early predictors of posttraumatic stress disorder. *Biological Psychiatry, 53,* 789–795.

Bryant, R. A. (2007). Does dissociation further our understanding of PTSD? *Journal of Anxiety Disorders, 21,* 183–191.

Bryant, R. A., & Guthrie, R. M. (2007). Maladaptive self-appraisals before trauma exposure predict posttraumatic stress disorder. *Journal of Consulting and Clinical Psychology, 75,* 812–815.

Bryant, R. A., & Harvey, A. G. (1995). Processing threatening information in posttraumatic stress disorder. *Journal of Abnormal Psychology, 104,* 537–541.

Bryant, R. A., & Harvey, A. G.

(1998). Relationship between acute stress disorder and post-traumatic stress disorder following mild traumatic brain injury. *American Journal of Psychiatry, 155*, 625–629.

Bryant, R. A., Moulds, M. L., Guthrie, R. M., Dang, S. T., & Nixon, R. D. V. (2003). Imaginal exposure alone and imaginal exposure with cognitive restructuring in treatment of posttraumatic stress disorder. *Journal of Consulting and Clinical Psychology, 71*, 706–712.

Bryant, R. A., Moulds, M. L., & Nixon, R. V. D. (2003). Cognitive behavior therapy of acute stress disorder: A four-year follow-up. *Behaviour Research and Therapy, 41*, 489–494.

Bryant, R. A., Moulds, M. L., Nixon, R. D. V., Mastrodomenico, J., Felmingham, K., & Hopwood, S. (2006). Hypnotherapy and cognitive behavior therapy of acute stress disorder: A 3-year follow-up. *Behaviour Research and Therapy, 44*, 1331–1335.

Buckley, T. C., Blanchard, E. B., & Hickling, E. J. (2002). Automatic and strategic processing of threat stimuli: A comparison between PTSD, panic disorder, and nonanxiety controls. *Cognitive Therapy and Research, 26*, 97–115.

Buckley, T. C., Blanchard, E. B., & Neill, W. T. (2000). Information processing and PTSD: A review of the empirical literature. *Clinical Psychology Review, 28*, 1041–1065.

Buller, R., Maier,W., & Benkert, O. (1986). Clinical subtypes of panic disorder: Their descriptive and prospective validity. *Journal of Affective Disorders, 11*, 105–114.

Buller, R., Maier, W., Goldenberg, I. M., Lavori, P. W., & Benkert, O. (1991). Chronology of panic and avoidance, age of onset in panic disorder, and prediction of treatment response: A report from the Cross-National Collaborative Panic Study. *European Archives of Psychiatry and Clinical Neuroscience, 240*, 163–168.

Burke, K. C., Burke, J. D., Regier, D. A., & Rae, D. S. (1990). Age at onset of selected mental disorders in five community populations. *Archives of General Psychiatry, 47*, 511–518.

Burke, M., & Mathews, A. (1992). Autobiographical memory and clinical anxiety. *Cognition and Emotion, 6*, 23–35.

Burns, G. L., Formea, G. M., Keortge, S., & Sternberger, L. G. (1995). The utilization of nonpatient samples in the study of obsessive–compulsive disorder. *Behaviour Research and Therapy, 33*, 133–144.

Burns, G. L., Keortge, S. G., Formea, G. M., & Sternberger, L. G. (1996). Revision of the Padua Inventory of Obsessive Compulsive Disorder Symptoms: Distinctions between worry, obsessions and compulsions. *Behaviour Research and Therapy, 34*, 163–173.

Butler, G. (2007). *Overcoming social anxiety and shyness self-help course: A 3-part programme based on cognitive behavioural techniques. Part one: Understanding social anxiety.* London: Robinson.

Butler, A. C., Chapman, J. F., Forman, E. M., & Beck, A. T. (2006). The empirical status of cognitive-behavioral therapy: A review of meta-analyses. *Clinical Psychology Review, 26*, 17–31.

Butler, G., Fennell, M., Robson, P., & Gelder, M. (1991). Comparison of behavior therapy and cognitive behavior therapy in the treatment of generalized anxiety disorder. *Journal of Consulting and Clinical Psychology, 59*, 167–175.

Butler, G., & Hope, T. (2007). *Managing your mind: The mental fitness guide.* Oxford, UK: Oxford University Press.

Butler, G., & Mathews, A. (1983). Cognitive processes in anxiety. *Advances in Behaviour Research and Therapy, 5*, 51–62.

Butler, G., & Mathews, A. (1987). Anticipatory anxiety and risk perception. *Cognitive Therapy and Research, 11*, 551–565.

Butler, G., & Wells, A. (1995). Cognitive-behavioral treatments: Clinical applications. In R. G. Heimberg, M. R. Liebowitz, D. A. Hope, & F. R. Schneier (Eds.), *Social phobia: Diagnosis, assessment, and treatment* (pp. 310–333). New York: Guilford Press.

Butler, G., Wells, A., & Dewick, H. (1995). Differential effects of worry and imagery after exposure to a stressful stimulus: A pilot study. *Behavioural and Cognitive Psychotherapy, 23*, 45–56.

Calamari, J. E., Cohen, R. J., Rector, N. A., Szacun-Shimizu, K., Riemann, B. C., & Norberg, M. M. (2006). Dysfunctional belief-based obsessive–compulsive disorder subgroups. *Behaviour Research and Therapy, 44*, 1347–1360.

Calamari, J. E., Hale, L. R., Heffelfinger, S. K., Janeck, S., Lau, J. J., Weerts, M. A., et al. (2001). Relations between anxiety sensitivity and panic symptoms in nonreferred children and adolescents. *Journal of Behavior Therapy and Experimental Psychiatry, 32*, 117–136.

Calamari, J. E., & Janeck, A. S. (1997). *Negative intrusive thoughts in obsessive–compulsive disorder: Appraisal and response differences.* Poster presented at the Anxiety Disorders Association of America National Convention, New Orleans, LA.

Calamari, J. E., Wiegartz, P. S., Riemann, B. C., Cohen, R. J., Greer, A., Jacobi, D. M., et al. (2004). Obsessive–compulsive disorder subtypes: An attempted replication and extension of a symptom-based taxonomy. *Behaviour Research and Therapy, 42*, 647–670.

Calvocoressi, L., Lewis, B., Harris, M., Trufan, S. J., Goodman, W. K., McDougle, C. J., et al. (1995). Family accommodation in obsessive–compulsive disorder. *American Journal of Psychiatry, 152*, 441–443.

Canadian Community Health Survey: Mental health and well-being. (2003, September 3). *The Daily*, Statistics Canada.

Canli, T., Sivers, H., Whitfield, S. L., Gotlib, I. H., & Gabrieli, J. D. E. (2002). Amygdala response to happy faces as a function of extraversion. *Science, 296*, p. 2191. (Abstract)

Canli, T., Zhao, Z., Desmond, J. E., Kang, E., Gross, J., & Gabrieli, J. D. E. (2001). An fMRI study of personality influences on brain reactivity to emotional stimuli. *Behavioral Neuroscience, 115*, 33–42.

Canon, W. B. (1927). *Bodily changes in pain, hunger, fear and rage: An account of recent searches into the function of emotional excitement.* New York: Appleton and Company.

Cantor, N. (1990). From thought to behavior: "Having" and "doing" in the study of personality and cognition. *American Psychologist, 45*, 735–750.

Cantor, N., Norem, J., Langston, C., Zirkel, S., Fleeson, W., & Cook-Flannagan, C. (1991). Life tasks and daily life experience. *Journal of Personality, 59*, 425–451.

Carleton, R. N., Collimore, K. C., & Asmundson, G. J. G. (2007).

Social anxiety and fear of negative evaluation: Construct validity of the BFNE-II. *Journal of Anxiety Disorders, 21*, 131–141.

Carr, A. T. (1974). Compulsive neurosis: A review of the literature. *Psychological Bulletin, 81*, 311–318.

Carr, R. E., Lehrer, P. M., Rausch, L., & Hochron, S. M. (1994). Anxiety sensitivity and panic attacks in an asthmatic population. *Behaviour Research and Therapy, 32*, 411–418.

Carter, M. M., Suchday, S., & Gore, K. L. (2001). The utility of the ASI factors in predicting response to voluntary hyperventilation among nonclinical participants. *Journal of Anxiety Disorders, 15*, 217–230.

Carter, R. M., Wittchen, H.-U., Pfister, H., & Kessler, R. C. (2001). One-year prevalence of subthreshold and threshold DSM-IV generalized anxiety disorder in a nationally representative sample. *Depression and Anxiety, 13*, 78–88.

Cartwright-Hatton, S., & Wells, A. (1997). Beliefs about worry and intrusions: The Meta-Cognitions Questionnaire and its correlates. *Journal of Anxiety Disorders, 11*, 279–296.

Carver, C. S., Scheier, M. F., & Weintraub, J. K. (1989). Assessing coping strategies: A theoretically based approach. *Journal of Personality and Social Psychology, 56*, 267–283.

Casey, L. M., Oei, T. P. S., & Newcombe, P. A. (2004). An integrated cognitive model of panic disorder: The role of positive and negative cognitions. *Clinical Psychology Review, 24*, 529–555.

Cassidy, K. L., McNally, R. J., & Zeitlin, S. B. (1992). Cognitive processing of trauma cues in rape vicitms with post-traumatic stress disorder. *Cognitive Therapy and Reserch, 16*, 283–295.

Cautela, J. R., & Groden, J. (1978). *Relaxation: A comprehensive manual for adults, children and children with special needs.* Champaign, IL: Research Press.

Ceschi, G., Van der Linden, M., Dunker, D., Perroud, A., & Brédart, S. (2003). Further exploration memory bias in compulsive washers. *Behaviour Research and Therapy, 41*, 737–748.

Chambless, D. L., Baker, M. J., Baucom, D. H., Beutler, L. E., Calhoun, K. S., Crits-Christoph, P., et al. (1998). Update on empirically

validated therapies II. *Clinical Psychologist, 51*, 3–16.

Chambless, D. L., Caputo, G. C., Bright, P., & Gallagher, R. (1984). Assessment of fear of fear in agoraphobics: The Body Sensations Questionnaire and the Agoraphobic Cognitions Questionnaire. *Journal of Consulting and Clinical Psychology, 52*, 1090–1097.

Chambless, D. L., Caputo, G. C., Jasin, S. E., Gracely, E. J., & Williams, C. (1985). The Mobility Inventory for Agoraphobia. *Behaviour Research and Therapy, 23*, 35–44.

Chambless, D. L., Fydrich, T., & Rodebaugh, T. L. (2006). Generalized social phobia and avoidant personality disorder: Meaningful distinction or useless duplication? *Depression and Anxiety, 10*, 1–12.

Chambless, D. L., & Gracely, E. J. (1989). Fear of fear and the anxiety disorders. *Cognitive Therapy and Research, 13*, 9–20.

Chambless, D. L., & Ollendick, T. H. (2001). Empirically supported psychological interventions: Controversies and evidence. *Annual Review of Psychology, 52*, 685–716.

Chambless, D. L., & Peterman, M. (2004). Evidence on cognitive-behavioral therapy for generalized anxiety disorder and panic disorder. In R. L. Leahy (Ed.), *Contemporary cognitive therapy: Theory, research, and practice* (pp. 86–115). New York: Guilford Press.

Chapman, T. F., Mannuzza, S., & Fyer, A. J. (1995). Epidemiological and family studies of social phobia. In R. G. Heimberg, M. R. Liebowitz, D. A. Hope, & F. R. Schneier (Eds.), *Social phobia: Diagnosis, assessment, and treatment* (pp. 21–40). New York: Guilford Press.

Chartier, M. J., Hazen, A. L., & Stein, M. B. (1998). Lifetime patterns of social phobia: A retrospective study of the course of social phobia in a nonclinical population. *Depression and Anxiety, 7*, 113–121.

Chartier, M. J., Walker, J. R., & Stein, M. B. (2001). Social phobia and potential childhood risk factors in a community sample. *Psychological Medicine, 31*, 307–315.

Chavira, D. A., Stein, M. B., & Malcarne, V. L. (2002). Scrutinizing the relationship between shyness

and social phobia. *Journal of Anxiety Disorders, 16*, 585–598.

Chelminski, I., & Zimmerman, M. (2003). Pathological worry in depressed and anxious patients. *Journal of Anxiety Disorders, 17*, 533–546.

Chen, E., Lewin, M. R., & Craske, M. G. (1996). Effects of state anxiety on selective processing of threatening information. *Cognition and Emotion, 10*, 225–240.

Chen, Y. P., Ehlers, A., Clark, D. M., & Mansell, W. (2002). Patients with generalized social phobia direct their attention away from faces. *Behaviour Research and Therapy, 40*, 677–687.

Cherian, A. E., & Frost, R. O. (2007). Treating compulsive hoarding. In M. M. Antony, C. Purdon, & L. J. Summerfeldt (Eds.), *Psychological treatment of obsessive–compulsive disorder: Fundamentals and beyond* (pp. 231–249). Washington, DC: American Psychological Association.

Chilcoat, H. D., & Breslau, N. (1998). Posttraumatic stress disorder and drug disorders: Testing causal pathways. *Archives of General Psychiatry, 55*, 913–917.

Chorpita, B. F., & Barlow, D. H. (1998). The development of anxiety: The role of control in the early environment. *Psychological Bulletin, 124*, 3–21.

Christensen, H., Hadzi-Pavlovic, D., Andrews, G., & Mattick, R. (1987). Behavior therapy and tricyclic medication in the treatment of obsessive–compulsive disorder: A quantitative review. *Journal of Consulting and Clinical Psychology, 55*, 701–711.

Clark, D. A. (2002). A cognitive perspective on OCD and depression: Distinct and related features. In R. O. Frost & G. S. Steketee (Eds.), *Cognitive approaches to obsessions and compulsions: Theory, assessment and treatment* (pp. 233–250). Oxford, UK: Elsevier Press.

Clark, D. A. (2004). *Cognitive behavior therapy for OCD.* New York: Guilford Press.

Clark, D. A. (2006a). Obsessive–compulsive disorder: The role of homework assignments. In N. Kazantzis & L. L'Abate (Eds.), *Handbook of homework assignments in psychotherapy: Research, practice and prevention.* New York: Springer.

Clark, D. A. (2006b). *Sensitivity and specificity analysis of the CBOCI* based on the validation sample. Unpublished manuscript, University of New Brunswick, Canada.

Clark, D. A., Antony, M. M., Beck, A. T., Swinson, R. P., & Steer, R. A. (2005). Screening for obsessive and compulsive symptoms: Validation of the Clark–Beck Obsessive–Compulsive Inventory. *Psychological Assessment, 17*, 132–143.

Clark, D. A., & Beck, A. T. (2002). *Manual for the Clark–Beck Obsessive Compulsive Inventory*. San Antonio, TX: Psychological Corporation.

Clark, D. A., & Beck, A. T. (2010). *Defeat fear and anxiety: A cognitive therapy workbook*. Manuscript in preparation, Department of Psychology, University of New Brunswick, Canada.

Clark, D. A., & Beck, A. T. (with Alford, B.). (1999). *Scientific foundations of cognitive theory and therapy of depression*. New York: Wiley.

Clark, D. A., Beck, A. T., & Beck, J. S. (1994). Symptom differences in major depression, dysthymia, panic disorder, and generalized anxiety disorder. *American Journal of Psychiatry, 151*, 205–209.

Clark, D. A., Beck, A. T., & Stewart, B. (1990). Cognitive specificity and positive–negative affectivity: Complementary or contradictory views on anxiety and depression? *Journal of Abnormal Psychology, 99*, 148–155.

Clark, D. A., & Claybourn, M. (1997). Process characteristics of worry and obsessive intrusive thoughts. *Behaviour Research and Therapy, 35*, 1139–1141.

Clark, D. A., & Guyitt, B. D. (2008). Pure obsessions: Conceptual misnomer or clinical anomaly? In J. S. Abramowitz, S. Taylor, & D. McKay (Eds.), *Obsessive-compulsive disorder: Subtypes and spectrum conditions* (pp. 53–75). Amsterdam, The Netherlands: Elsevier.

Clark, D. A., & O'Connor, K. (2005). Thinking is believing: Ego-dystonic intrusive thoughts in obsessive-compulsive disorder. In D. A. Clark (Ed.), *Intrusive thoughts in clinical disorders: Theory, research and treatment* (pp. 145–174). New York: Guilford Press.

Clark, D. A., Purdon, C., & Byers, E. S. (2000). Appraisal and control of sexual and non-sexual intrusive thoughts in university students.

Behaviour Research and Therapy, 38, 439–455.

Clark, D. A., Purdon, C., & Wang, A. (2003). The Meta-Cognitive Beliefs Questionnaire: Development of a measure of obsessional beliefs. *Behaviour Research and Therapy, 41*, 655–669.

Clark, D. A., Radomsky, A., Sica, C., & Simos, G. (2005). *Normal obsessions: A matter of interpretation?* Paper presented at the annual meeting of the European Association for Behavioural and Cognitive Therapies, Thessaloniki, Greece.

Clark, D. A., & Rhyno, S. (2005). Unwanted intrusive thoughts in nonclinical individuals: Implications for clinical disorders. In D. A. Clark (Ed.), *Intrusive thoughts in clinical disorders: Theory, research, and treatment* (pp. 1–29). New York: Guilford Press.

Clark, D. A., Steer, R. A., & Beck, A. T. (1994). Common and specific dimensions of self-reported anxiety and depression: Implications for the cognitive and tripartite models. *Journal of Abnormal Psychology, 103*, 645–654.

Clark, D. A., Steer, R. A., Beck, A. T., & Snow, D. (1996). Is the relationship between anxious and depressive cognitions and symptoms linear or curvilinear? *Cognitive Therapy and Research, 20*, 135–154.

Clark, D. B., Keske, U., Masia, C. L., Spaulding, S. A., Brown, C., Mammen, O., et al. (1997). Systematic assessment of social phobia in clinical practice. *Depression and Anxiety, 6*, 47–61.

Clark, D. B., Turner, S. M., Beidel, D. C., Donovan, J. E., Kirisci, L., & Jacob, R. G. (1994). Reliability and validity of the Social Phobia and Anxiety Inventory for adolescents. *Psychological Assessment, 6*, 135–140.

Clark, D. M. (1986a). A cognitive approach to panic. *Behaviour Research and Therapy, 24*, 461–470.

Clark, D. M. (1986b). Cognitive therapy for anxiety. *Behavioural Psychotherapy, 14*, 283–294.

Clark, D. M. (1988). A cognitive model of panic attacks. In S. Rachman & J. D. Maser (Eds.), *Panic:Psychological perspectives* (pp. 71–89). Hillsdale, NJ: Erlbaum.

Clark, D. M. (1993). Cognitive mediation of panic attacks induced

by biological challenge tests. *Advances in Behaviour Research and Therapy, 15*, 75–84.

Clark, D. M. (1996). Panic disorder: From theory to therapy. In P. M. Salkovskis (Ed.), *Frontiers of cognitive therapy* (pp. 318–344). New York: Guilford Press.

Clark, D. M. (1997). Panic disorder and social phobia. In D. M. Clark & C. G. Fairburn (Eds.), *Science and practice of cognitive behaviour therapy* (pp. 121–153). Oxford, UK: Oxford University Press.

Clark, D. M. (1999). Anxiety disorders: Why they persist and how to treat them. *Behaviour Research and Therapy, 37*(Suppl. 1), S5–S27.

Clark, D. M. (2001). A cognitive perspective on social phobia. In W. R. Crozier & L. E. Alden (Eds.), *International handbook of social anxiety: Concepts, research and interventions relating to the self and shyness* (pp. 405–430). New York: Wiley.

Clark, D. M., & Beck, A. T. (1988). Cognitive approaches. In C. Last & M. Hersen (Eds.), *Handbook of anxiety disorders* (pp. 362–385). Elmsford, NY: Pergamon Press.

Clark, D. M., & Ehlers, A. (1993). An overview of the cognitive theory and treatment of panic disorder. *Applied and Preventive Psychology, 2*, 131–139.

Clark, D. M., & Ehlers, A. (2004). Posttraumatic stress disorder: From cognitive theory to therapy. In R. L. Leahy (Ed.), *Contemporary cognitive therapy: Theory, research, and practice* (pp. 141–160). New York: Guilford Press.

Clark, D. M., Ehlers, A., Hackmann, A., McManus, F., Fennell, M., Grey, N., et al. (2006). Cognitive therapy versus exposure and applied relaxation in social phobia: A randomized controlled trial. *Journal of Consulting and Clinical Psychology, 74*, 568–578.

Clark, D. M., Ehlers, A., McManus, F., Hackmann, A., Fennell, M., Campbell, H., et al. (2003). Cognitive therapy versus fluoxetine in generalized social phobia: A randomized placebo-controlled trial. *Journal of Consulting and Clinical Psychology, 71*, 1058–1067.

Clark, D. M., & McManus, F. (2002). Information processing in social phobia. *Biological Psychiatry, 51*, 92–100.

Clark, D. M., & Salkovskis, P. M. (1986). *Cognitive treatment for panic attacks: Therapist's manual.* Unpublished manuscript, Department of Psychiatry, Oxford University, Warneford Hospital, Oxford, UK.

Clark, D. M., Salkovskis, P. M., & Chalkley, A. J. (1985). Respiratory control as a treatment for panic attacks. *Journal of Behavior Therapy and Experimental Psychiatry, 16,* 23–30.

Clark, D. M., Salkovskis, P. M., Gelder, M., Koehler, C., Martin, M., Anastasides, P., et al. (1988). Tests of a cognitive theory of panic. In I. Hand & H. U. Wittchen (Eds.), *Panic and phobias 2* (pp. 149–158). Berlin: Springer-Verlag.

Clark, D. M., Salkovskis, P. M., Hackmann, A., Middleton, H., Anastasiades, P., & Gelder, M. (1994). A comparison of cognitive therapy, applied relaxation and imipramine in the treatment of panic disorder. *British Journal of Psychiatry, 164,* 759–769.

Clark, D. M., Salkovskis, P. M., Hackman, A., Wells, A., Ludgate, J., & Gelder, M. (1999). Brief cognitive therapy for panic disorder: A randomized controlled trial. *Journal of Consulting and Clinical Psychology, 67,* 583–589.

Clark, D. M., Salkovskis, P. M., Öst, L.-G., Breitholtz, E., Koehler, K. A., Westling, B. E., et al. (1997). Misinterpretation of body sensations in panic disorder. *Journal of Consulting and Clinical Psychology, 65,* 203–213.

Clark, D. M., & Wells, A. (1995). A cognitive model of social phobia. In R. G. Heimberg, M. R. Liebowitz, D. A. Hope, & F. R. Schneier (Eds.), *Social phobia: diagnosis, assessment and treatment* (pp. 69–93). New York: Guilford Press.

Clark, L. A., Watson, D., & Mineka, S. (1994). Temperament, personality, and the mood and anxiety disorders. *Journal of Abnormal Psychology, 103,* 103–116.

Classen, C., Koopman, C., Hales, R., & Spiegel, D. (1998). Acute stress disorder as a predictor of posttraumatic stress symptoms. *American Journal of Psychiatry, 155,* 620–624.

Clerkin, E. M., Teachman, B. A., & Smith-Janik, S. B. (2008). Sudden gains in group cognitive-behavioral therapy for panic disorder. *Behaviour Research and Therapy, 46,* 1244–1250.

Cloitre, M., Cancienne, J., Heimberg, R. G., Holt, C. S., & Liebowitz, M. (1995). Memory bias does not generalize across anxiety disorders. *Behaviour Research and Therapy, 33,* 305–307.

Cloitre, M., Shear, M. K., Cancienne, J., & Zeitlin, S. B. (1994). Implicit and explicit memory for catastrophic associations to bodily sensation words in panic disorder. *Cognitive Therapy and Research, 18,* 225–240.

Cohen, R. J., & Calamari, J. E. (2004). Thought-focused attention and obsessive–compulsive symptoms: An evaluation of cognitive self-consciousness in a nonclinical sample. *Cognitive Therapy and Research, 28,* 457–471.

Coleman, S. S., Brod, M., Potter, L. P., Buesching, D. P., & Rowland, C. R. (2004). Cross-sectional 7-year follow-up of anxiety in primary care patients. *Depression and Anxiety, 19,* 105–111.

Coles, M. E., & Heimberg, R. G. (2002). Memory biases in the anxiety disorders: Current status. *Clinical Psychology Review, 22,* 587–627.

Coles, M. E., & Heimberg, R. G. (2005). Thought control strategies in generalized anxiety disorder. *Cognitive Therapy and Research, 29,* 47–56.

Coles, M. E., & Horng, B. (2006). A prospective test of cognitive vulnerability to obsessive compulsive disorder. *Cognitive Therapy and Research, 30,* 723–746.

Coles, M. E., Pietrefesa, A. S., Schofield, C. A., & Cook, L. M. (2008). Predicting changes in obsessive compulsive symptoms over a six month follow-up: A prospective test of cognitive models of obsessive compulsive disorder. *Cognitive Therapy and Research, 32,* 657–675.

Coles, M. E., Turk, C. L., & Heimberg, R. G. (2002). The role of memory perspective in social phobia: Immediate and delayed memories for role-played situations. *Behavioural and Cognitive Psychotherapy, 3,* 415–425.

Coles, M. E., Turk, C. L., Heimberg, R. G., & Fresco, D. M. (2001). Effects of varying levels of anxiety within social situations: Relationship to memory perspective and attributions in social phobia. *Behaviour Research and Therapy, 39,* 651–665.

Collins, K. A., Westra, H. A., Dozois, D. J. A., & Stewart, S. H. (2005). The validity of the brief version of the Fear of Negative Evaluation Scale. *Journal of Anxiety Disorders, 19,* 345–359.

Connor, K. M., & Davidson, J. R. T. (1998). Generalized anxiety disorder: Neurobiological and pharmacotherapeutic perspectives. *Biological Psychiatry, 44,* 1286–1294.

Conrad, A., & Roth, W. T. (2007). Muscle relaxation therapy for anxiety disorders: It works but how? *Journal of Anxiety Disorders, 21,* 243–264.

Constans, J. I. (2001). Worry propensity and the perception of risk. *Behaviour Research and Therapy, 39,* 721–729.

Constans, J. I., McCloskey, M. S., Vasterling, J. J., Brailey, K., & Mathews, A. (2004). Suppression of attentional bias in PTSD. *Journal of Abnormal Psychology, 113,* 315–323.

Constans, J. I., Penn, D. L., Ilen, G. H., & Hope, D. A. (1999). Intepretative biases for ambiguous stimuli in social anxiety. *Behaviour Research and Therapy, 37,* 643–651.

Conway, M., Howell, A., & Giannopoulos, C. (1991). Dysphoria and thought suppression. *Cognitive Therapy and Research, 15,* 153–166.

Coplan, J. D., & Lydiard, R. B. (1998). Brain circuits in panic disorder. *Biological Psychiatry, 44,* 1264–1276.

Corneil, W., Beaton, R., Murphy, S., Johnson, C., & Pike, K. (1999). Exposure to traumatic incidents and prevalence of posttraumatic stress symptomatology in urban firefighters in two countries. *Journal of Occupational Health Psychology, 4,* 131–141.

Coryell, W., Noyes, R., & House, J. D. (1986). Mortality among outpatients with anxiety disorders. *American Journal of Psychiatry, 143,* 508–510.

Costello, C. G. (1971). Anxiety and the persisting novelty of input from the autonomic nervous system. *Behavior Therapy, 2,* 321–333.

Costello, E. J., Mustillo, S., Erkanli, A., Keeler, G., & Angold, A. (2003). Prevalence and development of psychiatric disorders in childhood and adolescence. *Archives of General Psychiatry, 60,* 837–844.

Cottraux, J., Mollard, E., Bouvard,

M., Marks, I., Sluys, M., Nury, A. M., et al. (1990). A controlled study of fluvoxamine and exposure in obsessive–compulsive disorder. *International Clinical Psychopharmacology, 5,* 17–30.

Cottraux, J., Note, I., Yao, S. N., Lafont, S., Note, B., Mollard, E., et al. (2001). A randomized controlled trial of cognitive therapy versus intensive behavior therapy in obsessive compulsive disorder. *Psychotherapy and Psychosomatics, 70,* 288–297.

Covin, R., Ouimet, A. J., Seeds, P. M., & Dozois, D. J. A. (2008). A meta-analysis of CBT for pathological worry among clients with GAD. *Journal of Anxiety Disorders, 22,* 108–116.

Cox, B. J., Endler, N. S., Norton, G. R., & Swinson, R. P. (1991). Anxiety sensitivity and nonclinical panic attacks. *Behaviour Research and Therapy, 29,* 367–369.

Cox, B. J., Endler, N. S., Swinson, R. P., & Norton, G. R. (1992). Situations and specific coping strategies associated with clinical and nonclinical panic attacks. *Behaviour Research and Therapy, 30,* 67–69.

Cox, B. J., Enns, M. W., Walker, J. R., Kjernisted, K., & Pidlubny, S. R. (2001). Psychological vulnerabilities in patients with major depression vs. panic disorder. *Behaviour Research and Therapy, 39,* 567–573.

Cox, B. J., MacPherson, P. S. R., & Enns, M. W. (2005). Psychiatric correlates of childhood shyness in a nationally representative sample. *Behaviour Research and Therapy, 43,* 1019–1027.

Cox, B. J., Ross, L., Swinson, R. P., & Direnfeld, D. M. (1998). A comparison of social phobia outcome measures in cognitive-behavioral group therapy. *Behavior Modification, 22,* 285–297.

Craske, M. G. (2003). *Origins of phobias and anxiety disorders: Why more women than men?* Amsterdam, The Netherlands: Elsevier.

Craske, M. G., & Barlow, D. H. (1988). A review of the relationship between panic and avoidance. *Clinical Psychology Review, 8,* 667–685.

Craske, M. G., & Barlow, D. H. (2001). Panic disorder and agoraphobia. In D. H. Barlow (Ed.), *Clinical handbook of psychological disorders* (3rd ed., pp. 1–59). New York: Guilford Press.

Craske, M. G., & Barlow, D. H. (2006). *Mastery of your anxiety and worry: Workbook* (2nd ed.). Oxford, UK: Oxford University Press.

Craske, M. G., Farchione, T. J., Allen, L. B., Barrios, V., Stoyanova, M., & Rose, R. (2007). Cognitive behavioral therapy for panic disorder and comorbidity: More of the same or less of more? *Behaviour Research and Therapy, 45,* 1095–1109.

Craske, M. G., & Freed, S. (1995). Expectations about arousal and nocturnal panic. *Journal of Abnormal Psychology, 104,* 567–575.

Craske, M. G., Lang, A. J., Aikins, D., & Mystkowski, J. L. (2005). Cognitive behavioral therapy for nocturnal panic. *Behavior Therapy, 36,* 43–54.

Craske, M. G., Lang, A. J., Rowe, M., DeCola, J. P., Simmons, J., Mann, C., et al. (2002). Presleep attributions about arousal during sleep: nocturnal panic. *Journal of Abnormal Psychology, 111,* 53–62.

Craske, M. G., Lang, A. J., Tsao, J. C., Mystkowski, J., & Rowe, M. (2001). Reactivity to interoceptive cues in nocturnal panic. *Journal of Behavior Therapy and Experimental Psychiatry, 32,* 173–190.

Craske, M. G., Poulton, R., Tsao, J. C. I., & Plotkin, D. (2001). Paths to panic disorder/agoraphobia: An exploratory analysis from age 3 to 21 in an unselected birth cohort. *Journal of the American Academy of Child and Adolescent Psychiatry, 40,* 556–563.

Craske, M. G., Rachman, S. J., & Tallman, K. (1986). Mobility, cognitions, and panic. *Journal of Psychopathology and Behavioral Assessment, 8,* 199–210.

Craske, M. G., Rapee, R. M., & Barlow, D. H. (1988). The significance of panic-expectancy for individual patterns of avoidance. *Behavior Therapy, 19,* 577–592.

Craske, M. G., Rapee, R. M., Jackel, L., & Barlow, D. H. (1989). Qualitative dimensions of worry in DSM-III-R generalized anxiety disorder subjects and nonanxious subjects. *Behaviour Research and Therapy, 27,* 397–402.

Craske, M. G., & Rowe, M. K. (1997). Nocturnal panic. *Clinical Psychology: Science and Practice, 4,* 153–174.

Craske, M. G., Sanderson, W. C., & Barlow, D. H. (1987). The rela-

tionships among panic, fear, and avoidance. *Journal of Anxiety Disorders, 1,* 153–160.

Creamer, M., Burgess, P., & McFarlane, A. C. (2001). Post-traumatic stress disorder: Findings from the Australian National Survey of Mental Health and Well-Being. *Psychological Medicine, 31,* 1237–1247.

Creamer, M., Foran, J., & Bell, R. (1995). The Beck Anxiety Inventory in a nonclinical sample. *Behaviour Research and Therapy, 33,* 477–485.

Crino, R. D., & Andrews, G. (1996). Obsessive–compulsive disorder and Axis I comorbidity. *Journal of Anxiety Disorders, 10,* 37–46.

Cromer, K. R., Schmidt, N. B., & Murphy, D. L. (2007). An investigation of traumatic life events and obsessive–compulsive disorder. *Behaviour Research and Therapy, 45,* 1683–1691.

Cuthbert, B. N., Lang, P. J., Strauss, C., Drobes, D., Patrick, C. J., & Bradley, M. M. (2003). The psychophysiology of anxiety disorder: Fear memory imagery. *Psychophysiology, 40,* 407–422.

Dalgleish, T. (2004). Cognitive approaches to posttraumatic stress disorder: The evolution of multirepresentational theorizing. *Psychological Bulletin, 130,* 228–260.

Dalgleish, T., Cameron, C. M., Power, M. J., & Bond, A. (1995). The use of an emotional priming paradigm with clinically anxious patients. *Cognitive Therapy and Research, 19,* 69–89.

Daly, J. A., Vangelisti, A. L., & Lawrence, S. G. (1989). Self-focused attention and public speaking anxiety. *Personality and Individual Differences, 10,* 903–913.

Davey, G. C. L. (1993). A comparison of three worry questionnaires. *Behaviour Research and Therapy, 31,* 51–56.

Davey, G. C. L. (1994). Worrying, social problem-solving abilities, and social problem-solving confidence. *Behaviour Research and Therapy, 32,* 327–330.

Davey, G. C. L. (1997). A conditioning model of phobias. In G. C. L. Davey (Ed.), *Phobias: A handbook of theory, research and treatment* (pp. 301–322). Chichester, UK: Wiley.

Davey, G. C. L. (2006). The Catastrophizing Interview procedure. In G. C. L. Davey & A. Wells

(Eds.), *Worry and its psychological disorders: Theory, assessment and treatment* (pp. 157–176). Chichester, UK: Wiley.

Davey, G. C. L., Hampton, J., Farrell, J., & Davidson, S. (1992). Some characteristics of worrying: Evidence for worrying and anxiety as separate constructs. *Personality and Individual Differences, 13,* 133–147.

Davey, G. C. L., Jubb, M., & Cameron, C. (1996). Catastrophic worrying as a function of changes in problem-solving confidence. *Cognitive Therapy and Research, 20,* 333–344.

Davey, G. C. L., Tallis, F., & Capuzzo, N. (1996). Beliefs about the consequences of worrying. *Cognitive Therapy and Research, 20,* 499–520.

Davidson, J. R. T., Foa, E. B., Huppert, J. D., Keefe, F. J., Franklin, M. E., Compton, J. S., et al. (2004). Fluoxetine, comprehensive cognitive behavioral therapy, and placebo in generalized social phobia. *Archives of General Psychiatry, 61,* 1005–1013.

Davidson, P. R., & Parker, K. C. H. (2001). Eye movement desensitization and reprocessing (EMDR): A meta-analysis. *Journal of Consulting and Clinical Psychology, 69,* 305–316.

Davies, M. I., & Clark, D. M. (1998a). Thought suppression produces a rebound effect with analogue post-traumatic intrusions. *Behaviour Research and Therapy, 36,* 571–582.

Davies, M. I., & Clark, D. M. (1998b). Predictors of analogue post-traumatic intrusive cognitions. *Behavioural and Cognitive Psychotherapy, 26,* 303–314.

Davis, M. (1998). Are different parts of the extended amygdala involved in fear versus anxiety? *Biological Psychiatry, 44,* 1239–1247.

Deacon, B., & Abramowitz, J. S. (2005). The Yale–Brown Obsessive Compulsive Scale: Factor analysis, construct validity, and suggestions for refinement. *Journal of Anxiety Disorders, 19,* 573–585.

Deacon, B., & Abramowitz, J. S. (2006a). Anxiety sensitivity and its dimensions across the anxiety disorders. *Journal of Anxiety Disorders, 20,* 837–857.

Deacon, B., & Abramowitz, J. S. (2006b). A pilot study of two-day cognitive-behavioral therapy for panic disorder. *Behaviour Research and Therapy, 44,* 807–817.

Deacon, B. J., Lickel, J., & Abramowitz, J. S. (2008). Medical utilization across the anxiety disorders. *Journal of Anxiety Disorders, 22,* 344–350.

de Bruin, G. O., Muris, P., & Rassin, E. (2007). Are there specific metacognitions associated with vulnerability to symptoms of worry and obsessional thoughts? *Personality and Individual Differences, 42,* 689–699.

de Jong, P. J. (2002). Implicit self-esteem and social anxiety: Differential self-favoring effects in high and low anxious individuals. *Behaviour Research and Therapy, 40,* 501–508.

de Jong, P. J., & Merckelbach, H. (2000). Phobia-relevant illusory correlations: The role of phobic responsivity. *Journal of Abnormal Psychology, 109,* 597–601.

de Jong, P. J., Merckelbach, H., & Arntz, A. (1995). Covariation bias in phobic women: The relationship between a prior expectancy, on-line expectancy, autonomic responding, and a posteriori contingency judgment. *Journal of Abnormal Psychology, 104,* 55–62.

de Jong, P. J., van den Hout, M. A., Rietbrock, H., & Huijding, J. (2003). Dissociations between implicit and explicit attitudes toward phobic stimuli. *Cognition and Emotion, 17,* 521–545.

Demal, U., Lenz, G., Mayrhofer, A., Zapotoczky, H.-G., & Zirrerl, W. (1993). Obsessive–compulsive disorder and depression: A retrospective study on course and interaction. *Psychopathology, 26,* 145–150.

Derryberry, D., & Reed, M. A. (2002). Anxiety-related attentional biases and their regulation by attentional control. *Journal of Abnormal Psychology, 111,* 225–236.

DeRubeis, R. J., & Crits-Christoph, P. (1998). Empirically supported individual and group psychological treatments for adult mental disorders. *Journal of Consulting and Clinical Psychology, 66,* 37–52.

de Silva, P. (2003). The phenomenology of obsessive–compulsive disorder. In R. G. Menzies & P. de Silva (Eds.), *Obsessive–compulsive disorder: Theory, research and treatment* (pp. 21–36). Chichester, UK: Wiley.

Diaferia, G., Sciuto, G., Perna, G., Bernardeschi, L., Battaglia, M., Rusmini, S., et al. (1993). DSM-III-R personality disorders in panic disorder. *Journal of Anxiety Disorders, 7,* 153–161.

Diefenbach, G. J., Abramowitz, J. S., Norberg, M. M., & Tolin, D. F. (2007). Changes in quality of life following cognitive-behavioral therapy for obsessive–compulsive disorder. *Behaviour Research and Therapy, 45,* 3060–3068.

Diefenbach, G. J., McCarthy-Lazelere, M. E., Williamson, D. A., Mathews, A., Manguno-Mire, G. M., & Bentz, B. G. (2001). Anxiety, depression, and the content of worries. *Depression and Anxiety, 14,* 247–250.

Di Nardo, P. A., & Barlow, D. H. (1990). Syndrome and symptom co-occurrence in the anxiety disorders. In J. D. Maser & C. R. Cloninger (Eds.), *Comorbidity of mood and anxiety disorders* (pp. 205–230). Washington, DC: American Psychiatric Press.

Dodge, C. S., Hope, D. A., Heimberg, R. G., & Becker, R. E. (1988). Evaluation of the Social Interaction Self-Statement Test with a social phobic population. *Cognitive Therapy and Research, 12,* 211–222.

Dohrenwand, B. P., Turner, J. B., Turse, N. A., Lewis-Fernandez, R., & Yager, T. J. (2008). War-related posttraumatic stress disorder in black, Hispanic, and majority white Vietnam veterans: The roles of exposure and vulnerability. *Journal of Traumatic Stress, 21,* 133–141.

Dorfan, N. M., & Woody, S. R. (2006). Does threatening imagery sensitize distress during contaminant exposure? *Behaviour Research and Therapy, 44,* 395–413.

Doron, G., & Kyrios, M. (2005). Obsessive compulsive disorder: A review of possible specific internal representations within a broader cognitive theory. *Clinical Psychology Review, 25,* 415–432.

Doron, G., Kyrios, M., & Moulding, R. (2007). *Sensitive domains of self-concept in obsessive compulsive disorder (OCD): Further evidence for a multidimensional model of cognitive vulnerability in OCD.* Unpublished manuscript, University of Melbourne, Australia.

Dozois, D. J., Dobson, K. S., & Ahnberg, J. L. (1998). A psychometric evaluation of the Beck Depression Inventory—II. *Psychological Assessment, 10,* 83–89.

Dozois, D. J. A., & Westra, H. A. (2004). The nature of anxiety and depression: Implications for prevention. In D. J. A. Dozois & K. S. Dobson (Eds.), *The prevention of anxiety and depression: Theory, research and practice* (pp. 9–41). Washington, DC: American Psychological Press.

Dugas, M. J., Buhr, K., & Ladouceur, R. (2004). The role of intolerance of uncertainty in etiology and maintenance. In R. G. Heimberg, C. L. Turk, & D. S. Mennin (Eds.), *Generalized anxiety disorder: Advances in research and practice* (pp. 143–163). New York: Guilford Press.

Dugas, M. J., Freeston, M. H., & Ladouceur, R. (1997). Intolerance of uncertainty and problem orientation in worry. *Cognitive Therapy and Research, 21,* 593–606.

Dugas, M. J., Freeston, M. H., Ladouceur, R., Rhéaume, J., Provencher, M., & Boisvert, J.-M. (1998). Worry themes in primary GAD, secondary GAD, and other anxiety disorders. *Journal of Anxiety Disorders, 12,* 253–261.

Dugas, M. J., Gagnon, F., Ladouceur, R., & Freeston, M. H. (1998). Generalized anxiety disorder: A preliminary test of a conceptual model. *Behaviour Research and Therapy, 36,* 215–226.

Dugas, M. J., Gosselin, P., & Ladouceur, R. (2001). Intolerance of uncertainty and worry: Investigating specificity in a nonclinical sample. *Cognitive Therapy and Research, 25,* 551–558.

Dugas, M. J., Ladouceur, R., Léger, E., Freeston, M. H., Langlois, F., Provencher, M. D., et al. (2003). Group cognitive-behavioral therapy for generalized anxiety disorder: Treatment outcome and long-term follow-up. *Journal of Consulting and Clinical Psychology, 71,* 821–825.

Dugas, M. J., Letarte, H., Rhéaume, J., Freeston, M. H., & Ladouceur, R. (1995). Worry and problem solving: Evidence of a specific relationship. *Cognitive Therapy and Research, 19,* 109–120.

Dugas, M. J., Merchand, A., & Ladouceur, R. (2005). Further validation of a cognitive-behavioral model of generalized anxiety disorder: Diagnostic and symptom specificity. *Journal of Anxiety Disorders, 19,* 329–343.

DuHamel, K. N., Ostroff, J., Ashman, T., Winkel, G., Mundy, E. A., Keane, T. M., et al. (2004). Construct validity of the Posttraumatic Stress Disorder Checklist in cancer survivors: Analyses based on two samples. *Psychological Assessment, 16,* 255–266.

Duke, D., Krishnan, M., Faith, M., & Storch, E. A. (2006). The psychometric properties of the Brief Fear of Negative Evaluation Scale. *Journal of Anxiety Disorders, 20,* 807–817.

Dunmore, E., Clark, D. M., & Ehlers, A. (1999). Cognitive factors involved in the onset and maintenance of posttraumatic stress disorder (PTSD) after physical or sexual assault. *Behaviour Research and Therapy, 37,* 809–829.

Dunmore, E., Clark, D. M., & Ehlers, A. (2001). A prospective investigation of the role of cognitive factors in persistent posttraumatic stress disorder (PTSD) after physical or sexual assault. *Behaviour Research and Therapy, 39,* 1063–1084.

Dupuy, J.-B., Beaudoin, S., Rhéaume, J., Ladouceur, R., & Dugas, M. J. (2001). Worry: Daily self-report in clinical and non-clinical populations. *Behaviour Research and Therapy, 39,* 1249–1255.

Dupuy, J.-B., & Ladouceur, R. L. (2008). Cognitive processes of generalized anxiety disorder in comorbid generalized anxiety disorder and major depressive disorder. *Journal of Anxiety Disorders, 22,* 505–514.

Durham, R. C., Chambers, J. A., MacDonald, R. R., Power, K. G., & Major, K. (2003). Does cognitive-behavioural therapy influence the long-term outcome of generalized anxiety disorder?: An 8–14 year follow-up of two clinical trials. *Psychological Medicine, 33,* 499–509.

Durham, R. C., Chambers, J. A., Power, K. G., Sharp, D. M., MacDonald, R. R., Major, K. A., et al. (2005). Long-term outcome of cognitive behavior therapy clinical trials in central Scotland. *Health Technology Assessment, 9,* 1–174.

Durham, R. C., Fisher, P. L., Dow, M. G. T., Sharp, D., Power, K. G., Swan, J. S., et al. (2004). Cognitive behaviour therapy for good and poor prognosis generalized anxiety disorder: A clinical effectiveness study. *Clinical Psychology and Psychotherapy, 11,* 145–157.

Durham, R. C., Fisher, P. L., Treliv-

ing, L. R., Hau, C. M., Richard, K., & Stewart, J. B. (1999). One year follow-up of cognitive therapy, analytic psychotherapy and anxiety management training for generalized anxiety disorder: Symptom change, medication usage and attitudes to treatment. *Behavioural and Cognitive Psychotherapy, 27,* 19–35.

Durham, R. C., Murphy, T., Allan, T., Richard, K., Treliving, L. A., & Fenton, G. W. (1994). Cognitive therapy, analytic psychotherapy and anxiety management training for generalized anxiety disorder. *British Journal of Psychiatry, 165,* 315–323.

Durham, R. C., & Turvey, A. A. (1987). Cognitive therapy vs. behavior therapy in the treatment of chronic generalized anxiety. *Behaviour Research and Therapy, 25,* 229–234.

Dyck, I. R., Phillips, K. A., Warshaw, M. G., Dolan, R. T., Shea, M. T., Stout, R. L., et al. (2001). Patterns of personality pathology in patients with generalized anxiety disorder, panic disorder with and without agoraphobia, and social phobia. *Journal of Personality Disorders, 15,* 60–71.

D'Zurilla, T. J, & Nezu, A. M. (2007). *Problem-solving therapy: A positive approach to clinical intervention* (3rd ed.). New York: Springer.

Easterbrook, J. A. (1959). The effect of emotion on cue utilization and the organization of behavior. *Psychological Review, 66,* 183–201.

Eaton, W. W., Dryman, A., & Weissman, M. M. (1991). Panic and phobia. In L. N. Robins & D. A. Regier (Eds.), *Psychiatric disorders in America: The Epidemiologic Catchment Area Study* (pp. 155–179). New York: Free Press.

Eaton, W. W., Kessler, R. C., Wittchen, H.-U., & Magee, W. J. (1994). Panic and panic disorder in the United States. *American Journal of Psychiatry, 151,* 413–420.

Eddy, K. T., Dutra, L., Bradley, R., & Westen, D. (2004). A multidimensional meta-analysis of psychotherapy and pharmacotherapy for obsessive–compulsive disorder. *Clinical Psychology Review, 24,* 1011–1030.

Edelmann, R. J. (1992). *Anxiety: Theory, research and intervention in clinical and health psychology.* Chichester, UK: Wiley.

Edwards, M. S., Burt, J. S., & Lipp,

O. V. (2006). Selective processing of masked and unmasked verbal threat material in anxiety: Influence of an immediate acute stressor. *Cognition and Emotion, 20,* 812–835.

Ehlers, A. (1995). A 1-year prospective study of panic attacks: Clinical course and factors associated with maintenance. *Journal of Abnormal Psychology, 104,* 164–172.

Ehlers A., & Breuer, P. (1992). Increased cardiac awareness in panic disorder. *Journal of Abnormal Psychology, 101,* 371–382.

Ehlers, A., Breuer, P., Dohn, D., & Fiegenbaum, W. (1995). Heartbeat perception and panic disorder: Possible explanations for discrepant findings. *Behaviour Research and Therapy, 33,* 69–76.

Ehlers, A., & Clark, D. M. (2000). A cognitive model of posttraumatic stress disorder. *Behaviour Research and Therapy, 38,* 319–345.

Ehlers, A., Clark, D. M., Hackmann, A., McManus, F., & Fennell, M. (2005). Cognitive therapy for posttraumatic stress disorder: Development and evaluation. *Behaviour Research and Therapy, 43,* 413–431.

Ehlers, A., Clark, D. M., Hackmann, A., McManus, F., Fennell, M., Herbert, C., et al. (2003). A randomized controlled trial of cognitive therapy, a self-help booklet, and repeated assessments as early interventions for posttraumatic stress disorder. *Archives of General Psychiatry, 60,* 1024–1032.

Ehlers, A., Margraf, J., Davies, S., & Roth, W. T. (1988). Selective processing of threat cues in subjects with panic attacks. *Cognition and Emotion, 2,* 201–219.

Ehlers, A., & Steil, R. (1995). Maintenance of intrusive memories in posttraumatic stress disorder: A cognitive approach. *Behavioural and Cognitive Psychotherapy, 23,* 217–249.

Ehntholt, K. A., Salkovskis, P. M., & Rimes, K. A. (1999). Obsessive–compulsive disorder, anxiety disorders, and self-esteem: An exploratory study. *Behaviour Research and Therapy, 37,* 771–781.

Ehring, T., Ehlers, A., & Glucksman, E. (2006). Contribution of cognitive factors to the prediction of post-traumatic stress disorder, phobia and depression after motor vehicle accidents. *Behaviour Research and Therapy, 44,* 1699–1716.

Eifert, G. H., Zvolensky, M. J., & Lejuez, C. W. (2000). Heart-focused anxiety and chest pain: A conceptual and clinical review. *Clinical Psychology: Science and Practice, 7,* 403–417.

Ekman, P. (1999). Basic emotions. In T. Dalgleish & M. Power (Eds.), *Handbook of cognition and emotion* (pp. 45–60). Chichester, UK: Wiley.

Elliott, D. M. (1997). Traumatic events: Prevalence and delayed recall in the general population. *Journal of Consulting and Clinical Psychology, 65,* 811–820.

Elsesser, K., Sartory, G., & Tackenberg, A. (2004). Attention, heart rate, and startle response during exposure to trauma-relevant pictures: A comparison of recent trauma victims and patients with posttraumatic stress disorder. *Journal of Abnormal Pscyhology, 113,* 289–301.

Elting, D. T., & Hope, D. A. (1995). Cognitive assessment. In R. G. Heimberg, M. R. Liebowitz, D. A. Hope, & F. R. Schneier (Eds.), *Social phobia: Diagnosis, assessment and treatment* (pp. 232–258). New York: Guilford Press.

Emmelkamp, P. M. G., & Aardema, A. (1999). Metacognition, specific obsessive–compulsive beliefs and obsessive–compulsive behaviour. *Clinical Psychology and Psychotherapy, 6,* 139–145.

Emmelkamp, P. M. G., van Oppen, P., & van Balkom, A. J. L. M. (2002). Cognitive changes in patients with obsessive compulsive rituals treated with exposure in vivo and response prevention. In R. O. Frost & G. S. Steketee (Eds.), *Cognitive approaches to obsessions and compulsions: Theory, assessment and treatment* (pp. 392–401). Oxford, UK: Elsevier Press.

Emmons, R. A. (1986). Personal strivings: An approach to personality and subjective well-being. *Journal of Personality and Social Psychology, 51,* 1058–1068.

Engelhard, I. M., van den Hout, M. A., Kindt, M., Arntz, A., & Schouten, E. (2003). Peritraumatic dissociation and posttraumatic stress after pregnancy loss: A prospective study. *Behaviour Research and Therapy, 41,* 67–78.

Eriksson, C. B., Vande Kemp, H., Gorsuch, R., Hoke, S., & Foy, D. W. (2001). Trauma exposure and PTSD symptoms in international relief and development personnel.

Journal of Traumatic Stress, 14, 205–212.

Eysenck, H. J. (1979). The conditioning model of neurosis. *Behavioral and Brain Sciences, 2,* 155–199.

Eysenck, H. J., & Eysenck, S. B. G. (1975). *Manual of the Eysenck Personality Questionnaire (Junior & Adult).* Sevenoaks, UK: Hodder and Stoughton.

Eysenck, H. J., & Rachman, S. (1965). *The causes and cures of neurosis.* San Diego, CA: Knapp.

Eysenck, M. W. (1992). *Anxiety: The cognitive perspective.* Hove, UK: Erlbaum.

Eysenck, M. W., & Byrne, A. (1994). Implicit memory bias, explicit memory bias, and anxiety. *Cognition and Emotion, 8,* 415–431.

Eysenck, M. W., Mogg, K., May, J., Richards, A., & Mathews, A. (1991). Bias in interpretation of ambiguous sentences related to threat in anxiety. *Journal of Abnormal Psychology, 100,* 144–150.

Falsetti, S. A., Monnier, J., & Resnick, H. S. (2005). Intrusive thoughts in posttraumatic stress disorder. In D. A. Clark (Ed.), *Intrusive thoughts in clinical disorders: Theory, research, and treatment* (pp. 30–53). New York: Guilford Press.

Fama, J., & Wilhelm, S. (2005). Formal cognitive therapy: A new treatment for OCD. In J. S. Abramowitz & A. C. Houts (Eds.), *Concepts and controversies in obsessive-compulsive disorder* (pp. 263–281). New York: Springer.

Faravelli, C., & Pallanti, S. (1989). Recent life events and panic disorder. *American Journal of Psychiatry, 146,* 622–626.

Faravelli, C., Pallanti, S., Biondi, F., Paterniti, S., & Scarpato, M. A. (1992). Onset of panic disorder. *American Journal of Psychiatry, 149,* 827–828.

Faravelli, C., Paterniti, S., & Scarpato, A. (1995). Five-year prospective, naturalistic follow-up study of panic disorder. *Comprehensive Psychiatry, 36,* 271–277.

Fava, G. A., Zielezny, M., Savron, G., & Grandi, S. (1995). Long-term effects of behavioral treatment for panic disorder with agoraphobia. *British Journal of Psychiatry, 166,* 87–92.

Feeny, N. C., & Foa, E. B. (2006). Cognitive vulnerability to PTSD. In L. B. Alloy & J. H. Riskind (Eds.), *Cognitive vulnerability* to emotional disorders (pp. 285–301). Mahwah, NJ: Erlbaum.

Fehm, L., & Hoyer, J. (2004). Measuring thought control strategies: The Thought Control Questionnaire and a look beyond. Cognitive Therapy and Research, 28, 105–117.

Fenigstein, A., Scheier, M. F., & Buss, A. H. (1975). Public and private self-consciousness: Assessment and theory. Journal of Consulting and Clinical Psychology, 43, 522–527.

Ferrier, S., & Brewin, C. (2005). Feared identity and obsessive-compulsive disorder. Behaviour Research and Therapy, 43, 1363–1374.

Feske, U., & Chambless, D. L. (1995). Cognitive behavioral versus exposure only treatment for social phobia: A meta-analysis. Behavior Therapy, 26, 695–720.

Feske, U., & Chambless, D. L. (2000). A review of assessment measures for obsessive–compulsive disorder. In W. K. Goodman, M. V. Rudorfor, & J. D. Maser (Eds.), Obsessive–compulsive disorder: Contemporary issues in treatment (pp. 157–182). Mahwah, NJ: Erlbaum.

Field, A. P., Psychol, C., & Morgan, J. (2004). Post-event processing and the retrieval of autobiographical memories in socially anxious individuals. Journal of Anxiety Disorders, 18, 647–663.

Field, E. L., Norman, P., & Barton, J. (2008). Cross-sectional and prospective associations between cognitive appraisals and posttraumatic stress disorder symptoms following stroke. Behaviour Research and Therapy, 46, 62–70.

Fields, L., & Prinz, R. J. (1997). Coping and adjustment during childhood and adolescence. Clinical Psychology Review, 17, 937–976.

First, M. B., Spitzer, R. L., Gibbon, M., & Williams, J. B. W. (1997). Structured Clinical Interview for DSM-IV Axis I Disorders (SCID-I)—Clinical Version. Washington, DC: American Psychiatric Press.

First, M. B., Spitzer, R. L., Gibbon, M., & Williams, J. B. W. (2002). Structured Clinical Interview for DSM-IV Axis I Disorders, Research Version, Non-patient Edition (SCID-I/NP). New York: Biometrics Research, New York State Psychiatric Institute.

Fisher, P. L. (2006). The efficacy of psychological treatments for generalized anxiety disorder? In G. C. L. Davey & A. Wells (Eds.), Worry and its psychological disorders: Theory, assessment and treatment (pp. 359–377). Chichester, UK: Wiley.

Fisher, P. L., & Durham, R. C. (1999). Recovery rates in generalized anxiety disorder following psychological therapy: An analysis of clinically significant change in the STAI-T across outcome studies since 1990. Psychological Medicine, 29, 1425–1434.

Fisher, P. L., & Wells, A. (2005). Experimental modification of beliefs in obsessive–compulsive disorder: A test of the metacognitive model. Behaviour Research and Therapy, 43, 821–829.

Flavell, J. H. (1979). Metacognition and cognitive monitoring: A new area of cognitive-developmental inquiry. American Psychologist, 34, 906–911.

Foa, E. B. (1979). Failure in treating obsessive compulsives. Behaviour Research and Therapy, 17, 169–176.

Foa, E. B., Abramowitz, J. S., Franklin, M. E., & Kozak, M. J. (1999). Feared consequences, fixity of belief, and treatment outcome in patients with obsessive–compulsive disorder. Behavior Therapy, 30, 717–724.

Foa, E. B., Amir, N., Gershuny, B., Molnar, C., & Kozak, M. J. (1997). Implicit and explicit memory in obsessive–compulsive disorder. Journal of Anxiety Disorders, 11, 119–129.

Foa, E. B., Cashman, L., Jaycox, L., & Perry, K. (1997). The validation of a self-report measure of posttraumatic stress disorder: The Posttraumatic Diagnostic Scale. Psychological Assessment, 9, 445–451.

Foa, E. B., Davidson, J. R. T., & Frances, A. (1999). The expert consensus guideline series: Treatment of posttraumatic stress disorder. Journal of Clinical Psychiatry, 60(Suppl. 16), 6–76.

Foa, E. B., Ehlers, A., Clark, D. M., Tolin, D. F., & Orsillo, S. M. (1999). The Posttraumatic Cognitions Inventory (PTCI): Development and validation. Psychological Assessment, 11, 303–314.

Foa, E. B., Franklin, M. E., & Kozak, M. J. (1998). Psychosocial treatments for obsessive–compulsive disorder: Literature review. In R. P. Swinson, M. M. Antony, S. Rachman, & M. A. Richter (Eds.), Obsessive–compulsive disorder: Theory, research and treatment (pp. 258–276). New York: Guilford Press.

Foa, E. B., Franklin, M. E., Perry, K. J., & Herbert, J. D. (1996). Cognitive biases in generalized social phobia. Journal of Abnormal Psychology, 105, 433–439.

Foa, E. B., Hembree, E. A., Feeny, N. C., Cahill, S. P., Rauch, S. A. M., Riggs, D. S., et al. (2005). Randomized trial of prolonged exposure for posttraumatic stress disorder with and without cognitive restructuring: Outcome at academic and community clinics. Journal of Consulting and Clinical Psychology, 73, 953–964.

Foa, E. B., Huppert, J. D., Leiberg, S., Hajcak, G., Langner, R., Kichic, R., et al. (2002). The Obsessive-Compulsive Inventory: Development and validation of a short version. Psychological Assessment, 14, 485–496.

Foa, E. B., Ilai, D., McCarthy, P. R., Shoyer, B., & Murdock, T. (1993). Information processing in obsessive–compulsive disorder. Cognitive Therapy and Research, 17, 173–189.

Foa, E. B., & Kozak, M. J. (1985). Treatment of anxiety disorders: Implications for psychopathology. In A. H. Tuma & J. Maser (Eds.), Anxiety and the anxiety disorders (pp. 421–461). Hillsdale, NJ: Erlbaum.

Foa, E. B., & Kozak, M. J. (1986). Emotional processing of fear: Exposure to corrective information. Psychological Bulletin, 99, 20–35.

Foa, E. B., & Kozak, M. J. (1995). DSM-IV field trial: Obsessive-compulsive disorder. American Journal of Psychiatry, 152, 90–96.

Foa, E. B., & Kozak, M. J. (1996). Psychological treatment for obsessive–compulsive disorder. In M. R. Mavissakalian & R. F. Prien (Eds.), Long-term treatments of anxiety disorders (pp. 285–309). Washington, DC: American Psychiatric Press.

Foa, E. B., & Kozak, M. J. (1997). Mastery of obsessive–compulsive disorder: Client workbook. San Antonio, TX: Psychological Corporation.

Foa, E. B., Kozak, M. J., Salkovskis,

P. M., Coles, M. E., & Amir, N. (1998). The validation of a new obsessive–compulsive disorder scale: The Obsessive–Compulsive Inventory. *Psychological Assessment, 10*, 206–214.

Foa, E. B., Liebowitz, M. R., Kozak, M. J., Davies, S., Campeas, R., Franklin, M. E., et al. (2005). Randomized, placebo-controlled trial of exposure and ritual prevention, clomipramine, and their combination in the treatment of obsessive–compulsive disorder. *American Journal of Psychiatry, 162*, 151–161.

Foa, E. B., & McNally, R. J. (1986). Sensitivity to feared stimuli in obsessive-compulsives: A dichotic listening analysis. *Cognitive Therapy and Research, 10*, 477–485.

Foa, E. B., & McNally, R. J. (1996). Mechanisms of change in exposure therapy. In R. M. Rapee (Ed.), *Current controversies in the anxiety disorders* (pp. 329–343). New York: Guilford Press.

Foa, E. B., & Rauch, S. A. M. (2004). Cognitive changes during prolonged exposure versus prolonged exposure plus cognitive restructuring in female assault survivors with posttraumatic stress disorder. *Journal of Consulting and Clinical Psychology, 72*, 879–884.

Foa, E. B., & Rothbaum, B. O. (1998). *Treating the trauma of rape: Cognitive-behavioral therapy for PTSD*. New York: Guilford Press.

Foa, E. B., Rothbaum, B. O., Riggs, D. S., & Murdock, T. B. (1991). Treatment of posttraumatic stress disorder in rape victims: A comparison between cognitive-behavioral procedures and counseling. *Journal of Consulting and Clinical Psychology, 59*, 715–723.

Foa, E. B., Sacks, M. B., Tolin, D. F., Prezworski, A., & Amir, N. (2002). Inflated perception of responsibility for harm in OCD patients with and without checking compulsions: A replication and extension. *Journal of Anxiety Disorders, 16*, 443–453.

Foa, E. B., Steketee, G., Grayson, J. B., & Doppelt, H. G. (1983). Treatment of obsessive–compulsives: When do we fail? In E. B. Foa & P. M. G. Emmelkamp (Eds.), *Failures in behavior therapy* (pp. 10–34). New York: Wiley.

Folkman, S., & Moskowitz, J. T. (2004). Coping: Pitfalls and promise. *Annual Review of Psychology, 55*, 745–774.

Forrester, E., Wilson, C., & Salkovskis, P. M. (2002). The occurrence of intrusive thoughts transforms meaning in ambiguous situations: An experimental study. *Behavioural and Cognitive Psychotherapy, 30*, 143–152.

Fox, E. (1993). Attentional bias in anxiety: Selective or not? *Behaviour Research and Therapy, 31*, 487–493.

Fox, E. (1994). Attentional bias in anxiety: A defective inhibition hypothesis. *Cognition and Emotion, 8*, 165–195.

Fox, E. (1996). Selective processing of threatening words in anxiety: The role of awareness. *Cognition and Emotion, 10*, 449–480.

Franklin, J. A., & Andrews, G. (1989). Stress and the onset of agoraphobia. *Australian Psychologist, 24*, 203–219.

Franklin, M. E., Abramowitz, J. S., Bux, D. A., Zoellner, L. A., & Feeny, N. C. (2002). Cognitive-behavioral therapy with and without medication in the treatment of obsessive–compulsive disorder. *Professional Psychology: Research and Practice, 33*, 162–168.

Franklin, M. E., Abramowitz, J. S., Kozak, M. J., Levitt, J. T., & Foa, E. B. (2000). Effectiveness of exposure and ritual prevention for obsessive–compulsive disorder: Randomized compared with nonrandomized samples. *Journal of Consulting and Clinical Psychology, 68*, 594–602.

Franklin, M. E., Riggs, D. S., & Pai, A. (2005). Obsessive–compulsive disorder. In M. M. Antony, D. R. Ledley, & R. G. Heimberg (Eds.), *Improving outcomes and preventing relapse in cognitive-behavioral therapy* (pp. 128–173). New York: Guilford Press.

Frazier, P. A. (2003). Perceived control and distress following sexual assault: A longitudinal test of a new model. *Journal of Personality and Social Psychology, 84*, 1257–1269.

Freeston, M. H., & Ladouceur, R. (1997a). What do patients do with their obsessive thoughts? *Behaviour Research and Therapy, 35*, 335–348.

Freeston, M. H., & Ladouceur, R. (1997b). *The cognitive behavioral treatment of obsessions: A treatment manual*. Unpublished manuscript, École de psychologie, Université Laval, Québec, Canada.

Freeston, M. H., & Ladouceur, R. (1999). Exposure and response prevention for obsessional thoughts. *Cognitive and Behavioral Practice, 6*, 362–383.

Freeston, M. H., Ladouceur, R., Gagnon, F., Thibodeau, N., Rhéaume, J., Letarte, H., et al. (1997). Cognitive-behavioral treatment of obsessive thoughts: A controlled study. *Journal of Consulting and Clinical Psychology, 65*, 405–413.

Freeston, M. H., Ladouceur, R., Rhéaume, J., Letarte, H., Gagnon, F., & Thibodeau, N. (1994). Self-report of obsessions and worry. *Behaviour Research and Therapy, 32*, 29–36.

Freeston, M. H., Ladouceur, R., Thibodeau, N., & Gagnon, F. (1991). Cognitive intrusions in a non-clinical population: I. Response style, subjective experience, and appraisal. *Behaviour Research and Therapy, 29*, 585–597.

Freeston, M. H., Ladouceur, R., Thibodeau, N., & Gagnon, F. (1992). Cognitive intrusions in a non-clinical population: II. Associations with depressive, anxious, and compulsive symptoms. *Behaviour Research and Therapy, 30*, 263–271.

Freeston, M. H., Léger, E., & Ladouceur, R. (2001). Cognitive therapy of obsessive thoughts. *Cognitive and Behavioral Practice, 8*, 61–78.

Freeston, M. H., Rhéaume, J., Letarte, H., Dugas, M., & Ladouceur, R. (1994). Why do people worry? *Personality and Individual Differences, 17*, 791–802.

Fresco, D. M., Coles, M. E., Heimberg, R. G., Liebowitz, M. R., Hami, S., Stein, M. B., et al. (2001). The Liebowitz Social Anxiety Scale: A comparison of the psychometric properties of self-report and clinician-administered formats. *Psychological Medicine, 31*, 1025–1035.

Fresco, D. M., Heimberg, R. G., Mennin, D. S., & Turk, C. L. (2002). Confirmatory factor analysis of the Penn State Worry Questionnaire. *Behaviour Research and Therapy, 40*, 313–323.

Fresco, D. M., Mennin, D. S., Heimberg, R. G., & Turk, C. L. (2003). Using the Penn State Worry Questionnaire to identify individuals with generalized anxiety disorder: A receiver operating characteristic analysis. *Journal of Behavior Therapy and Experimental Psychiatry, 34,* 283–291.

Freud, S. (1955). Analysis of a phobia in a five-year-old boy. In J. Strachey (Ed., & Trans.), *The standard edition of the complete psychological works of Sigmund Freud* (Vol. 10, pp. 3–149). London: Hogarth Press. (Original work published 1909)

Frewen, P. A., Dozois, D. J. A., & Lanius, R. A. (2008). Neuroimaging studies of psychological interventions for mood and anxiety disorders: Empirical findings and methodological review. *Clinical Psychology Review, 28,* 228–246.

Friedman, B. H., & Thayer, J. F. (1998). Anxiety and autonomic flexibility: A cardiovascular approach. *Biological Psychology, 47,* 243–263.

Friedman, M. J., Resick, P. A., & Keane, T. M. (2007). PTSD: Twenty-five years of progress and challenges. In M. J. Freidman, T. M. Keane, & P. A. Resick (Eds.), *Handbook of PTSD: Science and practice* (pp. 3–18). New York: Guilford Press.

Friedman, S., Smith, L., Fogel, D., Paradis, C., Viswanathan, R., Ackerman, R., et al. (2002). The incidence and influence of early traumatic life events in patients with panic disorder: A comparison with other psychiatric outpatients. *Journal of Anxiety Disorders, 16,* 259–272.

Friedman, S., Smith, L. C., Halpern, B., Levine, C., Paradis, C., Viswanathan, R., et al. (2003). Obsessive–compulsive disorder in a multi-ethnic urban outpatient clinic: Initial presentation and treatment outcome with exposure and ritual prevention. *Behavior Therapy, 34,* 397–410.

Frijda, N. H. (1986). *The emotions.* Cambridge, UK: Cambridge University Press.

Frost, R. O., Novara, C., & Rhéaume, J. (2002). Perfectionism in obsessive compulsive disorder. In R. O. Frost & G. Steketee (Eds.), *Cognitive approaches to obsessions and compulsions: Theory, assessment and treatment* (pp. 92–105). Oxford, UK: Elsevier.

Frost, R. O., & Steketee, G. (Eds.). (2002). *Cognitive approaches to obsessions and compulsions: Theory, assessment, and treatment.* Amsterdam, The Netherlands: Elsevier.

Fyer, M. R., Uy, J., Martinez, J., Goetz, R., Klein, D. F., Fyer, A., et al. (1987). CO_2 challenge of patients with panic disorder. *American Journal of Psychiatry, 144,* 1080–1082.

Fydrich, T., Dowdall, D., & Chambless, D. L. (1992). Reliability and validity of the Beck Anxiety Inventory. *Journal of Anxiety Disorders, 6,* 55–61.

Galea, S., Ahern, J., Resnick, H., Kilpatrick, D., Bucuvalas, M., Gold, J., et al. (2002). Psychological sequelae of the September 11 terrorist attacks in New York City. *New England Journal of Medicine, 346,* 982–987.

Galea, S., Brewin, C. R., Gruber, M., Jones, R. T., King, D. W., King, L. A., et al. (2007). Exposure to hurricane-related stress and mental illness after Hurricane Katrina. *Archives of General Psychiatry, 64,* 1427–1434.

Galea, S., Viahov, D., Resnick, H., Ahern, J., Susser, E., Gold, J., et al. (2003). Trends of probable posttraumatic stress disorder in New York City after the September 11 terrorist attacks. *American Journal of Epidemiology, 158,* 514–524.

Gardenswartz, C. A., & Craske, M. G. (2001). Prevention of panic disorder. *Behavior Therapy, 32,* 725–737.

Gardner, C. R., Tully, W. R., & Hedgecock, C. J. R. (1993). The rapidly expanding range of neuronal benzodiazepine receptor ligands. *Progressive Neurobiology, 40,* 1–61.

Garner, M., Mogg, K., & Bradley, B. P. (2006). Fear-relevant selective associations and social anxiety: Absence of a positive bias. *Behaviour Research and Therapy, 44,* 201–217.

Gaskell, S. L., Wells, A., & Calam, R. (2001). An experimental investigation of thought suppression and anxiety in children. *British Journal of Clinical Psychology, 40,* 45–56.

Gater, R., Tansella, M., Korten, A., Tiemens, B. G., Mavreas, V. G., & Olatawura, M. O. (1998). Sex differences in the prevalence and detection of depressive and anxiety disorders in general health care settings: Report from the World Health Organization Collaborative Study on Psychological Problems in General Health Care. *Archives of General Psychiatry, 55,* 405–413.

Geller, D. A. (1998). Juvenile obsessive–compulsive disorder.

In M. A. Jenicke, L. Baer, & W. E. Minichiello (Eds.), *Obsessive-compulsive disorders: Practical management* (3rd ed., pp. 44–64). St. Louis: Mosby.

Genest, M., Bowen, R. C., Dudley, J., & Keegan, D. (1990). Assessment of strategies for coping with anxiety: Preliminary investigations. *Journal of Anxiety Disorders, 4,* 1–14.

George, L., & Stopa, L. (2008). Private and public self-awareness in social anxiety. *Journal of Behavior Therapy and Experimental Psychiatry, 39,* 57–72.

Geraerts, E., Merckelbach, H., Jelicic, M., & Smeets, E. (2006). Long term consequences of suppression of anxious thoughts and repressive coping. *Behaviour Research and Therapy, 44,* 1451–1460.

Germer, C. K. (2005). Anxiety disorders: Befriending fear. In C. K. Germer, R. D. Siegel, & P. R. Fulton (Eds.), *Mindfulness and psychotherapy* (pp. 152–172). New York: Guilford Press.

Gershuny, B. S., & Sher, K. J. (1998). The relation between personality and anxiety: Findings from a 3-year prospective study. *Journal of Abnormal Psychology, 107,* 252–262.

Gibb, B. E., Chelminski, I., & Zimmerman, M. (2007). Childhood emotional, physical, and sexual abuse, and diagnoses of depressive and anxiety disorders in adult psychiatric outpatients. *Depression and Anxiety, 24,* 256–263.

Gilbert, P. (2000). The relationship of shame, social anxiety and depression: The role of the evaluation of social rank. *Clinical Psychology and Psychotherapy, 7,* 174–189.

Gilboa-Schechtman, E., Foa, E. B., & Amir, N. (1999). Attentional biases for facial expressions in social phobias: The face-in-the-crowd paradigm. *Cognition and Emotion, 13,* 305–318.

Gillis, M. M., Haaga, D. A. F., & Ford, G. T. (1995). Normative values for the Beck Anxiety Inventory, Fear Questionnaire, Penn State Worry Questionnaire, and Social Phobia and Anxiety Inventory. *Psychological Assessment, 7,* 450–455.

Gladstone, G. L., Parker, G. B., Michell, P. B., Malhi, G. S., Wilhem, K. A., & Austin, M.-P. (2005). A Brief Measure of Worry Severity (BMWS): Personality and clinical correlates of severe worriers. *Journal of Anxiety Disorders, 19*, 877–892.

Glass, C. R., Merluzzi, T. V., Biever, J. L., & Larsen, K. H. (1982). Cognitive assessment of social anxiety: Development and validation of a self-statement questionnaire. *Cognitive Therapy and Research, 6*, 37–55.

Goisman, R. M., Warshaw, M. G., Peterson, L. G., Rogers, M. P., Cuneo, P., Hunt, M. F., et al. (1994). Panic, agoraphobia, and panic disorders with agoraphobia: Data from a multicenter anxiety disorders study. *Journal of Nervous and Mental Disease, 182*, 72–79.

Gökalp, P. G., Tükel, R., Solmaz, D., Demir, T., Kiziltan, E., Demir, D., et al. (2001). Clinical features and co-morbidity of social phobics in Turkey. *European Psychiatry, 16*, 115–121.

Goldfried, M. R., & Davison, G. (1976). *Clinical behavior therapy*. New York: Holt, Rinehart and Winston.

Goodman, W. K., Price, L. H., Rasmussen, S. A., Mazure, C., Fleischmann, R. L., Hill, C. L., et al. (1989a). The Yale–Brown Obsessive Compulsive Scale: I. Development, use, and reliability. *Archives of General Psychiatry, 46*, 1006–1011.

Goodman, W. K., Price, L. H., Rasmussen, S. A., Mazure, C., Delgado, P., Heninger, G. R., et al. (1989b). The Yale–Brown Obsessive Compulsive Scale: II. Validity. *Archives of General Psychiatry, 46*, 1012–1016.

Goodwin, R. D. (2002). Anxiety disorders and the onset of depression among adults in the community. *Psychological Medicine, 32*, 1121–1124.

Gortner, E.-M., Rude, S. S., & Pennebaker, J. W. (2006). Benefits of expressive writing in lowering rumination and depressive symptoms. *Behavior Therapy, 37*, 292–303.

Gosselin, P., Ladouceur, R., Morin, C. M., Dugas, M. J., & Baillargeon, L. (2006). Benzodiazepine discontinuation among adults with GAD: A randomized trial of cognitive-behavioral therapy. *Journal of Consulting and Clinical Psychology, 74*, 908–919.

Gotlib, I. H., Kasch, K. L., Traill, S., Joormann, J., Arnow, B. A., & Johnson, S. L. (2004). Coherence and specificity of information-processing biases in depression and social phobia. *Journal of Abnormal Psychology, 113*, 386–398.

Gotlib, I. H., Krasnoperova, E., Joormann, J., & Yue, D. N. (2004). Attentional biases for negative interpersonal stimuli in clinical depression. *Journal of Abnormal Psychology, 113*, 127–135.

Gould, R. A., Otto, M. W., & Pollack, M. H. (1995). A meta-analysis of treatment outcome for panic disorder. *Clinical Psychology Review, 15*, 819–844.

Gould, R. A., Otto, M. W., Pollack, M. H., & Yap, L. (1997). Cognitive behavioral and pharmacological treatment of generalized anxiety disorder: A preliminary meta-analysis. *Behavior Therapy, 28*, 285–305.

Gould, R. A., Safren, S. A., Washington, D. O., & Otto, M. W. (2004). A meta-analytic review of cognitive-behavioral treatments. In R. G. Heimberg, C. L. Turk, & D. S. Mennin (Eds.), *Generalized anxiety disorder: Advances in research and practice* (pp. 248–264). New York: Guilford Press.

Grabill, K., Merlo, L., Duke, D., Harford, K.-L., Keeley, M. L., Geffken, G. R., et al. (2008). Assessment of obsessive–compulsive disorder: A review. *Journal of Anxiety Disorders, 22*, 1–17.

Grant, B. F., Hasin, D. S., Stinson, F. S., Dawson, D. A., Chou, S. P., Ruan, W. J., et al. (2005). Co-occurrence of 12-month mood and anxiety disorders and personality disorders in the US: Results from the National Epidemiologic Survey on Alcohol and Related Conditions. *Journal of Psychiatric Research, 39*, 1–9.

Grant, B. F., Stinson, F. S., Dawson, D. A., Chou, P., Dufour, M. C., Compton, W., et al. (2004). Prevalance and co-occurrence of substance use disorders and independent mood and anxiety disorders: Results from the National Epidemiologic Survey on Alcohol and Related Conditions. *Archives of General Psychiatry, 61*, 807–816.

Grant, D. M., & Beck, J. G. (2006). Attentional biases in social anxiety and dysphoria: Does comorbidity make a difference? *Journal of Anxiety Disorders, 20*, 520–529.

Gray, J. A. (1987). *The psychology of fear and stress* (2nd ed.). Cambridge, UK: Cambridge University Press.

Gray, J. A. (1999). Cognition, emotion, conscious experience and the brain. In T. Dalgleish & M. Power (Eds.), *Handbook of cognition and emotion* (pp. 83–102). Chichester, UK: Wiley.

Gray, J. A., & McNaughton, N. (1996). The neuropsychology of anxiety: Reprise. In D. A. Hope (Ed.), *Nebraska symposium on motivation: Vol. 43. Perspectives on anxiety, panic, and fear* (pp. 61–134). Lincoln: University of Nebraska Press.

Greenberg, M. S., & Alloy, L. B. (1989). Depression versus anxiety: Processing of self- and other-referent information. *Cognition and Emotion, 3*, 207–223.

Greenberg, P. E., Sisitsky, T., Kessler, R. C., Finkelstein, S. N., Berndt, E. R., Davidson, J. R. T., et al. (1999). The economic burden of anxiety disorders in the 1990s. *Journal of Clinical Psychiatry, 60*, 427–435.

Greenberg, R. L. (1989). Panic disorder and agoraphobia. In J. M. G. Williams & A. T. Beck (Eds.), *Cognitive therapy in clinical practice: An illustrative casebook* (pp. 25–49). London: Croom Helm.

Greenwald, A. G., McGhee, D. E., & Schwartz, J. L. K. (1998). Measuring individual differences in implicit cognition: The Implicit Association Test. *Journal of Personality and Social Psychology, 74*, 1464–1480.

Grey, S., & Mathews, A. (2000). Effects of training on interpretation of emotional ambiguity. *Quarterly Journal of Experimental Psychology, 53A*, 1143–1162.

Griffin, M. G., Uhlmansiek, M. H., Resick, P. A., & Mechanic, M. B. (2004). Comparison of the Posttraumatic Stress Disorder Scale versus the Clinician-Administered Posttraumatic Stress Disorder Scale in domestic violence survivors. *Journal of Traumatic Stress, 17*, 497–503.

Grillon, C. (2002). Startle reactivity and anxiety disorders: Aversive conditioning, context, and neurobiology. *Biological Psychiatry, 52*, 958–975.

Gross, J. J., & Levenson, R. W. (1997). Hiding feelings: The acute effects of inhibiting negative and positive emotion. *Journal of Abnormal Psychology, 106*, 95–103.

Gross, P. R., & Eifert, G. H. (1990). Delineating generalized anxiety: A preliminary investigation. *Journal of Psychopathology and Behavioral Assessment, 12*, 345–358.

Guthrie, R., & Bryant, R. (2000). Attempting suppression of traumatic memories over extended periods in acute stress disorder. *Behaviour Research and Therapy, 38*, 899–907.

Guy, W. (1976). *NCDEU assessment manual for psychopharmacology* (DHSS Publication No. ADM-91-338). Washington, DC: U.S. Department of Health, Education, and Welfare.

Hackmann, A., Surawy, C., & Clark, D. M. (1998). Seeing yourself through others' eyes: A study of spontaneously occurring images on social phobia. *Behaviourial and Cognitive Psychotherapy, 26*, 3–12.

Haines, A. P., Imeson J. D., & Meade, T. W. (1987). Phobic anxiety and ischaemic heart disease. *British Medical Journal, 295*, 297–299.

Hajcak, G., Huppert, J. D., Simmons, R. F., & Foa, E. B. (2004). Psychometric properties of the OCI-R in a college sample. *Behaviour Research and Therapy, 42*, 115–123.

Halligan, S. L., Clark, D. M., & Ehlers, A. (2002). Cognitive processing, memory, and the development of PTSD symptoms: Two experimental analogue studies. *Journal of Behavior Therapy and Experimental Psychiatry, 33*, 73–89.

Halligan, S. L., Michael, T., Clark, D. M., & Ehlers, A. (2003). Post-traumatic stress disorder following assault: The role of cognitive processing, trauma memory, and appraisals. *Journal of Consulting and Clinical Psychology, 71*, 419–431.

Hamilton, M. (1959). The assessment of anxiety states by rating. *British Journal of Medical Psychology, 32*, 50–55.

Hamilton, M. (1960). A rating scale for depression. *Journal of Neurology, Neurosurgery and Psychiatry, 23*, 56–61.

Hammen, C. (1988). Depression and cognitions about personal stressful life events. In L. B. Alloy (Ed.), *Cognitive processes in depression* (pp. 77–108). New York: Guilford Press.

Hankin, B. L., Abramson, L. Y., & Siler, M. (2001). A prospective test of the hopelessness theory of depression in adolescence. *Cognitive Therapy and Research, 25*, 607–632.

Hansson, L. (2002). Quality of life in depression and anxiety. *International Review of Psychiatry, 14*, 185–189.

Hardy, A., & Brewin, C. R. (2005). The role of thought suppression in the development of obsessions. *Behavioural and Cognitive Psychotherapy, 33*, 61–69.

Hare, T. A., Tottenham, N., Davidson, M. C., Glover, G. H., & Casey, B. J. (2005). Contributions of amygdala and striatal activity in emotional regulation. *Biological Psychiatry, 57*, 624–632.

Hariri, A. R., Mattay, V. S., Tessitore, A., Fera, F., & Weinberger, D. R. (2003). Neocortical modulation of the amygdala response to fearful stimuli. *Biological Psychiatry, 53*, 494–501.

Harvey, A. G. (2003). The attempted suppression of presleep cognitive activity in insomnia. *Cognitive Therapy and Research, 27*, 593–602.

Harvey, A. G. (2005). Unwanted intrusive thoughts in insomnia. In D. A. Clark (Ed.), *Intrusive thoughts in clinical disorders: Theory, research, and treatment* (pp. 86–118). New York: Guilford Press.

Harvey, A. G., & Bryant, R. A. (1998a). The effect of attempted thought suppression in acute stress disorder. *Behaviour Research and Therapy, 36*, 583–590.

Harvey, A. G., & Bryant, R. A. (1998b). The relationship between acute stress disorder and posttraumatic stress disorder: A prospective evaluation of motor vehicle accident survivors. *Journal of Consulting and Clinical Psychology, 66*, 507–512.

Harvey, A. G., & Bryant, R. A. (1999). The role of anxiety in attempted thought suppression following exposure to distressing or neutral stimuli. *Cognitive Therapy and Research, 23*, 39–52.

Harvey, A. G., & Bryant, R. A. (2002). Acute stress disorder: A synthesis and critique. *Psychological Bulletin, 128*, 886–902.

Harvey, A. G., Bryant, R. A., & Tarrier, N. (2003). Cognitive behavior therapy for posttraumatic stress disorder. *Clinical Psychology Review, 23*, 501–522.

Harvey, A. G., Ehlers, A., & Clark, D. M. (2005). Learning history in social phobia. *Behavioural and Cognitive Psychotherapy, 33*, 257–271.

Harvey, J. M., Richards, J. C., Dziadosz, T., & Swindell, A. (1993). Misinterpretation of ambiguous stimuli in panic disorder. *Cognitive Therapy and Research, 17*, 235–248.

Haslam, N., Williams, B. J., Kyrios, M., McKay, D., & Taylor, S. (2005). Subtyping obsessive–compulsive disorder: A taxometric analysis. *Behavior Therapy, 36*, 381–391.

Hauri, P. J., Friedman, M., & Ravaris, C. L. (1989). Sleep in patients with spontaneous panic attacks. *Sleep, 12*, 323–337.

Hayes, S. C. (2004). Acceptance and commitment therapy and the new behavior therapies: Mindfulness, acceptance, and relationship. In S. C. Hayes, V. M. Follette, & M. M. Linehan (Eds.), *Mindfulness and acceptance: Expanding the cognitive-behavioral traition* (pp. 1–29). New York: Guilford Press.

Hayes, S. C., Follette, V. M., & Linehan, M. M. (Eds.). (2004). *Mindfulness and acceptance: Expanding the cognitive-behavioral tradition*. New York: Guilford Press.

Hayes, S. C., & Strosahl, K. D. (Eds.). (2004). *A practical guide to acceptance and commitment therapy*. New York: Springer.

Hayes, S. C., Strosahl, K. D., Buting, K., Twohig, M., & Wilson, K. G. (2004). What is acceptance and commitment therapy? In S. C. Hayes & K. D. Strosahl (Eds.), *A practical guide to acceptance and commitment therapy* (pp. 3–29). New York: Springer.

Hayes, S. C., Strosahl, K. D., & Wilson, K. G. (1999). *Acceptance and commitment therapy: An experiential approach to behavior therapy*. New York: Guilford Press.

Hayes, S. C., Strosahl, K., Wilson, K. G., Bissett, R. T., Pistorello, J., Toarmino, D., et al. (2004). Measuring experiential avoidance: A preliminary test of a working model. *Psychological Record, 54*, 553–578.

Hayward, C., Killen, J. D., Kraemer, H. C., Blair-Greiner, A., Strachowski, D., Cunning, D., et al. (1997). Assessment and phenomenology of nonclinical panic attacks in adolescent girls. *Journal of Anxiety Disorders, 11*, 17–32.

Hayward, P., Ahmad, T., & Wardle, J. (1994). Into the dangerous world: An *in vivo* study of information processing in agoraphobics. *British Journal of Clinical Psychology, 33,* 307–315.

Hazlett-Stevens, H., & Borkovec, T. D. (2004). Interpretative cues and ambiguity in generalized anxiety disorder. *Behaviour Research and Therapy, 42,* 881–892.

Hazlett-Stevens, H., Zucker, B. G., & Craske, M. G. (2002). The relationship of thought–action fusion to pathological worry and generalized anxiety disorder. *Behaviour Research and Therapy, 40,* 1199–1204.

Headland, K., & McDonald, B. (1987). Rapid audio-tape treatment of obsessional rumination: A case report. *Behavioural Psychotherapy, 15,* 188–192.

Heckelman, L. R., & Schneier, F. R. (1995). Diagnostic issues. In R. G. Heimberg, M. R. Liebowitz, D. A. Hope, & F. R. Schneier (Eds.), *Social phobia: Diagnosis, assessment, and treatment* (pp. 3–20). New York: Guilford Press.

Heimberg, R. G. (1996). Social phobia, avoidant personality disorder and the multiaxial conceptualization of interpersonal anxiety. In P. M. Salkovskis (Ed.), *Trends in cognitive and behavioural therapies* (pp. 43–61). Chichester, UK: Wiley.

Heimberg, R. G., & Becker, R. E. (2002). *Cognitive-behavioral group therapy for social phobia: Basic mechanisms and clinical strategies.* New York: Guilford Press.

Heimberg, R. G., Horner, K. J., Juster, H. R., Safren, S. A., Brown, E. J., Schneier, F. R., et al. (1999). Psychometric properties of the Liebowitz Social Anxiety Scale. *Psychological Medicine, 29,* 199–212.

Heimberg, R. G., & Juster, H. R. (1995). Cognitive-behavioral treatments: Literature review. In R. G. Heimberg, M. R. Liebowitz, D. A. Hope, & F. R. Schneier (Eds.), *Social phobia: Diagnosis, assessment, and treatment* (pp. 261–309). New York: Guilford Press.

Heimberg, R. G., Klosko, J. S., Dodge, C. S., Shadick, R., Becker, R. E., & Barlow, D. H. (1989). Anxiety disorders, depression, and attributional style: A further test of the specificity of depressive attributions. *Cognitive Therapy and Research, 13,* 21–36.

Heimberg, R. G., Liebowitz, M. R., Hope, D. A., Schneier, F. R., Holt, C. S., Welkowitz, L. A., et al. (1998). Cognitive behavioral group therapy vs. phenelzine therapy for social phobia: 12–week outcome. *Archives of General Psychiatry, 55,* 1133–1141.

Heimberg, R. G., Makris, G. S., Juster, H. R., Öst, L.-G., & Rapee, R. M. (1997). Social phobia: A preliminary cross-national comparison. *Depression and Anxiety, 5,* 130–133.

Heimberg, R. G., & Turk, C. L. (2002). Assessment of social phobia. In R. G. Heimberg & R. E. Becker (Eds.), *Cognitive-behavioral group therapy for social phobia: Basic mechanisms and clinical strategies* (pp. 107–126). New York: Guilford Press.

Heinrichs, N., & Hofmann, S. G. (2001). Information processing in social phobia: A critical review. *Clinical Psychology Review, 21,* 751–770.

Heinrichs, N., & Hofmann, S. G. (2004). Encoding processes in social anxiety. *Journal of Behavior Therapy and Experimental Psychiatry, 35,* 57–74.

Heiser, N. A., Turner, S. M., & Beidel, D. C. (2003). Shyness: Relationship to social phobia and other psychiatric disorders. *Behaviour Research and Therapy, 41,* 209–221.

Heldt, E., Manfro, G. G., Kipper, L., Blaya, C., Isolan, L., & Otto, M. W. (2006). One-year follow-up of pharmacotherapy-resistant patients with panic disorder treated with cognitive-behavior therapy: Outcome and predictors of remission. *Behaviour Research and Therapy, 44,* 657–665.

Hembree, E. A., & Foa, E. B. (2004). Promoting cognitive changes in posttraumatic stress disorder. In M. A. Reinecke & D. A. Clark (Eds.), *Cognitive therapy across the lifespan: Evidence and practice* (pp. 231–257). Cambridge, UK: Cambridge University Press.

Henderson, L., & Zimbardo, P. (2001). Shyness, social anxiety, and social phobia. In S. G. Hofmann & P. M. DiBartolo (Eds.), *From social anxiety to social phobia: Multiple perspectives* (pp. 46–64). Boston: Allyn & Bacon.

Henning, E. R., Turk, C. L., Mennin, D. S., Fresco, D. M., & Heimberg, R. G. (2007). Impairment and quality of life in individuals with generalized anxiety disorder. *Depression and Anxiety, 24,* 342–349.

Herbert, J. D., Hope, D. A., & Bellack, A. S. (1992). Validity of the distinction between generalized social phobia and avoidant personality disorder. *Journal of Abnormal Psychology, 101,* 332–339.

Herbert, J. D., Rheingold, A. A., Gaudiano, B. A., & Myers, V. H. (2004). Standard versus extended cognitive behavior therapy for social anxiety disorder: A randomized-controlled trial. *Behavioural and Cognitive Psychotherapy, 32,* 131–147.

Hermann, C., Ofer, J., & Flor, H. (2004). Covariation bias for ambiguous social stimuli in generalized social phobia. *Journal of Abnormal Psychology, 113,* 646–653.

Hettema, J. M., Kuhn, J. W., Prescott, C. A., & Kendler, K. (2006). The impact of generalized anxiety disorder and stressful life events on risk for major depressive episodes. *Psychological Medicine, 36,* 789–795.

Hettema, J. M., Neale, M. C., & Kendler, K. S. (2001). A review and meta-analysis of the genetic epidemiology of anxiety disorders. *American Journal of Psychiatry, 158,* 1568–1578.

Hewitt, P. L., & Norton, G. R. (1993). The Beck Anxiety Inventory: A psychometric analysis. *Psychological Assessment, 5,* 408–412.

Hibbert, G. A. (1984). Ideational components of anxiety: Their origin and content. *British Journal of Psychiatry, 144,* 618–624.

Hinrichsen, H., & Clark, D. M. (2003). Anticipatory processing in social anxiety: Two pilot studies. *Journal of Behavior Therapy and Experimental Psychiatry, 34,* 205–218.

Hirsch, C. R., & Clark, D. M. (2004). Information-processing bias in social phobia. *Clinical Psychology Review, 24,* 799–825.

Hirsch, C. R., Clark, D. M., & Mathews, A. (2006). Imagery and interpretations in social phobia: Support for the combined cognitive biases hypothesis. *Behavior Therapy, 37,* 223–236.

Hirsch, C. R., Clark, D. M., Williams, R., & Morrison, J. A. (2005). Interview anxiety: Taking the perspective of a confident other changes inferential processing. *Behavioural and Cognitive Psychotherapy, 33,* 1–12.

Hirsch, C.R., Hayes, S., & Mathews,

A. (2009). Looking on the bright side: Accessing benign meanings reduces worry. *Journal of Abnormal Psychology, 118*, 44–54.

Hirsch, C. R., & Mathews, A. (1997). Interpretative inferences when reading about emotional events. *Behaviour Research and Therapy, 35*, 1123–1132.

Hirsch, C. R., & Mathews, A. (2000). Impaired positive inferential bias in social phobia. *Journal of Abnormal Psychology, 109*, 705–712.

Hirsch, C. R., Meynen, T., & Clark, D. M. (2004). Negative self-imagery in social anxiety contaminates social interactions. *Memory, 12*, 496–506.

Hiss, H., Foa, E. B., & Kozak, M. J. (1994). Relapse prevention program for treatment of obsessive-compulsive disorder. *Journal of Consulting and Clinical Psychology, 62*, 801–808.

Hochn-Saric, R., McLeod, D. R., Funderburk, F., & Kowalski, P. (2004). Somatic symptoms and physiological responses in generalized anxiety disorder and panic disorder. *Archives of General Psychiatry, 61*, 913–921.

Hodgson, R. J., & Rachman, S. J. (1977). Obsessional compulsive complaints. *Behaviour Research and Therapy, 15*, 389–395.

Hoffman, D. L., Dukes, E. M., & Wittchen, H.-U. (2008). Human and economic burden of generalized anxiety disorder. *Depression and Anxiety, 25*, 72–90.

Hofmann, S. G. (2004a). The cognitive model of panic. In M. A. Reinecke & D. A. Clark (Eds.), *Cognitive therapy across the lifespan: Evidence and practice* (pp. 117–137). Cambridge, UK: Cambridge University Press.

Hofmann, S. G. (2004b). Cognitive mediation of treatment change in social phobia. *Journal of Consulting and Clinical Psychology, 72*, 392–399.

Hofmann, S. G. (2005). Perception of control over anxiety mediates the relation between catastrophic thinking and social anxiety in social phobia. *Behaviour Research and Therapy, 43*, 885–895.

Hofmann, S. G., & Asmundson, G. J. G. (2008). Acceptance and mindfulness-based therapy: New wave or old hat? *Clinical Psychology Review, 28*, 1–16.

Hofmann, S. G., & Barlow, D. H. (2002). Social phobia (social anxiety disorder). In D. H. Barlow (Ed.), *Anxiety and its disorders: The nature and treatment of anxiety and panic* (2nd ed., pp. 454–476). New York: Guilford Press.

Hofmann, S. G., Ehlers, A., & Roth, W. T. (1995). Conditioning theory: A model for the etiology of public speaking anxiety? *Behaviour Research and Therapy, 33*, 567–571.

Hofmann, S. G., Schulz, S. M., Meuret, A. E., Moscovitch, D. A., & Suvak, M. (2006). Sudden gains during therapy of social phobia. *Journal of Consulting and Clinical Psychology, 74*, 687–697.

Hoge, C. W., Auchterlonie, J. L., & Milliken, C. S. (2006). Mental health problems, use of mental health services, and attrition from military service after returning from deployment to Iraq or Afghanistan. *Journal of the American Medical Association, 295*, 1023–1032.

Hohagen, F., Winkelmann, G., Rasche-Rauchle, H., Hand, I., König, A., Münchau, N., et al. (1998). Combination of behavior therapy with fluvoxamine in comparison with behavior therapy and placebo: Results of a multicentre study. *British Journal of Psychiatry, 173*(Suppl. 35), 71–78.

Holaway, R. M., Heimberg, R. G., & Coles, M. E. (2006). A comparison of intolerance of uncertainty in analogue obsessive–compulsive disorder and generalized anxiety disorder. *Journal of Anxiety Disorders, 20*, 158–174.

Holaway, R. M., Rodebaugh, T. L., & Heimberg, R. G. (2006). The epidemiology of worry and generalized anxiety disorder. In G. C. L. Davey & A. Wells (Eds.), *Worry and its psychological disorders: Theory, assessment and treatment* (pp. 4–20). Chichester, UK: Wiley.

Hollifield, M., Hewage, C., Gunawardena, C. N., Kodituwakku, P., Bopagoda, K., & Weerarathnege, K. (2008). Symptoms and coping in Sri Lanka 20–21 months after the 2004 tsunami. *British Journal of Psychiatry, 192*, 39–44.

Hollon, S. D., Stewart, M. O., & Strunk, D. (2006). Enduring effects for cognitive behavior therapy in the treatment of depression and anxiety. *Annual Review of Psychology, 57*, 285–315.

Holloway, W., & McNally, R. J. (1987). Effects of anxiety sensitivity on the response to hyperventilation. *Journal of Abnormal Psychology, 96*, 330–334.

Holmes, E. A., Arntz, A., & Smucker, M. R. (2007). Imagery rescripting in cognitive behavior therapy: Images, treatment techniques and outcomes. *Journal of Behavior Therapy and Experimental Psychiatry, 38*, 297–305.

Holmes, E. A., Mathews, A., Dalgleish, T., & Mackintosh, B. (2006). Positive interpretation training: Effects of mental imagery versus verbal training on positive mood. *Behavior Therapy, 37*, 237–247.

Holt, C. S., Heimberg, R. G., & Hope, D. A. (1992). Avoidant personality disorder and the generalized subtype of social phobia. *Journal of Abnormal Psychology, 101*, 318–325.

Holt, P. E., & Andrews, G. (1989). Hyperventilations and anxiety in panic disorder, social phobia, GAD and normal controls. *Behaviour Research and Therapy, 27*, 453–460.

Holwerda, T. J., Schoevers, R. A., Dekker, J., Deeg, D. J. H., Jonker, C., & Beekman, A. T. F. (2007). The relationship between generalized anxiety disorder, depression and mortality in old age. *International Journal of Geriatric Psychiatry, 22*, 241–249.

Hope, D. A., Heimberg, R. G., Juster, H. R., & Turk, C. L. (2000). *Managing social anxiety: A cognitive-behavioral therapy approach. Client workbook.* Oxford, UK: Oxford University Press.

Hope, D. A., Heimberg, R. G., & Turk, C. L. (2006). *Managing social anxiety: A cognitive-behavioral therapy approach.* Oxford, UK: Oxford University Press.

Hope, D. A., Laguna, L. B., Heimberg, R. G., & Barlow, D. H. (1996–1997). Realtionship between ADIS Clinician's Severity Rating and self-report measures among social phobics. *Depression and Anxiety, 4*, 120–125.

Hope, D. A., Rapee, R. M., Heimberg, R. G., & Dombeck, M. J. (1990). Representations of the self in social phobia: Vulnerability to social threat. *Cognitive Therapy and Research, 14*, 177–189.

Höping, W., & de Jong-Meyer, R. (2003). Differentiating unwanted intrusive thoughts from thought suppression: What does the White

Bear Suppression Inventory measure? *Personality and Individual Differences, 34,* 1049–1055.

Horowitz, M. J. (2001). *Stress response syndromes* (4th ed.). Northvale, NJ: Aronson.

Horowitz, M. J., Wilner, N., & Alvarez, W. (1979). Impact of Event Scale: A measure of subjective stress. *Psychosomatic Medicine, 41,* 209–218.

Horwath, E., Johnson, J., & Hornig, C. D. (1993). Epidemiology of panic disorder in African-Americans. *American Journal of Psychiatry, 150,* 465–469.

Howell, A., & Conway, M. (1992). Mood and the suppression of positive and negative self-referent thoughts. *Cognitive Therapy and Research, 16,* 535–555.

Hoyer, J., Becker, E. S., Neumer, S., Soeder, U., & Margraf, J. (2002). Screening for anxiety in an epidemiological sample: Predictive accuracy of questionnaires. *Journal of Anxiety Disorders, 16,* 113–134.

Hoyer, J., Becker, E. S., & Roth, W. T. (2001). Characteristics of worry in GAD patients, social phobics, and controls. *Depression and Anxiety, 13,* 89–96.

Hudson, J. L., & Rapee, R. M. (2004). From anxious temperament to disorder: An etiological model. In R. G. Heimberg, C. L. Turk, & D. S. Mennin (Eds.), *Generalized anxiety disorder: Advances in research and practice* (pp. 51–74). New York: Guilford Press.

Hunt, C., Slade, T., & Andrews, G. (2004). Generalized anxiety disorder and major depression disorder comorbidity in the National Survey of Mental Health and Well-Being. *Depression and Anxiety, 20,* 23–31.

Hunt, S., Wisocki, P., & Yanko, J. (2003). Worry and use of coping strategies among older and younger adults. *Journal of Anxiety Disorders, 17,* 547–560.

Huppert, J. D., Walther, M. R., Hajcak, G., Yadin, E., Foa, E. B., Simpson, H. B., et al. (2007). The OCI R: Validation of the subscales in a clinical sample. *Journal of Anxiety Disorders, 21,* 394–406.

Ikin, J. F., Sim, M. R., McKenzie, D. P., Horsley, K. W. A., Wilson, E. J., Moore, M. R., et al. (2007). Anxiety, post-traumatic stress disorder and depression in Korean War veterans 50 years after the war.

British Journal of Psychiatry, 190, 475–483.

IMS. (2004). Liptor leads the way in 2003. Retrieved May 31, 2004, from *www.ims-global.com.*

Ingham, J. G., Kreitman, N. B., Miller, P. McC., Sashidharan, S. P., & Surtees, P. G. (1986). Self-esteem, vulnerability and psychiatric disorder in the community. *British Journal of Psychiatry, 148,* 375–385.

Ingram, R. E. (1990). Attentional nonspecificity in depressive and generalized anxious affective states. *Cognitive Therapy and Research, 14,* 25–35.

Ingram, R. E., Kendall, P. C., Smith, T. W., Donnell, C., & Ronan, K. (1987). Cognitive specificity in emotional disorders. *Journal of Personality and Social Psychology, 53,* 734–742.

Ingram, R. E., Miranda, J., & Segal, Z. V. (1998). *Cognitive vulnerability to depression.* New York: Guilford Press.

Ingram, R. E., & Price, J. M. (2001). The role of vulnerability in understanding psychopathology. In R. E. Ingram & J. M. Price (Eds.), *Vulnerability to psychopathology: Risks across the lifespan* (2nd ed., pp. 3–19). New York: Guilford Press.

Ishiyama, F. I. (1984). Shyness: Anxious social sensitivity and self-isolation tendency. *Adolescence, 19,* 903–911.

Izard, C. E. (1991). *The psychology of emotions.* New York: Plenum Press.

Jacobsen, L. K., Southwick, S. M., & Kosten, T. R. (2001). Substance use disorders in patients with posttraumatic stress disorder: A review of the literature. *American Journal of Psychiatry, 158,* 1184–1190.

Jacobson, E. (1968). *Progressive relaxation: A physiological and clinical investigation of muscular states and their significance in psychology and medical practice.* Chicago: University of Chicago Press.

Janeck, A. S., & Calamari, J. E. (1999). Thought suppression in obsessive–compulsive disorder. *Cognitive Therapy and Research, 23,* 497–509.

Janeck, A. S., Calamari, J. E., Riemann, B. C., & Heffelfinger, S. K. (2003). Too much thinking about thinking?: Metacognitive differences in obsessive–compulsive

disorder. *Journal of Anxiety Disorders, 17,* 181–195.

Janoff-Bulman, R. (1989). Assumptive worlds and the stress of traumatic events: Applications of schema construct. *Social Cognition, 7,* 113–136.

Janoff-Bulman, R. (1992). *Shattered assumptions: Towards a new psychology of trauma.* New York: Free Press.

Jenkins, R., Lewis, G., Bebbington, P., Brugha, T., Farrell, M., Gill, B., et al. (1997). The National Psychiatric Morbidity Surveys of Great Britain: Initial findings from the Household Survey. *Psychological Medicine, 27,* 775–789.

Jeon, H. J., Suh, T., Lee, H. J., Hahm, B.-J., Lee, J.-J., Cho, S.-J., et al. (2007). Partial versus full PTSD in the Korean community: Prevalence, duration, correlates, comorbidity, and dysfunction. *Depression and Anxiety, 24,* 577–585.

John, O. P., & Gross, J. J. (2004). Healthy and unhealthy emotion regulation: Personality processes, individual differences, and life span development. *Journal of Personality, 72,* 1301–1333.

Johnson, J. G., Cohen, P., Kasen, S., & Brook, J. S. (2006). Personality disorders evident by early adulthood and risk for anxiety disorders during middle childhood. *Journal of Anxiety Disorders, 20,* 408–426.

Johnson, J. G., & Miller, S. M. (1990). Attributional, life-event, and affective predictors of onset of depression, anxiety, and negative attributional style. *Cognitive Therapy and Research, 14,* 417–430.

Joiner, T. E., Steer, R. A., Beck, A. T., Schmidt, N. B., Rudd, M. D., & Catanzaro, S. J. (1999). Physiological hyperarousal: Construct validity of a central aspect of the tripartite model of depression and anxiety. *Journal of Abnormal Psychology, 108,* 290–298.

Jolly, J. B., Dyck, M. J., Kramer, T. A., & Wherry, J. N. (1994). Integration of positive and negative affectivity and cognitive content-specificity: Improved discrimination of anxious and depressive symptoms. *Journal of Abnormal Psychology, 103,* 544–552.

Jolly, J. B., & Dykman, R. A. (1994). Using self-report data to differentiate anxious and depressive symptoms in adolescents: Cognitive content-specificity and global distress? *Cognitive Therapy and Research, 18,* 25–37.

Jolly, J. B., & Kramer, T. A. (1994). The hierarchical arrangement of internalizing cognitions. *Cognitive Therapy and Research, 18,* 1–14.

Jones, M. K., & Menzies, R. G. (1998). Danger ideation reduction therapy (DIRT) for obsessive–compulsive washers: A controlled trial. *Behaviour Research and Therapy, 36,* 959–970.

Jones, W. H., Briggs, S. R., & Smith, T. G. (1986). Shyness: Conceptualization and measurement. *Journal of Personality and Social Psychology, 51,* 629–639.

Joorman, J., & Stöber, J. (1997). Measuring facets of worry: A LISREL analysis of the Worry Domains Questionnaire. *Personality and Individual Differences, 23,* 827–837.

Julien, D., O'Connor, K. P., & Aardema, F. (2007). Intrusive thoughts, obsessions, and appraisals in obsessive–compulsive disorder: A critical review. *Clinical Psychology Review, 27,* 366–383.

Julien, D., O'Connor, K. P., Aardema, F., & Todorov, C. (2006). The specificity of belief domains in obsessive–compulsive subtypes. *Personality and Individual Differences, 41,* 1205–1216.

Kabat-Zinn, J. (1990). *Full catastrophe living: Using the wisdom of your body and mind to face stress, pain, and illness.* New York: Bantam Dell.

Kabat-Zinn, J. (2005). *Coming to our senses: Healing ourselves and the world through mindfulness.* New York: Hyperion.

Kabat-Zinn, J., Massion, A. O., Kristeller, J., Peterson, L. G., Fletcher, K. E., Pbert, L., et al. (1992). Effectiveness of a meditation-based stress reduction program in the treatment of anxiety disorders. *American Journal of Psychiatry, 149,* 936–943.

Kaler, M. E., Frazier, P. A., Anders, S. L., Tashiro, T., Tomich, P., Tennen, H., et al. (2008). Assessing the psychometric properties of the World Assumptions Scale. *Journal of Traumatic Stress, 21,* 326–332.

Kamieniecki, G. W., Wade, T., & Tsourtos, G. (1997). Interpretative bias for benign sensations in panic disorder with agoraphobia. *Journal of Anxiety Disorders, 11,* 141–156.

Kampman, M., Keijsers, G. P. J., Ver-

braak, M. J. P. M., Näring, G., & Hoogduin, C. A. L. (2002). The emotional Stroop: A comparison of panic disorder patients, obsessive–compulsive patients, and normal controls, in two experiments. *Journal of Anxiety Disorders, 16,* 425–441.

Kangas, M., Henry, J. L., & Bryant, R. A. (2005). The relationship between acute stress disorder and posttraumatic stress disorder following cancer. *Journal of Consulting and Clinical Psychology, 73,* 360–364.

Karajgi, B., Rifkin, A., Doddi, S., & Kolli, R. (1990). The prevalence of anxiety disorders in patients with chronic obstructive pulmonary disease. *American Journal of Psychiatry, 147,* 200–201.

Karno, M., Golding, J. M., Sorenson, S. B., & Burnam, A. (1988). The epidemiology of obsessive–compulsive disorder in five US communities. *Archives of General Psychiatry, 45,* 1094–1099.

Kashani, J. H., & Orvaschel, H. (1990). A community study of anxiety in children and adolescents. *American Journal of Psychiatry, 147,* 313–318.

Kashdan, T. B., Barrios, V., Forsyth, J. P., & Steger, M. F. (2006). Experiential avoidance as a generalized psychological vulnerability: Comparisons with coping and emotion regulation strategies. *Behaviour Research and Therapy, 44,* 1301–1320.

Kaspi, S. P., McNally, R. J., & Amir, N. (1995). Cognitive processing of emotional information in posttraumatic stress disorder. *Cognitive Therapy and Research, 19,* 433–444.

Katerndahl, D. A. (1993). Panic and prolapse: Meta-analysis. *Journal of Nervous and Mental Disease, 181,* 539–544.

Katerndahl, D. A., & Realini, J. P. (1993). Lifetime prevalence of panic states. *American Journal of Psychiatry, 150,* 246–249.

Katerndahl, D. A., & Realini, J. P. (1995). Where do panic attack sufferers seek care? *Journal of Family Practice, 40,* 237–243.

Katerndahl, D. A., & Realini, J. P. (1997). Comorbid psychiatric disorders in subjects with panic attacks. *Journal of Nervous and Mental Disease, 185,* 669–674.

Katon, W., Hall, M. L., Russo, J., Cormier, L., Hollifield, M.,

Vitaliano, P. P., et al. (1988). Chest pain: Relationship of psychiatric illness to coronary arteriographic results. *American Journal of Medicine, 84,* 1–9.

Katon, W., Vitaliano, P. P., Russo. J., Cormier, L., Anderson, K., & Jones, M. (1986). Panic disorder: Epidemiology in primary care. *The Journal of Family Practice, 23,* 233–239.

Kazantzis, N., Deane, F. P., & Ronan, K. R. (2000). Homework assignments in cognitive and behavioral therapy: A meta-analysis. *Clinical Psychology: Science and Practice, 7,* 189–202.

Kazantzis, N., & L'Abate, L. (Eds.). (2006). *Handbook of homework assignments in psychotherapy: Research, practice, and prevention.* New York: Springer.

Keane, T. M., & Barlow, D. H. (2002). Posttraumatic stress disorder. In D. H. Barlow (Ed.), *Anxiety and its disorders: The nature and treatment of anxiety and panic* (2nd ed., pp. 418–453). New York: Guilford Press.

Keane, T. M., Brief, D. J., Pratt, E. M., & Miller, M. W. (2007). Assessment of PTSD and its comorbidities in adults. In M. J. Freidman, T. M. Keane, & P. A. Resick (Eds.), *Handbook of PTSD: Science and practice* (pp. 279–305). New York: Guilford Press.

Keane, T. M., Caddell, J. M., & Taylor, K. L. (1988). Mississippi Scale for Combat-Related Posttraumatic Stress Disorder: Three studies in reliability and validity. *Journal of Consulting and Clinical Psychology, 56,* 85–90.

Keane, T. M., Kolb, L. C., Kaloupek, D. G., Orr, S. P., Blanchard, E. B., Thomas, R. G., et al. (1998). Utility of psychophysiological measurement in the diagnosis of posttraumatic stress disorder: Results from a Department of Veterans Affairs cooperative study. *Journal of Consulting and Clinical Psychology, 66,* 914–923.

Keller, M. B. (2003). The lifelong course of social anxiety disorder: A clinical perspective. *Acta Psychiatrica Scandinavica, 108*(Suppl. 417), 85–94.

Kelly, A. E., & Kahn, J. H. (1994). Effects of suppression of personal intrusive thoughts. *Journal of Personality and Social Psychology, 66,* 998–1006.

Kelly, M. M., Forsyth, J. P., & Karekla, M. (2006). Sex differences in response to a panicogenic challenge procedure: An experimental evaluation of panic vulnerability in a non-clinical sample. *Behaviour Research and Therapy, 44,* 1421–1430.

Ken, W. L., Paller, A., & Zinbarg, R. E. (2008). Conscious intrusion of threat information via unconscious priming in anxiety. *Cognition and Emotion, 22,* 44–62.

Kenardy, J., & Taylor, C. B. (1999). Expected versus unexpected panic attacks: A naturalistic prospective study. *Journal of Anxiety Disorders, 13,* 435–445.

Kenardy, J. A., Dow, M. G. T., Johnston, D. W., Newman, M. G., Thomson, A., & Taylor, C. B. (2003). A comparison of delivery methods of cognitive-behavioral therapy for panic disorder: An international multicenter trial. *Journal of Consulting and Clinical Psychology, 71,* 1068–1075.

Kendall, P. C., & Ingram, R. E. (1989). Cognitive-behavioral perspectives: Theory and research in depression and anxiety. In P. C. Kendall & D. Watson (Eds.), *Anxiety and depression: Distinctive and overlapping features* (pp. 27–53). San Diego: Academic Press.

Kendler, K. S., Heath, A. C., Martin, N. G., & Eaves, L. J. (1987). Symptoms of anxiety and symptoms of depression: Same genes, different environments? *Archives of General Psychiatry, 44,* 451–457.

Kendler, K. S., Hettema, J. M., Butera, F., Gardner, C. O., & Prescott, C. A. (2003). Life event dimensions of loss, humiliation, entrapment, and danger in the prediction of onsets of major depression and generalized anxiety. *Archives of General Psychiatry, 60,* 789–796.

Kendler, K. S., Myers, J., & Prescott, C. A. (2002). The etiology of phobias: An evaluation of the stress–diathesis model. *Archives of General Psychiatry, 59,* 242–248.

Kendler, K. S., Neale, M. C., Kessler, R. C., Heath, A. C., & Eaves, L. J. (1992a). Major depression and generalized anxiety disorder: Same genes, (partly) different environments? *Archives of General Psychiatry, 49,* 716–722.

Kendler, K. S., Neale, M. C., Kessler, R. C., Heath, A. C., & Eaves, L. J. (1992b). The genetic epidemiology of phobia in women: The interrelationship of agoraphobia, social

phobia, situational phobia, and simple phobia. *Archives of General Psychiatry, 49,* 273–281.

Kendler, K. S., Walters, E. E., Neale, M. C., Kessler, R. C., Heath, A. C., & Eaves, L. J. (1995). The structure of the genetic and environmental risk factors for six major psychiatric disorders in women. *Archives of General Psychiatry, 52,* 374–383.

Kessler, R. C., Berglund, P., Demler, O., Robertson, M. S., & Walters, E. E. (2005). Lifetime prevalence and age-of-onset distributions of DSM-IV disorders in the National Comorbidity Survey Replication. *Archives of General Psychiatry, 62,* 593–602.

Kessler, R. C., Chiu, W. T., Demler, O., & Walters, E. E. (2005). Prevalence, severity, and comorbidity of 12-month DSM-IV disorders in the National Comorbidity Survey Replication. *Archives of General Psychiatry, 62,* 617–627.

Kessler, R. C., Davis, C. G., & Kendler, K. S. (1997). Childhood adversity and adult psychiatric disorder in the US National Comorbidity Survey. *Psychological Medicine, 27,* 1101–1119.

Kessler, R. C., & Frank, R. (1997). The impact of psychiatric disorders on work loss days. *Psychological Medicine, 27,* 861–873.

Kessler, R. C., Herringa, S., Lakoma, M. D., Petukhova, M., Rupp, A. E., Schoenbaum, M., et al. (2008). Individual and societal effects of mental disorders on earnings in the United States: Results from the National Comorbidity Survey Replication. *American Journal of Psychiatry, 165,* 703–711.

Kessler, R. C., McGonagle, K. A., Shanyang, Z., Nelson, B., Hughes, M., Eshleman, S., et al. (1994). Lifetime and 12-month prevalence of DSM-III-R psychiatric disorders in the United States. *Archives of General Psychiatry, 51,* 8–19.

Kessler, R. C., Nelson, C. B., McGonagle, K. A., Liu, J., Swartz, M., & Blazer, D. G. (1996). Comorbidity of DSM-III-R major depressive disorder in the general population: Results from the US National Comorbidity Survey. *British Journal of Psychaitry, 168 (suppl. 30),* 17–30.

Kessler, R. C., Sonnega, A., Bromet, E., Hughes, M., & Nelson, C. B. (1995). Posttraumatic stress disorder in the National Comorbidity

Survey. *Archives of General Psychiatry, 52,* 1048–1060.

Kessler, R. C., Stein, M. B., & Berglund, P. (1998). Social phobia subtypes in the National Comorbidity Survey. *American Journal of Psychiatry, 155,* 613–619.

Kessler, R. C., Walters, E. E., & Wittchen, H.-U. (2004). Epidemiology. In R. G. Heimberg, C. L. Turk, & D. S. Mennin (Eds.), *Generalized anxiety disorder: Advances in research and practice* (pp. 29–50). New York: Guilford Press.

Khan, A. A., Jacobson, K. C., Gardner, C. O., Prescott, C. A., & Kendler, K. S. (2005). Personality and comorbidity of common psychiatric disorders. *British Journal of Psychiatry, 186,* 190–196.

Khawaja, N. G., & Oei, T. P. S. (1992). Development of a catastrophic cognition questionnaire. *Journal of Anxiety Disorders, 6,* 305–318.

Khawaja, N. G., & Oei, T. P. S. (1998). Catastrophic cognitions in panic disorder with and without agoraphobia. *Clinical Psychology Review, 18,* 341–365.

Khawaja, N. G., Oei, T. P. S., & Baglioni, A. J. (1994). Modification of the Catastrophic Cognitions Questionnaire (CCQ-M) for normals and patients: Exploratory and LISERAL analyses. *Journal of Psychopathology and Behavioral Assessment, 16,* 325–342.

Kilpatrick, D. G., Ruggiero, K. J., Acierno, R., Saunders, B. E., Resnick, H. S., & Best, C. L. (2003). Violence and risk of PTSD, major depression, substance abuse/dependence, and comorbidity: Results from the National Survey of Adolescents. *Journal of Consulting and Clinical Psychology, 71,* 692–700.

Kimbrel, N. A. (2008). A model of the development and maintenance of generalized social phobia. *Clinical Psychology Review, 28,* 592–612.

Kircanski, K., Craske, M. G., & Bjork, R. A. (2008). Thought suppression enhances memory bias for threat material. *Behaviour Research and Therapy, 46,* 5–27.

Kline, P. (1968). Obsessional traits, obsessional symptoms and anal eroticism. *British Journal of Medical Psychology, 41,* 299–304.

Klinger, E. (1975). Consequences of commitment to and disengagement from incentives. *Psychological Review, 82,* 1–25.

Kobak, K. A., Greist, J. H., Jefferson, J. W., Katzelnick, D. J., & Henk, H. J. (1998). Behavioral versus pharmacological treatments of obsessive compulsive disorder: A meta-analysis. *Psychopharmacology, 136,* 205–216.

Kobak, K. A., Reynolds, W. M., & Greist, J. H. (1993). Development and validation of a computer-administered version of the Hamilton Anxiety Scale. *Psychological Assessment, 5,* 487–492.

Kocovski, N. L., & Endler, N. S. (2000). Social anxiety, self-regulation, and fear of negative evaluation. *European Journal of Personality, 14,* 347–358.

Kocovski, N. L., Endler, N. S., Rector, N. A., & Flett, G. L. (2005). Ruminative coping and post-event processing in social anxiety. *Behaviour Research and Therapy, 43,* 971–984.

Kocovski, N. L., & Rector, N. A. (2008). Post-event processing in social anxiety disorder: Idiosyncratic priming in the course of CBT. *Cognitive Therapy and Research, 32,* 23–36.

Koenen, K. C., Stellman, S. D., Sommer, J. F., & Stellman, J. M. (2008). Persisting posttraumatic stress disorder symptoms and their relationship to functioning in Vietnam veterans: A 14-year follow-up. *Journal of Traumatic Stress, 21,* 49–57.

Koenen, K. C., Stellman, J. M., Stellman, S. D., & Sommer, J. F. (2003). Risk factors for course of posttraumatic stress disorder among Vietnam veterans: A 14-year follow-up of American Legionnaires. *Journal of Consulting and Clinical Psychology, 71,* 980–986.

Koerner, N., & Dugas, M. J. (2006). A cognitive model of generalized anxiety disorder: The role of intolerance of uncertainty. In G. C. L. Davey & A. Wells (Eds.), *Worry and its psychological disorders: Theory, assessment and treatment* (pp. 202–216). Chichester, UK: Wiley.

Kollman, D. M., Brown, T. A., Liverant, G. I., & Hofmann, S. G. (2006). A taxometric investigation of the latent structure of social anxiety disorder in outpatients with anxiety and mood disorders. *Depression and Anxiety, 23,* 190–199.

Kolts, R. L., Robinson, A. M., & Tracy, J. J. (2004). The relationship of sociotropy and autonomy to posttraumatic cognitions and PTSD symptomatology in trauma survivors. *Journal of Clinical Psychology, 60,* 53–63.

Koren, D., Arnon, I., & Klein, E. (1999). Acute stress response and posttraumatic stress disorder in traffic accident victims: A one-year prospective, follow-up study. *American Journal of Psychiatry, 156,* 367–373.

Koster, E. H. W., Crombez, G., Verschuere, B., & De Houwer, J. (2004). Selective attention to threat in the dot probe paradigm: Differentiating vigilance and difficulty to disengage. *Behaviour Research and Therapy, 42,* 1183–1192.

Koster, E. H. W., Crombez, G., Verschuere, B., Van Damme, S., & Wiersema, J. R. (2006). Components of attentional bias to threat in high trait anxiety: Facilitated engagement, impaired disengagement, and attentional avoidance. *Behaviour Research and Therapy, 44,* 1757–1771.

Koster, E. H. W., Rassin, E., Crombez, G., & Näring, G. W. B. (2003). The paradoxical effects of suppressing anxious thoughts during imminent threat. *Behaviour Research and Therapy, 41,* 1113–1120.

Kozak, M. J. (1999). Evaluating treatment efficacy for obsessive–compulsive disorder: Caveat practitioner. *Cognitive and Behavioral Practice, 6,* 422–426.

Kozak, M. J., & Coles, M. E. (2005). Treatment for OCD : Unleashing the power of exposure. In J. S. Abramowitz & A. C. Houts (Eds.), *Concepts and controversies in obsessive–compulsive disorder* (pp. 283–304). New York: Springer.

Kozak, M. J., & Foa, E. B. (1997). *Mastery of obsessive–compulsive disorder: A cognitive behavioral approach. Therapist guide.* San Antonio, TX: Psychological Corporation.

Kozak, M. J., Foa, E. B., & McCarthy, P. R. (1988). Obsessive–compulsive disorder. In C. G. Last & M. Hersen (Eds.), *Handbook of anxiety disorders* (pp. 87–108). New York: Pergamon Press.

Kozak, M. J., Liebowitz, M. R., & Foa, E. B. (2000). Cognitive behavior therapy and pharmacotherapy for obsessive–compulsive disorder: The NIMH-Sponsored Collaborative Study. In W. K. Goodman, M. V. Rudorfor, & J. D. Maser (Eds.), *Obsessive–compulsive disorder: Contemporary issues in treatment* (pp. 501–530). Mahwah, NJ: Erlbaum.

Krochmalik, A., Jones, M. K., & Menzies, R. G. (2001). Danger ideation reduction therapy (DIRT) for treatment-resistant compulsive washing. *Behaviour Research and Therapy, 39,* 897–912.

Kroeze, S., & van den Hout, M. (2000a). Selective attention for cardiac information in panic patients. *Behaviour Research and Therapy, 38,* 63–72.

Kroeze, S., & van den Hout, M. (2000b). Selective attention for hyperventilatory sensations in panic disorder. *Journal of Anxiety Disorders, 14,* 563–581.

Kroeze, S., van der Does, W., Schot, R., Sterk, P. J., Spinhoven, P., & van den Aardweg, J. G. (2005). Automatic negative evaluation of suffocation sensations in individuals with suffocation fear. *Journal of Abnormal Psychology, 114,* 466–470.

Krueger, R. F. (1999). The structure of common mental disorders. *Archives of General Psychiatry, 56,* 921–926.

Kulka, R. A., Schlenger, W. E., Fairbank, J. A., Hough, R. L., Jordon, B. K., Marmar. C. R., et al. (1990). *Trauma and the Vietnam War generation: Report of findings from the National Vietnam Veterans Readjustment Study.* New York: Brunner/Mazel.

Kushner, M. G., Abrams, K., & Borchardt, C. (2000). The relationship between anxiety disorders and alcohol use disorders: A review of major perspectives and findings. *Clinical Psychology Review, 20,* 149–171.

Kushner, M. G., Sher, K. J., & Beitman, B. D. (1990). The relation between alcohol problems and the anxiety disorders. *American Journal of Psychiatry, 147,* 685–695.

Kushner, M. G., Sher, K. J., & Erickson, D. J. (1999). Prospective analysis of the relation between DSM-III anxiety disorders and alcohol use disorders. *American Journal of Psychiatry, 156,* 723–732.

Kyrios, M., & Iob, M. (1998). Automatic and strategic processing in obsessive–compulsive disorder: Attentional bias, cognitive avoidance or more complex phenomena?

Journal of Anxiety Disorders, 12, 271–292.

Ladouceur, R., Dugas, M. J., Freeston, M. H., Léger, E., Gagnon, F., & Thibodeau, N. (2000). Efficacy of a cognitive-behavioral treatment for generalized anxiety disorder: Evaluation in a controlled clinical trial. *Journal of Consulting and Clinical Psychology, 68*, 957–964.

Ladouceur, R., Dugas, M. J., Freeston, M. H., Rhéaume, J., Blais, F., Boisvert, J.-M., et al. (1999). Specificity of generalized anxiety disorder symptoms and processes. *Behavior Therapy, 30*, 191–207.

Ladouceur, R., Freeston, M. H., Fournier, S., Dugas, M. J., & Doucet, C. (2002). The social basis of worry in three samples: High-school students, university students, and older adults. *Behavioural and Cognitive Psychotherapy, 30*, 427–438.

Ladouceur, R., Freeston, M. H., Rheaume, J., Dugas, M. J., Gagnon, F., Thibodeau, N., et al. (2000). Strategies used with intrusive thoughts: A comparison of OCD patients with anxious and community controls. *Journal of Abnormal Psychology, 109*, 179–187.

Ladouceur, R., Léger, E., Rhéaume, J., & Dubé, D. (1996). Correction of inflated responsibility in the treatment of obsessive–compulsive disorder. *Behaviour Research and Therapy, 34*, 767–774.

Ladouceur, R., Rhéaume, J., Freeston, M. H., Aublet, F., Jean, K., Lachange, S., et al. (1995). Experimental manipulations of responsibility: An analogue test for models of obsessive–compulsive disorder. *Behaviour Research and Therapy, 33*, 937–946.

Landon, T. M., & Barlow, D. H. (2004). Cognitive-behavioral treatment for panic disorder: Current status. *Journal of Psychiatric Practice, 10*, 211–225.

Lang, P. J. (1979). A bio-informational theory of emotional imagery. *Psychophysiology, 16*, 495–512.

Lang, P. J., Bradley, M. M., & Cuthbert, B. N. (1998). Emotion, motivation, and anxiety: Brain mechanisms and psychophysiology. *Biological Psychiatry, 44*, 1248–1263.

Lang, P. J., Levin, D. N., Miller, G. A., & Kozak, M. J. (1983). Fear behavior, fear imagery, and the psychophysiology of emotion: The problem of affective response integration. *Journal of Abnormal Psychology, 92*, 279–306.

Langlois, F., Freeston, M. H., & Ladouceur, R. (2000a). Differences and similarities between obsessive intrusive thoughts and worry in a non-clinical population: Study 1. *Behaviour Research and Therapy, 38*, 157–173.

Langlois, F., Freeston, M. H., & Ladouceur, R. (2000b). Differences and similarities between obsessive intrusive thoughts and worry in a non-clinical population: Study 2. *Behaviour Research and Therapy, 38*, 175–189.

Laposa, J. M., & Alden, L. E. (2003). Posttraumatic stress disorder in the emergency room: Exploration of a cognitive model. *Behaviour Research and Therapy, 41*, 49–65.

Laposa, J. M., & Alden, L. E. (2006). An analogue study of intrusions. *Behaviour Research and Therapy, 44*, 925–946.

Larsen, K. E., Schwartz, S. A., Whiteside, S. P., Khandker, M., Moore, K. M., & Abramowitz, J. S. (2006). Thought control strategies used by parents reporting postpartum obsessions. *Journal of Cognitive Psychotherapy: An International Quarterly, 20*, 435–445.

Lauterbach, D., & Vrana, S. (2001). The relationship among personality variables, exposure to traumatic events, and severity of posttraumatic stress symptoms. *Journal of Traumatic Stress, 14*, 29–45.

Lavy, E., van Oppen, P., & van den Hout, M. (1994). Selective processing of emotional information in obsessive compulsive disorder. *Behaviour Research and Therapy, 32*, 243–246.

Lazarus, R. S., & Folkman, S. (1984). *Stress, appraisal, and coping.* New York: Springer.

Leahy, R. L. (2001). *Overcoming resistance in cognitive therapy.* New York: Guilford Press.

Leahy, R. L. (2003). *Cognitive therapy techniques: A practitioner's guide.* New York: Guilford Press.

Leahy, R. L. (2005). *The worry cure: Seven steps to stop worry from stopping you.* New York: Harmony Books.

Leahy, R. L. (2009). *Anxiety free: Unravel your fears before they unravel you.* Carlsbad, CA: Hay House.

Leary, M. R. (1983). A brief version of the Fear of Negative Evaluation Scale. *Personality and Social Psychology Bulletin, 9*, 371–375.

Ledley, D. R., Fresco, D. M., & Heimberg, R. G. (2006). Cognitive vulnerability to social anxiety disorder. In L. B. Alloy & J. H. Riskind (Eds.), *Cognitive vulnerability to emotional disorders* (pp. 251–283). Mahwah, NJ: Erlbaum.

Ledley, D. R., Huppert, J. D., Foa, E. B., Davidson, J. R. T., Keefe, F. J., & Potts, N. L. S. (2005). Impact of depressive symptoms on the treatment of generalized social anxiety disorder. *Depression and Anxiety, 22*, 161–167.

LeDoux, J. E. (1989). Cognitive–emotional interactions in the brain. *Cognition and Emotion, 3*, 267–289.

LeDoux, J. E. (1996). *The emotional brain: The mysterious underpinnings of emotional life.* New York: Simon & Schuster.

LeDoux, J. E. (2000). Emotion circuits in the brain. *Annual Review of Neuroscience, 23*, 155–184.

Ledwidge, B. (1978). Cognitive behavior modification: A step in the wrong direction? *Psychological Bulletin, 85*, 353–375.

Lee, C., Gavriel, H., Drummond, P., Richards, J., & Greenwald, R. (2002). Treatment of PTSD: Stress inoculation training with prolonged exposure compared to EMDR. *Journal of Clinical Psychology, 58*, 1071–1089.

Lee, H.-J., & Kwon, S.-M. (2003). Two different types of obsession: Autogenous obsessions and reactive obsessions. *Behaviour Research and Therapy, 41*, 11–29.

Lee, K. A., Vaillant, G. E., Torrey, W. C., & Elder, G. H. (1995). A 50-year prospective study of the psychological sequeale of World War II combat. *American Journal of Psychiatry, 152*, 516–522.

Lees, A., Mogg, K., & Bradley, B. P. (2005). Health anxiety, anxiety sensitivity, and attentional biases for pictoral and linguistic health-threat cues. *Cognition and Emotion, 19*, 453–462.

Lensi, P., Cassano, G. B., Correddu, G., Ravagli, S., Kunovac, J. L., & Akiskal, H. S. (1996). Obsessive–compulsive disorder: Familial-developmental history, symptomatology, comorbidity and course with special reference to gender-related differences. *British Journal of Psychiatry, 169*, 101–107.

Lenze, E. J., Mulsant, B. H., Shear,

M. K., Schulberg, H. C., Dew, M. A., Begley, A. E., et al. (2000). Comorbid anxiety disorders in depressed elderly patients. *American Journal of Psychiatry, 157,* 722–728.

Leon, A. C., Portera, L., & Weissman, M. M. (1995). The social cost of anxiety disorders. *British Journal of Psychiatry, 166*(Suppl. 27), 19–22.

Leskin, G. A., & Sheikh, J. I. (2002). Lifetime trauma history and panic disorder: findings from the National Comorbidity Survey. *Journal of Anxiety Disorders, 16,* 599–603.

Levenson, M. R., Aldwin, C. M., Bossé, R., & Spiro, A. (1988). Emotionality and mental health: Longitudinal findings from the Normative Aging Study. *Journal of Abnormal Psychology, 97,* 94–96.

Lévesque, J., Eugene, F., Joanette, Y., Paquette, V., Mensour, B., Beaudoin, G., et al. (2003). Neural circuitry underlying voluntary suppression of sadness. *Biological Psychiatry, 53,* 502–510.

Levitt, J. T., Brown, T. A., Orsillo, S. M., & Barlow, D. H. (2004). The effects of acceptance versus suppression of emotion on subjective and psychophysiological response to carbon dioxide challenge in patients with panic disorder. *Behavior Therapy, 35,* 747–766.

Leyfer, O. T., Ruberg, J. L., & Woodruff-Borden, J. (2006). Examination of the utility of the Beck Anxiety Inventory and its factors as a screener for anxiety disorders. *Journal of Anxiety Disorders, 20,* 444–458.

Lieb, R., Wittchen, H.-U., Höfler, M., Fuetsch, M., Stein, M. B., & Merikangas, K. R. (2000). Parental psychopathology, parenting styles and the risk of social phobia in offspring: A prospective-longitudinal community study. *Archives of General Psychiatry, 57,* 859–866.

Liebowitz, M. R. (1987). Social phobia. *Modern Problems in Pharmacopsychiatry, 22,* 141–173.

Liebowitz, M. R., Gorman, J. M., Fyer, A. J., Levitt, M., Dillon, D., Levy, G., et al. (1985). Lacate provocation of panic attacks: II. Biochemical and physiological findings. *Archives of General Psychiatry, 42,* 709–719.

Liebowitz, M. R., Heimberg, R. G., Fresco, D. M., Travers, J., & Stein, M. B. (2000). Social phobia or social anxiety disorder: What's in the name? [Letter to the editor]. *Archives of General Psychiatry, 57,* 191–192.

Liebowitz, M. R., Heimberg, R. G., Schneier, F. R., Hope, D. A., Davies, S., Holt, C. S., et al. (1999). Cognitive-behavioral group therapy versus phenelzine in social phobia: Long term outcome. *Depression and Anxiety, 10,* 89–98.

Lilienfeld, S. O. (1996). Anxiety sensitivity is not distinct from trait anxiety. In R. M. Rapee (Ed.), *Current controversies in the anxiety disorders* (pp. 228–244). New York: Guilford Press.

Lilienfeld, S. O., Jacob, R. G., & Turner, S. M. (1989). Comment on Holloway and McNally's (1987) "Effects of anxiety sensitivity on the response to hyperventilation." *Journal of Abnormal Psychology, 98,* 100–102.

Lim, S.-L., & Kim, J.-H. (2005). Cognitive processing of emotional information in depression, panic, and somatoform disorder. *Journal of Abnormal Psychology, 114,* 50–61.

Lindsay, W. R., Gamsu, C. V., McLaughlin, E., Hood, E. M., & Espie, C. A. (1987). A controlled trial of treatments for generalized anxiety. *British Journal of Clinical Psychology, 26,* 3–15.

Lint, D. W., Taylor, C. B., Fried-Behar, L., & Kenardy, J. (1995). Does ischemia occur with panic attacks? *American Journal of Psychiatry, 152,* 1678–1680.

Lissek, S., Powers, A. S., McClure, E. B., Phelps, E. A., Woldehawariat, G., Grillon, C., et al. (2005). Classical fear conditioning in the anxiety disorders: A meta-analysis. *Behaviour Research and Therapy, 43,* 1391–1424.

Litz, B. T., Miller, M. W., Ruef, A. M., & McTeague, L. M. (2002). Exposure to trauma in adults. In M. M. Antony & D. H. Barlow (Eds.), *Handbook of assessment and treatment planning for psychological disorders* (pp. 215–258). New York: Guilford Press.

Litz, B. T., Orsillo, S. M., Kaloupek, D., & Weathers, F. (2000). Emotional processing in posttraumatic stress disorder. *Journal of Abnormal Psychology, 109,* 26–39.

Lohr, J. M., Olatunji, B. O., & Sawchuk, C. N. (2007). A functional analysis of danger and safety signals in anxiety disorders. *Clinical Psychology Review, 27,* 114–126.

Longley, S. L., Watson, D., Noyes, R., & Yoder, K. (2006). Panic and phobic anxiety: Associations among neuroticism, physiological hyperarousal, anxiety sensitivity, and three phobias. *Journal of Anxiety Disorders, 20,* 718–739.

Lopatka, C., & Rachman, S. (1995). Perceived responsibility and compulsive checking: An experimental analysis. *Behaviour Research and Therapy, 33,* 673–684.

Lovibond, P. F., & Lovibond, S. H. (1995a). The structure of negative emotional states: Comparison of the Depression Anxiety Stress Scales (DASS) with the Beck Depression and Anxiety Inventories. *Behaviour Research and Therapy, 33,* 335–343.

Lovibond, S. H., & Lovibond, P. F. (1995b). *Manual for the Depression Anxiety Stress Scales.* Sydney, Australia: Psychology Foundation Monograph.

Lucock, M. P., & Salkovskis, P. M. (1988). Cognitive factors in social anxiety and its treatment. *Behaviour Research and Therapy, 26,* 297–302.

Lundh, L.-G., & Öst, L.-G. (1997). Explicit and implicit memory bias in social phobia: The role of subdiagnostic type. *Behaviour Research and Therapy, 35,* 305–317.

Lundh, L.-G., Thulin, U., Czyzykow, S., & Öst, L.-G. (1998). Recognition bias for safe faces in panic disorder with agoraphobia. *Behaviour Research and Therapy, 36,* 323–337.

Lundh, L.-G., Wikström, J., Westerlund, J., & Öst, L.-G. (1999). Preattentive bias for emotional information in panic disorder with agoraphobia. *Journal of Abnormal Psychology, 108,* 222–232.

Luoma, J. B., & Hayes, S. C. (2003). Cognitive defusion. In W. O'Donohue, J. E. Fisher, & S. C. Hayes (Eds.), *Cognitive behavior therapy: Applying empirically supported techniques in your practice* (pp. 71–78). Hoboken, NJ: Wiley.

Luten, A. G., Ralph, J. A., & Mineka, S. (1997). Pessimistic attributional style: Is it specific to depression versus anxiety versus negative affect? *Behaviour Research and Therapy, 35,* 703–719.

Luu, P., Tucker, D. M., & Derryberry, D. (1998). Anxiety and the motivational basis of working memory.

Cognitive Therapy and Research, 22, 577–594.

Lyons, L. (2004, April 6). Teens and terrorism: Fear subsiding, but slowly. *The Gallup Organization.* Retrieved January 11, 2005, from *www.gallup.com.*

Ma, S., & Teasdale, J. D. (2004). Mindfulness-based cognitive therapy for depression: Replication and exploration of differential relapse prevention effects. *Journal of Consulting and Clinical Psychology, 72*, 31–40.

Mackintosh, B., Mathews, A., Yiend, J., Ridgeway, V., & Cook, E. (2006). Induced biases in emotional interpretation influence stress vulnerability and endure despite changes in context. *Behavior Therapy, 37*, 209–222.

MacLeod, A. K., & Byrne, A. (1996). Anxiety, depression, and the anticipation of future positive and negative experiences. *Journal of Abnormal Psychology, 105*, 286–289.

MacLeod, A. K., Williams, J. M. G., & Bekerian, D. A. (1991). Worry is reasonable: The role of explanations in pessimism about future personal events. *Journal of Abnormal Psychology, 100*, 478–486.

MacLeod, C. (1999). Anxiety and anxiety disorders. In T. Dalgleish & M. Power (Eds.), *Handbook of cognition and emotion* (pp. 447–477). Chichester, UK: Wiley.

MacLeod, C., Campbell, L., Rutherford, E., & Wilson, E. (2004). The causal status of anxiety-linked attentional and interpretative bias. In J. Yiend (Ed.), *Cognition, emotion and psychopathology: Theoretical, empirical and clinical directions* (pp. 172–189). Cambridge, UK: Cambridge University Press.

MacLeod, C., & Cohen, I. L. (1993). Anxiety and the interpretation of ambiguity: A text comprehension study. *Journal of Abnormal Psychology, 102*, 238–247.

MacLeod, C., & Hagan, R. (1992). Individual differences in the selective processing of threatening information, and emotional responses to a stressful life event. *Behaviour Research and Therapy, 30*, 151–161.

MacLeod, C., Koster, E.H.W., & Fox, E. (2009). Whither cognitive bias modification research? Commentary on the special section articles. *Journal of Abnormal Psychology, 118*, 89–99.

MacLeod, C., Mathews, A., & Tata, P. (1986). Attentional bias in emotional disorders. *Journal of Abnormal Psychology, 95*, 15–20.

MacLeod, C., & McLaughlin, K. (1995). Implicit and explicit memory bias in anxiety: A conceptual replication. *Behaviour Research and Therapy, 33*, 1–14.

MacLeod, C., & Rutherford, E. M. (1992). Anxiety and the selective processing of emotional information: Mediating roles of awareness, trait and state variables, and personal relevance of stimulus materials. *Behaviour Research and Therapy, 30*, 479–491.

MacLeod, C., & Rutherford, E. (2004). Information-processing approaches: Assessing the selective functioning of attention, interpretation, and retrieval. In R. G. Heimberg, C. L. Turk, & D. S. Mennin (Eds.), *Generalized anxiety disorder: Advances in research and practice* (pp. 109–142). New York: Guilford Press.

MacLeod, C., Rutherford, E., Campbell, L., Ebsworthy, G., & Holker, L. (2002). Selective attention and emotional vulnerability: Assessing the causal basis of their association through the experimental manipulation of attentional bias. *Journal of Abnormal Psychology, 111*, 107–123.

Magee, W. J. (1999). Effects of negative life experiences on phobia onset. *Social Psychiatry and Psychiatric Epidemiology, 34*, 343–351.

Magee, W. J., Eaton, W. W., Wittchen, H.-U., McGonagle, K. A., & Kessler, R. C. (1996). Agoraphobia, simple phobia, and social phobia in the National Comorbidity Survey. *Archives of General Psychiatry, 53*, 159–168.

Magee, J. C., & Teachman, B. A. (2007). Why did the white bear return?: Obsessive–compulsive symptoms and attributions for unsuccessful thought suppression. *Behaviour Research and Therapy, 45*, 2884–2898.

Magee, J. C., & Zinbarg, R. E. (2007). Suppressing and focusing on a negative imagery memory in social anxiety: Effects on unwanted thoughts and mood. *Behaviour Research and Therapy, 45*, 2836–2849.

Maier, W., Buller, R., Philipp, M., & Heuser, I. (1988). The Hamilton Anxiety Scale: Reliability, validity and sensitivity to change in anxiety and depressive disorders. *Journal of Affective Disorders, 14*, 61–68.

Malan, J. R., Norton, G. R., & Cox, B. J. (1990). *Nonclinical panickers: A critical review.* Paper presented at the annual convention of the Canadian Psychological Association, Ottawa.

Maller, R. G., & Reiss, S. (1992). Anxiety sensitivity in 1984 and panic attacks in 1987. *Journal of Anxiety Disorders, 6*, 241–247.

Maltby, N. (2001). Evaluation of a brief preventative treatment for panic disorder (Doctoral dissertation, University of Connecticut). *Dissertation Abstracts International, 62*, 4226.

Maltby, N., Mayers, M. F., Allen, G. J., & Tolin, D. F. (2005). Anxiety sensitivity: Stability in prospective research. *Journal of Anxiety Disorders, 19*, 708–716.

Mancini, F., D'Olimpio, F., & Cieri, L. (2004). Manipulation of responsibility in non-clinical subjects: Does expectation of failure exacerbate obsessive-compulsive behaviors? *Behaviour Research and Therapy, 42*, 449–457.

Mannuzza, S., Schneier, F. R., Chapman, T. F., Liebowitz, M. R., Klein, D. F., & Fyer, A. J. (1995). Generalized social phobia: Reliability and validity. *Archives of General Psychiatry, 52*, 230–237.

Mansell, W. (2000). Conscious appraisal and the modification of automatic processes in anxiety. *Behavioural and Cognitive Psychotherapy, 28*, 99–120.

Mansell, W., & Clark, D. M. (1999). How do I appear to others?: Social anxiety and processing of the observable self. *Behaviour Research and Therapy, 37*, 419–434.

Mansell, W., Clark, D. M., & Ehlers, A. (2003). Internal versus external attention in social anxiety: An investigation using a novel paradigm. *Behaviour Research and Therapy, 41*, 555–572.

Mansell, W., Clark, D. M., Ehlers, A., & Chen, Y.-P. (1999). Social anxiety and attention away from emotional faces. *Cognition and Emotion, 13*, 673–690.

Marcaurelle, R., Bélanger, C., & Marchand, A. (2003). Marital relationship and the treatment of panic disorder with agoraphobia: A critical review. *Clinical Psychology Review, 23*, 247–276.

March, J. S., Frances, A., Carpenter, D., & Kahn, D. A. (1997). Expert consensus guideline for treatment of obsessive–compulsive disorder. *Journal of Clinical Psychiatry, 58*(Suppl. 4), 5–72.

Marciniak, M. D., Lage, M. J., Dunayevich, E., Russell, J. M., Bowman, L., Landbloom, R. P., et al. (2005). The cost of treating anxiety: The medical and demographic correlates that impact total medical costs. *Depression and Anxiety, 21*, 178–184.

Marciniak, M., Lage, M. J., Landbloom, R. P., Dunayevich, E., & Bowman, L. (2004). Medical and productivity costs of anxiety disorders: Case control study. *Depression and Anxiety, 19*, 112–120.

Marcus, S. C., Olfson, M., Pincus, H. A., Shear, M. K., & Zarin, D. A. (1997). Self-reported anxiety, general medical conditions, and disability bed days. *American Journal of Psychiatry, 154*, 1766–1768.

Margraf, J., & Schneider, S. (1991, November). *Outcome and active ingredients of cognitive-behavioral treatments for panic disorder.* Paper presented at the 25th Annual Meeting of the Association for the Advancement of Behavior Therapy, New York.

Markowitz, L. J., & Borton, J. L. S. (2002). Suppression of negative self-referent and neutral thoughts: A preliminary investigation. *Behavioural and Cognitive Psychotherapy, 30*, 271–277.

Marks, I. M. (1970). The classification of phobic disorders. *British Journal of Psychiatry, 116*, 377–386.

Marks, I. M. (1987). *Fears, phobias, and rituals: Panic, anxiety and their disorders.* New York: Oxford University Press.

Marks, I. M., & Gelder, M. G. (1966). Different ages of onset in varieties of phobia. *American Journal of Psychiatry, 123*, 218–221.

Marks, I. M., Hodgson, R., & Rachman, S. (1975). Treatment of chronic obsessive–compulsive neurosis by *in vivo* exposure: A two year follow-up and issues in treatment. *British Journal of Psychiatry, 127*, 349–364.

Marks, I., Lovell, K., Noshirvani, H., Livanou, M., & Thrasher, S. (1998). Treatment of posttraumatic stress disorder by exposure and/or cognitive restructuring. *Archives of General Psychiatry, 55*, 317–325.

Marshall, J. R., & Lipsett, S. (1994). *Social phobia: From shyness to stage fright.* New York: Basic Books.

Martin, M., Williams, R. M., & Clark, D. M. (1991). Does anxiety lead to selective processing of threat-related information? *Behaviour Research and Therapy, 29*, 147–160.

Martinsen, E. W., Raglin, J. S., Hoffart, A., & Friis, S. (1998). Tolerance of intensive exercise and high levels of lactate in panic disorder. *Journal of Anxiety Disorders, 12*, 333–342.

Maser, J. D., & Cloninger, C. R. (1990). Comorbidity of anxiety and mood disorders: Introduction and overview. In J. D. Maser & C. R. Cloninger (Eds.), *Comorbidity of mood and anxiety disorders* (pp. 3–12). Washington, DC: American Psychiatric Press.

Massion, A. O., Dyck, I. R., Shea, T., Phillips, K. A., Warshaw, M. G., & Keller, M. B. (2002). Personality disorders and time to remission in generalized anxiety disorder, social phobia, and panic disorder. *Archives of General Psychiatry, 59*, 434–440.

Massion, A. O., Warshaw, M. G., & Keller, M. B. (1993). Quality of life and psychiatric morbidity in panic disorder and generalized anxiety disorder. *American Journal of Psychiatry, 150*, 600–607.

Mathews, A. (1990). Why worry?: The cognitive function of worry. *Behaviour Research and Therapy, 28*, 455–468.

Mathews, A. (2006). Towards an experimental cognitive science of CBT. *Behavior Therapy, 37*, 314–318.

Mathews, A., & Klug, F. (1993). Emotionality and interference with color-naming in anxiety. *Behaviour Research and Therapy, 31*, 57–62.

Mathews, A., & Mackintosh, B. (1998). A cognitive model of selective processing in anxiety. *Cognitive Therapy and Research, 22*, 539–560.

Mathews, A., & Mackintosh, B. (2000). Induced emotional interpretation bias and anxiety. *Journal of Abnormal Psychology, 109*, 602–615.

Mathews, A., & MacLeod, C. (1985). Selective processing of threat cues in anxiety states. *Behaviour Research and Therapy, 23*, 563–569.

Mathews, A., & MacLeod, C. (1986).

Discrimination of threat cues without awareness in anxiety states. *Journal of Abnormal Psychology, 95*, 131–138.

Mathews, A., & MacLeod, C. (1994). Cognitive approaches to emotion and emotional disorders. *Annual Review of Psychology, 45*, 25–50.

Mathews, A., & MacLeod, C. (2002). Induced processing biases have causal effects on anxiety. *Cognition and Emotion, 16*, 331–354.

Mathews, A., & MacLeod, C. (2005). Cognitive vulnerability to emotional disorders. *Annual Review of Clinical Psychology, 1*, 167–195.

Mathews, A., May, J., Mogg, K., & Eysenck, M. (1990). Attentional bias in anxiety: Selective search or defective filtering? *Journal of Abnormal Psychology, 99*, 166–173.

Mathews, A., & Milroy, R. (1994). Effects of priming and suppression of worry. *Behaviour Research and Therapy, 32*, 843–850.

Mathews, A., Mogg, K., Kentish, J., & Eysenck, M. (1995). Effect of psychological treatment on cognitive bias in generalized anxiety disorder. *Behaviour Research and Therapy, 33*, 293–303.

Mathews, A., Mogg, K., May, J., & Eysenck, M. (1989). Implicit and explicit memory bias in anxiety. *Journal of Abnormal Psychology, 98*, 236–240.

Mathews, A., Richards, A., & Eysenck, M. (1989). Interpretation of homophones related to threat in anxiety states. *Journal of Abnormal Psychology, 98*, 31–34.

Mathews, A., Ridgeway, V., Cook, E., & Yiend, J. (2007). Inducing a benign interpretational bias reduces trait anxiety. *Journal of Behavior Therapy and Experimental Psychiatry, 38*, 225–236.

Mathews, A., Ridgeway, V., & Williamson, D. A. (1996). Evidence for attention to threatening stimuli in depression. *Behaviour Research and Therapy, 34*, 695–705.

Matthews, G., & Funke, G. J. (2006). Worry and information-processing. In G. C. L. Davey & A. Wells (Eds.), *Worry and its psychological disorders: Theory, assessment and treatment* (pp. 51–67). Chichester, UK: Wiley.

Mattia, J. I., Heimberg, R. G., & Hope, D. A. (1993). The revised Stroop color-naming task in social phobics. *Behaviour Research and Therapy, 31*, 305–313.

Mattick, R. P., & Clarke, J. C. (1998).

Development and validation of measures of social phobia scrutiny fear and social interaction anxiety. *Behaviour Research and Therapy, 36,* 455–470.

Mattick, R. P., & Peters, L. (1988). Treatment of severe social phobia: Effects of guided exposure with and without cognitive restructuring. *Journal of Consulting and Clinical Psychology, 56,* 251–260.

Mauss, I. B., Wilhelm, F. H., & Gross, J. J. (2004). Is there less to social anxiety than meets the eye?: Emotion experience, expression, and bodily responding. *Cognition and Emotion, 18,* 631–662.

May, R. (1953). *Man's search for himself.* New York: Norton.

Mayo, P. R. (1989). A further study of the personality-congruent recall effect. *Personality and Individual Differences, 10,* 247–252.

Mayou, R., Bryant, B., & Ehlers, A. (2001). Prediction of psychological outcomes one year after a motor vehicle accident. *American Journal of Psychiatry, 158,* 1231–1238.

McCann, I. L., Sakheim, D. K., & Abrahamson, D. J. (1988). Trauma and victimization: A model of psychological adaptation. *Counseling Psychologist, 16,* 531–594.

McDonagh, A., Friedman, M., McHugo, G., Ford, J., Sengupta, A., Mueser, K., et al. (2005). Randomized trial of cognitive-behavioral therapy for chronic posttraumatic stress disorder in adult female survivors of childhood sexual abuse. *Journal of Consulting and Clinical Psychology, 73,* 515–524.

McFall, M. E., Smith, D. E., Roszell, D. K., Tarver, D. J., & Malas, K. L. (1990). Convergent validity of measures of PTSD in Vietnam combat veterans. *American Journal of Psychiatry, 147,* 645–648.

McFarlane, A. C. (1998). Epidemiological evidence about the relationship between PTSD and alcohol abuse: The nature of the association. *Addictive Behaviors, 23,* 813–825.

McGlinchey, J. B., & Zimmerman, M. (2007). Examing a dimensional representation of depression and anxiety disorders' comorbidity in psychiatric outpatients with item response modeling. *Journal of Abnormal Psychology, 116,* 464–474.

McKay, D., Abramowitz, J. S., Calamari, J. E., Kyrios, M., Radomsky, A., Sookman, D., et al. (2004). A critical evaluation of obsessive–compulsive disorder subtypes: Symptoms versus mechanisms. *Clinical Psychology Review, 24,* 283–313.

McKeon, J., Roa, B., & Mann, A. (1984). Life events and personality traits in obsessive–compulsive neurosis. *British Journal of Psychiatry, 144,* 185–189.

McKinnon, A. C., Nixon, R. D. V., & Brewer, N. (2008). The influence of data-driven processing on perceptions of memory quality and intrusive symptoms in children following traumatic events. *Behaviour Research and Therapy, 46,* 766–775.

McLaren, S., & Crowe, S. F. (2003). The contribution of perceived control of stressful life events and thought suppression to the symptoms of obsessive–compulsive disorder in both non-clinical and clinical samples. *Journal of Anxiety Disorders, 17,* 389–403.

McLean, A., & Broomfield, N. M. (2007). How does thought suppression impact upon beliefs about uncontrollability of worry? *Behaviour Research and Therapy, 45,* 2938–2949.

McLean, L. M., & Gallop, R. (2003). Implications of childhood sexual abuse for adult borderline personality disorder and complex posttraumatic stress disorder. *American Journal of Psychiatry, 160,* 369–371.

McLean, P. D., Whittal, M. L., Sochting, I., Koch, W. J., Paterson, R., Thordarson, D. S., et al. (2001). Cognitive versus behavior therapy in the group treatment of obsessive–compulsive disorder. *Journal of Consulting and Clinical Psychology, 69,* 205–214.

McManus, F., Clark, D. M., & Hackmann, A. (2000). Specificity of cognitive biases in social phobia and their role in recovery. *Behavioural and Cognitive Psychotherapy, 28,* 201–209.

McNally, R. J. (1994). *Panic disorder: A critical analysis.* New York: Guilford Press.

McNally, R. J. (1995). Automaticity and the anxiety disorders. *Behaviour Research and Therapy, 33,* 747–754.

McNally, R. J. (1996). Anxiety sensitivity is distinguishable from trait anxiety. In R. M. Rapee (Ed.), *Current controversies in the anxiety disorders* (pp. 214–227). New York: Guilford Press.

McNally, R. J. (1999). Anxiety sensitivity and information-processing biases for threat. In S. Taylor (Ed.), *Anxiety sensitivity: Theory, research, and treatment of the fear of anxiety* (pp. 183–198). Mahwah, NJ: Erlbaum.

McNally, R. J. (2001). Vulnerability to anxiety disorders in adulthood. In R. E. Ingram & J. M. Price (Eds.), *Vulnerability to psychopathology: Risk across the lifespan* (pp. 304–321). New York: Guilford Press.

McNally, R. J. (2002). Anxiety sensitivity and panic disorder. *Biological Psychiatry, 52,* 938–946.

McNally, R. J. (2003a). Progress and controversy in the study of posttraumatic stress disorder. *Annual Review of Psychology, 54,* 229–252.

McNally, R. J. (2003b). Psychological mechanisms in acute response to trauma. *Biological Psychiatry, 53,* 779–788.

McNally, R. J. (2007a). Mechanisms of exposure therapy: How neuroscience can improve psychological treatment for anxiety disorders. *Clinical Psychology Review, 27,* 750–759.

McNally, R. J. (2007b). Can we solve the mysteries of the National Vietnam Veternas Readjustment Study? *Journal of Anxiety Disorders, 21,* 192–200.

McNally, R. J., & Amir, N. (1996). Perceptual implicit memory for trauma-related information in post-traumatic stress disorder. *Cognition and Emotion, 10,* 551–556.

McNally, R. J., Amir, N., & Lipke, H. J. (1996). Subliminal processing of threat cues in posttraumatic stress disorder? *Journal of Anxiety Disorders, 10,* 115–128.

McNally, R. J., Amir, N., Louro, C. E., Lukach, B. M., Riemann, B. C., & Calamari, J. E. (1994). Cognitive processing of idiographic emotional information in panic disorder. *Behaviour Research and Therapy, 32,* 119–122.

McNally, R. J., & Eke, M. (1996). Anxiety sensitivity, suffocation fear, and breath-holding duration as predictors of response to carbon dioxide challenge. *Journal of Abnormal Psychology, 105,* 146–149.

McNally, R. J., & Foa, E. B. (1987). Cognition and agoraphobia: Bias in the interpretation of threat. *Cognitive Therapy and Research, 11,* 567–581.

McNally, R. J., & Heatherton, T. F. (1993). Are covariation biases attributable to a priori expectancy biases? *Behaviour Research and Therapy, 31,* 653–658.

McNally, R. J., Hornig, C. D., & Donnell, C. A. (1995). Clinical versus nonclinical panic: A test of suffocation false alarm theory. *Behaviour Research and Therapy, 33,* 127–131.

McNally, R. J., Kaspi, S. P., Riemann, B. C., & Zeitlin, S. B. (1990). Selective processing of threat cues in posttraumatic stress disorder. *Journal of Abnormal Psychology, 99,* 398–402.

McNally, R. J., Malcarne, V. L., & Hansdottir, I. (2001). Vulnerability to anxiety disorders across the lifespan. In R. E. Ingram & J. M. Price (Eds.), *Vulnerability to psychopathology: Risk across the lifespan* (pp. 322–325). New York: Guilford Press.

McNally, R. J., Metzger, L. J., Lasko, N. B., Clancy, S. A., & Pitman, R. K. (1998). Directed forgetting of trauma cues in adult survivors of childhood sexual abuse with and without posttraumatic stress disorder. *Journal of Abnormal Psychology, 107,* 596–601.

McNally, R. J., Riemann, B. C., & Kim, E. (1990). Selective processing of threat cues in panic disorder. *Behaviour Research and Therapy, 28,* 407–412.

McNally, R. J., Riemann, B. C., Louro, C. E., Lukach, B. M., & Kim, E. (1992). Cognitive processing of emotional information in panic disorder. *Behaviour Research and Therapy, 30,* 143–149.

McNeil, D. W. (2001). Terminology and evolution of the constructs in social anxiety and social phobia. In S. G. Hofmann & P. M. DiBartolo (Eds.), *From social anxiety to social phobia: Multiple perspectives* (pp. 8–19). Boston: Allyn & Bacon.

Meiser-Stedman, R., Dalgleish, T., Smith, P., Yule, W., & Glucksman, E. (2007). Diagnostic, demographic, memory quality, and cognitive variables associated with acute stress disorder in children and adolescents. *Journal of Abnormal Psychology, 116,* 65–79.

Mellings, T. M. B., & Alden, L. E. (2000). Cognitive processes in social anxiety: The effects of self-focus, rumination and anticipatory processing. *Behaviour Research and Therapy, 38,* 243–257.

Mellman, T. A., & Uhde, T. W. (1989). Sleep panic attacks: New clinical findings and theoretical implications. *American Journal of Psychiatry, 146,* 1204–1207.

Melzer, D., Tom, B. D. M., Brugha, T. S., Fryers, T., & Meltzer, H. (2002). Common mental disorder symptom counts in populations: Are there distinct case groups above epidemiological cut-offs? *Psychological Medicine, 32,* 1195–1201.

Mendlowicz, M. V., & Stein, M. B. (2000). Quality of life in individuals with anxiety disorders. *American Journal of Psychiatry, 157,* 669–682.

Mennin, D. S., Fresco, D. M., Heimberg, R. G., Schneier, F. R., Davies, S. O., & Liebowitz, M. R. (2002). Screening for social anxiety disorder in the clinical setting: Using the Liebowitz Social Anxiety Scale. *Journal of Anxiety Disorders, 16,* 661–673.

Mennin, D. S., Heimberg, R. G., & Turk, C. L. (2004). Clinical presentation and diagnostic features. In R. G. Heimberg, C. L. Turk, & D. S. Mennin (Eds.), *Generalized anxiety disorder: Advances in research and practice* (pp. 3–28). New York: Guilford Press.

Mennin, D. S., Turk, C. L., Heimberg, R. G., & Carmin, C. N. (2004). Regulation of emotion in generalized anxiety disorder. In M. A. Reinecke & D. A. Clark (Eds.), *Cognitive therapy across the lifespan: Evidence and practice* (pp. 60–89). Cambridge, UK: Cambridge University Press.

Menzies, R. G., Harris, L. M., Cumming, S. R., & Einstein, D. A. (2000). The relationship between inflated personal responsibility and exaggerated danger expectancies in obsessive–compulsive concerns. *Behaviour Research and Therapy, 38,* 1029–1037.

Merikangas, K. R., Mehta, R. L., Molnar, B. E., Walters, E. E., Swendsen, J. D., Aguilar-Gaziola, S., et al. (1998). Comorbidity of substance use disorders with mood and anxiety disorders: Results of the International Consortium in Psychiatric Epidemiology. *Addictive Behaviors, 23,* 893–907.

Merikangas, K. R., Zhang, H., Avenevoli, S., Acharyya, S., Neuenschwander, M., & Angst, J. (2003). Longitudinal trajectories of depression and anxiety in a prospective community study: The Zurich

Cohort Study. *Archives of General Psychiatry, 60,* 993–1000.

Metalsky, G. I., Halberstadt, L. J., & Abramson, L. Y. (1987). Vulnerability to depressive mood reactions: Toward a more powerful test of the diathesis–stress and causal mediation components of the reformulated theory of depression. *Journal of Personality and Social Psychology, 52,* 386–393.

Meuret, A. E., Ritz, T., Wilhelm, F. H., & Roth, W. T. (2005). Voluntary hyperventilation in the treatment of panic disorder: Functions of hyperventilation, their implications for breathing training, and recommendations for standardization. *Clinical Psychology Review, 25,* 285–306.

Meuret, A. E., Wilhelm, F. H., Ritz, T., & Roth, W. T. (2003). Breathing training for treating panic disorder: Useful intervention or impediment? *Behavior Modification, 27,* 731–754.

Meyer, T. J., Miller, M. L., Metzger, R. L., & Borkovec, T. D. (1990). Development and validation of the Penn State Worry Questionnaire. *Behaviour Research and Therapy, 28,* 487–495.

Miller, M. W., & Litz, B. T. (2004). Emotional-processing in posttraumatic stress disorder: II. Startle reflex modulation during picture processing. *Journal of Abnormal Psychology, 113,* 451–463.

Miller, P. R. (2001). Inpatient diagnostic assessments: 2. Interrater reliability and outcomes of structured vs. unstructured interviews. *Psychiatry Research, 105,* 265–271.

Miller, P. R. (2002). Inpatient diagnostic assessments: 3. Causes and effects of diagnostic imprecision. *Psychiatry Research, 111,* 191–197.

Miller, P. R., Dasher, R., Collins, R., Griffiths, P., & Brown, F. (2001). Inpatient diagnostic assessments: 1. Accuracy of structured vs. unstructured interviews. *Psychiatry Research, 105,* 255–264.

Milliken, C. S., Auchterlonie, J. L., & Hoge, C. W. (2007). Longitudinal assessment of mental health problems among active and reserve component soldiers returning from the Iraq war. *Journal of the American Medical Association, 298,* 2141–2148.

Milosevic, I., & Radomsky, A. S. (2008). Safety behavior does not necessarily interfere with exposure therapy. *Behaviour Research and Therapy, 46,* 1111–1118.

Mineka, S. (1979). The role of fear in theories of avoidance learning, flooding, and extinction. *Psychological Bulletin, 86,* 985–1010.

Mineka, S. (2004). The positive and negative consequences of worry in the aetiology of generalized anxiety disorder: A learning theory perspective. In J. Yiend (Ed.), *Cognition, emotion and psychopathology: Theoretical, empirical and clinical directions* (pp. 29–48). Cambridge, UK: Cambridge University Press.

Mineka, S., & Kihlstrom, J. F. (1978). Unpredictable and uncontrollable events: A new perspective on experimental neurosis. *Journal of Abnormal Psychology, 87,* 256–271.

Mineka, S., Watson, D., & Clark, L. A. (1998). Comorbidity of anxiety and unipolar mood disorders. *Annual Review of Psychology, 49,* 377–412.

Mitte, K. (2005). Meta-analysis of cognitive-behavioral treatments for generalized anxiety disorder: A comparison with pharmacotherapy. *Psychological Bulletin, 131,* 785–795.

Mizes, J. S., Landolf-Fritsche, B., & Grossman-McKee, D. (1987). Patterns of distorted cognitions in phobic disorders: An investigation of clinically severe simple phobias, social phobias, and agoraphobics. *Cognitive Therapy and Research, 11,* 583–592.

Mofitt, T. E., Harrington, H., Caspi, A., Kim-Cohen, J., Goldberg, D., Gregory, A. M., et al. (2007). Depression and generalized anxiety disorder: Cumulative and sequential comorbidity in a birth cohort followed prospectively to age 32 years. *Archives of General Psychiatry, 64,* 651–660.

Mogg, K., & Bradley, B. P. (1998). A cognitive-motivational analysis of anxiety. *Behaviour Research and Therapy, 36,* 809–848.

Mogg, K., & Bradley, B. P. (1999a). Selective attention and anxiety: A cognitive-motivational perspective. In T. Dalgleish & M. Power (Eds.), *Handbook of cognition and emotion* (pp. 145–170). Chichester, UK: Wiley.

Mogg, K., & Bradley, B. P. (1999b). Some methodological issues in assessing attentional biases for threatening faces in anxiety: A replication study using a modified version of the probe detection task. *Behaviour Research and Therapy, 37,* 595–604.

Mogg, K., & Bradley, B. P. (2002). Selective orienting of attention to masked threat faces in social anxiety. *Behaviour Research and Therapy, 40,* 1403–1414.

Mogg, K., & Bradley, B. P. (2004). A cognitive-motivational perspective on the processing of threat information and anxiety. In J. Yiend (Ed.), *Cognition, emotion, and psychopathology* (pp. 68–85). Cambridge, UK: Cambridge University Press.

Mogg, K., Bradley, B. P., Miles, F., & Dixon, R. (2004). Time course of attentional bias for threat scenes: Testing the vigilance–avoidance hypothesis. *Cognition and Emotion, 18,* 689–700.

Mogg, K., Bradley, B. P., Millar, N., & White, J. (1995). A follow-up study of cognitive bias in generalized anxiety disorder. *Behaviour Research and Therapy, 33,* 927–935.

Mogg, K., Bradley, B. P., Miller, T., Potts, H., Glenwright, J., & Kentish, J. (1994). Interpretation of homophones related to threat: Anxiety or response bias effects? *Cognitive Therapy and Research, 18,* 461–477.

Mogg, K., Bradley, B., & Williams, R. (1995). Attentional bias in anxiety and depression: The role of awareness. *British Journal of Clinical Psychology, 34,* 17–36.

Mogg, K., Bradley, B. P., Williams, R., & Mathews, A. (1993). Subliminal processing of emotional information in anxiety and depression. *Journal of Abnormal Psychology, 102,* 304–311.

Mogg, K., & Marden, B. (1990). Processing of emotional information in anxious subjects. *British Journal of Clinical Psychology, 29,* 227–229.

Mogg, K., & Mathews, A. (1990). Is there a self-referent mood-congruent recall bias in anxiety? *Behaviour Research and Therapy, 28,* 91–92.

Mogg, K., Mathews, A., Bird, C., & Macgregor-Morris, R. (1990). Effects of stress and anxiety on the processing of threat stimuli. *Journal of Personality and Social Psychology, 59,* 1230–1237.

Mogg, K., Mathews, A., & Eysenck, M. (1992). Attentional bias to threat in clinical anxiety states. *Cognition and Emotion, 6,* 149–159.

Mogg, K., Mathews, A., May, J., Grove, M., Eysenck, M., & Weinman, J. (1991). Assessment of cognitive bias in anxiety and depression using a colour perception task. *Cognition and Emotion, 5,* 221–238.

Mogg, K., Mathews, A., & Wienman, J. (1987). Memory bias in clinical anxiety. *Journal of Abnormal Psychology, 96,* 94–98.

Mogg, K., Mathews, A., & Weinman, J. (1989). Selective processing of threat cues in anxiety states: A replication. *Behaviour Research and Therapy, 27,* 317–323.

Mogg, K., McNamara, J., Powys, M., Rawlinson, H., Seiffer, A., & Bradley, B. P. (2000). Selective attention to threat: A test of two cognitive models of anxiety. *Cognition and Emotion, 14,* 375–399.

Mogg, K., Philipott, P., & Bradley, B. P. (2004). Selective attention to angry faces in clinical social phobia. *Journal of Abnormal Psychology, 113,* 160–165.

Mohlman, J. (2004). Psychosocial treatment of late-life generalized anxiety disorder: Current status and future directions. *Clinical Psychology Review, 24,* 149–169.

Mohlman, J., & Zinbarg, R. E. (2000). The structure and correlates of anxiety sensitivity in older adults. *Psychological Assessment, 12,* 440–446.

Molina, A., & Borkovec, T. D. (1994). The Penn State Worry Questionnaire: Psychometric properties and associated characteristics. In G. C. L. Davey & F. Tallis (Eds.), *Worrying: Perspectives on theory, assessment and treatment* (pp. 265–283). Chichester, UK: Wiley.

Molina, S., Borkovec, T. D., Peasley, C., & Person, D. (1998). Content analysis of worrisome streams of consciousness in anxious and dysphoric participants. *Cognitive Therapy and Research, 22,* 109–123.

Monson, C. M., & Friedman, M. J. (2006). Back to the future of understanding trauma: Implications for cognitive-behavioral therapies for trauma. In V. M. Follette & J. I. Ruzek (Eds.), *Cognitive-behavioral therapies for trauma* (2nd ed., pp. 1–13). New York: Guilford Press.

Montorio, I., Wetherell, J., & Nuevo, R. (2006). Beliefs about worry in community-dwelling older adults. *Depression and Anxiety, 23,* 466–473.

Moore, E. L., & Abramowitz, J. S. (2007). The cognitive mediation of thought-control strategies. *Behaviour Research and Therapy, 45,* 1949–1955.

Moras, K., Di Nardo, P. A., & Barlow, D. H. (1992). Distinguishing anxiety and depression: Reexamination of the reconstructed Hamilton Scales. *Psychological Assessment, 4,* 224–227.

Morillo, C., Belloch, A., & Garcia-Soriano, G. (2007). Clinical obsessions in obsessive–compulsive patients and obsession-relevant intrusive thoughts in non-clinical, depressed and anxious patients: Where are the differences? *Behaviour Research and Therapy, 45,* 1319–1333.

Morgan, I. A., Matthews, G., & Winton, M. (1995). Coping and personality as predictors of post-traumatic intrusions, numbing, avoidance and general distress: A study of victims of the Perth Flood. *Behavioural and Cognitive Psychotherapy, 23,* 251–264.

Morgan, J., & Banerjee, R. (2008). Post-event processing and autobiographical memory in social anxiety: The influence of negative feedback and rumination. *Journal of Anxiety Disorders, 22,* 1190–1204.

Morris, A., Baker, B., Devins, G. M., & Shapiro, C. M. (1997). Prevalence of panic disorder in cardiac outpatients. *Canadian Journal of Psychiatry, 42,* 185–190.

Morris, E. P., Stewart, S. H., & Ham, L. S. (2005). The relationship between social anxiety disorder and alcohol use disorders: A critical review. *Clinical Psychology Review, 25,* 734–760.

Morris, J. S., Öhman, A., & Dolan, R. J. (1998). Conscious and unconscious emotional learning in the human amygdala. *Nature, 393,* 467–470.

Mörtberg, E., Karlsson, A., Fyring, C., & Sundin, Ö. (2006). Intensive cognitive-behavioral group treatment (CBGT) of social phobia: A randomized controlled study. *Journal of Anxiety Disorders, 20,* 646–660.

Moulding, R., & Kyrios, M. (2006). Anxiety disorders and control related beliefs: The exemplar of obsessive–compulsive disorder (OCD). *Clinical Psychology Review, 26,* 573–583.

Mowrer, O. H. (1939). A stimulus–response analysis of anxiety and its role as a reinforcing agent. *Psychological Review, 46,* 553–565.

Mowrer, O. H. (1953). Neurosis, psychotherapy, and two-factor learning theory. In O. H. Mowrer (Ed.), *Psychotherapy theory and research* (pp. 140–149). New York: Ronald Press.

Mowrer, O. H. (1960). *Learning theory and behavior.* New York: Wiley.

Mueser, K. T., Rosenberg, S. D., Xie, H., Hamblen, J. L., Jankowski, M. K., Bolton, E. E., et al. (2008). A randomized controlled trial of cognitive-behavioral treatment for posttraumatic stress disorder in severe mental illness. *Journal of Consulting and Clinical Psychology, 76,* 259–271.

Muller, J., & Roberts, J. E. (2005). Memory and attention in obsessive–compulsive disorder: A review. *Journal of Anxiety Disorders, 19,* 1–28.

Mumford, D. B., Nazir, M., Jilani, F.-M., & Yar Baig, I. (1996). Stress and psychiatric disorder in the Hindu Kush: A community survey of mountain villages in Chitral, Pakistan. *British Journal of Psychiatry, 168,* 299–307.

Muris, P., Merckelbach, H., & Clavan, M. (1997). Abnormal and normal compulsions. *Behaviour Research and Therapy, 35,* 249–252.

Muris, P., Merckelbach, H., van den Hout, M., & de Jong, P. (1992). Suppression of emotional and neutral material. *Behaviour Research and Therapy, 30,* 639–642.

Muris, P., & van der Heiden, S. (2006). Anxiety, depression, and judgments about the probability of future negative and positive events in children. *Journal of Anxiety Disorders, 20,* 252–261.

Murphy, R., Hirsch, C. R., Mathews, A., Smith, K., & Clark, D. M. (2007). Facilitating a benign interpretation bias in a high socially anxious population. *Behaviour Research and Therapy, 45,* 1517–1529.

Mussgay, L., & Rüddel, H. (2004). Autonomic dysfunctions in patients with anxiety throughout therapy. *Journal of Psychophysiology, 18,* 27–37.

Myers, S. G., & Wells, A. (2005). Obsessive–compulsive symptoms: The contribution of metacognitions and responsibility. *Journal of Anxiety Disorders, 19,* 806–817.

Myhr, G., & Payne, K. (2006). Cost-effectiveness of cognitive-behavioural therapy for mental disorders: Implications for public health care funding policy in Canada. *Canadian Journal of Psychiatry, 51,* 662–670.

Najavits, L. M. (2002). *Seeking safety: A treatment manual for PTSD and substance abuse.* New York: Guilford Press.

National Institute of Clinical Excellence (NICE). (2005). *Posttraumatic stress disorder: The management of PTSD in adults and children in primary and secondary care.* Clinical Guideline 26. London: National Collaborating Centre for Mental Health. Retrieved July 24, 2008, from *www.nice.org.uk/CG026NICEguideline.*

National Institute of Mental Health (NIMH). (2001). *Facts about anxiety disoders.* Retrieved January 13, 2005, from *www.nimh.nih.gov/publicat/adfacts.cfm.*

National Institute of Mental Health (NIMH). (2003). *The numbers count: Mental disorders in America.* Retrieved March 10, 2003, from *www.nimh.nih.gov/publicat/numbers.cfm*

Nay, W. T., Thorpe, G. L., Robertson-Nay, R., Hecker, J. E., & Sigmon, S. T. (2004). Attentional bias to threat and emotional response to biological challenge. *Journal of Anxiety Disorders, 18,* 609–627.

Newman, D. L., Moffitt, T. E., Silva, P. A., Caspi, A., Magdol, L., & Stanton, W. R. (1996). Psychiatric disorder in a birth cohort of young adults: Prevalence, comorbidity, clinical significance, and new case incidence from ages 11 to 21. *Journal of Consulting and Clinical Psychology, 64,* 552–562.

Newman, M. G., Zuellig, A. R., Kachin, K. E., Constantino, M. J., Przeworski, A., Erickson, T., et al. (2002). Preliminary reliability and validity of the Generalized Disorder Questionnaire–IV: A revised self-report diagnostic measure of generalized anxiety disorder. *Behavior Therapy, 33,* 215–233.

Newman, S. C., & Bland, R. C. (1994). Life events and the 1-year prevalence of major depressive episode, generalized anxiety disorder, and panic disorder in a community sample. *Comprehensive Psychiatry, 35,* 76–82.

Newth, S., & Rachman, S. (2001).

The concealment of obsessions. *Behaviour Research and Therapy, 39*, 457–464.

Neziroglu, F., Stevens, K. P., McKay, D., & Yaryura-Tobia, J. A. (2001). Predictive validity of the Overvalued Ideas Scale: Outcome in obsessive–compulsive and body dysmorphic disorders. *Behaviour Research and Therapy, 39*, 745–756.

Nielssen, O., & Large, M. (2008). A proposal for a new disorder to replace PTSD in DSM-V. *British Journal of Psychiatry, 192*. [Electronic letters. Retrieved September 4, 2008, from *bjp.rcpsych.org/cgi/eletters/192/1/3*.

Nitschke, J. B., Heller, W., Imig, J. C., McDonald, R. P., & Miller, G. A. (2001). Distinguishing dimensions of anxiety and depression. *Cognitive Therapy and Research, 25*, 1–22.

Noorbala, A. A., Bagheri Yazdi, S. A., Yasamy, M. T., & Mohammad, K. (2004). Mental health survey of the adult population in Iran. *British Journal of Psychiatry, 184*, 70–73.

Norberg, M. M., Calamari, J. E., Cohen, R. J., & Riemann, B. C. (2008). Quality of life in obsessive–compulsive disorder: An evaluation of impairment and a preliminary analysis of the ameliorating effects of treatment. *Depression and Anxiety, 25*, 248–259.

Norris, F. H. (1992). Epidemiology of trauma: Frequency and impact of different potentially traumatic events on different demographic groups. *Journal of Consulting and Clinical Psychology, 60*, 409–418.

Norris, F. H. (2005). *Psychosocial consequences of natural disasters in developing countries: What does past research tell us about the potential effects of the 2004 tsunami?* Retrieved January 14, 2005, from *www. ncptsd.org.*

Norris, F. H., & Hamblen, J. L. (2004). Standardized self-report measures of civilian trauma and PTSD. In J. Wilson & T. M. Keane (Eds.), *Assessing psychological trauma and PTSD* (2nd ed., pp. 63–102). New York: Guilford Press.

Norris, F. H., & Slone, L. B. (2007). The epidemiology of trauma and PTSD. In M. J. Freidman, T. M. Keane, & P. A. Resick (Eds.), *Handbook of PTSD: Science and practice* (pp. 78–98). New York: Guilford Press.

North, C. S., Nixon, S. J., Shariat, S., Mallonee, S., McMillen, J. C., Spitznagel, E. L., et al. (1999). Psychiatric disorders among survivors of the Oklahoma City bombing. *Journal of the American Medical Association, 282*, 755–762.

Norton, G. R., Cox, B. J., & Malan, J. (1992). Nonclinical panickers: A critical review. *Clinical Psychology Review, 12*, 121–139.

Norton, G. R., Dorward, J., & Cox, B. J. (1986). Factors associated with panic attacks in nonclinical subjects. *Behavior Therapy, 17*, 239–252.

Norton, G. R., Harrison, B., Hauch, J., & Rhodes, L. (1985). Characteristics of people with infrequent panic attacks. *Journal of Abnormal Psychology, 94*, 216–221.

Noyes, R., Clancy, J., Woodman, C., Holt, C. S., Suelzer, M., Christiansen, J., et al. (1993). Environmental factors related to the outcome of panic disorder: A seven-year follow-up study. *Journal of Nervous and Mental Disease, 181*, 529–538.

Noyes, R., & Hoehn-Saric, R. (1998). *The anxiety disorders.* Cambridge, UK: Cambridge University Press.

Nunn, J. D., Stevenson, R. J., & Whalan, G. (1984). Selective memory effects in agoraphobic patients. *British Journal of Clinical Psychology, 23*, 195–201.

O'Banion, K., & Arkowitz, H. (1977). Social anxiety and selective memory for affective information about the self. *Social Behavior and Personality, 5*, 321–328.

Obsessive Compulsive Cognitions Working Group (OCCWG). (1997). Cognitive assessment of obsessive–compulsive disorder. *Behaviour Research and Therapy, 35*, 667–681.

Obsessive Compulsive Cognitions Working Group (OCCWG). (2001). Development and initial validation of the Obsessive Beliefs Questionnaire and the Interpretation of Intrusions Inventory. *Behaviour Research and Therapy, 39*, 987–1006.

Obsessive Compulsive Cognitions Working Group (OCCWG). (2003). Psychometric validation of the Obsessive Beliefs Questionnaire and the Interpretation of Intrusions Inventory: Part I. *Behaviour Research and Therapy, 41*, 863–878.

Obsessive Compulsive Cognitions Working Group (OCCWG). (2005). Psychometric validation of the Obsessive Beliefs Questionnaire and Interpretation of Intrusions Inventory: Part 2. Factor analyses and testing a brief version. *Behaviour Research and Therapy, 43*, 1527–1542.

O'Connor, K. P. (2002). Intrusions and inferences in obsessive compulsive disorder. *Clinical Psychology and Psychotherapy, 9*, 38–46.

O'Connor, K. P., Aardema, F., Bouthillier, D., Fournier, S., Guay, S., Robillard, S., et al. (2005). Evaluation of an interference-based approach to treating obsessive–compulsive disorder. *Cognitive Behaviour Therapy, 34*, 148–163.

O'Connor, K., Aardema, F., & Pélissier, M.-C. (2005). *Beyond reasonable doubt: Reasoning processes in obsessive–compulsive disorder and related disorders.* Chichester, UK: Wiley.

O'Connor, K., Freeston, M. H., Gareau, D., Careau, Y., Dufont, M. J., Aardema, F., et al. (2005). Group versus individual treatment in obsessions without compulsions. *Clinical Psychology and Psychotherapy, 12*, 87–96.

O'Connor, K. P., & Robillard, S. (1999). A cognitive approach to the treatment of primary inferences in obsessive–compulsive disorder. *Journal of Cognitive Psychotherapy: An International Quarterly, 13*, 359–375.

O'Connor, K., Todorov, C., Robillard, S., Borgeat, F., & Brault, M. (1999). Cognitive-behaviour therapy and medication in the treatment of obsessive–compulsive disorder: A controlled study. *Canadian Journal of Psychiatry, 44*, 64–71.

O'Donnell, M. L., Elliott, P., Wolfgang, B. J., & Creamer, M. (2007). Posttraumatic appraisals in the development and persistence of posttraumatic stress symptoms. *Journal of Traumatic Stress, 20*, 173–182.

Oei, T. P. S., Llamas, M., & Devilly, G. J. (1999). The efficacy and cognitive processes of cognitive behaviour therapy in the treatment of panic disorder with agoraphobia. *Behavioural and Cognitive Psychotherapy, 27*, 63–88.

Offord, D. R., Boyle, M. H., Campbell, D., Goering, P., Lin, E., Wong, M., et al. (1996). One-year prevalence of psychiatric disorder in Ontarians 15 to 64 years of age. *Canadian Journal of Psychiatry, 41*, 559–561.

Öhman, A. (2000). Fear and anxiety: Evolutionary, cognitive, and clinical perspectives. In M. Lewis & J. M. Haviland-Jones (Eds.), *Handbook of emotions* (2nd ed., pp. 573–593). New York: Guilford Press.

Öhman, A., & Mineka, S. (2001). Fears, phobias, and preparedness: Toward an evolved module of fear and fear learning. *Psychological Review, 108*, 483–522.

Öhman, A., & Wiens, S. (2004). The concept of an evolved fear module and cognitive theories of anxiety. In A. S. R. Manstead, N. Frijda, & A. Fischer (Eds.), *Feelings and emotions: The Amsterdam Symposium* (pp. 58–80). Cambridge, UK: Cambridge University Press.

Okasha, A., Saad, A., Khalil, A. H., El Dawla, A. S., & Yehia, N. (1994). Phenomenology of obsessive–compulsive disorder: A transcultural study. *Comprehensive Psychiatry, 35*, 191–197.

Olatunji, B. O., Cisler, J. M., & Tolin, D. F. (2007). Quality of life in the anxiety disorders: A meta-analytic review. *Clinical Psychology Review, 27*, 572–581.

Olfson, M., Broadhead, E., Weissman, M. M., Leon, A. C., Farber, L., Hoven, C., et al. (1996). Subthreshold psychiatric symptoms in a primary care group practice. *Archives of General Psychiatry, 53*, 880–886.

Olfson, M., Fireman, B., Weissman, M. M., Leo, A. C., Sheehan, D. V., Kathol, R., et al. (1997). Mental disorders and disability among patients in a primary care group practice. *American Journal of Psychiatry, 154*, 1734–1740.

Olfson, M., Shea, S., Feder, A., Fuentes, M., Nomura, Y., Gameroff, M., & et al. (2000). Prevalence of anxiety, depression and substance use disorders in an urban general medicine practice. *Archives of Family Medicine, 9*, 876–883.

Oquendo, M. A., Friend, J. M., Halberstam, B., Brodsky, B. S., Burke, A. K., Grunebaum, M. F., et al. (2003). Association of comorbid posttraumatic stress disorder and major depression with greater risk for suicidal behavior. *American Journal of Psychiatry, 160*, 580–582.

Orsillo, S. M. (2001). Measures for social phobia. In M. M. Antony, S. M. Orsillo, & L. Roemer (Eds.), *Practitioner's guide to empirically based measures of anxiety* (pp. 165–187). New York: Kluwer Academic/Plenum.

Orsillo, S. M., Roemer, L., Lerner, J. B., & Tull, M. T. (2004). Acceptance, mindfulness, and cognitive-behavioral therapy: Comparisons, contrasts, and application to anxiety. In S. C. Hayes, V. M. Follette, & M. M. Linehan (Eds.), *Mindfulness and acceptance: Expanding the cognitive-behavioral tradition* (pp. 66–95). New York: Guilford Press.

Osman, A., Barrios, F. X., Haupt, D., King, K., Osman, J. R., & Slavens, S. (1996). The Social Phobia and Anxiety Inventory: Further validation in two nonclinical samples. *Journal of Psychopathology and Behavioral Assessment, 18*, 35–47.

Osman, A., Gutierrez, P. M., Barrios, F. X., Kopper, B. A., & Chiros, C. E. (1998). The Social Phobia and Social Interaction Anxiety Scales: Evaluation of psychometric properties. *Journal of Psychopathology and Behavioral Assessment, 20*, 249–264.

Öst, L.-G. (1987a). Applied relaxation: Description of a coping technique and review of controlled studies. *Behaviour Research and Therapy, 25*, 397–409.

Öst, L.-G. (1987b). Age of onset in different phobias. *Journal of Abnormal Psychology, 96*, 223–229.

Öst, L.-G. (2008). Efficacy of the third wave of behavioral therapies: A systematic review and meta-analysis. *Behaviour Research and Therapy, 46*, 296–321.

Öst, L.-G., & Breitholz, E. (2000). Applied relaxation vs. cognitive therapy in the treatment of generalized anxiety disorder. *Behaviour Research and Therapy, 38*, 777–790.

Öst, L.-G., & Csatlos, P. (2000). Probability ratings in claustrophobic patients and normal controls. *Behaviour Research and Therapy, 38*, 1107–1116.

Öst, L.-G.,Thulin,U., & Ramnerö, J. (2004). Cognitive behavior therapy vs. exposure in vivo in the treatment of panic disorder with agoraphobia. *Behaviour Research and Therapy, 42*, 1105–1127.

Öst, L.-G., & Westling, B. E. (1995). Applied relaxation vs. cognitive behavior therapy in the treatment of panic disorder. *Behaviour Research and Therapy, 33*, 145–158.

Ottaviani, R., & Beck, A. T. (1987). Cognitive aspects of panic disorder. *Journal of Anxiety Disorders, 1*, 15–28.

Otto, M. W., Pollack, M. H., & Maki, K. M. (2000). Empirically supported treatments for panic disorder: Costs, benefits, and stepped care. *Journal of Consulting and Clinical Psychology, 68*, 556–563.

Otto, M. W., Pollack, M. H., Maki, K. M., Gould, R. A., Worthington, J. J., Smoller, J. W., et al. (2001). Childhood history of anxiety disorders among adults with social phobia: Rates, correlates, and comparisons with patients with panic disorder. *Depression and Anxiety, 14*, 209–213.

Ouimette, P. C., Brown, P. J., & Najavitis, L. M. (1998). Course and treatment of patients with both substance use and posttraumatic stress disorders. *Addictive Behaviors, 23*, 785–795.

Ozer, E. J., Best, S. R., Lipsey, T. L., & Weiss, D. S. (2003). Predictors of posttraumatic stress disorder and symptoms in adults: A meta-analysis. *Psychological Bulletin, 129*, 52–73.

Palmieri, P. A., Weathers, F. W., Difede, J., & King, D. W. (2007). Confirmatory factor analysis of the PTSD Checklist and the Clinician-Administered PTSD Scale in disaster workers exposed to the World Trade Center Ground Zero. *Journal of Abnormal Psychology, 116*, 329–341.

Panasetis, P., & Bryant, R. A. (2003). Peritraumatic versus persistent dissociation in acute stress disorder. *Journal of Traumatic Stress, 16*, 563–566.

Papageorgiou, C., & Wells, A. (1998). Effects of attention training on hypochondriasis: A brief case series. *Psychological Medicine, 28*, 193–200.

Papageorgiou, C., & Wells, A. (1999). Process and meta-cognitive dimensions of depressive and anxious thoughts and relationships with emotional intensity. *Clinical Psychology and Psychotherapy, 6*, 156–162.

Papageorgiou, C., & Wells, A. (2004). Nature, functions, and beliefs about depressive rumination. In C.

Papageorgiou & A. Wells (Eds.), *Depressive rumination: Nature, theory and treatment* (pp. 3–20). Chichester, UK: Wiley.

Parkinson, L., & Rachman, S. (1981a). Part II. The nature of intrusive thoughts. *Advances in Behaviour Research and Therapy, 3,* 101–110.

Parkinson, L., & Rachman, S. (1981b). Part III. Intrusive thoughts: The effects of an uncontrived stress. *Advances in Behaviour Research and Therapy, 3,* 111–118.

Pauli, P., Dengler, W., & Wiedemann, G. (2005). Implicit and explicit memory processes in panic patients as reflected in behavioral and electrophysiological measures. *Journal of Behavior Therapy and Experimental Psychiatry, 36,* 111–127.

Pauli, P., Dengler, W., Wiedeman, G., Flor, H., Montoya, P., Birbaumer, N., et al. (1997). Behavioral and neurophysiological evidence for altered processing of anxiety-related words in panic disorder. *Journal of Abnormal Psychology, 106,* 213–220.

Pauli, P., Marguardt, C., Hartl, L., Nutzinger, D. O., Hölzl, R., & Strain, F. (1991). Anxiety induced by cardiac perception in patients with panic attacks: A field study. *Behaviour Research and Therapy, 29,* 137–145.

Pauli, P., Montoya, P., & Martz, G.-E. (1996). Covariation bias in panic-prone individuals. *Journal of Abnormal Psychology, 105,* 658–662.

Paunovic, N., Lundh, L.-G., & Öst, L. (2002). Attentional and memory bias for emotional information in crime vicitms with acute post-traumatic stress disorder (PTSD). *Journal of Anxiety Disorders, 16,* 675–692.

Paunovic, N., & Öst, L.-G. (2001). Cognitive-behavior therapy vs exposure therapy in the treatment of PTSD in refugees. *Behaviour Research and Therapy, 39,* 1183–1197.

Pearlman, L. A (2001). Treatment of persons with complex PTSD and other trauma-related disruptions of the self. In J. P. Wilson, M. J. Friedman, & J. D. Lindy (Eds.), *Treating psychological trauma and PTSD* (pp. 205–236). New York: Guilford Press.

Pennebaker, J. W. (1993). Social mechanisms of constraint. In D. M. Wegner & J. W. Pennebaker

(Eds.), *Handbook of mental control* (pp. 200– 219). Upper Saddle River, NJ: Prentice-Hall.

Pennebaker, J. W. (1997). Writing about emotional experiences as a therapeutic process. *Psychological Science, 8,* 162–166.

Perna, G., Barbini, B., Cocchi, S., Bertani, A., & Gasperini, M. (1995). 35% CO_2 challenge in panic and mood disorders. *Journal of Affective Disorders, 33,* 189–194.

Perna, G., Casolari, A., Bussi, R., Cucchi, M., Arancio, C., & Bellodi, L. (2004). Comparison of 35% carbon dioxide reactivity between panic disorder and eating disorder. *Psychiatry Research, 125,* 277–283.

Persons, J. B. (1989). *Cognitive therapy in practice: A case formulation approach.* New York: Norton.

Persons, J. B., & Davidson, J. (2001). Cognitive-behavioral case formulation. In K. S. Dobson (Ed.), *Handbook of cognitive-behavioral therapies* (2nd ed., pp. 86–110). New York: Guilford Press.

Peters, L. (2000). Discriminant validity of the Social Phobia and Anxiety Inventory (SPAI), the Social Phobia Scale (SPS) and the Social Interaction Anxiety Scale (SIAS). *Behaviour Research and Therapy, 38,* 943–950.

Peters, L., Issakidis, C., Slade, T., & Andrews, G. (2006). Gender differences in the prevalence of DSM-IV and ICD-10 PTSD. *Psychological Medicine, 36,* 81–89.

Pineles, S. L., & Mineka, S. (2005). Attentional biases to internal and external sources of potential threat in social anxiety. *Journal of Abnormal Psychology, 114,* 314–318.

Pineles, S. L., Shipherd, J. C., Welch, L. P., & Yovel, I. (2007). The role of attentional biases in PTSD: Is it interference or facilitation? *Behaviour Research and Therapy, 45,* 1903–1913.

Pinto-Gouveia, J., Castilho, P., Galhardo, A., & Cunha, M. (2006). Early maladaptive schemas and social phobia. *Cognitive Therapy and Research, 30,* 571–584.

Piotrkowiski, C. S., & Brannen, S. J. (2002). Exposure, threat appraisal, and lost confidence as predictors of PTSD symptoms following September 11, 2001. *American Journal of Orthopsychiatry, 72,* 476–485.

Pitman, R. K. (1987). Pierre Janet on obsessive–compulsive disorder (1903): Review and commentary.

Archives of General Psychiatry, 44, 226–232.

Plehn, K., & Peterson, R. A. (2002). Anxiety sensitivity as a predictor of the development of panic symptoms, panic attacks, and panic disorder: A prospective study. *Journal of Anxiety Disorders, 16,* 455–474.

Plutchik, R. (2003). *Emotions and life: Perspectives from psychology, biology, and evolution.* Washington, DC: American Psychological Association.

Pollard, C. A. (2007). Treatment readiness, ambivalence, and resistance. In M. M. Antony, C. Purdon, & L. J. Summerfeldt (Eds.), *Psychological treatment of obsessive-compulsive disorder: Fundamentals and beyond* (pp. 61–77). Washington, DC: American Psychological Association.

Pollard, C. A., Henderson, J. G., Frank, M., & Margolis, R. B. (1989). Help-seeking patterns of anxiety-disordered individuals in the general population. *Journal of Anxiety Disorders, 3,* 131–138.

Pollard, C. A., Pollard, H. J., & Corn, K. J. (1989). Panic onset and major events in the lives of agoraphobics: A test of contiguity. *Journal of Abnormal Psychology, 98,* 318–321.

Pollock, R. A., Carter, A. S., Amir, N., & Marks, L. E. (2006). Anxiety sensitivity and auditory percepton of heartbeat. *Behaviour Research and Therapy, 44,* 1739–1756.

Power, K., McGoldrick, T., Brown, K., Buchanan, R., Sharp, D., Swanson, V., et al. (2002). A controlled comparison of eye movement desensitization and reprocessing versus exposure plus cognitive restructuring versus waiting list in the treatment of post-traumatic stress disorder. *Clinical Psychology and Psychotherapy, 9,* 299–318.

Pratt, E. M., Brief, D. J., & Keane, T. M. (2006). Recent advances in psychological assessment of adults with posttraumatic stress disorder. In V. M. Follette & J. I. Ruzek (Eds.), *Cognitive-behavioral therapies for trauma* (2nd ed., pp. 34–61). New York: Guilford Press.

Pribor, E. F., & Dinwiddie, S. H. (1992). Psychiatric correlates of incest in childhood. *American Journal of Psychiatry, 149,* 52–56.

Pruzinsky, T., & Borkovec, T. D. (1990). Cognitive and personality characteristics of worriers. *Behav-*

iour Research and Therapy, 28, 507–512.

Purdon, C. (1999). Thought suppression and psychopathology. *Behaviour Research and Therapy, 37,* 1029–1054.

Purdon, C. (2001). Appraisal of obsessional thought recurrences: Impact on anxiety and mood state. *Behavior Therapy, 32,* 47–64.

Purdon, C., & Clark, D. A. (1993). Obsessive intrusive thoughts in nonclinical subjects: Part I. Content and relation with depressive, anxious and obsessional symptoms. *Behaviour Research and Therapy, 31,* 713–720.

Purdon, C. L., & Clark, D. A. (1994a). Obsessive intrusive thoughts in nonclinical subjects: Part II. Cognitive appraisal, emotional response and thought control strategies. *Behaviour Research and Therapy, 32,* 403–410.

Purdon, C. L., & Clark, D. A. (1994b). Perceived control and appraisal of obsessional intrusive thoughts: A replication and extension. *Behavioural and Cognitive Psychotherapy, 22,* 269–285.

Purdon, C., & Clark, D. A. (2000). White bears and other elusive phenomena: Assessing the relevance of thought suppression for obsessional phenomena. *Behavior Modification, 24,* 425–453.

Purdon, C. L., & Clark, D. A. (2001). Suppression of obsession-like thoughts in nonclinical individuals: Part I. Impact on thought frequency, appraisal and mood state. *Behaviour Research and Therapy, 39,* 1163–1181.

Purdon, C. L., & Clark, D. A. (2002). The need to control thoughts. In R. O. Frost & G. Steketee (Eds.), *Cognitive approaches to obsessions and compulsions: Theory, assessment and treatment* (pp. 29–43). Oxford, UK: Elsevier.

Purdon, C. L., & Clark, D. A. (2005). *Overcoming obsessive thoughts: How to gain control of your OCD.* Oakland, CA: New Harbinger.

Purdon, C. L., Gifford, S., & Antony, M. M. (2007). *Thought dismissability in OCD vs. panic: Predictors and impact.* Paper presented at the annual meeting of the Canadian Psychological Association, Ottawa.

Purdon, C. L., & Rowa, K. (2002). *Thought control strategies in OCD: Motivation, success and impact.* Paper presented at the

annual convention of the Anxiety Disorders Association of America, Austin, TX.

Purdon, C., Rowa, K., & Antony, M. M. (2005). Thought suppression and its effects on thoughts frequency, appraisal and mood state in individuals with obsessive–compulsive disorder. *Behaviour Research and Therapy, 43,* 93–108.

Purdon, C., Rowa, K., & Antony, M. M. (2007). Diary records of thought suppression attempts by individuals with obsessive–compulsive disorder. *Behavioural and Cognitive Psychotherapy, 35,* 47–59.

Pynoos, R. S., Goenjian, A., Tashjian, M., Karakashian, M., Manjikian, R., Manjikian, R., et al. (1993). Post-traumatic stress reactions in children after the 1988 Armenian earthquake. *British Journal of Psychiatry, 163,* 239–247.

Qin, J., Mitchell, K. J., Johnson, M. K., Krystal, J. H., Southwick, S. M., Rasmusson, A. M., et al. (2003). Reactions to and memories for the September 11, 2001, terrorist attacks in adults with posttraumatic stress disorder. *Applied Cognitive Psychology, 17,* 1081–1097.

Rachman, S. (1976). The passing of the two-stage theory of fear and avoidance: Fresh possibilities. *Behaviour Research and Therapy, 14,* 125–131.

Rachman, S. (1977). The conditioning theory of fear-acquisition: A critical examination. *Behaviour Research and Therapy, 15,* 375–387.

Rachman, S. (1981). Part I. Unwanted intrusive cognitions. *Advances in Behaviour Research and Therapy, 3,* 89–99.

Rachman, S. J. (1983). Obstacles to the successful treatment of obsessions. In E. B. Foa & P. M. G. Emmelkamp (Ed.), *Failures in behavior therapy* (pp. 35–57). New York: Wiley.

Rachman, S. (1984a). Agoraphobia: A safety-signal perspective. *Behaviour Research and Therapy, 22,* 59–70.

Rachman, S. (1984b). The experimental analysis of agoraphobia. *Behaviour Research and Therapy, 22,* 631–640.

Rachman, S. J. (1985). An overview of clinical and research issues in obsessional-compulsive disorders. In M. Mavissakalian, S. M. Turner, & L. Michelson (Eds.), *Obsessive–*

compulsive disorder: Psychological and pharmacological treatment (pp. 1–47). New York: Plenum.

Rachman, S. J. (1993). Obsessions, responsibility and guilt. *Behaviour Research and Therapy, 31,* 149–154.

Rachman, S. J. (1997). A cognitive theory of obsessions. *Behaviour Research and Therapy, 35,* 793–802.

Rachman, S. J. (1998). A cognitive theory of obsessions: Elaborations. *Behaviour Research and Therapy, 36,* 385–401.

Rachman, S. J. (2003). *The treatment of obsessions.* Oxford, UK: Oxford University Press.

Rachman, S. J. (2004). *Anxiety* (2nd ed.). East Sussex, UK: Psychology Press.

Rachman, S. J. (2006). *Fear of contamination: Assessment and treatment.* Oxford, UK: Oxford University Press.

Rachman, S., Cobb, J., Grey, S., McDonald, B., Mawson, D., Sartory, G., et al. (1979). The behavioural treatment of obsessional–compulsive disorders, with and without clomipramine. *Behaviour Research and Therapy, 17,* 467–478.

Rachman, S. J., & de Silva, P. (1978). Abnormal and normal obsessions. *Behaviour Research and Therapy, 16,* 233–248.

Rachman, S. J., & Hodgson, R. J. (1980). *Obsessions and compulsions.* Englewood Cliffs, NJ: Prentice-Hall.

Rachman, S., & Levitt, K. (1985). Panics and their consequences. *Behaviour Research and Therapy, 23,* 585–600.

Rachman, S., Levitt, K., & Lopatka, C. (1987). Panic: The links between cognitions and bodily symptoms: I. *Behaviour Research and Therapy, 25,* 411–423.

Rachman, S., Levitt, K., & Lopatka, C. (1988). Experimental analyses of panic: III. Claustrophobic subjects. *Behaviour Research and Therapy, 26,* 41–52.

Rachman, S., & Lopatka, C. (1986). Match and mismatch in the perception of fear: I. *Behaviour Research and Therapy, 24,* 387–393.

Rachman, S., Lopatka, C., & Levitt, K. (1988). Experimental analysis of panic: II. Panic patients. *Behaviour Research and Therapy, 26,* 33–40.

Rachman, S. J., & Shafran, R. (1998). Cognitive and behavioral features of obsessive–compulsive disorder. In R. P. Swinson, M. M. Antony, S. Rachman, & M. A. Richter (Eds.), *Obsessive–compulsive disorder: Theory, research and treatment* (pp. 51–78). New York: Guilford Press.

Rachman, S., Shafran, R., Mitchell, D., Trant, J., & Teachman, B. (1996). How to remain neutral: An experimental analysis of neutralization. *Behaviour Research and Therapy, 34,* 889–898.

Rachman, S. J., Shafran, R., & Riskind, J. H. (2006). Cognitive vulnerability to obsessive–compulsive disorders. In L. B. Alloy & J. H. Riskind (Eds.), *Cognitive vulnerability to emotional disorders* (pp. 235–249). Mahwah, NJ: Erlbaum.

Radomsky, A. S., & Rachman, S. (1999). Memory bias in obsessive–compulsive disorder (OCD). *Behaviour Research and Therapy, 37,* 605–618.

Radomsky, A. S., Rachman, S., & Hammond, D. (2001). Memory bias, confidence and responsibility in compulsive checking. *Behaviour Research and Therapy, 39,* 813–822.

Radomsky, A. S., Rachman, S., & Hammond, D. (2002). Panic termination and the post-panic period. *Journal of Anxiety Disorders, 16,* 97–111.

Radomsky, A. S., & Taylor, S. (2005). Subtyping OCD: Prospects and problems. *Behavior Therapy, 36,* 371–379.

Rapee, R. M. (1986). Differential response to hyperventilation in panic disorder and generalized anxiety disorder. *Journal of Abnormal Psychology, 95,* 24–28.

Rapee, R. M. (1991). Generalized anxiety disorder: A review of clinical features and theoretical concepts. *Clinical Psychology Review, 11,* 419–440.

Rapee, R. M. (1995a). Psychological factors influencing the affective response to biological challenge procedures in panic disorder. *Journal of Anxiety Disorders, 9,* 59–74.

Rapee, R. M. (1995b). Descriptive psychopathology of social phobia. In R. G. Heimberg, M. R. Liebowitz, D. A. Hope, & F. R. Schneier (Eds.), *Social phobia: Diagnosis, assessment, and treatment* (pp. 41–66). New York: Guilford Press.

Rapee, R. M. (1997). Perceived threat and perceived control as predictors of the degree of fear in physical and social situations. *Journal of Anxiety Disorders, 11,* 455–461.

Rapee, R. M., Ancis, J. R., & Barlow, D. H. (1988). Emotional reactions to physiological sensations: Panic disorder patients and non-clinical Ss. *Behaviour Research and Therapy, 26,* 265–269.

Rapee, R. M., Brown, T. A., Antony, M. M., & Barlow, D. H. (1992). Response to hyperventilation and inhalation of 5.5% carbon dioxide-enriched air across the DSM-III-R anxiety disorders. *Journal of Abnormal Psychology, 101,* 538–552.

Rapee, R. M., Craske, M. G., & Barlow, D. H. (1994–1995). Assessment instrument for panic disorder that includes fear of sensation-producing activities: The Albany Panic and Phobia Questionnaire. *Anxiety, 1,* 114–122.

Rapee, R. M., Craske, M. G., Brown, T. A., & Barlow, D. H. (1996). Measurement of perceived control over anxiety-related events. *Behavior Therapy, 27,* 279–293.

Rapee, R. M., & Heimberg, R. G. (1997). A cognitive-behavioral model of anxiety in social phobia. *Behaviour Research and Therapy, 35,* 741–756.

Rapee, R. M., & Lim, L. (1992). Discrepancy between self- and observer ratings of performance in social phobics. *Journal of Abnormal Psychology, 101,* 728–731.

Rapee, R. M., McCallum, S. L., Melville, L. F., Ravenscroft, H., & Rodney, J. M. (1994). Memory bias in social phobia. *Behaviour Research and Therapy, 32,* 89–99.

Rapee, R. M., & Medoro, L. (1994). Fear of physical sensations and trait anxiety as mediators of the response to hyperventilation in nonclinical subjects. *Journal of Abnormal Psychology, 103,* 693–699.

Rapee, R. M., Sanderson, W. C., & Barlow, D. H. (1988). Social phobia features across the DSM-III-R anxiety disorders. *Journal of Psychopathology and Behavioral Assessment, 10,* 287–299.

Rapee, R. M., & Spence, S. H. (2004). The etiology of social phobia: Empirical evidence and an initial model. *Clinical Psychology Review, 24,* 737–767.

Rasinski, K. A., Berktold, J., Smith, T. W., & Albertson, B. L. (2002). *America recovers: A follow-up to a national study of public response to the September 11th terrorist attacks.* Unpublished manuscript, National Association for Research (NORC), University of Chicago.

Rasmussen, A., Rosenfeld, B., Reeves, K., & Keller, A. S. (2007). The effects of torture-related injuries on long-term psychological distress in a Punjabi Sikh sample. *Journal of Abnormal Psychology, 116,* 734–740.

Rasmussen, S. A., & Eisen, J. L. (1992). The epidemiology and clinical features of obsessive compulsive disorder. *Psychiatric Clinics of North America, 15,* 743–758.

Rasmussen, S. A., & Eisen, J. L. (1998). The epidemiology and clinical features of obsessive–compulsive disorder. In M. A. Jenike & W. E. Minichiello (Eds.), *Obsessive-compulsive disorders: Practical management* (pp. 12–43). St. Louis: Mosby.

Rasmussen, S. A., & Tsuang, M. T. (1986). Clinical characteristics and family history in DSM-III obsessive–compulsive disorder. *American Journal of Psychiatry, 143,* 317–322.

Rassin, E. (2005). *Thought suppression.* Amsterdam, The Netherlands: Elsevier.

Rassin, E., & Diepstraten, P. (2003). How to suppress obsessive thoughts. *Behaviour Research and Therapy, 41,* 97–103.

Rassin, E., Diepstraten, P., Merckelbach, H., & Muris, P. (2001). Thought–action fusion and thought suppression in obsessive-compulsive disorder. *Behaviour Research and Therapy, 39,* 757–764.

Rassin, E., Mercekelbach, H., & Muris, P. (2000). Paradoxical and less paradoxical effects of thought suppression: A critical review. *Clinical Psychology Review, 20,* 973–995.

Rassin, E., Merchelback, H., Muris, P., & Spaan, V. (1999). Thought-fusion as a causal factor in the development of intrusions. *Behaviour Research and Therapy, 37,* 231–237.

Rassin, E., & Muris, P. (2006). Abnormal and normal obsessions: A reconsideration. *Behaviour Research and Therapy, 45,* 1065–1070.

Rassovsky, Y., Kushner, M. G.,

Schwarze, N. J., & Wangensteen, O. D. (2000). Psychological and physiological predictors of response to carbon dioxide challenge in individuals with panic disorder. *Journal of Abnormal Psychology, 109*, 616–623.

Rauch, S. L., Savage, C. R., Alpert, N. M., Fishman, A. J. ., & Jenike, M. A. (1997). The functional neuroimaging of anxiety: A study of three disorders using positron emission tomography and symptom provocation. *Biological Psychiatry, 42*, 446–452.

Reardon, J. M., & Williams, N. L. (2007). The specificity of cognitive vulnerabilities to emotional disorders: Anxiety sensitivity, looming vulnerability and explanatory style. *Journal of Anxiety Disorders, 21, 625–643.*

Rector, N. A., Szacun-Shimizu, K., & Leybman, M. (2007). Anxiety sensitivity within the anxiety disorders: Disorder-specific sensitivities and depression comorbidity. *Behaviour Research and Therapy, 45*, 1967–1975.

Regier, D. A., Burke, J. D., & Burke, K. C. (1990). Comorbidity of affective and anxiety disorders in the NIMH Epidemiologic Catchment Area Program. In J. D. Maser & C. R. Cloninger (Eds.), *Comorbidity of mood and anxiety disorders* (pp. 113–122). Washington, DC: American Psychiatric Press.

Regier, D. A., Narrow, W. E., Rae, D. S., Manderscheid, R. W., Locke, B. Z., & Goodwin, F. K. (1993). The de facto US mental and addictive disorders service system. *Archives of General Psychiatry, 50*, 85–94.

Reiss, S. (1991). Expectancy model of fear, anxiety, and panic. *Clinical Psychology Review, 11*, 141–153.

Reiss, S. (1997). Trait anxiety: It's not what you think it is. *Journal of Anxiety Disorders, 11*, 201–214.

Reiss, S., & McNally, R. J. (1985). Expectancy model of fear. In S. Reiss, & R. R. Bootzin (Eds.), *Theoretical issues in behavior therapy* (pp. 107–121). Orlando, FL: Academic Press.

Reiss, S., Peterson, R. A., Gursky, D. M., & McNally, R. J. (1986). Anxiety sensitivity, anxiety frequency and the prediction of fearfulness. *Behaviour Research and Therapy, 24*, 1–8.

Renaud, J. M., & McConnell, A. R. (2002). Organization of the self-concept and the suppression of self-relevant thoughts. *Journal of Experimental Social Psychology, 38*, 79–86.

Renneberg, B., Chambless, D. L., & Gracely, E. J. (1992). Prevalence of SCID-diagnosed personality disorders in agoraphobic outpatients. *Journal of Anxiety Disorders, 6*, 111–118.

Rescorla, R. A. (1988). Pavlovian conditioning: It's not what you think it is. *American Psychologist, 43*, 151–160.

Resick, P. A., Galovski, T. E., Uhlmansiek, M. O., Scher, C. D., Clum, G. A., & Young-Xu, Y. (2008). A randomized clinical trial to dismantle components of cognitive processing therapy for posttraumatic stress disorder in female victims of interpersonal violence. *Journal of Consulting and Clinical Psychology, 76*, 243–258.

Resick, P. A., Monson, C. M., & Rizvi, S. L. (2008). Posttraumatic stress disorder. In D. H. Barlow (Ed.), *Clinical handbook of psychological disorders: A step-by-step treatment manual* (4th ed., pp. 65–122). New York: Guilford Press.

Resick, P. A., Nishith, P., Weaver, T. L., Astin, M. C., & Feuer, C. A. (2002). A comparison of cognitive-processing therapy with prolonged exposure and a waiting condition for the treatment of chronic posttraumatic stress disorder in female rape victims. *Journal of Consulting and Clinical Psychology, 70*, 867–879.

Resick, P. A., & Schnicke, M. K. (1992). Cognitive processing therapy for sexual assault victims. *Journal of Consulting and Clinical Psychology, 60*, 748–756.

Resnick, H. S., Kilpatrick, D. G., Dansky, B. S., Saunders, B. E., & Best, C. L. (1993). Prevalence of civilian trauma and posttraumatic stress disorder in a representative national sample of women. *Journal of Consulting and Clinical Psychology, 61*, 984–991.

Rhéaume, J., Freeston, M. H., Léger, E., & Ladouceur, R. (1998). Bad luck : An underestimated factor in the development of obsessive–compulsive disorder. *Clinical Psychology and Psychotherapy, 5*, 1–12.

Rhéaume, J., & Ladouceur, R. (2000). Cognitive and behavioural treatments of checking behaviours: An examination of individual cognitive change. *Clinical Psychology and Psychotherapy, 7*, 118–127.

Rice, D. P., & Miller, L. S. (1998). Health economics and cost implications of anxiety and other mental disorders in the United States. *British Journal of Psychiatry, 173*(Suppl. 34), 4–9.

Richards, A., & French, C. C. (1991). Effects of encoding and anxiety on implicit and explicit memory performance. *Personality and Individual Differences, 12*, 131–139.

Richards, A., French, C. C., Johnson, W., Naparstek, J., & Williams, J. (1992). Effects of mood manipulation and anxiety on performance of an emotional Stroop task. *British Journal of Psychology, 83*, 479–491.

Ries, B. J., McNeil, D. W., Boone, M. L., Turk, C. L., Carter, L. E., & Heimberg, R. G. (1998). Assessment of contemporary social phobia verbal report instruments. *Behaviour Research and Therapy, 36*, 983–994.

Riggs, D. S., Cahill, S. P., & Foa, E. B. (2006). Prolonged exposure treatment of posttraumatic stress disorder. In V. M. Follette & J. I. Ruzek (Eds.), *Cognitive-behavioral therapies for trauma* (2nd ed., pp. 65–95). New York: Guilford Press.

Rinck, M., & Becker, E. S. (2005). A comparison of attentional biases and memory biases in women with social phobia and major depression. *Journal of Abnormal Psychology, 114*, 62–74.

Rinck, M., Becker, E. S., Kellermann, J., & Roth, W. T. (2003). Selective attention in anxiety: Distraction and enhancement in visual search. *Depression and Anxiety, 18*, 18–28.

Riskind, J. H. (1997). Looming vulnerability to threat: A cognitive paradigm for anxiety. *Behaviour Research and Therapy, 35*, 685–702.

Riskind, J. H., & Alloy, L. B. (2006). Cognitive vulnerability to emotional disorders: Theory and research design/methodology. In L. B. Alloy & J. H. Riskind (Eds.), *Cognitive vulnerability to emotional disorders* (pp. 1–29). Mahwah, NJ: Erlbaum.

Riskind, J. H., Beck, A. T., Berchick, R. J., Brown, G., & Steer, R. A. (1987). Reliability of DSM-III diagnosis for major depression and generalized anxiety disorder using the Structured Clinical Interview for DSM-III. *Archives of General Psychiatry, 44*, 817–820.

Riskind, J. H., Kelly, K., Harman, W., Moore, R., & Gaines, H. S. (1992). The loomingness of danger: Does it discriminate focal phobia and general anxiety from depression? *Cognitive Therapy and Research, 16*, 603–622.

Riskind, J. H., & Maddux, J. E. (1993). Loomingness, helplessness, and fearfulness: An integration of harm-looming and self-efficacy models of fear. *Journal of Social and Clinical Psychology, 12*, 73–89.

Riskind, J. H., Moore, R., & Bowley, L. (1995). The looming of spiders: The fearful perceptual distortion of movement and menace. *Behaviour Research and Therapy, 33*, 171–178.

Riskind, J. H., & Williams, N. L. (1999). Specific cognitive content of anxiety and catastrophizing: Looming vulnerability and the looming maladaptive style. *Journal of Cognitive Psychotherapy: An International Quarterly, 13*, 41–54.

Riskind, J. H., & Williams, N. L. (2005). The looming cognitive style and generalized anxiety disorder: Distinctive danger schemas and cognitive phenomenology. *Cognitive Therapy and Research, 29*, 7–27.

Riskind, J. H., & Williams, N. L. (2006). A unique vulnerability common to all anxiety disorders: The looming maladaptive style. In L. B. Alloy & J. H. Riskind (Eds.), *Cognitive vulnerability to emotional disorders* (pp. 175–206). Mahwah, NJ: Erlbaum.

Riskind, J. H., Williams, N. L., Gessner, T. L., Chrosniak, L. D., & Cortina, J. M. (2000). The looming maladaptive style: Anxiety, danger, and schematic processing. *Journal of Personality and Social Psychology, 79*, 837–852.

Robertson-Ny, R., Strong, D. R., Nay, W. T., Beidel, D. C., & Turner, S. M. (2007). Development of an abbreviated Social Phobia and Anxiety Inventory (SPAI) using item response theory: The SPAI-23. *Psychological Assessment, 19*, 133–145.

Robichaud, M., & Dugas, M. J. (2005). Negative problem orientation (Part II): construct validity and specificity to worry. *Behav-*

iour Research and Therapy, 43, 403–412.

Robichaud, M., & Dugas, M. J. (2006). A cognitive-behavioral treatment targeting intolerance of uncertainty. In G. C. L. Davey & A. Wells (Eds.), *Worry and its psychological disorders: Theory, assessment and treatment* (pp. 289–304). Chichester, UK: Wiley.

Rodebaugh, T. L., Holaway, R. M., & Hemiberg, R. G. (2004). The treatment of social anxiety disorder. *Clinical Psychology Review, 24*, 883–908.

Rodebaugh, T. L., Woods, C. M., Thissen, D. M., Heimberg, R. G., Chambless, D. L., & Rapee, R. M. (2004). More information from fewer questions: The factor structure and item properties of the original and Brief Fear of Negative Evaluation Scale. *Psychological Assessment, 16*, 169–181.

Rodriguez, B. F., Bruce, S. E., Pagano, M. E., & Keller, M. B. (2005). Relationships among psychosocial functioning, diagnostic comorbidity, and the recurrence of generalized anxiety disorder, panic disorder, and major depression. *Journal of Anxiety Disorders, 19*, 752–766.

Rodriguez, B. F., Pagano, M. E., & Keller, M. B. (2007). Psychometric characteristics of the Mobility Inventory in a longitudinal study of anxiety disorders: Replicating and exploring a three component solution. *Journal of Anxiety Disorders, 21*, 752–761.

Roemer, L. (2001). Measures for anxiety and related constructs. In M. M. Antony, S. M. Orsillo, & L. Roemer (Eds.), *Practitioner's guide to empirically based measures of anxiety* (pp. 49–83). New York: Kluwer Academic/Plenum Press.

Roemer, L., & Borkovec, T. D. (1993). Worry: Unwanted cognitive activity that controls somatic experience. In D. M. Wegner & J. W. Pennebaker (Eds.), *Handbook of mental control* (pp. 220–238). Upper Saddle River, NJ: Prentice-Hall.

Roemer, L., & Borkovec, T. D. (1994). Effects of suppressing thoughts about emotional material. *Journal of Abnormal Psychology, 103*, 467–474.

Roemer, L., Borkovec, M., Posa, S., & Borkovec, T. D. (1995). A self-report diagnostic measure of generalized anxiety disorder. *Journal*

of Behavior Therapy and Experimental Psychiatry, 26, 345–350.

Roemer, L., Litz, B. T., Orsillo, S. M., & Wagner, A. W. (2001). A preliminary investigation of the role of strategic withholding of emotions in PTSD. *Journal of Traumatic Stress, 14*, 149–156.

Roemer, L., Molina, S., Litz, B. T., & Borkovec, T. D. (1996–1997). Preliminary investigation of the role of previous exposure to potentially traumatizing events in generalized anxiety disorder. *Depression and Anxiety, 4*, 134–138.

Roemer, L., & Orsillo, S. M. (2007). An open trial of an acceptance-based behavior therapy for generalized anxiety disorder. *Behavior Therapy, 38*, 72–85.

Roemer, L., Orsillo, S. M., & Barlow, D. H. (2002). Generalized anxiety disorder. In D. H. Barlow (Ed.), *Anxiety and its disorders: The nature and treatment of anxiety and panic* (2nd ed., pp. 477–515). New York: Guilford Press.

Rogers, M. P., White, K., Warshaw, M. G., Yonkers, K. A., Rodriguez-Villa, F., Chang, G., et al. (1994). Prevalence of medical illness in patients with anxiety disorders. *International Journal of Psychiatry in Medicine, 24*, 83–96.

Rohner, J.-C. (2002). The time course of visual threat processing: High trait anxious individuals eventually avert their gaze from angry faces. *Cognition and Emotion, 16*, 837–844.

Rohner, J.-C. (2004). Memory-based attentional biases: Anxiety is linked to threat avoidance. *Cognition and Emotion, 18*, 1027–1054.

Romano, E., Tremblay, R. E., Vitaro, F., Zoccolillo, M., & Pagani, L. (2001). Prevalence of psychiatric diagnoses and the role of perceived impairment: Findings from an adolescent community sample. *Journal of Child Psychology and Psychiatry, 42*, 451–461.

Rosen, G. M., & Lilienfeld, S. O. (2008). Posttraumatic stress disorder: An empirical evaluation of core assumptions. *Clinical Psychology Review, 28*, 837–868.

Rosen, G. M., Spitzer, R. L., & McHugh, P. R. (2008). Problems with the posttraumatic stress disorder diagnosis and its future in DSM-V. *British Journal of Psychiatry, 192*, 3–4.

Roth, S., Newman, E., Pelcovitz, D., van der Kolk, B., & Mandel, F. S.

(1997). Complex PTSD in victims exposed to sexual and physical abuse: Results from the DSM-IV field trial for posttraumatic stress disorder. *Journal of Traumatic Stress, 10*, 539–555.

Roth, W. T., Wilhelm, F. H., & Pettit, D. (2005). Are current theories of panic falsifiable? *Psychologica Bulletin, 131*, 171–192.

Rothbaum, B. O., Foa, E. B., Riggs, D., Murdock, T., & Walsh, W. (1992). A prospective examination of post-traumatic stress disorder in rape victims. *Journal of Traumatic Stress, 5*, 455–475.

Rouf, K., Fennell, M., Westbrook, D., Cooper, M., & Bennett-Levy, J. (2004). Devising effective behavioural experiments. In J. Bennett-Levy, G. Butler, M. Fennell, A. Hackmann, M. Mueller, & D. Westbrook (Eds.), *Oxford guide to behavioural experiments in cognitive therapy* (pp. 20–58). Oxford, UK: Oxford University Press.

Rowa, K., Antony, M. M., & Swinson, R. P. (2007). Exposure and response prevention. In M. M. Antony, C. Purdon, & L. J. Summerfeldt (Eds.), *Psychological treatment of obsessive–compulsive disorder: Fundamentals and beyond* (pp. 79–109). Washington, DC: American Psychological Association.

Rowa, K., & Purdon, C. (2003). Why are certain intrusive thoughts more upsetting than others? *Behavioural and Cognitive Psychotherapy, 31*, 1–11.

Rowa, K., Purdon, C., Summerfeldt, L. J., & Antony, M. M. (2005). Why are some obsessions more upsetting than others? *Behaviour Research and Therapy, 43*, 1453–1465.

Roy-Byrne, P. P., Mellman, T. A., & Uhde, T. W. (1988). Biologic findings in panic disorder: Neuroendocrine and sleep-related abnormalities. *Journal of Anxiety Disorders, 2*, 17–29.

Roy-Byrne, P. P., Stang, P., Wittchen, H.-U., Ustun, B., Walters, E. E., & Kessler, R. C. (2000). Lifetime panic-depression comorbidity in the National Comorbidity Survey: Association with symptoms, impairment, course and help-seeking. *British Journal of Psychiatry, 176*, 229–235.

Rubin, G. J., Brewin, C. R., Greenberg, N., Hughes, J. H., Simpson, J., & Wessely, S. (2007). Enduring consequences of terrorism: 7-month follow-up survey of reactions to the bombings in London on 7 July 2005. *British Journal of Psychiatry, 190*, 350–356.

Rubin, G. J., Brewin, C. R., Greenberg, N., Simpson, J., & Wessely, S. (2005). Psychological and behavioral reactions to the bombings in London on 7 July 2005: Cross-sectional survey of a representative sample. *British Medical Journal, 331*, 606–611.

Ruggiero, K. J., Del Ben, K., Scotti, J. R., & Rabalais, A. E. (2003). Psychometric properties of the PTSD Checklist—Civilian Version. *Journal of Traumatic Stress, 16*, 495–502.

Ruscio, A. M. (2002). Delimiting the boundaries of generalized anxiety disorder: Differentiating high worriers with and without GAD. *Journal of Anxiety Disorders, 16*, 377–400.

Ruscio, A. M., & Borkovec, T. D. (2004). Experience and appraisal of worry among high worriers with and without generalized anxiety disorder. *Behaviour Research and Therapy, 42*, 1469–1482.

Ruscio, A. M., Borkovec, T. D., & Ruscio, J. (2001). A taxometric investigation of the latent structure of worry. *Journal of Abnormal Psychology, 110*, 413–422.

Ruscio, A. M., Brown, T. A., Chiu, W. T., Sareen, J., Stein, M. B., & Kessler, R. C. (2007). Social fears and social phobia in the USA: Results from the National Comorbidity Survey Replication. *Psychological Medicine, 38*, 15–28.

Ruscio, A. M., Chiu, W. T., Roy-Byrne, P., Stang, P. E., Stein, D. J., Wittchen, H.-U., et al. (2007). Broadening the definition of generalized anxiety disorder: Effects on prevalence and associations with other disorders in the National Comorbidity Survey Replication. *Journal of Anxiety Disorders, 21*, 662–676.

Ruscio, A. M., Ruscio, J., & Keane, T. M. (2002). The latent structure of posttraumatic stress disorder: A taxometric investigation of reactions to extreme stress. *Journal of Abnormal Psychology, 111*, 290–301.

Rutherford, E. M., MacLeod, C., & Campbell, L. W. (2004). Negative selectivity effects and emotional selectivity effects in anxiety: Differential attentional correlates of state and trait variables. *Cognition and Emotion, 18*, 711–720.

Rutledge, P. C. (1998). Obsessionality and the attempted suppression of unpleasant personal intrusive thoughts. *Behaviour Research and Therapy, 36*, 403–416.

Rutledge, P. C., Hancock, R. A., & Rutledge, J. H. (1996). Predictors of thought rebound. *Behaviour Research and Therapy, 34*, 555–562.

Rutledge, P. C., Hollenberg, D., & Hancock, R. A. (1993). Individual differences in the Wegner rebound effect: Evidence for a moderator variable in thought rebound following thought suppression. *Psychological Reports, 72*, 867–880.

Rygh, J. L., & Sanderson, W. C. (2004). *Treating generalized anxiety disorder: Evidenced-based strategies, tools, and techniques.* New York: Guilford Press.

Sachs, E., Rosenfeld, B., Lhewa, D., Rasmussen, A., & Keller, A. (2008). Entering exile: Trauma, mental health, and coping among Tibetan refugees arriving in Dharamsala, India. *Journal of Traumatic Stress, 21*, 199–208.

Safren, S. A., Heimberg, R. G., Brown, E. J., & Holle, C. (1996–1997). Quality of life in social phobia. *Depression and Anxiety, 4*, 126–133.

Safren, S. A., Heimberg, R. G., Lerner, J., Henin, A., Warman, M., & Kendall, P. C. (2000). Differentiating anxious and depressive self-statements: Combined factor structure of the Anxious Self-Statements Questionnaire and the Automatic Thoughts Questionnaire—Revised. *Cognitive Therapy and Research, 24*, 327–344.

Salemink, E., van den Hout, M., & Kindt, M. (2007a). Trained interpretative bias: Validity and effects on anxiety. *Journal of Behavior Therapy and Experimental Psychiatry, 38*, 212–224.

Salemink, E., van den Hout, M., & Kindt, M. (2007b). Trained interpretative bias and anxiety. *Behaviour Research and Therapy, 45*, 329–340.

Salge, R. A., Beck, J. G., & Logan, A. C. (1988). A community survey of panic. *Journal of Anxiety Disorders, 2*, 157–167.

Salkovskis, P. M. (1983). Treatment of obsessional patient using habituation to audiotaped ruminations.

British Journal of Clinical Psychology, 22, 311–313.

Salkovskis, P. M. (1985). Obsessional–compulsive problems: A cognitive-behavioural analysis. *Behaviour Research and Therapy, 23,* 571–583.

Salkovskis, P. M. (1988). Phenomenology, assessment, and the cognitive model of panic. In S. Rachman & J. D. Maser (Eds.), *Panic: Psychological perspectives* (pp. 111–136). Hillsdale, NJ: Erlbaum.

Salkovskis, P. M. (1989). Cognitive-behavioural factors and the persistence of intrusive thoughts in obsessional problems. *Behaviour Research and Therapy, 27,* 677–682.

Salkovskis, P. M. (1996a). The cognitive approach to anxiety: Threat beliefs, safety-seeking behavior, and the special case of health anxiety obsessions. In P. M. Salkovskis (Ed.), *Frontiers of cognitive therapy* (pp. 48–74). New York: Guilford Press.

Salkovskis, P. M. (1996b). Avoidance behavior is motivated by threat belief: A possible resolution of the cognitive-behavior debate. In P. M. Salkovskis (Ed.), *Trends in cognitive and behavioral therapies* (pp. 25–41). Chichester, UK: Wiley.

Salkovskis, P. M. (1999). Understanding and treating obsessive-compulsive disorder. *Behaviour Research and Therapy, 37,* S29–S52.

Salkovskis, P. M., & Bass, C. (1997). Hypochondriasis. In D. M. Clark & C. G. Fairburn (Eds.), *Science and practice of cognitive behaviour therapy* (pp. 313–339). Oxford, UK: Oxford University Press.

Salkovskis, P. M., Clark, D. M., & Gelder, M. G. (1996). Cognition-behaviour links in the persistence of panic. *Behaviour Research and Therapy, 34,* 453–458.

Salkovskis, P. M., Clark, D. M., & Hackman, A. (1991). Treatment of panic attacks using cognitive therapy without exposure or breathing retraining. *Behaviour Research and Therapy, 29,* 161–166.

Salkovskis, P. M., Clark, D. M., Hackmann, A., Wells, A., & Gelder, M. G. (1999). An experimental investigation of the role of safety-seeking behaviours in the maintenance of panic disorder with agoraphobia. *Behaviour Research and Therapy, 37,* 559–574.

Salkovskis, P. M., & Forrester, E. (2002). Responsibility. In R. O. Frost & G. Steketee (Eds.), *Cognitive approaches to obsessions and compulsions: Theory, assessment and treatment* (pp. 45–61). Oxford, UK: Elsevier Science.

Salkovskis, P. M., & Freeston, M. H. (2001). Obsessions, compulsions, motivation, and responsibility for harm. *Australian Journal of Psychology, 53,* 1–6.

Salkovskis, P. M., Hackmann, A., Wells, A., Gelder, M. G., & Clark, D. M. (2006). Belief disconfirmation versus habituation approaches to situational exposure in panic disorder with agoraphobia: A pilot study. *Behaviour Research and Therapy, 45,* 877–885.

Salkovskis, P. M., & Harrison, J. (1984). Abnormal and normal obsessions: A replication. *Behaviour Research and Therapy, 22,* 1–4.

Salkovskis, P. M., Jones, D. O., & Clark, D. M. (1986). Respiratory control in the treatment of panic attacks: Replication and extension with concurrent measurement of behaviour and $_pCO_2$, *British Journal of Psychiatry, 148,* 526–532.

Salkovskis, P., Shafran, R., Rachman, S., & Freeston, M. H. (1999). Multiple pathways to inflated responsibility beliefs in obsessional problems: Possible origins and implications for therapy and research. *Behaviour Research and Therapy, 37,* 1055–1072.

Salkovskis, P. M., Thorpe, S. J., Wahl, K., Wroe, A. L., & Forrester, E. (2003). Neutralizing increases discomfort associated with obsessional thoughts: An experimental study with obsessional patients. *Journal of Abnormal Psychology, 112,* 709–715.

Salkovskis, P. M., & Wahl, K. (2004). Treating obsessional problems using cognitive-behavioural therapy. In M. Reinecke & D. A. Clark (Eds.), *Cognitive therapy across the lifespan: Theory, research and practice* (pp. 138–171). Cambridge, UK: Cambridge University Press.

Salkovskis, P. M., & Warwick, H. M. C. (1988). Cognitive therapy of obsessive–compulsive disorder. In C. Perris, I. M. Blackburn, & H. Perris (Eds.), *Cognitive psychotherapy: Theory and practice* (pp. 376–395). Berlin: Springer-Verlag.

Salkovskis, P. M., Westbrook, D., Davis, J., Jeavons, A., & Gledhill, A. (1997). Effects of neutralizing on intrusive thoughts: An experiment investigating the etiology of obsessive–compulsive disorder. *Behaviour Research and Therapy, 35,* 211–219.

Salkovskis, P. M., Wroe, A. L., Gledhill, A., Morrison, N., Forrester, E., Richards, C., et al. (2000). Responsibility attitudes and interpretations are characteristic of obsessive compulsive disorder. *Behaviour Research and Therapy, 38,* 347–372.

Salvador-Carulla, L., Seguí, J., Fernández-Cano, P., & Canet, J. (1995). Costs and effects in panic disorder. *British Journal of Psychiatry, 166*(Suppl. 27), 23–28.

Sanavio, E. (1988). Obsessions and compulsions: The Padua Inventory. *Behaviour Research and Therapy, 26,* 169–177.

Sanderson, W. C., Rapee, R. M., & Barlow, D. H. (1989). The influence of an illusion of control on panic attacks via inhalation of 5.5% carbon dioxide-enriched air. *Archives of General Psychiatry, 46,* 157–162.

Sanderson, W. C., Wetzler, S., Beck, A. T., & Betz, F. (1994). Prevalence of personality disorders among patients with anxiety disorders. *Psychiatry Research, 51,* 167–174.

Sareen, J., Cox, B. J., Clara, I., & Asmundson, G. J. G. (2005). The relationship between anxiety disorders and physical disorders in the U. S. National Comorbidity Survey. *Depression and Anxiety, 21,* 193–202.

Sartorius, N., Ustun, T. B., Lecrubier, Y., & Wittchen, H.-U. (1996). Depression comorbid with anxiety: Results from the WHO study on psychological disorders in primary health care. *British Journal of Psychiatry, 168*(Suppl. 30), 38–43.

Saunders, B. E., Villeponteaux, L. A., Lipovsky, J. A., Kilpatrick, D. G., & Veronen, L. J. (1992). Child sexual assault as a risk factor for mental disorders among women: A community survey. *Journal of Interpersonal Violence, 7,* 189–204.

Sbrana, A., Bizzarri, J. V., Rucci, P., Gonnelli, C., Doria, M. R., Spagnolli, S., et al. (2005). The spectrum of substance use in mood and anxiety disorders. *Comprehensive Psychiatry, 46,* 6–13.

Schacter, D. L. (1990). Introduction

to "Implicit memory: Multiple perspectives." *Bulletin of the Psychonomic Society, 28,* 338–340.

Schatzberg, A. F., Samson, J. A., Rothschild, A. J., Bond, T. C., & Regier, D. A. (1998). McLean Hospital Depression Research Facility: Early-onset phobic disorders and adult-onset major depression. *British Journal of Psychiatry, 173*(Suppl. 34), 29–34.

Schmidt, N. B., & Cook, J. H. (1999). Effects of anxiety sensitivity on anxiety and pain during a cold pressor challenge in patients with panic disorder. *Behaviour Research and Therapy, 37,* 313–323.

Schmidt, N. B., Eggleston, A. M., Woolaway-Bickel, K., Fitzpatrick, K. K., Vasey, M. W., & Richey, J. A. (2007). Anxiety sensitivity amelioration training (ASAT): A longitudinal primary prevention program targeting cognitive vulnerability. *Journal of Anxiety Disorders, 21,* 302–319.

Schmidt, N. B., Forsyth, J. P., Santiago, H. T., & Trakowski, J. H. (2002). Classification of panic attack subtypes in patients and normal controls in response to biological challenge: Implications for assessment and treatment. *Journal of Anxiety Disorders, 16,* 625–638.

Schmidt, N. B., & Joiner, T. E. (2002). Structure of the Anxiety Sensitivity Index: Psychometrics and factor structure in a community sample. *Journal of Anxiety Disorders, 16,* 33–49.

Schmidt, N. B., Lerew, D. R., & Jackson, R. J. (1997). Prospective evaluation of anxiety sensitivity in the pathogenesis of panic: Replication and extension. *Journal of Abnormal Psychology, 108,* 532–537.

Schmidt, N. B., Lerew, D. R., & Jackson, R. J. (1999). The role of anxiety sensitivity in the pathogenesis of panic: Prospective evaluation of spontaneous panic attacks during acute stress. *Journal of Abnormal Psychology, 106,* 355–364.

Schmidt, N. B., Lerew, D. R., & Joiner, T. E. (2000). Prospective evaluation of the etiology of anxiety sensitivity: Test of a scar model. *Behaviour Research and Therapy, 38,* 1083–1095.

Schmidt, N. B., Lerew, D. R., & Trakowski, J. H. (1997). Body vigilance in panic disorder: Evaluating attention to bodily perturbations.

Journal of Consulting and Clinical Psychology, 65, 214–220.

Schmidt, N. B., & Mallot, M. (2006). Evaluating anxiety sensitivity and other fundamental sensitivities predicting anxiety symptoms and fearful response to a biological challenge. *Behaviour Research and Therapy, 44,* 1681–1688.

Schmidt, N. B., Maner, J. K., & Zvolensky, M. J. (2007). Reactivity to challenge with carbon dioxide as a prospective predictor of panic attacks. *Psychiatry Research, 151,* 173–176.

Schmidt, N.B., Richey, J.A., Buckner, J.D., & Timpano, K.R. (2009). Attention training for generalized social anxiety disorder. *Journal of Abnormal Psychology, 118,* 5–14.

Schmidt, N. B., Richey, J. A., & Fitzpatrick, K. K. (2006). Discomfort intolerance: Development of a construct and measure relevant to panic disorder. *Journal of Anxiety Disorders, 20,* 263–280.

Schmidt, N.B., Richey, A., Wollaway-Bickel, K., & Maner, J. K. (2006). Differential effects of safety in extinction of anxious responding to a CO_2 challenge in patients with panic disorder. *Journal of Abnormal Psychology, 115,* 341–350.

Schmidt, N. B., & Woolaway-Bickel, K. (2006). Cognitive vulnerability to panic disorder. In L. B. Alloy & J. H. Riskind (Eds.), *Cognitive vulnerability to emotional disorders* (pp. 207–234). Mahwah, NJ: Erlbaum.

Schmidt, N. B., Woolaway-Bickel, K., Trakowski, J., Santiago, H., Storey, J., Koselka, M., & Cook, J. (2000). Dismantling cognitive-behavioral treatment for panic disorder: Questioning the utility of breathing retraining. *Journal of Consulting and Clinical Psychology, 68,* 417–424.

Schneider, R., & Schulte, D. (2007). Panic patients reveal idiographic associations between anxiety symptoms and catastrophes in a semantic priming task. *Behaviour Research and Therapy, 45,* 211–223.

Schneier, F. R., Johnson, J., Hornig, C. D., Liebowitz, M. R., & Weissman, M. M. (1992). Social phobia: Comorbidity and morbidity in the epidemiologic sample. *Archives of General Psychiatry, 49,* 282–288.

Schniering, C. A., & Rapee, R. M. (2004). The relationship between

automatic thoughts and negative evaluation in children and adolescents: A test of the cognitive content-specificity hypothesis. *Journal of Abnormal Psychology, 113,* 464–470.

Schnurr, P. P., Freidman, M. J., Foy, D. W., Shea, T., Hsieh, F. Y., Lavori, P. W., et al. (2003). Randomized trial of trauma-focused group therapy for posttraumatic stress disorder: Results from a Department of Veterans Affairs Cooperative Study. *Archives of General Psychiatry, 60,* 481–489.

Schoevers, R. A., Beekman, A. T. F., Deeg, D. J. H., Jonker, C., & van Tilburg, W. (2003). Comorbidity and risk-patterns of depression, generalized anxiety disorder and mixed anxiety-depression in later life: Results from the AMSTEL study. *International Journal of Geriatric Psychiatry, 18,* 994–1001.

Schuurmans, J., Comijs, H. C., Beekman, A. T. F., de Beurs, E., Deeg, D. J. H., Emmelkamp, P. M. G., et al. (2005). The outcome of anxiety disorders in older people at 6-year follow-up: Results from the Longitudinal Aging Study Amsterdam. *Acta Psychiatrica Scandinavica, 111,* 420–428.

Scott, E. L., Eng, W., & Heimberg, R. G. (2002). Ethnic differences in worry in a nonclinical population. *Depression and Anxiety, 15,* 79–82.

See, J., MacLeod, C., & Bridle, R. (2009). The reduction of anxiety vulnerability through the modification of attentional bias: A real-world study using a home-based cognitive bias modification procedure. *Journal of Abnormal Psychology, 118,* 65–75.

Seedat, S., Njenga, C., Vythilingum, B., & Stein, D. J. (2004). Trauma exposure and post-traumatic stress symptoms in urban African schools. *British Journal of Psychiatry, 184,* 169–175.

Segal, Z. V., Teasdale, J. D., & Williams, J. M. G. (2005). Mindfulness-based cognitive therapy: Theoretical rationale and empirical status. In S. C. Hayes, V. M. Follette, & M. M. Linehan (Eds.), *Mindfulness and acceptance: Expanding the cognitive-behavioral tradition* (pp. 45–65). New York: Guilford Press.

Segal, Z. V., Williams, J. M. G., & Teasdale, J. D. (2002). *Mindful-*

ness-based cognitive therapy for depression. New York: Guilford Press.

Segerstrom, S. C., Tsao, J. C. I., Alden, L. E., & Craske, M. G. (2000). Worry and rumination: Repetitive thoughts as a concomitant and predictor of negative mood. Cognitive Therapy and Research, 24, 671–688.

Seligman, M. E. P., & Johnston, J. C. (1973). A cognitive theory of avoidance learning. In J. McGuigan & B. Lumsden (Eds.), Contemporary approaches to conditioning and learning (pp. 69–110). New York: Wiley.

Sexton, K. A., & Dugas, M. J. (2008). The Cognitive Avoidance Questionnaire: Validation of the English translation. Journal of Anxiety Disorders, 22, 355–370.

Shafran, R. (1997). The manipulation of responsibility in obsessive–compulsive disorder. British Journal of Clinical Psychology, 36, 397–407.

Shafran, R. (2003). Obsessive–compulsive disorder in children and adolescents. In R. G. Menzies & P. de Silva (Eds.), Obsessive–compulsive disorder: Theory, research and treatment (pp. 311–320). Chichester, UK: Wiley.

Shafran, R. (2005). Cognitive-behavioral models of OCD. In J. S. Abramowitz & A. C. Houts (Eds.), Concepts and controversies in obsessive–compulsive disorder (pp. 229–252). New York: Springer.

Shafran, R., Thordarson, D. S., & Rachman, S. J. (1996). Thought-action fusion in obsessive compulsive disorder. Journal of Anxiety Disorders, 10, 379–391.

Shalev, A. Y. (2002). Acute stress reactions in adults. Biological Psychiatry, 51, 532–543.

Shapiro, D. H., Schwartz, C. E., & Astin, J. A. (1996). Controlling ourselves, controlling our world: Psychology's role in understanding positive and negative consequences of seeking and gaining control. American Psychologist, 51, 1213–1230.

Shear, M. K., & Maser, J. D. (1994). Standardized assessment for panic disorder research: A conference report. Archives of General Psychiatry, 51, 346–354.

Sherbourne, C. D., Wells, K. B., & Judd, L. L. (1996). Functioning and well-being of patients with panic disorder. American Journal of Psychiatry, 153, 213–218.

Sherbourne, C. D., Wells, K. B., Meredith, L. S., Jackson, C. A., & Camp, P. (1996). Comorbid anxiety disorder and the functioning and well-being of chronically ill patients of general medical providers. Archives of General Psychiatry, 53, 889–895.

Shipherd, J. C., & Beck, J. G. (1999). The effects of suppressing trauma-related thoughts on women with rape-related posttraumaic stress disorder. Behaviour Research and Therapy, 37, 99–112.

Shipherd, J. C., Street, A. E., & Resick, P. A. (2006). Cognitive therapy for posttraumatic stress disorder. In V. M. Follette & J. I. Ruzek (Eds.), Cognitive-behavioral therapies for trauma (pp. 96–116). New York: Guilford Press.

Sibrava, N. J., & Borkovec, T. D. (2006). The cognitive avoidance theory of worry. In G. C. L. Davey & A. Wells (Eds.), Worry and its psychological disorders: Theory, assessment and treatment (pp. 239–256). Chichester, UK: Wiley.

Sica, C., Coradeschi, D., Sanavio, E., Dorz, S., Manchisi, D., & Novara, C. (2004). A study of the psychometric properties of the Obsessive Beliefs Inventory and Interpretations of Intrusions Inventory on clinical Italian individuals. Journal of Anxiety Disorders, 18, 291–307.

Siegel, L., Jones, W. C., & Wilson, J. O. (1990). Economic and life consequences experienced by a group of individuals with panic disorder. Journal of Anxiety Disorders, 4, 201–211.

Siev, J., & Chambless, D. L. (2007). Specificity of treatment effects: Cognitive therapy and relaxation for generalized anxiety and panic disorders. Journal of Consulting and Clinical Psychology, 75, 513–522.

Silver, R. C., Holman, E. A., McIntosh, D. N., Poulin, M., & Gil-Rivas, V. (2002). Nationwide longitudinal study of psychological responses to September 11. Journal of the American Medical Association, 288, 1235–1244.

Simms, L. J., Watson, D., & Doebbeling, B. N. (2002). Confirmatory factor analysis of posttraumatic stress symptoms in deployed and nondeployed veterans of the Gulf War. Journal of Abnormal Psychology, 111, 637–647.

Simon, N. M., Otto, M. W., Korbly, N. B., Peters, P. M., Nicolaou, D. C., & Pollack, M. H. (2002). Quality of life in social anxiety disorder compared with panic disorder and the general population. Psychiatric Services, 53, 714–718.

Simpson, J. R., Öngür, D., Akbudak, E., Conturo, T. E., Ollinger, J. M., Snyder, A. Z., et al. (2000). The emotional modulation of cognitive processing: An fMRI study. Journal of Cognitive Neuroscience, 12(Suppl. 2), 157–170.

Sinha, S. S., Mohlman, J., & Gorman, J. M. (2004). Neurobiology. In R. G. Heimberg, C. L. Turk, & D. S. Mennin (Eds.), Generalized anxiety disorder: Advances in research and practice (pp. 187–216). New York: Guilford Press.

Skoog, G., & Skoog, I. (1999). A 40-year follow-up of patients with obsessive–compulsive disorder. Archives of General Psychiatry, 56, 121–127.

Sleath, B., & Rubin, R. H. (2002). Gender, ethnicity, and physician–patient communication about depression and anxiety in primary care. Patient Education and Counseling, 48, 243–252.

Sloan, T., & Telch, M. J. (2002). The effects of safety-seeking behavior and guided threat reappraisal on fear reduction during exposure: An experimental investigation. Behaviour Research and Therapy, 40, 235–251.

Smári, J., Birgisdóttir, A. B., & Brynjólfsdóttir, B. (1995). Obsessive–compulsive symptoms and suppression of personally relevant unwanted thoughts. Personality and Individual Differences, 18, 621–625.

Smoller, J. W., Pollack, M. H., Wassertheil-Smoller, S., Jackson, R. D., Oberman, A., Wong, N. D., et al. (2007). Panic attacks and risk of incident cardiovascular events among postmenopausal women in the Women's Health Initiative Observatioal Study. Archives of General Psychiatry, 64, 1153–1160.

Smyth, J. M. (1998). Written emotional expression: Effect sizes, outcome types, and moderating variables. Journal of Consulting and Clinical Psychology, 66, 174–184.

Smyth, L. (1999). Overcoming posttraumatic stress disorder: Thera-

pist protocol. Oakland, CA: New Harbinger.

Sokol, L., Beck, A. T., Greenberg, R. L., Wright, F. D., & Berchick, R. J. (1989). Cognitive therapy of panic disorder: A nonpharmacological alternative. *Journal of Nervous and Mental Disease, 177,* 711–716.

Solomon, Z., & Mikulincer, M. (2007). Posttraumatic intrusive, avoidance, and social dysfunctioning: A 20-year longitudinal study. *Journal of Consulting and Clinical Psychology, 75,* 316–324.

Somerville, L. H., Kim, H., Johnstone, T., Alexander, A. L., & Whalen, P. J. (2004). Human amygdala responses during presentation of happy and neutral faces: Correlations with state anxiety. *Biological Psychiatry, 55,* 897–903.

Somoza, E., Steer, R. A., Beck, A. T., & Clark, D. A. (1994). Differentiating major depression and panic disorder by self-report and clinical rating scales: ROC analysis and information theory. *Behaviour Research and Therapy, 32,* 771–782.

Sookman, D., & Pinard, G. (2002). Overestimation of threat and intolerance of uncertainty in obsessive compulsive disorder. In R. O. Frost & G. Steketee (Eds.), *Cognitive approaches to obsessions and compulsions: Theory, assessment and treatment* (pp. 63–89). Oxford, UK: Elsevier Press.

Sookman, D., Pinard, G., & Beck, A. T. (2001). Vulnerability schemas in obsessive–compulsive disorder. *Journal of Cognitive Psychotherapy: An International Quarterly, 15,* 109–130.

Spector, I. P., Pecknold, J. C., & Libman, E. (2003). Selective attention bias related to the noticeability aspect of anxiety symptoms in generalized social phobia. *Journal of Anxiety Disorders, 17,* 517–531.

Spielberger, C. D. (1985). Anxiety, cognition and affect: A state-trait perspective. In A. H. Tuma & J. Maser (Eds.), *Anxiety and the anxiety disorders* (pp. 171–182). Hillsdale, NJ: Erlbaum.

Spielberger, C. D., Gorsuch, R. L., & Lushene, R. (1970). *STAI manual.* Palo Alto, CA: Consulting Psychologists Press.

Spielberger, C. D., Gorsuch, R. L., Lushene, R., Vagg, P. R., & Jacobs, G. A. (1983). *Manual for the State-Trait Anxiety Inventory: STAI (Form Y).* Palo Alto, CA: Consulting Psychologists Press.

Spitzer, R. L., First, M. B., & Wakefield, J. C. (2007). Saving PTSD from itself in DSM-V. *Journal of Anxiety Disorders, 21,* 233–241.

Stangier, U., Esser, F., Leber, S., Risch, A. K., & Heidenreich, T. (2006). Interpersonal problems in social phobia versus unipolar depression. *Depression and Anxiety, 23,* 418–421.

Stangier, U., Heidenreich, T., Peitz, M., Lauterbach, W., & Clark, D. M. (2003). Cognitive therapy for social phobia: Individual versus group treatment. *Behaviour Research and Therapy, 41,* 991–1007.

Stangier, U., Heidenreich, T., & Schermelleh-Engel, K. (2006). Safety behaviors and social performance in patients with generalized social phobia. *Journal of Cognitive Psychotherapy: An International Quarterly, 20,* 17–31.

Stanley, M. A., Beck, J. G., Novy, D. M., Averill, P. M., Swann, A. C., Diefenach, G. J., et al. (2003). Cognitive-behavioral treatment of late-life generalized anxiety disorder. *Journal of Consulting and Clinical Psychology, 71,* 309–319.

Stanley, M. A., & Turner, S. M. (1995). Current status of pharmacological and behavioral treatment of obsessive–compulsive disorder. *Behavior Therapy, 26,* 163–186.

Starcevic, V., & Berle, D. (2006). Cognitive specificity of anxiety disorders: A review of selected key constructs. *Depression and Anxiety, 23,* 51–61.

Startup, M., Makgekgenene, L., & Webster, R. (2007). The role of self-blame for trauma as assessed by the Postraumatic Cognitions Inventory (PTCI): A self-protective cognition? *Behaviour Research and Therapy, 45,* 395–403.

St. Clare, T. (2003). Assessment procedures. In R. G. Menzies & P. de Silva (Eds.), *Obsessive–compulsive disorder: Theory, research and treatment* (pp. 239–257). Chichester, UK: Wiley.

Steer, R. A., Beck, A. T., Clark, D. A., & Beck, J. S. (1994). Psychometric properties of the Cognitions Checklist with psychiatric outpatients and university students. *Psychological Assessment, 6,* 67–70.

Steer, R. A., Ranieri, W., Beck, A. T., & Clark, D. A. (1993). Further evidence for the validity of the Beck Anxiety Inventory with psychiatric outpatients. *Journal of Anxiety Disorders, 7,* 195–205.

Steil, R., & Ehlers, A. (2000). Dysfunctional meaning of posttraumatic intrusions in chronic PTSD. *Behaviour Research and Therapy, 38,* 537–558.

Stein, M. B., Baird, A., & Walker, J. R. (1996). Social phobia in adults with stuttering. *American Journal of Psychiatry, 153,* 278–280.

Stein, M. B., Goldin, P. R., Sareen, J., Eyler Zorrilla, L. T., & Brown, G. G. (2002). Increased amygdala activation to angry and contemptuous faces in generalized social phobia. *Archives of General Psychiatry, 59,* 1027–1034.

Stein, M. B., Torgrud, L. J., & Walker, J. R. (2000). Social phobia symptoms, subtypes, and severity: Findings from a community survey. *Archives of General Psychiatry, 57,* 1046–1052.

Stein, M. B., Walker, J. R., Anderson, G., Hazen, A. L., Ross, C. A., Eldridge, G., & Forde, D. R. (1996). Childhood physical and sexual abuse in patients with anxiety disorders and in a community sample. *American Journal of Psychiatry, 153,* 275–277.

Stein, M. B., Walker, J. R., & Forde, D. R. (1994). Setting diagnostic thresholds for social phobia: Considerations from a community survey of social anxiety. *American Journal of Psychiatry, 151,* 408–412.

Stein, M. B., Walker, J. R., Hazen, A. L., & Forde, D. R. (1997). Full and partial posttraumatic stress disorder: Findings from a community survey. *American Journal of Psychiatry, 154,* 1114–1119.

Steiner, M., Allgulander, C., Ravindran, A., Kosar, H., Burt, T., & Austin, C. (2005). Gender differences in clinical presentation and response to sertraline treatment for generalized anxiety disorder. *Human Psychopharmacology and Clinical Experiments, 20,* 3–13.

Steketee, G. S. (1993). *Treatment of obsessive–compulsive disorder.* New York: Guilford Press.

Steketee, G. S. (1999). *Overcoming obsessive–compulsive disorder: A behavioral and cognitive protocol for the treatment of OCD.* Oakland, CA: New Harbinger.

Steketee, G. ., & Barlow, D. H. (2002). Obsessive–compulsive disorder. In D. H. Barlow (Ed.), *Anxi-*

ety and its disorders: The nature and treatment of anxiety and panic (2nd ed., pp. 516–550). New York: Guilford Press.

Steketee, G., & Frost, R. O. (2007). Compulsive hoarding and acquiring: Therapist guide. Oxford, UK: Oxford University Press.

Steketee, G. S., Frost, R. O., & Bogart, K. (1996). The Yale–Brown Obsessive Compulsive Scale: Interview versus self-report. Behaviour Research and Therapy, 34, 675–684.

Steketee, G., Frost, R. O., & Cohen, I. (1998). Beliefs in obsessive-compulsive disorder. Journal of Anxiety Disorders, 12, 525–537.

Stemberger, R. T., Turner, S. M., Beidel, D. C., & Calhoun, K. S. (1995). Social phobia: An analysis of possible developmental factors. Journal of Abnormal Psychology, 104, 526–531.

Sternberg, R. J. (1996). Cognitive psychology. Fort Worth, TX: Harcourt Brace College Publishers.

Stewart, W. F., Linet, M. S., & Celentano, D. D. (1989). Migraine headaches and panic attacks. Psychosomatic Medicine, 51, 559–569.

Stöber, J. (1998). Reliability and validity of two widely-used worry questionnaires: Self-report and self-peer convergences. Personality and Individual Differences, 24, 887–890.

Stöber, J., & Joorman, J. (2001). A short form of the Worry Domains Questionnaire: Construction and factorial validation. Personality and Individual Differences, 31, 591–598.

Stopa, L., & Clark, D. M. (1993). Cognitive processes in social phobia. Behaviour Research and Therapy, 31, 255–267.

Stopa, L., & Clark, D. M. (2000). Social phobia and interpretation of social events. Behaviour Research and Therapy, 38, 273–283.

Story, T. J., & Craske, M. G. (2008). Response to false physiological feedback in individuals with panic attacks and elevated anxiety sensitivity. Behaviour Research and Therapy, 46, 1001–1008.

Story, T. J., Zucker, B. G., & Craske, M. G. (2004). Secondary prevention of anxiety disorders. In D. J. A. Dozois & K. S. Dobson (Eds.), The prevention of anxiety and depression: Theory, research, and practice (pp. 131–160). Washing-

ton, DC: American Psychological Association Press.

Stravynski, A. (2007). Fearing others: The nature and treatment of social phobia. Cambridge, UK: Cambridge University Press.

Stravynski, A., Bond, S., & Amado, D. (2004). Cognitive causes of social phobia: A critical appraisal. Clinical Psychology Review, 24, 421–440.

Street, L. L., Craske, M. G., & Barlow, D. H. (1989). Sensation, cognitions, and the perception of cues associated with expected and unexpected panic attacks. Behaviour Research and Therapy, 27, 189–198.

Stroop, J. R. (1935). Studies of interference in serial verbal reactions Journal of Experimental Psychology, 18, 643–662.

Suarez, L., & Bell-Dolan, D. (2001). The relationship of child worry to cognitive biases: Threat interpretation and likelihood of event occurrence. Behavior Therapy, 32, 425–442.

Summerfeldt, L. J., & Antony, M. M. (2002). Structured and semistructured diagnostic interviews. In M. M. Antony & D. H. Barlow (Eds.), Handbook of assessment and treatment planning for psychological disorders (pp. 3–37). New York: Guilford Press.

Summerfeldt, L. J., Huta, V., & Swinson, R. P. (1998). Personality and obsessive–compulsive disorder. In R. P. Swinson, M. M. Antony, S. Rachman, & M. A. Richter (Eds.), Obsessive–compulsive disorder: Theory, research and treatment (pp. 79–119). New York: Guilford Press.

Sutherland, K., & Bryant, R. A. (2008). Social problem solving and autobiographical memory in posttraumatic stress disorder. Behaviour Research and Therapy, 46, 154–161.

Sweeney, P. D., Anderson, K., & Bailey, S. (1986). Attributional style in depression: A meta-analytic review. Journal of Personality and Social Psychology, 50, 974–991.

Swoboda, H., Amering, M., Windhaber, J., & Katschnig, H. (2003). The long-term course of panic disorder: An 11 year follow-up. Journal of Anxiety Disorders, 17, 223–232.

Tallis, F. (1994). Obsessions, responsibility and guilt: Two case reports suggesting a common and specific

etiology. Behaviour Research and Therapy, 32, 143–145.

Tallis, F., Davey, G. C. L., & Bond, A. (1994). The Worry Domains Questionnaire. In G. C. L. Davey & F. Tallis (Eds.), Worrying: Perspectives on theory, assessment and treatment (pp. 285–297). Chichester, UK: Wiley.

Tallis, F., Eysenck, M., & Mathews, A. (1992). A questionnaire for the measurement of nonpathological worry. Personality and Individual Differences, 13, 161–168.

Tanaka-Matsumi, J., & Kameoka, V. A. (1986). Reliabilities and concurrent validity of popular self-report measures of depression, anxiety, and social desirability. Journal of Consulting and Clinical Psychology, 54, 328–333.

Tanielian, T., & Jaycox, L. H. (2008). Invisible wounds of war: Psychological and cognitive injuries, their consequence, and services to assist recovery. Santa Monica, CA: RAND Corporation.

Tanner, R. J., Stopa, L., & de Houwer, J. (2006). Implicit views of the self in social anxiety. Behaviour Research and Therapy, 44, 1397–1409.

Tarrier, N., & Sommerfield, C. (2004). Treatment of chronic PTSD by cognitive therapy and exposure: 5-year follow-up. Behavior Therapy, 35, 231–246.

Tarrier, N., Pilgrim, H., Sommerfield, C., Faragher, B., Reynolds, M., Graham, E., et al. (1999). A randomized trial of cognitive therapy and imaginal exposure in the treatment of chronic posttraumatic stress disorder. Journal of Consulting and Clinical Psychology, 67, 13–18.

Tata, P. R., Leibowitz, J. A., Prunty, M. J., Cameron, M., & Pickering, A. D. (1996). Attentional bias in obsessive compulsive disorder. Behaviour Research and Therapy, 34, 53–60.

Taylor, C. B., Sheikh, J., Agras, W. S., Roth, W. T., Margraf, J., Ehlers, A., et al. (1986). Ambulatory heart rate changes in patients with panic attacks. American Journal of Psychiatry, 143, 478–482.

Taylor, S. (1995a). Anxiety sensitivity: Theoretical perspectives and recent findings. Behaviour Research and Therapy, 33, 243–258.

Taylor, S. (1995b). Assessment of obsessions and compulsions: Reliability, validity, and sensitivity to treatment effects. *Clinical Psychology Review, 15*, 261–296.

Taylor, S. (1998). Assessment of obsessive–compulsive disorder. In R. P. Swinson, M. M. Antony, S. Rachman, & M. A. Richter (Eds.), *Obsessive–compulsive disorder: Theory, research and treatment* (pp. 229–257). New York: Guilford Press.

Taylor, S. (2000). *Understanding and treating panic disorder: Cognitive-behavioural approaches*. Chichester, UK: Wiley.

Taylor, S. (2006). *Clinician's guide to PTSD: A cognitive-behavioral approach*. New York: Guilford Press.

Taylor, S., Abramowitz, J. S., & McKay, D. (2007). Cognitive-behavioral models of obsessive–compulsive disorder. In M. M. Antony, C. Purdon, & L. J. Summerfeldt (Eds.), *Psychological treatment of obsessive–compulsive disorder: Fundamentals and beyond* (pp. 9–29). Washington, DC: American Psychological Association.

Taylor, S., Abramowitz, J. S., McKay, D., Calamari, J. E., Sookman, D., Kyrios, M., et al. (2006). Do dysfunctional beliefs play a role in all types of obsessive–compulsive disorder? *Journal of Anxiety Disorders, 20*, 85–97.

Taylor, S., Asmundson, G. J. G., & Carleton, R. N. (2006). Simple versus complex PTSD: A cluster analytic investigation. *Journal of Anxiety Disorders, 20*, 459–472.

Taylor, S., & Cox, B. J. (1998). An expanded Anxiety Sensitivity Index: Evidence for a hierarchic structure in a clinical sample. *Journal of Anxiety Disorders, 12*, 463–483.

Taylor, S., Koch, W. J., & McNally, R. J. (1992). How does anxiety sensitivity vary across the anxiety disorders? *Journal of Anxiety Disorders, 6*, 249–259.

Taylor, S., Koch, W. J., McNally, R. J., & Crockett, D. J. (1992). Conceptualizations of anxiety sensitivity. *Psychological Assessment, 4*, 245–250.

Taylor, S., Thordarson, D. S., Maxfield, L., Fedoroff, I. C., Lovell, K., & Ogrodniczuk, J. (2003). Comparative efficacy, speed, and adverse effects of three PTSD treatments: Exposure therapy, EMDR, and relaxation training. *Journal of Consulting and Clinical Psychology, 71*, 330–338.

Taylor, S., Zvolensky, M. J., Cox, B. J., Deacon, B., Heimberg, R. G., Ledley, D. R. et al. (2007). Robust dimensions of anxiety sensitivity: Development and initial validation of the Anxiety Sensitivity Index–3. *Psychological Assessment, 19*, 176–188.

Teachman, B. A., Gregg, A., & Woody, S. (2001). Implicit attitudes toward fear-relevant stimuli in individuals with snake and spider fears. *Journal of Abnormal Psychology, 110*, 226–235.

Teachman, B. A., Smith-Janik, S. B., & Saporito, J. (2007). Information processing biases and panic disorder: Relationships among cognitive and symptom variables. *Behaviour Research and Therapy, 45*, 1791–1811.

Teachman, B. A., & Woody, S. R. (2003). Automatic processing in spider phobia: Implicit fear associations over the course of treatment. *Journal of Abnormal Psychology, 112*, 100–109.

Teachman, B. A., & Woody, S. R. (2004). Staying tuned to research in implicit cognition: Relevance for clinical practice with anxiety disorders. *Cognitive and Behavioral Practice, 11*, 149–159.

Teachman, B. A., Woody, S. R., & Magee, J. C. (2006). Implicit and explicit appraisals of the importance of intrusive thoughts. *Behaviour Research and Therapy, 44*, 785–805.

Teasdale, J. D., Segal, Z. V., Williams, J. M. G., Ridgeway, V. A., Soulsby, J. M., & Lau, M. A. (2000). Prevention of relapse/recurrence in major depression by mindfulness-based cognitive therapy. *Journal of Consulting and Clinical Psychology, 68*, 615–623.

Tek, C., & Ulug, B. (2001). Religiosity and religious obsessions in obsessive–compulsive disorder. *Psychiatry Research, 104*, 99–108.

Telch, M. J., Lucas, J. A., & Nelson, P. (1989). Nonclinical panic in college students: An investigation of prevalence and symptomatology. *Journal of Abnormal Psychology, 98*, 300–306.

Telch, M. J., Lucas, R. A., Smits, J. A. J., Powers, M. B., Heimberg, R. G., & Hart, T. (2004). Appraisal of Social Concerns: A cognitive assessment instrument for social phobia. *Depression and Anxiety, 19*, 217–224.

Telch, M. J., Silverman, A., & Schmidt, N. B. (1996). Effects of anxiety sensitivity and perceived control on emotional responding to caffeine challenge. *Journal of Anxiety Disorders, 10*, 21–35.

Thayer, J. F., Friedman, B. H., & Borkovec, T. D. (1996). Autonomic characteristics of generalized anxiety disorder and worry. *Biological Psychiatry, 39*, 255–266.

Thordarson, D. S., Radomsky, A. S., Rachman, S., Shafran, R., Sawchuk, C. N., & Hakstian, A. R. (2004). The Vancouver Obsessional Compulsive Inventory (VOCI). *Behaviour Research and Therapy, 42*, 1289–1314.

Thordarson, D. S., & Shafran, R. (2002). Importance of thoughts. In R. O. Frost & G. Steketee (Eds.), *Cognitive approaches to obsessions and compulsions: Theory, assessment and treatment* (pp. 15–28). Oxford, UK: Elsevier.

Thyer, B. A. (1985). Audio-taped exposure therapy in a case of obsessional neurosis. *Journal of Behavior Therapy and Experimental Psychiatry, 16*, 271–273.

Thyer, B. A., & Himle, J. (1985). Temporal relationship between panic attack onset and phobic avoidance in agoraphobia. *Behaviour Research and Therapy, 23*, 607–608.

Tolin, D. F., Abramowitz, J. S., Brigidi, B. D., & Foa, E. B. (2003). Intolerance of uncertainty in obsessive–compulsive disorder. *Journal of Anxiety Disorders, 17*, 233–242.

Tolin, D. F., Abramowitz, J. S., Hamlin, C., Foa, E. B., & Synodi, D. S. (2002). Attributions for thought suppression failure in obsessive–compulsive disorder. *Cognitive Therapy and Research, 26*, 505–517.

Tolin, D. F., Abramowitz, J. S., Przeworski, A., & Foa, E. B. (2002). Thought suppression in obsessive–compulsive disorder. *Behaviour Research and Therapy, 40*, 1255–1274.

Tolin, D. F., & Steketee, G. (2007). General issues in psychological treatment for obsessive–compulsive disorder. In Antony, M. M., Purdon, C., & Summerfeldt, L. J. (Eds.), *Psychological treatment of obsessive–compulsive disor-*

der: *Fundamentals and beyond* (pp. 31–59). Washington, DC: American Psychological Association.

Tolin, D. F., Worhunsky, P., & Maltby, N. (2006). Are "obsessive" beliefs specific to OCD?: A comparison across anxiety disorders. *Behaviour Research and Therapy, 44*, 469–480.

Tomarken, A. J., Mineka, S., & Cook, M. (1989). Fear-relevant selective association and covariation bias. *Journal of Abnormal Psychology, 98*, 381–394.

Trinder, H., & Salkovskis, P. M. (1994). Personally relevant intrusions outside the laboratory: Long-term suppression increases intrusion. *Behaviour Research and Therapy, 32*, 833–842.

Trull, T. J., & Sher, K. J. (1994). Relationship between the five-factor model of personality and Axis I disorders in a non-clinical sample. *Journal of Abnormal Psychology, 103*, 350–360.

Tsao, J. C. I., Mystkowski, J. L., Zucker, B. G., & Craske, M. G. (2005). Impact of cognitive-behavioral therapy for panic disorder on comorbidity: A controlled investigation. *Behaviour Research and Therapy, 43*, 959–970.

Turgeon, L., Marchand, A., & Dupuis, G. (1998). Clinical features of panic disorder with agoraphobia: A comparison of men and women. *Journal of Anxiety Disorders, 12*, 539–553.

Turk, C. L., Heimberg, R. G., & Magee, L. (2008). Social anxiety disorder. In D. H. Barlow (Ed.), *Clinical handbook of psychological disorders: A step-by-step treatment manual* (4th ed., pp. 123–163). New York: Guilford Press.

Turk, C. L., Heimberg, R. S., & Mennin, D. S. (2004). Assessment. In R. G. Heimberg, C. L. Turk, & D. S. Mennin (Eds.), *Generalized anxiety disorder: Advances in research and practice* (pp. 219–247). New York: Guilford Press.

Turk, C. L., & Wolanin, A. T. (2006). Assessment of generalized anxiety disorder. In G. C. L. Davey & A. Wells (Eds.), *Worry and its psychological disorders: Theory, assessment and treatment* (pp. 137–155). Chichester, UK: Wiley.

Turner, S., Bowie, C., Dunn, G., Shapo, L., & Yule, W. (2003). Mental health of Kosovan Albanian ref-

ugees in the UK. *British Journal of Psychiatry, 182*, 444–448.

Turner, S. M., & Beidel, D. C. (1985). Empirically derived subtypes of social anxiety. *Behavior Therapy, 16*, 384–392.

Turner, S. M., & Beidel, D. C. (1989). Social phobia, clinical syndrome, diagnosis, and comorbidity. *Clinical Psychology Review, 9*, 3–18.

Turner, S. M., Beidel, D. C., Borden, J. W., Stanley, M. R., & Jacobs, R. G. (1991). Social phobia: Axis I and Axis II correlates. *Journal of Abnormal Psychology, 100*, 102–106.

Turner, S. M., Beidel, D. C., & Dancu, C. V. (1996). *SPAI: Social Phobia and Anxiety Inventory Manual.* North Tonawanda, NY: Multi-Health Systems.

Turner, S. M., Beidel, D. C., Dancu, C. V., & Keys, D. J. (1986). Psychopathology of social phobia and comparison to avoidant personality disorder. *Journal of Abnormal Psychology, 95*, 389–394.

Turner, S. M., Beidel, D. C., Dancu, C. V., & Stanley, M. A. (1989). An empirically derived inventory to measure social fears and anxiety: The Social Phobia and Anxiety Inventory. *Psychological Assessment: A Journal of Consulting and Clinical Psychology, 1*, 35–40.

Turner, S. M., Beidel, D. C., & Frueh, B. C. (2005). Multicomponent behavioral treatment for chronic combat-related posttraumatic stress disorder. *Behavior Modification, 29*, 39–69.

Turner, S. M., Beidel, D. C., & Larkin, K. T. (1986). Situational determinants of social anxiety in clinic and nonclinic samples: Physiological and cognitive correlates. *Journal of Consulting and Clinical Psychology, 54*, 523–527.

Turner, S. M., Beidel, D. C., & Townsley, R. M. (1990). Social phobia: Relationship to shyness. *Behaviour Research and Therapy, 28*, 497–505.

Turner, S. M., Beidel, D. C., & Townsley, R. M. (1992). Social phobia: A comparison of specific and generalized subtypes and avoidant personality disorder. *Journal of Abnormal Psychology, 101*, 326–331.

Turner, S. M., Johnson, M. R., Beidel, D. C., Heiser, N. A., & Lydiard, R. B. (2003). The Social Thoughts and Beliefs Scale: A new inventory for assessing cognitions in social

phobia. *Psychological Assessment, 15*, 384–391.

Turner, S. M., Stanley, M. A., Beidel, D. C., & Bond, L. (1989). The Social Phobia and Anxiety Inventory: Construct validity. *Journal of Psychopathology and Behavioral Assessment, 11*, 221–234.

Turner, J., & Lloyd, D. A. (2004). Stress burden and the lifetime incidence of psychiatric disorder in young adults. *Archives of General Psychiatry, 61*, 481–488.

Twohig, M. P., Hayes, S. C., & Masuda, A. (2006). Increasing willingness to experience obsessions: Acceptance and commitment therapy as a treatment for obsessive–compulsive disorder. *Behavior Therapy, 37*, 3–13.

Tylee, A. (2000). Depression in Europe: Experience from the DEPRES II survey. *European Neuropsychopharmacology, 10*(Suppl. 4), S445–S448.

Tyrer, P., Gunderson, J. G., Lyons, M., & Tohen, M. (1997). Special feature: Extent of comorbidity between mental state and personality disorders. *Journal of Personality Disorders, 11*, 242–259

Ullman, S. E., Filipas, H. H., Townsend, S. M., & Starzynski, L. L. (2007). Psychosocial correlates of PTSD symptom severity in sexual assault survivors. *Journal of Traumatic Stress, 20*, 821–831.

Uren, T. H., Szabó, M., & Lovibond, P. F. (2004). Probability and cost estimates for social and physical outcomes in social phobia and panic disorder. *Journal of Anxiety Disorders, 18*, 481–498.

U.S. Department of Veterans Affairs. (2003). *2001 National Survey of Veterans (NSV), final report.* Washington, DC: Author.

van Balkom, A. J. L. M., de Haan, E., van Oppen, P., Spinhoven, P., Hoogduin, K. A. L., & van Dyck, R. (1998). Cognitive and behavioral therapies alone versus in combination with fluvoxamine in the treatment of obsessive compulsive disorder. *Journal of Nervous and Mental Disease, 186*, 492–499.

van Balkom, A. J. L. M., Nauta, M. C. E., & Bakker, A. (1995). Meta-analysis on the treatment of panic disorder with agoraphobia: Review and re-examination. *Clinical Psychology and Psychotherapy, 2*, 1–14.

van Balkom, A. J. L. M., van Oppen,

P., Vermeulen, A. W. A., van Dyck, R., Nauta, M. C. E., & Vorst, H. C. M. (1994). A meta-analysis on the treatment of obsessive compulsive disorder: A comparison of antidepressants, behavior, and cognitive therapy. *Clinical Psychology Review, 14*, 359–381.

van der Does, A. J. W., Antony, M. M., Ehlers, A., & Barsky, A. J. (2000). Heartbeat perception in panic disorder: A reanalysis. *Behaviour Research and Therapy, 38*, 47–62.

van de Hout, M., Arntz, A., & Hoekstra, R. (1994). Exposure reduced agoraphobia but not panic, and cognitive therapy reduced panic but not agoraphobia. *Behaviour Research and Therapy, 32*, 447–451.

Van den Heuvel, O. A., Veltman, D. J., Groenewegen, H. J., Dolan, R. J., Cath, D. C., Boellaard, R., et al. (2004). Amygdala activity in obsessive–compulsive disorder with contamination fear: A study with oxygen-15 water positron emission tomography. *Psychiatry Research: Neuroimaging, 132*, 225–237.

van den Hout, M. A., & Griez, E. (1984). Panic symptoms after inhalation of carbon dioxide. *British Journal of Psychiatry, 144*, 503–507.

van den Hout, M., & Merckelbach, H. (1991). Classical conditioning: Still going strong. *Behavioural Psychotherapy, 19*, 59–79.

van der Molen, G. M., van den Hout, M. A., Vroemen, J., Lousberg, H., & Griez, E. (1986). Cognitive determinants of lactate-induced anxiety. *Behaviour Research and Therapy, 24*, 677–680.

van Ommeren, M. (2003). Validity issues in transcultural epidemiology. *British Journal of Psychiatry, 182*, 376–378.

van Oppen, P., & Arntz, A. (1994). Cognitive therapy for obsessive–compulsive disorder. *Behaviour Research and Therapy, 32*, 79–87.

van Oppen, P., de Haan, E., van Balkom, A. J. L. M., Spinhoven, P., Hoogduin, K., & van Dyck, R. (1995). Cognitive therapy and exposure *in vivo* in the treatment of obsessive compulsive disorder. *Behaviour Research and Therapy, 33*, 379–390.

van Oppen, P., Hoekstra, R. J., & Emmelkamp, P. M. G. (1995). The structure of obsessive–compulsive symptoms. *Behaviour Research and Therapy, 33*, 15–23.

van Velzen, C. J. M., Emmelkamp, P. M. G., & Scholing, A. (2000). Generalized social phobia versus avoidant personality disorder: Differences in psychopathology, personality traits, and social and occupational functioning. *Journal of Anxiety Disorders, 14*, 395–411.

Vasey, M. W., & Borkovec, T. D. (1992). A catastrophizing assessment of worrisome thoughts. *Cognitive Therapy and Research, 16*, 505–520.

Vassilopoulos, S. Ph. (2005). Social anxiety and the vigilance–avoidance pattern of attentional processing. *Behavioural and Cognitive Psychotherapy, 33*, 13–24.

Vassilopoulos, S. Ph. (2008). Coping strategies and anticipatory processing in high and low socially anxious individuals. *Journal of Anxiety Disorders, 22*, 98–107.

Vazquez-Barquero, J. L., Garcia, J., Simon, J. A., Iglesias, C., Montejo, J., Herran, A., et al. (1997). Mental health in primary care: An epidemiological study of morbidity and use of health. *British Journal of Psychiatry, 170*, 529–539.

Veale, D. (2007). Treating obsessive-compulsive disorder in people with poor insight and overvalued ideation. In M. M. Antony, C. Purdon, & L. J. Summerfeldt (Eds.), *Psychological treatment of obsessive-compulsive disorder: Fundamentals and beyond* (pp. 267–280). Washington, DC: American Psychological Association.

Verburg, K., Griez, E., Meijer, J., & Pols, H. (1995). Discrimination between panic disorder and generalized anxiety disorders by 35% carbon dioxide challenge. *American Journal of Psychiatry, 152*, 1081–1083.

Verkuil, B., Brosschot, J. F., & Thayer, J. F. (2007). Capturing worry in daily life: Are trait questionnaires sufficient? *Behaviour Research and Therapy, 45*, 1835–1844.

Vickers, K., & McNally, R. J. (2004). Panic disorder and suicide attempt in the National Comorbidity Survey. *Journal of Abnormal Psychology, 113*, 582–591.

Vlahov, D., Galea, S., Resnick, H., Ahern, J., Boscarino, J. A., Bucuvalas, M., et al. (2002). Increased use of cigarettes, alcohol, and marijuana among Manhattan, New York, residents after the September 11th terrorist attacks. *American Journal of Epidemiology, 155*, 988–996.

Vogt, D. S., King, D. W., & King, L. A. (2007). Risk pathways for PTSD: Making sense of the literature. In M. J. Freidman, T. M. Keane, & P. A. Resick (Eds.), *Handbook of PTSD: Science and practice* (pp. 99–115). New York: Guilford Press.

Vogt, D. S., Samper, R. E., King, D. W., King, L. A., & Martin, J. A. (2008). Deployment of stressors and posttraumatic stress symptomatology: Comparing active duty and National Guard/Reserve personnel from Gulf War I. *Journal of Traumatic Stress, 21*, 66–74.

Voncken, M. J., Alden, L. E., & Bögels, S. M. (2006). Hiding anxiety versus acknowledgment of anxiety in social interaction: Relationship with social anxiety. *Behaviour Research and Therapy, 44*, 1673–1679.

Voncken, M. J., Bögels, S. M., & de Vries, K. (2003). Interpretation and judgmental biases in social phobia. *Behaviour Research and Therapy, 41*, 1481–1488.

Vrana, S., & Lauterbach, D. (1994). Prevalance of traumatic events and posttraumatic psychological symptoms in a nonclinical sample of college students. *Journal of Traumatic Stress, 7*, 289–302.

Vrana, S. R., Roodman, A., & Beckham, J. C. (1995). Selective processing of trauma-relevant words in posttraumatic stress disorder. *Journal of Anxiety Disorders, 9*, 515–530.

Vriends, N., Becker, E. S., Meyer, A., Michael, T., & Margraf, J. (2007). Subtypes of social phobia: Are they of any use? *Journal of Anxiety Disorders, 21*, 59–75.

Vriends, N., Becker, E. S., Meyer, A., Williams, S. L., Lutz, R., & Margraf, J. (2007). Recovery from social phobia in the community and its predictors: Data from a longitudinal epidemiological study. *Journal of Anxiety Disorders, 21*, 320–337.

Wagner, R., Silvoe, D., Marnane, C., & Rouen, D. (2006). Delays in referral of patients with social phobia, panic disorder and generalized anxiety disorder attending a specialist anxiety clinic. *Journal of Anxiety Disorders, 20,* 363–371.

Walker, E. A., Katon, W., Russo, J., Ciechanowski, P., Newman, E., & Wagner, A. W. (2003). Health care costs associated with posttraumatic stress disorder symptoms in women. *Archives of General Psychiatry, 60,* 369–374.

Walters, K. S., & Hope, D. A. (1998). Analysis of social behavior in individuals with social phobia and nonanxious participants using a psychobiological model. *Behavior Therapy, 29,* 387–407.

Walters, K., Rait, G., Petersen, I., Williams, R., & Nazareth, I. (2008). Panic disorder and risk of new onset coronary heart disease, acute myocardial infarction, and cardiac mortality: Cohort study using the general practice research database. *European Heart Journal, 29,* 2981–2988.

Wang, A., & Clark, D. A. (2008). *The suppression of worry and its triggers in a nonclinical sample: Rebound and other negative effects.* Unpublished manuscript, Department of Psychology, University of New Brunswick, Canada.

Wang, P. S., Berglund, P., Olfson, M., Pincus, H. A., Wells, K. B., & Kessler, R. C. (2005). Failure and delay in initial treatment contact after first onset of mental disorders in the National Comorbidity Survey Replication. *Archives of General Psychiatry, 63,* 603–613.

Wang, P. S., Lane, M., Olfson, M., Pincus, H. A., Wells, K. B., & Kessler, R. C. (2005). Twelve-month use of mental health services in the United States: Result from the National Comorbidity Survey Replication. *Archives of General Psychiatry, 63,* 629–640.

Watkins, E. R. (2004). Appraisals and strategies associated with rumination and worry. *Behaviour Research and Therapy, 37,* 679–694.

Watkins, E. R. (2008). Constructive and unconstructive repetitive thought. *Psychological Bulletin, 134,* 163–206.

Watkins, E. R., Moulds, M., & Mackintosh, B. (2005). Comparisons between rumination and worry in a non-clinical population. *Behaviour Research and Therapy, 43,* 1577–1585.

Watson, D. (2005). Rethinking the mood and anxiety disorders: A quantitative hierarchical model for DSM-V. *Journal of Abnormal Psychology, 114,* 522–536.

Watson, D., & Clark, L. A. (1984). Negative affectivity: The disposition to experience aversive emotional states. *Psychological Bulletin, 96,* 465–490.

Watson, D., Clark, L. A., & Carey, G. (1988). Positive and negative affectivity and their relation to anxiety and depressive disorders. *Journal of Abnormal Psychology, 97,* 346–353.

Watson, D., Clark, L. A., & Harkness, A. R. (1994). Structures of personality and their relevance to psychopathology. *Journal of Abnormal Psychology, 103,* 18–31.

Watson, D., & Friend, R. (1969). Measurement of social-evaluative anxiety. *Journal of Consulting and Clinical Psychology, 33,* 448–457.

Weathers, F. W., Keane, T. M., & Davidson, J. R. T. (2001). Clinician-Administered PTSD Scale: A review of the first ten years of research. *Depression and Anxiety, 13,* 132–156.

Weathers, F. W., Ruscio, A. M., & Keane, T. M. (1999). Psychometric properties of nine scoring rules for the Clinician-Administered Posttraumatic Stress Disorder Scale. *Psychological Assessment, 11,* 124–133.

Weeks, J. W., Heimberg, R. G., Rodebaugh, T. L., & Norton, P. J. (2008). Exploring the relationship between fear of positive evaluation and social anxiety. *Journal of Anxiety Disorders, 22,* 386–400.

Weens, C. F., Hayward, C., Killen, J., & Taylor, C. B. (2002). A longitudinal investigation of anxiety sensitivity in adolescence. *Journal of Abnormal Psychology, 111,* 471–477.

Wegner, D. M. (1994). Ironic processes of mental control. *Psychological Review, 101,* 34–52.

Wegner, D. M., Schneider, D. J., Carter, S. R., & White, T. L. (1987). Paradoxical effects of thought suppression. *Journal of Personality and Social Psychology, 53,* 5–13.

Wegner, D. M., & Zanakos, S. (1994). Chronic thought suppression. *Journal of Personality, 62,* 615–640.

Weiller, E., Bisserbe, J.-C., Maier, W., & LeCrubier, Y. (1998). Prevalence and recognition of anxiety syndromes in five European primary care settings: A report from the WHO Study on Psychological Problems in General Health Care. *British Journal of Psychiatry, 173*(Suppl. 34), 18–23.

Weiss, D. S., & Marmar, C. R. (1997). The Impact of Event Scale—Revised. In J. P. Wilson & T. M. Keane (Eds.), *Assessing psychological trauma and PTSD* (pp. 399–411). New York: Guilford Press.

Weissman, M. M., Bland, R. C., Canino, G. J., Greenwald, S., Hwu, H.-G., Lee, C. K., et al. (1994). The cross national epidemiology of obsessive compulsive disorder. *Journal of Clinical Psychiatry, 55*(Suppl. 3), 5–10.

Weissman, M. M., Klerman, G. L., Markowitz, J. S., & Ouellette, R. (1989). Suicidal ideation and suicide attempts in panic disorder and attacks. *New England Journal of Medicine, 321,* 1209–1214.

Weissman, M. M., Markowitz, J. S., Ouellette, R., Greenwald, S., & Kahn, J. P. (1990). Panic disorder and cardiovascular/cerebrovascular problems: Results from a community survey. *American Journal of Psychiatry, 147,* 1504–1508.

Wells, A. (1994a). A multidimensional measure of worry: Development and preliminary validation of the Anxious Thoughts Inventory. *Anxiety, Stress and Coping, 6,* 289–299.

Wells, A. (1994b). Attention and the control of worry. In G. C. L. Davey & F. Tallis (Eds.), *Worrying: Perspectives on theory, assessment and treatment* (pp. 91–114). Chichester, UK: Wiley.

Wells, A. (1995). Meta-cognition and worry: A cognitive model of generalized anxiety disorder. *Behavioural and Cognitive Psychotherapy, 23,* 301–320.

Wells, A. (1997). *Cognitive therapy of anxiety disorders: A practice manual and conceptual guide.* Chichester, UK: Wiley.

Wells, A. (1999). A cognitive model of generalized anxiety disorder. *Behavior Modification, 23,* 526–555.

Wells, A. (2000). *Emotional disorders and metacognition: Innovative cognitive therapy.* Chichester, UK: Wiley.

Wells, A. (2004). A cognitive model of GAD: Metacognitions and pathological worry. In R. G. Heimberg, C. L. Turk, & D. S. Mennin (Eds.), *Generalized anxiety disorder: Advances in research and practice* (pp. 164–186). New York: Guilford Press.

Wells, A. (2005a). Worry, intrusive thoughts, and generalized anxiety disorder: The metacognitive theory and treatment. In D. A. Clark (Ed.), *Intrusive thoughts in clinical disorders: Theory, research, and treatment* (pp. 119–144). New York: Guilford Press.

Wells, A. (2005b). The metacognitive model of GAD: Assessment of meta-worry and relationship with DSM-IV generalized anxiety disorder. *Cognitive Therapy and Research, 29,* 107–121.

Wells, A. (2006). The metacognitive model of worry and generalized anxiety disorder. In G. C. L. Davey & A. Wells (Eds.), *Worry and its psychological disorders: Theory, assessment and treatment* (pp. 179–216). Chichester, UK: Wiley.

Wells, A. (2009). *Metacognitive therapy for anxiety and depression.* New York: Guilford Press.

Wells, A., & Bulter, G. (1997). Generalized anxiety disorder. In D. M. Clark & C. G. Fairburn (Eds.), *Science and practice of cognitive behaviour therapy* (pp. 155–178). Oxford, UK: Oxford University Press.

Wells, A., & Carter, K. (1999). Preliminary tests of a cognitive model of generalized anxiety disorder. *Behaviour Research and Therapy, 37,* 585–594.

Wells, A., & Carter, K. (2001). Further tests of a cognitive model of generalized anxiety disorder: Metacognitions and worry in GAD, panic disorder, social phobia, depression, and nonpatients. *Behavior Therapy, 32,* 85–102.

Wells, A., & Cartwright-Hatton, S. (2004). A short form of the Metacognitions Questionnaire: Properties of the MCQ-30. *Behaviour Research and Therapy, 42,* 385–396.

Wells, A., & Clark, D. M. (1997). Social phobia: A cognitive approach. In G. C. L. Davey (Ed.), *Phobias: A handbook of theory, research and treatment* (pp. 3–26). Chichester, UK: Wiley.

Wells, A., Clark, D. M., Salkovskis, P. M., Ludgate, J., Hackmann, A., & Gelder, M. (1995). Social pho-

bia: The role of in-situation safety behaviors in maintaining anxiety and negative beliefs. *Behavior Therapy, 26,* 153–161.

Wells, A., & Davies, M. I. (1994). The Thought Control Questionnaire: A measure of individual differences in the control of unwanted thoughts. *Behaviour Research and Therapy, 32,* 871–878.

Wells, A., & Matthews, G. (1994). *Attention and emotion: A clinical perspective.* Hove, UK: Erlbaum.

Wells, A., & Matthews, G. (2006). Cognitive vulnerability to anxiety disorders: An integration. In L. B. Alloy & J. H. Riskind (Eds.), *Cognitive vulnerability to emotional disorders* (pp. 303–325). Mahwah, NJ: Erlbaum.

Wells, A., & Morrison, A. P. (1994). Qualitative dimensions of normal worry and normal obsessions: A comparative study. *Behaviour Research and Therapy, 32,* 867–870.

Wells, A., & Papageorgiou, C. (1995). Worry and the incubation of intrusive images following stress. *Behaviour Research and Therapy, 33,* 579–583.

Wells, A., & Papageorgiou, C. (1998a). Relationships between worry, obsessive–compulsive symptoms, and meta-cognitive beliefs. *Behaviour Research and Therapy, 36,* 899–913.

Wells, A., & Papageorgiou, C. (1998b). Social phobia: Effects of external attention on anxiety, negative beliefs, and perspective taking. *Behavior Therapy, 29,* 357–370.

Wells, A., & Papageorgiou, C. (2001). Social phobic interoception: Effects of bodily information on anxiety, beliefs and self-processing. *Behaviour Research and Therapy, 39,* 1–11.

Wells, A., & Sembi, S. (2004). Metacognitive therapy for PTSD: A core treatment manual. *Cognitive and Behavioral Practice, 11,* 365–377.

Wells, A., White, J., & Carter, K. (1997). Attention training: Effects on anxiety and beliefs in panic and social phobia. *Clinical Psychology and Psychotherapy, 4,* 226–232.

Wenzel, A., Finstrom, N., Jordan, J., & Brendle, J. R. (2005). Memory and interpretation of visual representations of threat in socially anxious and nonanxious individuals. *Behaviour Research and Therapy, 43,* 1029–1044.

Wenzel, A., & Holt, C. S. (2002). Memory bias against threat in social phobia. *British Journal of Clinical Psychology, 41,* 73–79.

Wenzel, A., Jackson, L. C., & Holt, C. S. (2002). Social phobia and the recall of autobiographical memories. *Depression and Anxiety, 15,* 186–189.

Wenzel, A., Sharp, I. R., Brown, G. K., Greenberg, R. L., & Beck, A. T. (2006). Dysfunctional beliefs in panic disorder: The Panic Belief Inventory. *Behaviour Research and Therapy, 44,* 819–833.

Wenzel, A., Sharp, I. R., Sokol, L., & Beck, A. T. (2005). *An investigation of attentional fixation in panic disorder.* Unpublished manuscript, University of Pennsylvania, Philadelphia.

Wenzel, A., Werner, M. M., Cochran, C. K., & Holt, C. S. (2004). A differential pattern of autobiographical memory retrieval in social phobic and nonanxious individuals. *Behavioural and Cognitive Psychotherapy, 32,* 1–13.

Wenzlaff, R. M., & Wegner, D. M. (2000). Thought suppression. *Annual Review of Psychology, 51,* 59–91.

Wenzlaff, R. M., Wegner, D. M., & Roper, D. W. (1988). Depression and mental control: The resurgence of unwanted negative thoughts. *Journal of Personality and Social Psychology, 55,* 882–892.

Wetherell, J. L., Gatz, M., & Craske, M. G. (2003). Treatment of generalized anxiety disorder in older adults. *Journal of Consulting and Clinical Psychology, 71,* 31–40.

Wetherell, J. L., Roux, H. L., & Gatz, M. (2003). DSM-IV criteria for generalized anxiety disorder in older adults: Distinguishing the worried from the well. *Psychology and Aging, 18,* 622–627.

Whalley, M. G., & Brewin, C. R. (2007). Mental health following terrorist attacks. *British Journal of Psychiatry, 190,* 94–96.

Whitaker, A., Johnson, J., Shaffer, D., Rapoport, J. L., Kalikow, K., Walsh, T., et al. (1990). Uncommon troubles in young people: Prevalence estimates of selected psychiatric disorders in a non-referred adolescent population. *Archives of General Psychiatry, 47,* 487–496.

White, K. S., & Barlow, D. H. (2002). Panic disorder and agoraphobia. In D. H. Barlow (Ed.), *Anxiety and its disorders: The nature and treatment of anxiety and panic* (2nd ed., pp. 328–379). New York: Guilford Press.

White, K. S., Brown, T. A., Somers, T. J., & Barlow, D. H. (2006). Avoidance behavior in panic disorder: The moderating influence of perceived control. *Behaviour Research and Therapy, 44,* 147–157.

Whiteside, S. P., Port, J. D., & Abramowitz, J. S. (2004). A meta-analysis of functional neuroimaging in obsessive–compulsive disorder. *Psychiatry Research: Neuroimaging, 132,* 69–79.

Whittal, M. L., & McLean, P. D. (2002). Group cognitive behavioral therapy for obsessive compulsive disorder. In R. O. Frost & G. Steketee (Eds.), *Cognitive approaches to obsessions and compulsions: Theory, assessment, and treatment* (pp. 417–433). Amsterdam, The Netherlands: Elsevier Science.

Whittal, M. L., Thordarson, D. S., & McLean, P. D. (2005). Treatment of obsessive–compulsive disorder: Cognitive behavior therapy vs. exposure and response prevention. *Behaviour Research and Therapy, 43,* 1559–1576.

WHO World Mental Health Survey Consortium. (2004). Prevalence, severity, and unmet need for treatment of mental disorders in the World Health Organization world mental health surveys. *Journal of the American Medical Association, 291,* 2581–2590.

Widiger, T. A. (1992). Generalized social phobia versus avoidant personality disorder: A commentary on three studies. *Journal of Abnormal Psychology, 101,* 340–343.

Wiedemann, G., Pauli, P., & Dengler, W. (2001). A priori expectancy bias in patients with panic disorder. *Journal of Anxiety Disorders, 15,* 401–412.

Wilhelm. S., & Steketee, G. S. (2006). *Cognitive therapy for obsessive–compulsive disorder: A guide for professionals.* Oakland, CA: New Harbinger.

Williams, J. B. W., Gibbon, M., First, M. B., Spitzer, R. L., Davies, M., Borus, J., et al. (1992). The Structured Clinical Interview for DSM-III-R (SCID): Multisite test–retest reliability. *Archives of General Psychiatry, 49,* 630–636.

Williams, J. M. G., Watts, F. N., MacLeod, C., & Mathews, A. (1997). *Cognitive psychology and emotional disorders* (2nd ed.). Chichester, UK: Wiley.

Williams, M. G., Teasdale, J. D., Segal, Z. V., & Kabat-Zinn, J. (2007). *The mindful way through depression: Freeing yourself from chronic unhappiness.* New York: Guilford Press.

Williams, N. L., Shahar, G., Riskind, J. H., & Joiner, T. E. (2005). The looming maladaptive style predicts shared variance in anxiety disorder symptoms: Further support for a cognitive model of vulnerability to anxiety. *Journal of Anxiety Disorders, 19,* 157–175.

Williams, S. L., Williams, D. R., Stein, D. J., Seedat, S., Jackson, P. B., & Moomal, H. (2007). Multiple traumatic events and psychological distress: The South Africa Stress and Health Study. *Journal of Traumatic Stress, 20,* 845–855.

Wilson, E., & MacLeod, C. (2003). Contrasting two accounts of anxiety-linked attentional bias: Selective attention to varying levels of stimulus threat intensity. *Journal of Abnormal Psychology, 112,* 212–218.

Wilson, E. J., MacLeod, C., Mathews, A., & Rutherford, E. M. (2006). The causal role of interpretative bias in anxiety reactivity. *Journal of Abnormal Psychology, 115,* 103–111.

Wilson, J. K., & Rapee, R. M. (2004). Cognitive theory and therapy of social phobia. In M. A. Reinecke & D. A. Clark (Eds.), *Cognitive therapy across the lifespan: Evidence and practice* (pp. 258–292). Cambridge, UK: Cambridge University Press.

Wilson, J. K., & Rapee, R. M. (2005). The interpretation of negative social events in social phobia with versus without comorbid mood disorder. *Journal of Anxiety Disorders, 19,* 245–274.

Wilson, J. K., & Rapee, R. M. (2006). Self-concept certainty in social phobia. *Behaviour Research and Therapy, 44,* 113–136.

Wilson, J. P. (2004). PTSD and complex PTSD: Symptoms, syndromes, and diagnoses. In J. P. Wilson & T. M. Keane (Eds.), *Assessing psychological trauma and PTSD* (2nd ed., pp. 7–44). New York: Guilford Press.

Wilson, K. A., & Chambless, D. L. (2005). Cognitive therapy for obsessive–compulsive disorder. *Behaviour Research and Therapy, 43,* 1645–1654.

Wilson, K. G., Sandler, L. S., Asmundson, G. J. G., Ediger, J. M., Larsen, D. K., & Walker, J. R. (1992). Panic attacks in the nonclinical population: An empirical approach to case identification. *Journal of Abnormal Psychology, 101,* 460–468.

Wittchen, H.-U. (2002). Generalized anxiety disorder: Prevalence, burden, and cost to society. *Depression and Anxiety, 16,* 162–171.

Wittchen, H.-U., & Boyer, P. (1998). Screening for anxiety disorders: Sensitivity and specificity of the Anxiety Screening Questionnaire (ASQ-15). *British Journal of Psychiatry, 173*(Suppl. 34), 10–17.

Wittchen, H.-U., Reed, V., & Kessler, R. C. (1998). The relationship of agoraphobia and panic in a community sample of adolescents and young adults. *Archives of General Psychiatry, 55,* 1017–1024.

Wittchen, H.-U., Stein, M. B., & Kessler, R. C. (1999). Social fears and social phobia in a community sample of adolescents and young adults: Prevalence, risk factors and comorbidity. *Psychological Medicine, 29,* 309–323.

Wittchen, H.-U., Zhao, S., Kessler, R. C., & Eaton, W. W. (1994). DSM-III-R generalized anxiety disorder in the National Comorbidity Survey. *Archives of General Psychiatry, 51,* 355–364.

Wolpe, J. (1958). *Psychotherapy by reciprocal inhibition.* Stanford, CA: Stanford University Press.

Wolpe, J., & Lazarus, A. A. (1966). *Behavior therapy techniques: A guide to the treatment of neuroses.* New York: Pergamon Press.

Woods, C. M., Frost, R. O., & Steketee, G. (2002). Obsessive compulsive (OC) symptoms and subjective severity, probability, and coping ability estimates of future negative events. *Clinical Psychology and Psychotherapy, 9,* 104–111.

Woody, S. R., & Rachman, S. (1994). Generalized anxiety disorder (GAD) as an unsuccessful search for safety. *Clinical Psychology Review, 14,* 743–753.

Woody, S. R., Steketee, G., & Chambless, D. L. (1995). Reliability and validity of the Yale–Brown Obsessive–Compulsive Scale. *Behaviour Research and Therapy, 33,* 597–605.

Woody, S. R., Taylor, S., McLean, P.

D., & Koch, W. J. (1998). Cognitive specificity in panic and depression: Implications for comorbidity. *Cognitive Therapy and Research, 22,* 427–443.

World Health Organization. (1992). *The ICD-10 classification of mental and behavioural disorders: Clinical descriptions and diagnostic guidelines.* Geneva, Switzerland: Author.

Wroe, A. L., Salkovskis, P. M., & Richards, H. C. (2000). "Now I know it could happen, I have to prevent it": A clinical study of the specificity of intrusive thoughts and the decision to prevent harm. *Behavioural and Cognitive Psychotherapy, 28,* 63–70.

Wu, K. D., Clark, L. A., & Watson, D. (2006). Relations between obsessive–compulsive disorder and personality: Beyond Axis I–Axis II comorbidity. *Journal of Anxiety Disorders, 20,* 695–717.

Yiend, J., Mackintosh, B., & Mathews, A. (2005). Enduring consequences of experimentally induced biases in interpretation. *Behaviour Research and Therapy, 43,* 779–797.

Yonkers, K. A., Bruce, S. E., Dyck, I. R., & Keller, M. B. (2003). Chronicity, relapse, and illness: Course of panic disorder, social phobia, and generalized anxiety disorder. Findings in men and women from 8 years of follow-up. *Depression and Anxiety, 17,* 173–179.

Yonkers, K. A., Dyck, I. R., Warshaw, M., & Keller, M. B. (2000). Factors predicting the clinical course of generalized anxiety disorder. *British Journal of Psychiatry, 176,* 544–549.

Yonkers, K. A., Warshaw, M. G., Massion, A. O., & Keller, M. B. (1996). Phenomenology and course of generalized anxiety disorder. *British Journal of Psychiatry, 168,* 308–313.

Yonkers, K. A., Zlotnick, C., Allsworth, J., Warshaw, M., Shea, T., & Keller, M. B. (1998). Is the course of panic disorder the same in women and men? *American Journal of Psychiatry, 155,* 596–602.

York, D., Borkovec, T. D., Vasey, M., & Stern, R. (1987). Effects of worry and somatic anxiety induction on thoughts, emotion and physiological activity. *Behaviour Research and Therapy, 25,* 523–526.

Zatzick, D. F., Marmar, C. R., Weiss, D. S., Browner, W. S., Metzler, T. J., Golding, J. M., et al. (1997). Posttraumatic stress disorder and functioning and quality of life outcomes in a nationally representative sample of male Vietnam veterans. *American Journal of Psychiatry, 154,* 1690–1695.

Zatzick, D. F., Rivara, F. P., Nathens, A. B., Jurkovich, G. J., Wang, J., Fan, M.-Y., et al. (2007). A nationwide US study of post-traumatic stress after hospitalization for physical injury. *Psychological Medicine, 37,* 1469–1480.

Zebb, B. J., & Moore, M. C. (1999). Another look at the psychometric properties of the Anxiety Control Questionnaire. *Behaviour Research and Therapy, 37,* 1091–1103.

Zhang, W., Ross, J., & Davidson, J. R. T. (2004). Social anxiety disorder in callers to the Anxiety Disorders Association of America. *Depression and Anxiety, 20,* 101–106.

Zhong, J., Wang, A., Qian, M., Zhang, L., Gao, J., Yang, J., et al. (2008). Shame, personality, and social anxiety symptoms in Chinese and American nonclinical samples: A cross-cultural study. *Depression and Anxiety, 25,* 449–460.

Zinbarg, R. E., & Barlow, D. H. (1996). Structure of anxiety and the anxiety disorders: A hierarchical model. *Journal of Abnormal Psychology, 105,* 181–193.

Zinbarg, R. E., Barlow, D. H., & Brown, T. A. (1997). Hierarchical structure and general factor saturation of the Anxiety Sensitivity Index: Evidence and implications. *Psychological Assessment, 9,* 277–284.

Zlotnick, C., Johnson, J., Kohn, R., Vicente, B., Rioseco, P., & Saldivia, S. (2006). Epidemiology of trauma, post-traumatic stress disorder (PTSD) and co-morbid disorders in Chile. *Psychological Medicine, 36,* 1523–1533.

Zoellner, L. A., Sacks, M. B., & Foa, E. B. (2003). Directed forgetting following mood induction in chronic posttraumatic stress disorder patients. *Journal of Abnormal Psychology, 112,* 508–514.

Zolensky, M. J., Arrindell, W. A., Taylor, S., Bouvard, M., Cox, B. J., Stewart, S. H., et al. (2003). Anxiety sensitivity in six countries. *Behaviour Research and Therapy, 41,* 841–859.

Zvolensky, M. J., Feldner, M. T., Eifert, G. H., & Stewart, S. H. (2001). Evaluating differential predictions of emotional reactivity during repeated 20% carbon dioxide-enriched air challenge. *Cognition and Emotion, 15,* 767–786.

Zvolensky, M. J., Kotov, R., Antipova, A. V., & Schmidt, N. B. (2005). Diathesis stress model for panic-related distress: A test in a Russian epidemiological sample. *Behaviour Research and Therapy, 43,* 521–532.

Zvolensky, M. J., Leen-Feldner, E. W., Feldner, M. T., Bonn-Miller, M. O., Lejuez, C. W., Kahler, C. W., et al. (2004). Emotional responding to biological challenge as a function of panic disorder and smoking. *Journal of Anxiety Disorders, 18,* 19–32.

Zvolensky, M. J., Schmidt, N. B., Bernstein, A., & Keough, M. E. (2006). Risk-factor research and prevention programs for anxiety disorders: A translational research framework. *Behaviour Research and Therapy, 44,* 1219–1239.

Index

618   Index

G

GAD; *See* Generalized anxiety disorder
Gandhi, Mahatma, 388
Gender
  anxiety disorders and, 12
  GAD and, 395–396
  PTSD and, 503
  social phobia and, 342
  trauma prevalence and, 498
Generalized anxiety disorder; *see also* Worry
  acceptance and commitment therapy for, 224–225
  applied relaxation in treatment of, 265
  automatic thoughts in, 80t
  boundary issues in, 392
  case illustration of, 388–389
  catastrophic interpretations, desired outcome, and
    alternative interpretation, 212t
  challenging perceived vulnerability in, 188–189
  cognitive assessment and case formulation for
    case conceptualization in, 418–424, 418f
    diagnostic and symptom measure in, 415–417
  cognitive model of, 399–406, 400f
    attentional threat bias and, 404
    automatic processing phase of, 402–405
    elaborative processing phase of, 405–406
    empirical status of, 406–415
    evocative phase of, 401–402
    schemas characterizing, 402–404, 403t
    threat interpretation bias and, 404–405
  cognitive therapy of, 388–445
    assessment and case formulation in, 415–424
    cognitive restructuring in, 428–429
    cognitive restructuring of metacognitive beliefs
      in, 434
    components of, 425t
    constructive problem-solving training in, 436
    description of, 424–438
    diagnostic considerations in, 389–392
    differentiating productive *versus* unproductive
      worry in, 427–428, 427t
    education phase of, 424–426
    efficacy of, 438–440
    elaborative process of present in, 436–437
    forms for, 442–445
    goals for, 425t
    relaxation training in, 437–438
    repeated worry expression in, 431–432
    risk and uncertainty inoculation in, 435–436
    safety cue processing in, 432–433
    summary and conclusion, 440–441
    worry induction and decatastrophizing in,
      429–431
  comorbidity of, 397–398
    with depression, 391–392
    with PTSD, 505–506
  cost-benefit analysis in treatment of, 206–207
  course and impairment, 397
  as diagnostic enigma, 390–392
  DSM-IV core features of, 9

  DSM-IV diagnostic criteria for, 389, 390t, 392
  dysfunctional beliefs and, 118–119
  emotional Stroop evaluation of, 59
  epidemiology and clinical features, 395–399
  fear imagery script in treatment of, 249–250
  first apprehensive thoughts/images and, 141
  focus of negative anxiety interpretation in, 76t
  gender/ethnicity and, 395–396
  genetic factors in, 18
  hopelessness in, 79–80
  imaginal reprocessing in treatment of, 221–222
  implicit memory bias in, 70–71
  metacognitive intervention for, 219
  onset and age differences in, 396
  personality and life events and, 398–399
  prevalence of, 395
  problem-solving ability and, 414–415
  schemas in, 423–424
  schematic activation in, 402–404, 403t
  with social phobia, 344
  threat focus in, 182
  threat probability, severity, vulnerability, and safety
    estimates in, 185t
  as unsuccessful search for safety, 414
  worry about worry in, 76–77
  worry and, 93, 393–395
Generalized Anxiety Disorder Questionnaire-IV,
  415–416
Genetic factors, 17–21
  in social phobia, 345–346
  in vulnerability to anxiety, 103, 122
Goals, personal
  GAD and, 419–420
  and worry in GAD, 410
Graded *in vivo* exposure, for panic disorder, 319–
  320
Guilt, in PTSD, 497

H

Hamilton Rating Scale of Anxiety, 132
Harvard-Brown Anxiety Research Program, 397
Hayes, Steven, 223
Heart palpitations, exaggerated faulty appraisal and
    threat-oriented schema associated with,
    145t
Helplessness, heightened, 36t, 37–38
Hippocampal system, fear response and, 20–21
Homework assignments, *in vivo*, 258; *see also* In vivo
    exposures
Homework compliance, in cognitive interventions,
    198–200
Homophones, auditory presentation of, for assessing
    threat-biased interpretations, 86–87
Hopelessness, in depression *versus* GAD, 79–80
Hughes, Howard, 446
Hypersensitivity
  interoceptive (*see* Interoceptive hypersensitivity)
  stimulus, 7